BURTON'S
MICROBIOLOGY
FOR THE HEALTH SCIENCES

Cover art: Artificially colorized scanning electron micrograph of *Escherichia coli* bacteria and a peritoneal macrophage.

BURTON'S
MICROBIOLOGY
FOR THE HEALTH SCIENCES

EIGHTH EDITION

Paul G. Engelkirk, Ph.D., MT(ASCP)
President, Bio Med Ed
(Biomedical Educational Services)
Belton, Texas

Gwendolyn R. W. Burton, M.S., Ph.D,
Professor Emeritus of Biology and Microbiology
Science Department
Front Range Community College
Westminster, Colorado

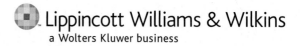
. Lippincott Williams & Wilkins
a Wolters Kluwer business

Acquisitions Editor: David B. Troy
Managing Editor: Kevin C. Dietz
Marketing Manager: Marisa A. O'Brien
Production Editor: Paula C. Williams
Designer: Risa J. Clow
Compositor: Maryland Composition, Inc.
Printer: RR Donnelley

351 West Camden Street
Baltimore, MD 21201

530 Walnut Street
Philadelphia, PA 19106

Printed in China
First Edition, 1979
Second Edition, 1983
Third Edition, 1988
Fourth Edition, 1992
Fifth Edition, 1996
Sixth Edition, 2000
Seventh Edition, 2004

Library of Congress Cataloging-in-Publication Data

Engelkirk, Paul G.
  Burton's microbiology for the health sciences / Paul G. Engelkirk, Gwendolyn R. W. Burton. --8th ed.
    p. ; cm.
  Rev. ed. of: Microbiology for the health sciences / Gwendolyn R. W.
Burton, Paul G. Engelkirk. 7th ed. c2004.
  Burton's name appears first on previous edition.
  Includes bibliographical references and index.
  ISBN:13 978-0-7817-7195-5
  ISBN:10 0-7817-7195-1 (alk. paper)
  1. Microbiology. 2. Medical microbiology. 3. Allied health personnel. 1. Burton, Gwendolyn R.W. (Gwendolyn R. Wilson).
Microbiology for the health sciences. II. Title. III. Title:
Microbiology for the health sciences.
  [DNLM: 1. Microbiology. 2. Allied Health Personnel. 3. Communicable Diseases. QW 4 E575b 2007]
  QR41.2.B88 2007
  616.9'041--dc22

               2006024929

08 09 10
5 6 7 8 9 10

IN MEMORIAM

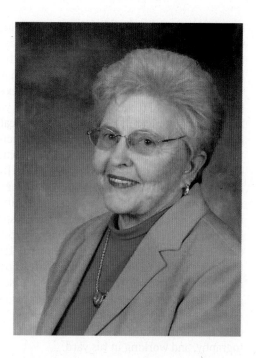

GWENDOLYN R. W. BURTON (1925–2006)
This book is dedicated to the memory of Gwendolyn R.W. Burton. During her lifetime, Gwen was many things to many people—wife, mother, grandmother, sister, microbiologist, author, teacher, mentor, colleague, and friend. During several decades of teaching and writing, she touched the lives of thousands of nursing students and students in other healthcare professions. Gwen was the sole author of this book through its first four editions—an extremely time- and energy-consuming task. She asked me to come aboard as coauthor on the fifth edition, and I have proudly served in that capacity for the past four editions. During my time in the Denver area, Gwen and I were active as officers in the Rocky Mountain Branch of the American Society for Microbiology. When it became apparent to her that I was planning to move away from the area, she graciously allowed me to serve as President of the Branch in her place. Gwen is deeply missed by all who knew her, but we find comfort in our belief that she has been reunited with her husband, Lynn, and other loved ones who passed on before her. Thank you so much, Gwen, for your friendship and your many contributions to society!

—PGE

ABOUT THE AUTHORS

Paul G. Engelkirk, Ph.D., MT(ASCP), is a former Professor of Biological Sciences in the Science Department at Central Texas College in Killeen, Texas, where he taught introductory microbiology to more than 200 nursing students per year. Before joining Central Texas College, he was an Associate Professor at the University of Texas Health Science Center in Houston, Texas, where he taught diagnostic microbiology to medical technology students for 7 years. Before that, Dr. Engelkirk served 22 years as an officer in the U.S. Army Medical Department, supervising a variety of immunology, clinical pathology, and microbiology laboratories in Germany, Vietnam, and the United States; he retired with the rank of Lieutenant Colonel. Dr. Engelkirk received his bachelor's degree (in Biology) from New York University and his master's and doctoral degrees (both in Microbiology and Public Health) from Michigan State University. He received additional medical technology and tropical medicine training at Walter Reed Army Hospital in Washington, D.C., and specialized training in anaerobic bacteriology, mycobacteriology, and virology at the Centers for Disease Control and Prevention in Atlanta, Georgia. Dr. Engelkirk is the author or coauthor of four microbiology textbooks, ten additional book chapters, five medical laboratory–oriented self-study courses, and many scientific articles. Dr. Engelkirk has been engaged in various aspects of clinical microbiology for more than 40 years and is a Past President of the Rocky Mountain Branch of the American Society for Microbiology. His hobbies include camping, hiking, kayaking, nature photography, and working in his yard.

Gwendolyn R. Wilson Burton, M.S., Ph.D., was retired Chairperson and Professor Emeritus of Biology and Microbiology of the Science Department at Front Range Community College, Westminster, Colorado, where she taught microbiology and human biology for 20 years. She also taught microbiology and immunology at the University of Denver and lectured at many colleges and high schools in the Denver area on sexually transmitted diseases. Dr. Burton received her bachelor's degree in Chemistry from Colorado State University, took graduate studies at the University of Oklahoma, and completed masters and doctoral degrees in Microbiology and Higher Education at the University of Denver. She developed 39 computer-interfaced videotaped microbiology lectures for individual study, and a series of self-paced learning materials for human biology students. Dr. Burton served as a state and international high school Science Fair Judge. As a delegate with the People-to-People Microbiology Delegation to the Peoples' Republic of China, she lectured on giardiasis at the medical schools in Beijing, Nanchang, and Guangzhou. Dr. Burton developed and began the widely recognized program for Hazardous Materials Technology Training at Front Range Community College, one of the first such programs at a community college in the nation. She was a member of the American Society for Microbiology and served as President of the Rocky Mountain Branch of that organization. Some of the honors presented to Dr. Burton include the Academic Excellence Science Award from the American Association of Community and Junior Colleges; Outstanding Educators of America; the World Safety Organization Special Recognition Award; and Distinguished Leadership Award for her many accomplishments in the educational fields of hazardous materials and microbiology. Dr. Burton was also a writer of poetry, short articles, and historical stories.

PREFACE

Microbiology—the study of microorganisms—is a fascinating subject. . .one that impacts our daily lives in a variety of ways. Microorganisms live on us and in us. They are necessary in many industries. They are essential for the cycling and recycling of elements such as carbon, oxygen, and nitrogen. They provide most of the oxygen in our atmosphere. They are used to clean up toxic wastes. They are used in genetic engineering and gene therapy. Many of them cause disease. In recent years, the public has been bombarded with news reports about microbe-associated medical problems such as bird flu, SARS, flesh-eating bacteria, mad cow disease, superbugs, black mold in buildings, West Nile virus, bioterrorism, anthrax, smallpox, meat recalls as a result of *E. coli* contamination, and epidemics of meningitis, hepatitis, influenza, tuberculosis, and diarrheal diseases.

Burton's Microbiology for the Health Sciences has been written with nurses and other healthcare professions foremost in the authors' minds. This book will provide students of these professions with vital microbiology information that will enable them to carry out their duties in an informed, safe, and efficient manner. This book is appropriate for use in any one-semester introductory microbiology course, whether for students of the healthcare professions or for science or biology majors. This book contains all of the core themes and concepts for an introductory microbiology course, as described by the American Society for Microbiology. Unlike many of the other introductory microbiology texts on the market, *all* of the material in this book can be covered in a single semester.

Chapters of special importance to students of the healthcare professions include those dealing with antibiotics and other antimicrobial agents, epidemiology and public health, hospital-acquired infections, infection control, how microorganisms cause disease, how our bodies protect us from pathogens and infectious diseases, and the major viral, bacterial, fungal, and parasitic diseases of humans.

The most obvious changes in the eighth edition are its increased use of color and increased trim size. Color illustrations appear throughout the book, rather than being grouped together in one location. The book is divided into eight major sections, containing a total of 18 chapters. Each chapter contains a chapter outline, Learning Objectives, a Review of Key Points (with the exception of Chapter 17), 10 multiple-choice self-assessment exercises, and information about the Student CD-ROM. The artwork has been expanded and updated to make it more useful and more appealing. Historical information, in the form of "Historical Notes," is spread throughout the book, and is presented in appropriate chapters.

The authors have made every attempt to create a student-friendly book. The book can be used by all types of students, including those with little or no science background and mature students returning to school after an absence of several years. It is written in a clear and concise manner. It contains more than 30 Study Aid boxes, which summarize important information and explain difficult concepts and similar-sounding terms. Clinically oriented tables (in the text) and Insight boxes (on the CD-ROM) are identified with a caduceus symbol. New terms are highlighted and defined in the text, and are included in a Glossary at the back of the book. Answers to self-assessment exercises contained in the book can be found in Appendix A. Appendix B contains a summary of key points about the most important bacterial pathogens discussed in the book. In the past, students have found this appendix to be especially helpful. Appendix C contains useful formulas for conversion of one type of unit to another (e.g., Fahrenheit to Celsius and vice versa).

Also new to the eighth edition are Student and Instructor CD-ROMs that provide a vast amount of supplemental information. The Student CD-ROM contains lists of new terms introduced in each chapter; many Insight boxes, which expand on important topics; and sections entitled "Increase Your Knowledge," "Microbiology—Hollywood Style," and "Critical Thinking." Also included on the Student CD-ROM are Case Studies (for Chapters 17 and 18), answers to the Self-Assessment Exercises found in the book, and an additional 20 Self-Assessment Exercises with answers. The

Instructor CD-ROM contains suggested laboratory exercises, suggested audiovisual aids, and answers to the various case studies and self-assessment exercises in the book and on the Student CD-ROM.

Although the book is intended primarily for individuals lacking a science background, it is not an easy text, because microbiology is not an easy topic. As students will discover, the concise nature of this book makes each sentence significant. Thus, the reader will be intellectually challenged to learn each new concept as it is presented. It is our hope that students will enjoy their study of microbiology and be motivated to further explore this exciting field, especially as it relates to their occupations. Many students who have used this textbook in their introductory microbiology course have gone on to become Infection Control Nurses, Epidemiologists, Clinical Laboratory Scientists (Medical Technologists), and Microbiologists.

We are deeply indebted to all of the people who helped with the writing, editing, and publication of this book. Special thanks to Dr. Janet Duben-Engelkirk for her constant support, to Dr. Patrick Hidy for providing many of the drawings, to Dr. Elmer Koneman for many of the illustrations, to Ms. Mary Ruth Beckham for valuable suggestions regarding the immunology chapter, and to David Troy, Kevin Dietz, Marisa O'Brien, and John Goucher from Lippincott Williams & Wilkins.

Paul G. Engelkirk, Ph.D., MT(ASCP)
Gwendolyn R. W. Burton, M.S., Ph.D.

User's Guide

In today's health careers, a thorough understanding of microbiology is more important than ever. Burtonís Microbiology for the Health Sciences, Eighth Edition not only provides the conceptual knowledge you'll need but also teaches you how to apply it. This User's Guide introduces you to the features and tools of this innovative textbook. Each feature is specifically designed to enhance your learning experience, preparing you for a successful career as a health professional.

CHAPTER OPENER FEATURES

The features that open each chapter are an introduction to guide you through the remainder of the lesson.

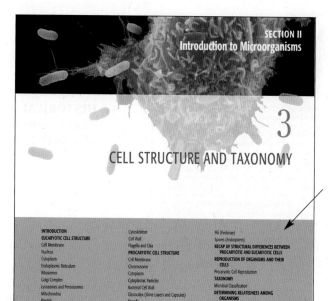

CHAPTER OUTLINE
Serves as a "roadmap" to the material ahead.

LEARNING OBJECTIVES
Highlight important concepts—helping you to organize and prioritize learning.

INTRODUCTION
Familiarizes you with the material covered in the chapter.

CHAPTER FEATURES

The following features appear throughout the body of the chapter. They're designed to hone critical thinking skills and judgment, build clinical proficiency, and promote comprehension and retention of the material.

STUDY AID BOXES
Summarize key information, explain difficult concepts and differentiate similar sounding terms.

○ STUDY AID

A Way to Remember the Sequence of Taxa From Kingdom to Species

Abbreviations and phrases are often helpful when trying to learn new material. A former student used the phrase "King David Came Over For Good Spaghetti" (KDCOFGS) to help her remember the sequence of taxa from Kingdom to Species. (K for Kingdom, D for Division, C for Class, O for Order, F for Family, G for Genus, and S for Species.) Or, if Phylum is preferred, rather than Division, King Philip can be substituted for King David. (KPCOFGS).

HISTORICAL NOTE

What's in a Name?

Sometimes, bacteria and other microorganisms are named for the person who discovered the organism. An interesting example is the name of the plague bacillus. The bacterium that causes plague was discovered in 1894 by Alexandre Emile Jean Yersin (1863–1943), a French bacteriologist of Swiss descent, who worked for many years at various Pasteur Institutes in Vietnam. Yersin originally named the organism *Bacillus pestis*, but in 1896 the name was changed to *Pasteurella pestis*, to honor Louis Pasteur, with whom Yersin had studied. Then, many years later, taxonomists changed the name to *Yersinia pestis* to honor Yersin—the person who discovered the organism. Other genera named for bacteriologists include *Bordetella* (Jules Bordet), *Escherichia* (Theodore Escherich), *Neisseria* (Albert Ludwig Neisser), and *Salmonella* (Daniel Elmer Salmon).

HISTORICAL NOTE BOXES
Provide insight into the history and development of microbiology and healthcare.

Clinical Procedure:

Proper Technique for Obtaining a Throat Swab Specimen

1. Using a tongue depressor to hold the patient's tongue down, observe the back of the throat and tonsillar area for localized areas of inflammation (redness) and exudate.

2. Remove a Dacron or calcium alginate swab from its packet.

3. Under direct observation, carefully but firmly rub the swab over any areas of inflammation or exudate or over the tonsils and posterior pharynx. Do not touch the cheeks, teeth, or gums with the swab as you withdraw it from the mouth.

4. Insert the swab back into its packet and crush the transport medium vial in the transport container.

5. Transport the swab to the laboratory as soon as possible. If transport will be delayed beyond 1 hour, refrigerate the swab.

CLINICAL PROCEDURE BOXES
Set forth step-by-step instructions for common procedures.

A Closer Look at *Streptococcus pneumoniae*

Streptococcus pneumoniae is also known as pneumo-coccus (pl., pneumococci). It is an encapsulated, α-hemolytic, catalase-negative, Gram-positive coccus, usually arranged in pairs (diplococci). In the laboratory, *S. pneumoniae* can be differentiated from other α-hemolytic *Streptococcus* species of human origin by using the P-disk (Optochin sensitivity) test; *S. pneumoniae* is Optochin-sensitive (killed by Optochin), whereas the other α-hemolytic streptococci are Optochin-resist-ant. *S. pneumoniae* is a facultative anaerobe and oppor-tunistic pathogen, found in low numbers as indigenous microflora of the upper respiratory tract. It is the most common cause of bacterial pneumonia in the world; the pneumonia it causes is often referred to as pneumococ-cal pneumonia. *S. pneumoniae* is also a common cause of meningitis (especially in the elderly) and causes about one third of U.S. cases of otitis media. Many strains of *S. pneumoniae* are penicillin-resistant and some strains are multidrug-resistant. A vaccine is available to prevent pneumococcal infections in the elderly.

A CLOSER LOOK BOXES
Amplify selected topics in the text with im-portant and intriguing facts and figures.

TEST PREPARATION FEATURES

These features help you review chapter content and test yourself before exams.

REVIEW OF KEY POINTS SECTION
Provides you with brief explanations of the chapterís main points.

REVIEW OF KEY POINTS

- Microorganisms, also called microbes, include viruses, bacteria, archaeans, certain algae, protozoa, and certain fungi.

- Because viruses are acellular (not composed of cells), they are often referred to as "infectious agents" or "in-fectious particles" rather than microorganisms.

- Microorganisms are ubiquitous, meaning that they are found virtually everywhere. Those that live on and in various parts of the human body are called our indige-nous microflora (or indigenous microbiota).

- Only a small percentage of known microbes cause disease. Those that do are called pathogens, and the diseases they cause are referred to as infectious diseases and microbial intoxications. Microorganisms that do not cause disease are called nonpathogens. Opportunistic pathogens do not cause disease under ordinary circumstances; however, they have the potential to cause disease if they gain access to the "wrong place" at the "wrong time."

SELF-ASSESSMENT EXERCISES
After studying this chapter, answer the following multiple-choice questions.

1. Which of the following individuals is considered to be the "Father of Microbiology?"
   a. Anton von Leeuwenhoek
   b. Louis Pasteur
   c. Robert Koch
   d. Rudolf Virchow

2. The microorganisms that usually live on or in a person are collectively referred to as:
   a. germs.
   b. indigenous microflora.
   c. nonpathogens.
   d. opportunistic pathogens.

3. Microorganisms that live on dead and decaying organic material are known as:
   a. indigenous microflora.
   b. parasites.
   c. pathogens.
   d. saprophytes.

4. The study of algae is called:
   a. algaeology.
   b. botany.
   c. mycology.
   d. phycology.

SELF-ASSESSMENT EXERCISES
Help you gauge your understanding of what you have learned.

ON THE CD-ROM BOX
Directs you to additional content and exercises
for review on the companion CD-ROM.

> **On the CD-ROM**
> - Insight: Additional Careers in Microbiology
> - Increase Your Knowledge
> - Microbiology—Hollywood Style
> - Critical Thinking
> - Additional Self-Assessment Exercises

BONUS CD-ROM

Packaged with this textbook, the CD-ROM is a powerful learning tool. It includes the
following features that help reinforce and review the material covered in the book:

- **Lists of New Terms Introduced in Each Chapter**
- **Answers to Text-Based Exercises**
- **Additional Self-Assessment Exercises**

Plus special Insight, Increase Your Knowledge, Microbiology-Hollywood Style, and
Critical Thinking sections provide additional information and exercises as well as fun
facts on selected topics from the text.

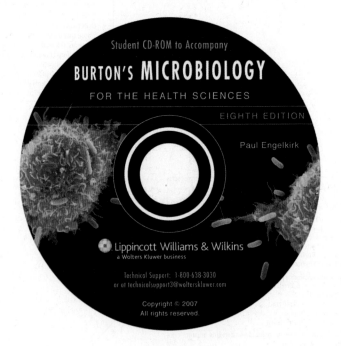

SECTION V   ENVIRONMENTAL MICROBIOLOGY

SECTION VI   MICROBIOLOGY IN HEALTHCARE
FACILITIES

BURTON'S
MICROBIOLOGY
FOR THE HEALTH SCIENCES

1

MICROBIOLOGY: THE SCIENCE

LEARNING OBJECTIVES

AFTER STUDYING THIS CHAPTER, YOU SHOULD BE
ABLE TO:
- Define microbiology, pathogen, nonpathogen, and
  opportunistic pathogen
- List several reasons why microorganisms are important
  (e.g., as a source of antibiotics)
- Explain the relationship between microorganisms and
  infectious diseases
- Differentiate between infectious diseases and microbial
  intoxications
- Outline some of the contributions of Leeuwenhoek,
  Pasteur, and Koch to microbiology
- Differentiate between biogenesis and abiogenesis
- Explain the germ theory of disease
- Outline Koch's postulates and cite some circumstances
  in which they may not apply
- Discuss two medically related fields of microbiology

INTRODUCTION

Welcome to the fascinating world of microbiology, where
you will learn about creatures so small that they cannot be
seen with the naked eye. In this chapter, you will discover
the effects that these organisms have on our daily lives and
the environment around us, and why knowledge of them is
of great importance to healthcare professionals. You will
learn that some of these tiny creatures are our friends,
whereas others are our enemies. You are about to embark
on an exciting journey. Enjoy the adventure!

What Is Microbiology?

A microbiology course is an advanced biology course. Ideally, students taking microbiology should have some background in biology. As you know, **biology** is the study of living organisms (from *bios,* referring to living organisms,
and *logy,* meaning "the study of"). *Micro* means very
small—anything so small that it must be viewed with a
microscope (an optical instrument used to observe very
small objects). Therefore, **microbiology is the study of very
small living organisms—organisms called *microorganisms* or *microbes*.** Microorganisms are said to be
ubiquitous, meaning they are virtually everywhere.

The various categories of microorganisms include
viruses, bacteria, archaeans, some algae, protozoa, and
some fungi (Fig. 1-1). These categories of microorganisms

are discussed in detail in Chapters 4 and 5. Because most scientists do not consider viruses to be living organisms, they are often referred to as "infectious agents" or "infectious particles," rather than microorganisms.

Your first introduction to microorganisms may have been when your mother warned you about "germs" (Fig.1-2). Although not a scientific term, "germs" are the microorganisms that cause disease. Your mother worried that you might become infected with these types of microorganisms. Disease-causing microorganisms are technically known as **pathogens** (Table 1-1). Actually, only about 3% of known microbes are capable of causing disease (i.e., only about 3% are pathogenic). Thus, the vast majority of known microorganisms are **nonpathogens**—microorganisms that do not cause disease. Some of the nonpathogens are beneficial to us and some have no effect on us at all. In newspapers and on television, we read and hear more about pathogens than we do about nonpathogens, but in this book you will learn about

both categories—the microorganisms that help us ("microbial allies") and those that harm us ("microbial enemies").

Why Study Microbiology?

Although they are very small, microorganisms play significant roles in our lives. Listed below are a few of the many reasons to take a microbiology course and to learn about microorganisms:

- We have, living on and in our bodies (e.g., on our skin and in our mouths and intestinal tract), approximately 10 times as many microorganisms as the total number of cells (i.e., epithelial cells, nerve cells, muscle cells, etc.) that make up our bodies (10 trillion cells × 10 = 100 trillion microbes). It has been estimated that perhaps as many as 500 to 1,000 different species of

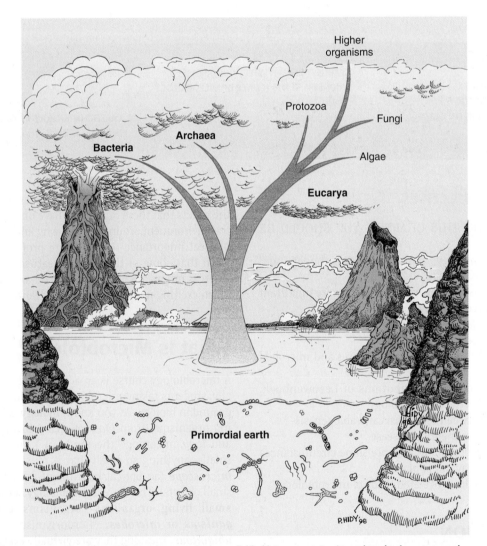

FIGURE 1-1. Family tree of microorganisms. Cellular microorganisms are divided into *eucaryotes* (organisms having a true nucleus, such as algae, fungi, and protozoa) and *procaryotes* (organisms lacking a true nucleus, such as archaeans and bacteria). Viruses are not considered to be cells (they are said to be acellular) and are, therefore, not included on this family tree. (The various categories of microorganisms are described in Chapters 4 and 5.)

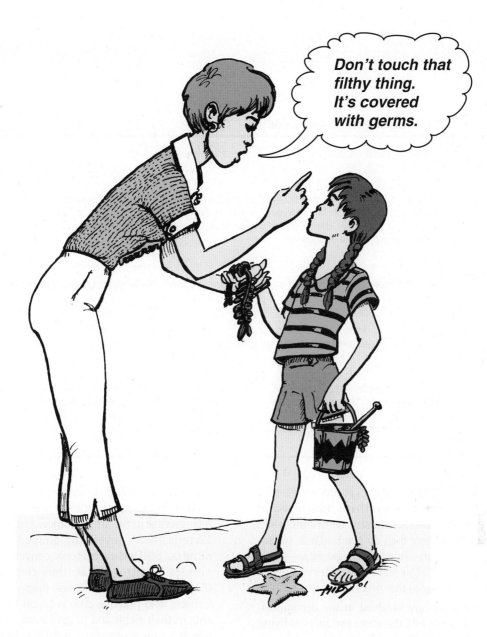

FIGURE 1-2. Germs. In all likelihood, your mother was your first microbiology instructor. Not only did she alert you to the fact that there were "invisible" critters in the world that could harm you, she also taught you the fundamentals of hygiene—like handwashing.

microorganisms live on and in us. Collectively, these microbes are known as our ***indigenous microflora*** (or indigenous microbiota) and, for the most part, they are beneficial to us. For example, the indigenous microflora inhibit the growth of pathogens in those areas of the body where they live by occupying space, depleting the food supply, and secreting materials (waste products, toxins, antibiotics, etc.) that may prevent or reduce the growth of pathogens. Indigenous microflora are discussed more fully in Chapter 10.

• Some of the organisms that colonize (inhabit) our bodies are known as ***opportunistic pathogens*** (or ***opportunists***). Although such organisms do not usually cause

us any problems, they have the potential to cause infections if they gain access to a part of our anatomy where they do not belong. For example, a bacterium called *Escherichia coli* (*E. coli*) lives in our intestinal tracts. This organism does not cause us any harm as long as it stays in our intestinal tract, but can cause disease if it gains access to our urinary bladder, bloodstream, or a wound. Other opportunistic pathogens strike when a person becomes run down, stressed out, or debilitated (weakened) as a result of some disease or condition. Opportunistic pathogens can be thought of as microorganisms awaiting the opportunity to cause disease.

• Microorganisms are essential for life on this planet as we

TABLE 1-1

Pathogens

CATEGORY	EXAMPLES OF DISEASES THEY CAUSE
Algae	A very rare cause of infections; intoxications (which result from ingestion of toxins)
Bacteria	Anthrax, botulism, cholera, diarrhea, diphtheria, ear and eye infections, food poisoning, gas gangrene, gonorrhea, hemolytic uremic syndrome (HUS), intoxications, Legionnaires' disease, leprosy, Lyme disease, meningitis, plague, pneumonia, Rocky Mountain spotted fever, scarlet fever, staph infections, strep throat, syphilis, tetanus, tuberculosis, tularemia, typhoid fever, typhus, urethritis, urinary tract infections, whooping cough
Fungi	Allergies, cryptococcosis, histoplasmosis, intoxications, meningitis, pneumonia, thrush, tinea (ringworm) infections, yeast vaginitis
Protozoa	African sleeping sickness, amebic dysentery, babesiosis, Chagas' disease, cryptosporidiosis, diarrhea, giardiasis, malaria, meningoencephalitis, pneumonia, toxoplasmosis, trichomoniasis
Viruses	Acquired immunodeficiency syndrome (AIDS), "bird flu," certain types of cancer, chickenpox, cold sores (fever blisters), common cold, dengue, diarrhea, encephalitis, genital herpes infections, German measles, hantavirus pulmonary syndrome (HPS), hemorrhagic fevers, hepatitis, infectious mononucleosis, influenza, measles, meningitis, mumps, pneumonia, polio, rabies, severe acute respiratory syndrome (SARS), shingles, smallpox, warts, yellow fever

know it. For example, some microbes produce oxygen by the process known as photosynthesis (discussed in Chapter 7). Actually, microorganisms contribute more oxygen to our atmosphere than do plants. Thus, organisms that require oxygen—humans, for example—owe a debt of gratitude to the algae and cyanobacteria (a group of photosynthetic bacteria) that produce oxygen.

- Many microorganisms are involved in the decomposition of dead organisms and the waste products of living organisms. Collectively, they are referred to as **decomposers** or **saprophytes.** By definition, a saprophyte is an organism that lives on dead or decaying organic matter. Imagine living in a world with no decomposers. Not a pleasant thought! Saprophytes aid in fertilization by returning inorganic nutrients to the soil. They break down dead and dying organic materials (plants and animals) into nitrates, phosphates, and other chemicals necessary for the growth of plants (Fig. 1-3).

- Some microorganisms are capable of decomposing industrial wastes (oil spills, for example). Thus, we can use microorganisms—genetically engineered microbes, in some cases—to clean up after ourselves. The use of microorganisms in this manner is called **bioremediation,** a topic discussed in more detail in Chapter 10. **Genetic engineering** is discussed briefly in this section and more fully in Chapter 7.

- Many microorganisms are involved in elemental cycles

(e.g., carbon, nitrogen, oxygen, sulfur, and phosphorous cycles). In the nitrogen cycle, certain bacteria convert nitrogen gas in the air to ammonia in the soil. Other soil bacteria then convert the ammonia to nitrites and nitrates. Still other bacteria convert the nitrogen in nitrates to nitrogen gas, thus completing the cycle (Fig. 1-4). Knowledge of these microbes is important to farmers who practice crop rotation to replenish nutrients in their fields and to gardeners who keep compost pits as a source of natural fertilizer. In both cases, dead organic material is broken down into inorganic nutrients (e.g., nitrates and phosphates) by microorganisms. The study of the relationships between microbes and the environment is called **microbial ecology.** Microbial ecology, the nitrogen cycle, and other elemental cycles are discussed more fully in Chapter 10.

- Algae and bacteria serve as food for tiny animals. Then, larger animals eat the smaller creatures, and so on. Thus, microbes serve as important links in food chains (Fig. 1-5). Microscopic organisms in the ocean, collectively referred to as **plankton,** serve as the starting point of many food chains. Tiny marine plants and algae are called **phytoplankton,** whereas tiny marine animals are called **zooplankton.**

- Some microorganisms live in the intestinal tracts of animals, where they aid in the digestion of food and, in some cases, produce substances that are of value to the

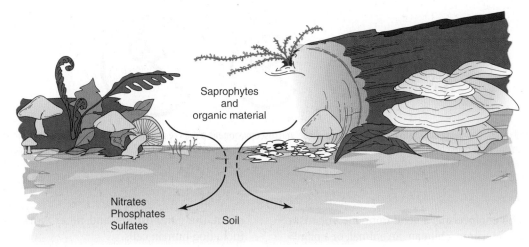

FIGURE 1-3. Saprophytes break down dead and decaying organic material into inorganic nutrients in the soil.

host animal. For example, the *E. coli* bacteria that live in the human intestinal tract produce vitamins K and B$_1$, which are absorbed and used by the human body. Although termites eat wood, they cannot digest wood. Fortunately for them, termites have cellulose-eating protozoa in their intestinal tracts that break down the wood that the termites consume into smaller molecules that the termites can use as nutrients.

- Many microorganisms are essential in various food and beverage industries, whereas others are used to produce certain enzymes and chemicals (Table 1-2). The use of

microorganisms in industry is called **biotechnology,** a topic discussed more fully in Chapter 10.

- Some bacteria and fungi produce antibiotics that are used to treat patients with infectious diseases. By definition, an **antibiotic** is a substance produced by a microorganism that is effective in killing or inhibiting the growth of other microorganisms. The use of microbes in the antibiotic industry is another example of biotechnology. Production of antibiotics by microorganisms is discussed in Chapters 9 and 10.
- Microbes are essential in the field of *genetic engineer-*

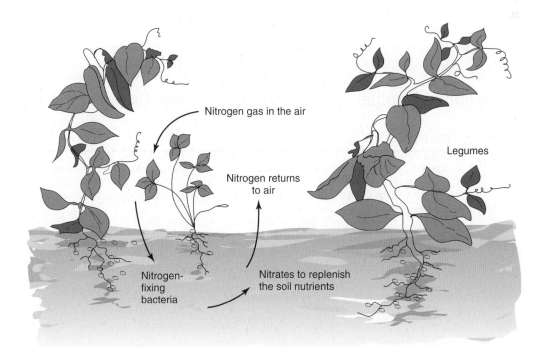

FIGURE 1-4. Nitrogen fixation. Nitrogen-fixing bacteria that live on or near the roots of legumes convert free nitrogen from the air into ammonia in the soil. Nitrifying bacteria then convert the ammonia into nitrites and nitrates, which are nutrients used by plants.

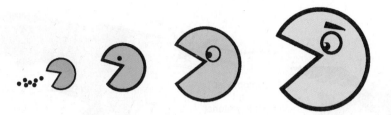

FIGURE 1-5. Food chain. Tiny living organisms such as bacteria, algae, microscopic aquatic plants (e.g., phytoplankton), and microscopic aquatic animals (e.g., zooplankton) are eaten by larger animals, which in turn are eaten by still larger animals, etc., until an animal in the chain is consumed by a human. Humans are at the top of the food chain.

ing. In genetic engineering, a gene from one organism (e.g., from a bacterium, a human, an animal, or a plant) is inserted into a bacterial or yeast cell. Because a gene contains the instructions for the production of a gene product (usually a protein), the cell that receives the new gene can now produce whatever product is coded for by that gene; so too can all of the cells that arise from the original cell. Microbiologists have engineered bacteria and yeasts to produce a variety of useful substances, such as insulin, various types of growth hormones, interferons, and materials for use as vaccines. Genetic engineering is discussed more fully in Chapter 7.

- For many years, microbes have been used as "cell models." The more that scientists learned about the structure and functions of microbial cells, the more they learned about cells in general. The intestinal bacterium *E. coli* is one of the most studied of all microbes. By studying *E. coli,* scientists have learned a great deal about the composition and inner workings of cells, including human cells.

- Finally, we come to diseases. Microorganisms cause two categories of diseases: infectious diseases and microbial intoxications (Fig. 1-6). An ***infectious disease*** results when a pathogen colonizes the body and subsequently causes disease. A ***microbial intoxication*** results when a person ingests a ***toxin*** (poisonous substance) that has been produced by a microorganism. Of the two categories, infectious diseases cause far more illnesses and deaths. Infectious diseases are the leading cause of death in the world and the third leading cause of death in the United States (after heart disease and cancer). Worldwide, infectious diseases cause about 50,000 deaths per day; the majority of deaths occur in developing countries. Anyone pursuing a career in a healthcare profession must be aware of infectious diseases, the pathogens that cause them, the sources of the pathogens, how these dis-

TABLE 1-2

Products Requiring Microbial Participation in the Manufacturing Process

CATEGORY	EXAMPLES
Foods	Acidophilus milk, bread, butter, buttermilk, chocolate, coffee, cottage cheese, cream cheese, fish sauces, green olives, kimchi (from cabbage), meat products (e.g., country-cured hams, sausage, salami), pickles, poi (fermented taro root), sauerkraut, sour cream, sourdough bread, soy sauce, various cheeses (e.g., cheddar, Swiss, Limburger, Camembert, Roquefort and other blue cheeses), vinegar, yogurt
Alcoholic beverages	Ale, beer, brandy, sake (rice wine), rum, sherry, vodka, whiskey, wine
Chemicals	Acetic acid, acetone, butanol, citric acid, ethanol, formic acid, glycerol, isopropanol, lactic acid
Antibiotics	Amphotericin B, bacitracin, cephalosporins, chloramphenicol, cycloheximide, cycloserine, erythromycin, griseofulvin, kanamycin, lincomycin, neomycin, novobiocin, nystatin, penicillin, polymyxin B, streptomycin, tetracycline

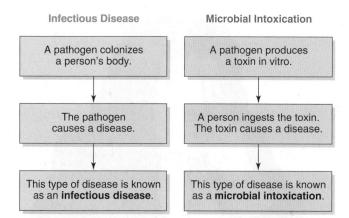

Infectious Disease	Microbial Intoxication
A pathogen colonizes a person's body.	A pathogen produces a toxin in vitro.
↓	↓
The pathogen causes a disease.	A person ingests the toxin. The toxin causes a disease.
↓	↓
This type of disease is known as an **infectious disease**.	This type of disease is known as a **microbial intoxication**.

FIGURE 1-6. The two categories of diseases caused by pathogens. Infectious diseases result when a pathogen colonizes (inhabits) the body and subsequently causes disease. Microbial intoxications result when a person ingests a toxin (poisonous substance) that has been produced by a microorganism in vitro (outside the body).

eases are transmitted, and how to protect yourself and your patients from these diseases. Physicians' assistants, nurses, dental assistants, laboratory technologists, respiratory therapists, orderlies, nurses' aides, and all others who are associated with patients and patient care must take precautions to prevent the spread of pathogens. Harmful microorganisms may be transferred from health workers to patients; from patient to patient; from contaminated mechanical devices, instruments, and syringes to patients; from contaminated bedding, clothes, dishes, and food to patients; and from patients to healthcare workers, hospital visitors, and other susceptible persons. To limit the spread of pathogens, sterile, aseptic, and antiseptic techniques (discussed in Chapter 12) are used everywhere in hospitals, nursing homes, operating rooms, and laboratories. In addition, the bioterrorist activities of recent years serve to remind us that everyone should have an understanding of the agents (pathogens) that are involved and how to protect ourselves from becoming infected. Bioterrorist and biological warfare agents are discussed in Chapter 11. Additional information about microbial intoxications can be found in CD-ROM Appendix 1 ("Microbial Intoxications").

First Microorganisms on Earth

Perhaps you have wondered how long microorganisms have existed on earth. Scientists tell us that the earth was formed about 4.5 billion years ago and, for the first 800 million to 1 billion years of earth's existence, there was no life on this planet. Fossils of primitive microorganisms (as many as 11 different types) found in ancient rock formations in northwestern Australia date back to about 3.5 billion years ago. By comparison, animals and humans are relative newcomers. Animals made their appearance on Earth between 900 and 650 million years ago (there is some disagreement in the scientific community about the exact date), and, in their present form, humans (*Homo sapiens*) have existed for only the past 100,000 years or so. Candidates for the first microorganisms on earth are archaeans and cyanobacteria; these microorganisms are discussed in Chapter 4.

Earliest Known Infectious Diseases

In all likelihood, infectious diseases of humans and animals have existed for as long as humans and animals have inhabited the planet. We know that human pathogens have existed for thousands of years because damage caused by them has been observed in the bones and internal organs of mummies and early human fossils. By studying mummies, scientists have learned that bacterial diseases, such as tuberculosis and syphilis, and parasitic worm infections, such as schistosomiasis, dracunculiasis (guinea worm infection), and tapeworm infections, have been around for a very long time.

The earliest known account of a "pestilence" occurred in Egypt about 3180 BC. This may represent the first recorded epidemic, although words like "pestilence" and "plague" were used without definition in early writings. Around 1900 BC, near the end of the Trojan War, the Greek army was decimated by an epidemic of what is thought to have been bubonic plague. The Ebers papyrus, describing epidemic fevers, was discovered in a tomb in Thebes, Egypt; it was written around 1500 BC. A disease thought to be smallpox occurred in China around 1122 BC. Epidemics of plague occurred in Rome in 790, 710, and 640 BC and in Greece around 430 BC.

In addition to the diseases already mentioned, there are early accounts of rabies, anthrax, dysentery, smallpox, ergotism, botulism, measles, typhoid fever, typhus fever, diphtheria, and syphilis. The syphilis story is quite interesting. It made its first appearance in Europe in 1493. Many people believe that syphilis was carried to Europe by Native Americans who were brought to Portugal by Christopher Columbus. The French called syphilis the Neapolitan disease; the Italians called it the French or Spanish disease; and the English called it the French pox. Other names for syphilis were Spanish, German, Polish, and Turkish pocks. The name "syphilis" was not given to the disease until 1530.

Pioneers in the Science of Microbiology

Bacteria and protozoa were the first microorganisms to be observed by humans. It then took about 200 years before a connection was established between microorganisms and infectious diseases. Among the most significant events in the early history of microbiology were the development of microscopes, bacterial staining procedures, techniques that enabled microorganisms to be cultured in the laboratory; and steps that could be taken to prove that specific microorganisms were responsible for specific infectious diseases. During the past 400 years, many individuals contributed to our present understanding of microorganisms. Three early microbiologists are discussed in this chapter; others are discussed at appropriate points throughout the book.

Anton van Leeuwenhoek (1632–1723)

Because Anton van Leeuwenhoek was the first person to see live bacteria and protozoa, he is sometimes referred to as the "Father of Microbiology," the "Father of Bacteriology," and the "Father of Protozoology." Interestingly, Leeuwenhoek was not a trained scientist. At various times in his life he was a fabric merchant, a surveyor, a wine assayer, and a minor city official in Delft, Holland. As a hobby, he ground tiny glass lenses, which he mounted in small metal frames, thus creating what today are known as single-lens microscopes or simple microscopes. During his lifetime, he made more than 500 of these microscopes. Leeuwenhoek's fine art of grinding lenses that would magnify an object to 200 to 300 times its size was lost at his death because he had not taught this skill to anyone during his lifetime. In one of the hundreds of letters that he sent to the Royal Society of London, he wrote:

My method for seeing the very smallest animalcules I do not impart to others; nor how to see very many animalcules at one time. This I keep for myself alone.

Apparently, Leeuwenhoek had an unquenchable curiosity, as he used his microscopes to examine almost anything he could get his hands on (Fig. 1-7). He examined scrapings from his teeth, water from ditches and ponds, water in which he had soaked peppercorns, blood, sperm, and even his own diarrheal stools; in many of these specimens he observed a variety of tiny living creatures, which he called "animalcules." Leeuwenhoek recorded his observations in the form of letters, which he sent to the Royal Society of London. The following passage is an excerpt from one of those letters (*Milestones in Microbiology,* edited by Thomas Brock. American Society for Microbiology, Washington, DC, 1961):

Tho my teeth are kept usually very clean, nevertheless when I view them in a Magnifying Glass, I find growing between them a little white matter as thick as wetted flower . . . I therefore took some of this flower and mixt it . . . with pure rain water wherein were no Animals . . . and then

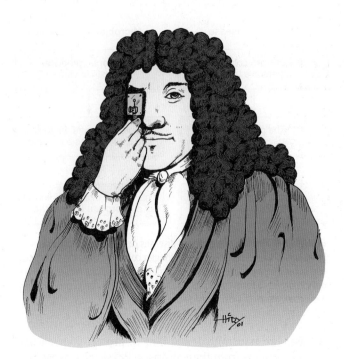

FIGURE 1-7. Anton van Leeuwenhoek using one of his single-lens microscopes.

to my great surprize perceived that the aforesaid matter contained very many small living Animals, which moved themselves very extravagantly . . . The number of these Animals in the scurf of a mans Teeth, are so many that I believe they exceed the number of Men in a kingdom. For upon the examination of a small parcel of it, no thicker than a Horse-hair, I found too many living Animals therein, that I guess there might have been 1000 in a quantity of matter no bigger than the 1/100 part of a sand.

Leeuwenhoek's letters finally convinced scientists of the late 17th century of the existence of microorganisms. Leeuwenhoek never speculated on the origin of these microbes, nor did he associate them with the cause of disease. Such relationships were not established until the work of Louis Pasteur and Robert Koch in the late 19th century.

The following quote is from Paul de Kruif's book, *Microbe Hunters,* Harcourt Brace, 1926:

[Leeuwenhoek] had stolen and peeped into a fantastic sub-visible world of little things, creatures that had lived, had bred, had battled, had died, completely hidden from and unknown to all men from the beginning of time. Beasts these were of a kind that ravaged and annihilated whole races

of men ten million times larger than they were themselves. Beings these were, more terrible than fire-spitting dragons or hydra-headed monsters. They were silent assassins that murdered babes in warm cradles and kings in sheltered places. It was this invisible, insignificant, but implacable—and sometimes friendly—world that Leeuwenhoek had looked into for the first time of all men of all countries.

Once scientists became convinced of the existence of tiny creatures that could not be observed with the naked eye, they began to speculate on their origin. On the basis of observation, many of the scientists of that time believed that life could develop spontaneously from inanimate substances, such as decaying corpses, soil, and swamp gases. The idea that life can arise spontaneously from nonliving material is called the theory of spontaneous generation or **abiogenesis.** For more than two centuries, from 1650 to 1850, this theory was debated and tested. Following the work of others, Louis Pasteur (discussed below) and John Tyndall (discussed in Chapter 3) finally disproved the theory of spontaneous generation and proved that life can only arise from preexisting life. This is called the theory of **biogenesis,** first proposed by a German scientist named Rudolf Virchow in 1858. Note that the theory of biogenesis does not speculate on the origin of life, a subject that has been discussed and debated for hundreds of years.

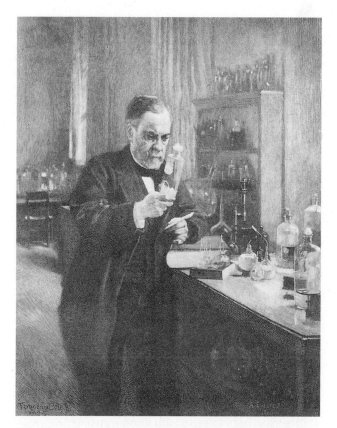

FIGURE 1-8. Pasteur in his laboratory. A 1925 wood engraving by Timothy Cole. (Zigrosser C. Medicine and the Artist [Ars Medica]. New York: Dover Publications, Inc., 1970. By permission of the Philadelphia Museum of Art.)

Louis Pasteur (1822–1895)

Louis Pasteur (Fig. 1-8), a French chemist, made numerous contributions to the newly emerging field of microbiology and, in fact, his contributions are considered by many people to be the foundation of the science of microbiology and a cornerstone of modern medicine. Listed below are some of his most significant contributions:

- While attempting to discover why wine becomes contaminated with undesirable substances, Pasteur discovered what occurs during alcoholic fermentation. (Fermentation is discussed in Chapter 7.) He also demonstrated that different types of microorganisms produce different fermentation products. For example, yeasts convert the glucose in grapes to ethyl alcohol (ethanol) by fermentation, but certain contaminating bacteria, such as *Acetobacter,* convert glucose to acetic acid (vinegar) by fermentation, thus, ruining the taste of the wine.

- Through his experiments, Pasteur dealt the fatal blow to the theory of spontaneous generation.

- Pasteur discovered forms of life that could exist in the absence of oxygen. He introduced the terms "aerobes" (organisms that require oxygen) and "anaerobes" (organisms that do not require oxygen).

- Pasteur developed a process (today known as pasteurization) to kill microbes that were causing wine to spoil—an economic concern to France's wine industry. **Pasteurization** can be used to kill pathogens in many types of liquids. Pasteur's process involved heating wine to $55°C^b$ and holding it at that temperature for several minutes; today, pasteurization is accomplished by heating liquids to 63° to 65°C for 30 minutes or to 73° to 75°C for 15 seconds. It should be noted that pasteurization does not kill *all* of the microorganisms in liquids—just the pathogens.

- Pasteur discovered the infectious agents that caused the silkworm diseases that were crippling the silk industry in France. He also discovered how to prevent such diseases.

- Pasteur made significant contributions to the germ theory of disease—the theory that specific microorganisms cause specific infectious diseases. For example, anthrax is caused by a specific bacterium (*Bacillus an-*

[b]"C" is an abbreviation for Celsius. Although Celsius is also referred to as centigrade, Celsius is preferred. Formulas for converting Celsius to Fahrenheit and vice versa can be found in Appendix C.

An Ethical Dilemma for Louis Pasteur

In July 1885, while he was developing a vaccine that would prevent rabies in dogs, Louis Pasteur faced an ethical decision. A 9-year-old boy, named Joseph Meister, had been bitten 14 times on the legs and hands by a rabid dog. At the time, it was assumed that virtually anyone who was bitten by a rabid animal would die. Meister's mother begged Pasteur to use his vaccine to save her son. Pasteur was a chemist, not a physician, and thus was not authorized to treat humans. Also, his experimental vaccine had never been administered to a human being. Nonetheless, 2 days after the boy had been bitten, Pasteur injected Meister with the vaccine in an attempt to save the boy's life. The boy survived, and Pasteur realized that he had developed a rabies vaccine that could be administered to a person after they had been infected with rabies virus.

To honor Pasteur and continue his work, especially in the development of a rabies vaccine, the Pasteur Institute was created in Paris in 1888. It became a clinic for rabies treatment, a research center for infectious diseases, and a teaching center. Many scientists who studied under Pasteur went on to make important discoveries of their own and create a vast international network of Pasteur Institutes. The first of the foreign institutes was founded in Saigon, Vietnam, which today is known as Ho Chi Minh City. One of the directors of that institute was Alexandre Emil Jean Yersin—a former student of Robert Koch and Louis Pasteur—who, in 1894, discovered the bacterium that causes plague.

thracis), whereas tuberculosis is caused by a different bacterium (*Mycobacterium tuberculosis*).

- Pasteur championed changes in hospital practices to minimize the spread of disease by pathogens.
- Pasteur developed vaccines to prevent chicken cholera, anthrax, and swine erysipelas (a skin disease). It was the development of these vaccines that made him famous in France. Before the vaccines, these diseases were decimating chickens, sheep, cattle, and pigs in that country—a serious economic problem.

- Pasteur developed a vaccine to prevent rabies in dogs and successfully used the vaccine to treat human rabies.

Robert Koch (1843–1910)

Robert Koch (Fig. 1-9), a German physician, made numerous contributions to the science of microbiology. Some of them are listed here:

- Koch made many significant contributions to the germ theory of disease. For example, he proved that the anthrax bacillus (*Bacillus anthracis*), which had been discovered earlier by other scientists, was truly the cause of anthrax. He accomplished this using a series of scientific steps which he and his colleagues had developed; these steps later became known as Koch's Postulates (described later in this chapter).

- Koch discovered that *Bacillus anthracis* produces spores, capable of resisting adverse conditions.

- Koch developed methods of fixing, staining, and photographing bacteria.

- Koch developed methods of cultivating bacteria on solid media. One of Koch's colleagues, R.J. Petri, invented a flat glass dish (now known as a **Petri dish**) in which to culture bacteria on solid media. It was Frau Hess—the wife of another of Koch's colleagues—who suggested the use of agar (a polysaccharide obtained from seaweed) as a solidifying agent. These methods enabled Koch to obtain pure cultures of bacteria. The term **pure culture** refers to a condition in which only one type of organism is growing on a solid culture medium or in a liquid culture medium in the laboratory; no other types of organisms are present.

- Koch discovered the bacterium (*Mycobacterium tuberculosis*) that causes tuberculosis and the bacterium (*Vibrio cholerae*) that causes cholera.

- Koch's work on tuberculin (a protein derived from *M. tuberculosis*) ultimately led to the development of a skin test valuable in diagnosing tuberculosis.

Koch's Postulates

During the mid- to late-1800s, Robert Koch and his colleagues established an experimental procedure to prove that a specific microorganism is the cause of a specific infectious disease. This scientific procedure, published in 1884, became known as ***Koch's Postulates*** (Fig. 1-10).

Koch's Postulates (paraphrased):

1. A particular microorganism must be found in all cases of the disease and must not be present in healthy animals or humans.

2. The microorganism must be isolated from the diseased animal or human and grown in pure culture in the laboratory.

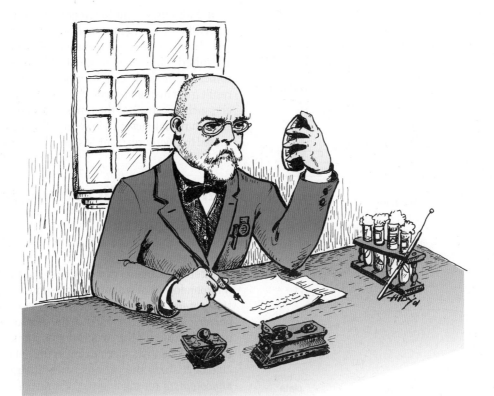

FIGURE 1-9. Robert Koch.

3. The same disease must be produced when microorganisms from the pure culture are inoculated into healthy susceptible laboratory animals.

4. The same microorganism must be recovered from the experimentally infected animals and grown again in pure culture.

After completing these steps, the microorganism is said to have fulfilled Koch's Postulates and has been proven to be the cause of that particular infectious disease. Koch's Postulates not only helped to prove the germ theory of disease, but also gave a tremendous boost to the development of microbiology by stressing laboratory culture and identification of microorganisms.

Exceptions to Koch's Postulates

Circumstances do exist in which Koch's Postulates cannot be fulfilled. Examples of such circumstances are as follows:

- To fulfill Koch's Postulates, it is necessary to grow (culture) the pathogen in the laboratory (*in vitro*[c]) in or on artificial culture media. However, certain pathogens will not grow on artificial media. Such pathogens include viruses, rickettsias (a category of bacteria), chlamydias (another category of bacteria), and the bac-

teria that cause leprosy and syphilis. Viruses, rickettsias, and chlamydias are called ***obligate intracellular pathogens*** (or *obligate intracellular parasites*) because they can only survive and multiply within living host cells. Such organisms can be grown in cell cultures (cultures of living human or animal cells of various types), embryonated chicken eggs, or certain animals (referred to as laboratory animals). In the laboratory, the leprosy bacterium (*Mycobacterium leprae*) is propagated in armadillos, and the spirochetes of syphilis (*Treponema pallidum*) grow well in the testes of rabbits and chimpanzees. Microorganisms having complex and demanding nutritional requirements are said to be ***fastidious*** (meaning fussy). Although certain fastidious organisms can be grown in the laboratory by adding special mixtures of vitamins, amino acids, and other nutrients to the culture media, others cannot be grown in the laboratory because no one has discovered what ingredient(s) to add to the medium to enable them to grow.

- To fulfill Koch's Postulates, it is necessary to infect laboratory animals with the pathogen being studied. However, many pathogens are species-specific, meaning that they infect only one species of animal. For example, some pathogens that infect humans will *only* infect humans. Thus, it is not always possible to find a laboratory animal that can be infected with a pathogen that causes human disease. Because human volunteers are difficult to obtain and ethical reasons limit their use, the researcher may

[c]The term ***in vitro*** refers to something that occurs outside the living body; the term often refers to something that occurs in the laboratory. The term ***in vivo*** refers to something that occurs within the living body.

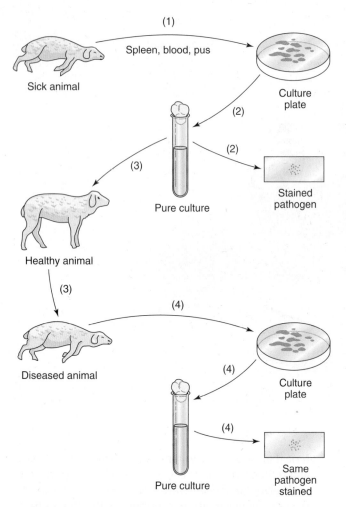

FIGURE 1-10. Koch's Postulates: proof of the germ theory of disease. (1) The microorganism must always be found in similarly diseased animals, but not in healthy ones. (2) The microorganism must be isolated from a diseased animal and grown in pure culture. (3) The isolated microorganism must cause the original disease when inoculated into a susceptible host. (4) The microorganism must be reisolated from the experimentally infected animals.

only be able to observe the changes caused by the pathogen in human cells that can be grown in the laboratory (called cell cultures).

- Some diseases, called synergistic infections, are caused not by one particular microorganism, but by the combined effects of two or more different microorganisms. Examples of such infections include acute necrotizing ulcerative gingivitis (ANUG; also known as "trench mouth") and bacterial vaginosis. It is very difficult to reproduce such synergistic infections in the laboratory.

- Another difficulty that is sometimes encountered while attempting to fulfill Koch's Postulates is that certain pathogens become altered when grown in vitro. Some become less pathogenic, whereas others become nonpathogenic. Thus, they will no longer infect animals after being cultured on artificial media.

It is also important to remember that not all diseases are caused by microorganisms. Many diseases, such as rickets and scurvy, result from dietary deficiencies. Some diseases are inherited because of an abnormality in the chromosomes, as in sickle cell anemia. Others, such as diabetes, result from malfunction of a body organ or system. Still others, such as cancer of the lungs and skin, are influenced by environmental factors. However, all infectious diseases are caused by microorganisms, as are all microbial intoxications.

Careers in Microbiology

A **microbiologist** is a scientist who studies microorganisms. He or she might have a bachelor's, master's, or doctoral degree in microbiology.

There are many career fields within the science of microbiology. For example, a person may specialize in the study of just one particular category of microorganisms. A **bacteriologist** is a scientist who specializes in **bacteriology**—the study of the structure, functions, and activities of bacteria. Scientists specializing in the field of **phycology** (or algology) study the various types of algae and are called **phycologists** (or algologists). **Protozoologists** explore the area of **protozoology**—the study of protozoa and their activities. Those who specialize in the study of fungi, or **mycology**, are called **mycologists**. **Virology** encompasses the study of viruses and their effects on living cells of all types. **Virologists** and cell biologists may become genetic engineers who transfer genetic material (deoxyribonucleic acid or DNA) from one cell type to another. Virologists may also study prions and viroids, acellular infectious agents that are even smaller than viruses (discussed in Chapter 4).

Other career fields in microbiology pertain more to applied microbiology—that is, how a knowledge of microbiology can be applied to different aspects of society, medicine, and industry. Two medically related career fields are discussed here; other microbiology career fields are discussed on the CD-ROM that accompanies this book. The scope of microbiology has broad, far-reaching effects on humans and their environment.

Medical and Clinical Microbiology

Medical microbiology is an excellent career field for individuals with interests in medicine and microbiology. The field of medical microbiology involves the study of pathogens, the diseases they cause, and the body's defenses against disease. This field is concerned with epidemiology, transmission of pathogens, disease-prevention measures, aseptic techniques, treatment of infectious diseases, immunology, and the production of vaccines to protect people and animals against infectious diseases. The complete or almost complete eradication of diseases like smallpox and polio, the safety of modern surgery, and the successful treatment of victims of infectious diseases are attributable to the many technological advances in this field. A branch of medical microbiology, called clinical or diagnostic microbiology, is concerned with the laboratory diagnosis of infectious diseases of humans. This is an excellent career field for individuals with interests in laboratory sciences and microbiology. Diagnostic microbiology and the clinical microbiology laboratory are discussed in Chapter 13.

REVIEW OF KEY POINTS

- Microorganisms, also called microbes, include viruses, bacteria, archaeans, certain algae, protozoa, and certain fungi.

- Because viruses are acellular (not composed of cells), they are often referred to as "infectious agents" or "infectious particles" rather than microorganisms.

- Microorganisms are ubiquitous, meaning that they are found virtually everywhere. Those that live on and in various parts of the human body are called our indigenous microflora (or indigenous microbiota).

- Only a small percentage of known microbes cause disease. Those that do are called pathogens, and the diseases they cause are referred to as infectious diseases and microbial intoxications. Microorganisms that do not cause disease are called nonpathogens. Opportunistic pathogens do not cause disease under ordinary circumstances; however, they have the potential to cause disease if they gain access to the "wrong place" at the "wrong time."

- Microorganisms play essential roles in various elemental cycles, such as the oxygen, carbon, nitrogen, phosphorous, and sulfur cycles. Photosynthetic algae and bacteria (such as cyanobacteria) produce much of the oxygen in our atmosphere.

- Decomposers and saprophytes play important roles by decomposing dead animals and plants and organic wastes. The use of microbes to clean up toxic wastes and other industrial waste products is known as bioremediation.

- Many microbes are used in various industries, such as food, beverage, chemical, and antibiotic industries. The use of microbes in industry is known as biotechnology.

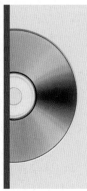

On the CD-ROM
- Insight: Additional Careers in Microbiology
- Increase Your Knowledge
- Microbiology—Hollywood Style
- Critical Thinking
- Additional Self-Assessment Exercises

SELF-ASSESSMENT EXERCISES

After studying this chapter, answer the following multiple-choice questions.

1. Which of the following individuals is considered to be the "Father of Microbiology?"
   a. Anton von Leeuwenhoek
   b. Louis Pasteur
   c. Robert Koch
   d. Rudolf Virchow

2. The microorganisms that usually live on or in a person are collectively referred to as:
   a. germs.
   b. indigenous microflora.
   c. nonpathogens.
   d. opportunistic pathogens.

3. Microorganisms that live on dead and decaying organic material are known as:
   a. indigenous microflora.
   b. parasites.
   c. pathogens.
   d. saprophytes.

4. The study of algae is called:
   a. algaeology.
   b. botany.
   c. mycology.
   d. phycology.

5. The field of parasitology involves the study of which of the following types of organisms?
   a. arthropods, bacteria, fungi, protozoa, and viruses
   b. arthropods, helminths, and certain protozoa
   c. bacteria, fungi, and protozoa
   d. bacteria, fungi, and viruses

6. Rudolf Virchow is given credit for proposing which of the following theories?
   a. abiogenesis
   b. biogenesis
   c. germ theory of disease
   d. spontaneous generation

7. Which of the following microorganisms are considered obligate intracellular pathogens?
   a. chlamydias, rickettsias, *Mycobacterium leprae,* and *Treponema pallidum*
   b. *Mycobacterium leprae* and *Treponema pallidum*
   c. *Mycobacterium tuberculosis* and viruses
   d. rickettsias, chlamydias, and viruses

8. Which of the following statements is true?
   a. Koch developed a rabies vaccine.
   b. Microorganisms are ubiquitous.
   c. Most microorganisms are harmful to humans.
   d. Pasteur conducted experiments that proved the theory of abiogenesis.

9. Which of the following are even smaller than viruses?
   a. chlamydias
   b. prions and viroids
   c. rickettsias
   d. cyanobacteria

10. Which of the following individuals introduced the terms "aerobes" and "anaerobes?"
    a. Anton von Leeuwenhoek
    b. Louis Pasteur
    c. Robert Koch
    d. Rudolf Virchow

2

MICROSCOPY

LEARNING OBJECTIVES

AFTER STUDYING THIS CHAPTER, YOU SHOULD BE ABLE TO:

- Explain the interrelationships among the following metric system units of length: centimeters, millimeters, micrometers, and nanometers
- State the metric units used to express the sizes of bacteria, protozoa, and viruses
- Compare and contrast the various types of microscopes, to include simple microscopes, compound light microscopes, and electron microscopes

INTRODUCTION

By definition, microorganisms are tiny organisms. But, how tiny are they? Generally, some type of microscope is required to see them; thus, microorganisms are said to be **microscopic.** Various types of microscopes are discussed in this chapter. The metric system will be discussed first, however, because metric system units of length are used to express the sizes of microorganisms and the resolving power of optical instruments.

Using the Metric System to Express the Sizes of Microorganisms

In microbiology, metric units (primarily micrometers and nanometers) are used to express the sizes of microorganisms. The basic unit of length in the metric system, the meter (m), is equivalent to approximately 39.4 inches and is, therefore, about 3.4 inches longer than a yard. A meter may be divided into 10 (10^1) equally spaced units called **decimeters**; or 100 (10^2) equally spaced units called **centimeters**; or 1,000 (10^3) equally spaced units called **millimeters**; or 1 million (10^6) equally spaced units called **micrometers**; or 1 billion (10^9) equally spaced units called **nanometers.** Interrelationships among these units are shown in Figure 2-1. Formulas that can be used to convert inches into centimeters, millimeters, etc., can be found in Appendix B ("Useful Conversions") at the back of the book.

It should be noted that the old terms "micron" (μ) and "millimicron" (mμ) have been replaced by the terms *micrometer* (μm) and *nanometer* (nm), respectively. An *angstrom* (Å) is 0.1 nanometer (0.1 nm). Using this scale, human red blood cells are about 7 mm in diameter.

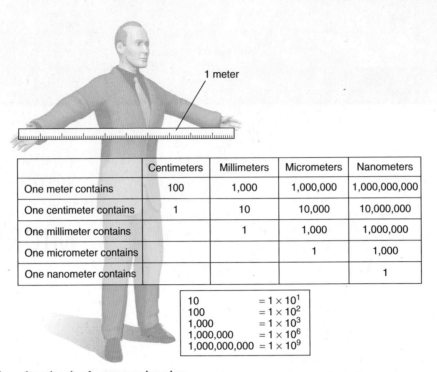

1 meter

	Centimeters	Millimeters	Micrometers	Nanometers
One meter contains	100	1,000	1,000,000	1,000,000,000
One centimeter contains	1	10	10,000	10,000,000
One millimeter contains		1	1,000	1,000,000
One micrometer contains			1	1,000
One nanometer contains				1

$$10 = 1 \times 10^1$$
$$100 = 1 \times 10^2$$
$$1,000 = 1 \times 10^3$$
$$1,000,000 = 1 \times 10^6$$
$$1,000,000,000 = 1 \times 10^9$$

FIGURE 2-1. Representations of metric units of measure and numbers.

The sizes of bacteria and protozoa are usually expressed in terms of micrometers. For example, a typical spherical bacterium (***coccus; pl., cocci***) is approximately 1 μm in diameter. About seven cocci could fit side-by-side across a human red blood cell. If the head of a pin was 1 mm (1,000 μm) in diameter, then 1,000 cocci could be placed side-by-side on the pinhead. A typical rod-shaped bacterium (***bacillus; pl., bacilli***) is about 1 μm wide × 3 μm long, although some bacilli are shorter and some form very long filaments. The sizes of viruses are expressed in terms of nanometers. Most of the viruses that cause human disease range in size from about 10 to 300 nm, although some (e.g., Ebola virus, a cause of hemorrhagic fever) can be as long as 1,000 nm (1 μm). Some very large protozoa reach a length of 2,000 μm (2 mm).

In the microbiology laboratory, the sizes of microorganisms are measured using an ocular micrometer, a tiny ruler within the eyepiece (ocular) of the compound light microscope. Before it can be used to measure objects, however, the ocular micrometer must first be calibrated, using a measuring device called a stage micrometer. Calibration must be performed for each of the objective lenses to determine the distance between the marks on the ocular micrometer. The ocular micrometer can then be used to measure lengths and widths of microbes and other objects on the specimen slide. The sizes of some microorganisms are shown in Table 2-1.

Microscopes

The human eye, a telescope, a pair of binoculars, a magnifying glass, and a microscope can all be thought of as various types of optical instruments. A microscope is an optical instrument that is used to observe tiny objects, often objects that cannot be seen at all with the unaided human eye. Each optical instrument has a limit as to what can be seen using that instrument. This limit is referred to as the ***resolving power*** or *resolution* of the instrument. Resolving power is discussed in more detail later in the chapter. Table 2-2 contains the resolving powers for various optical instruments.

Simple Microscopes

A ***simple microscope*** is defined as a microscope containing only one magnifying lens. Actually, a magnifying glass could be considered a simple microscope. Images seen when using a magnifying glass usually appear about 3 to 20 times larger than the object's actual size. During the late 1600s, Anton van Leeuwenhoek, who was discussed in Chapter 1, used simple microscopes to observe many tiny objects, including bacteria and protozoa (Fig. 2-2). Because of his unique ability to grind glass lenses, scientists believe that Leeuwenhoek's simple microscopes had a maximum magnifying power of about 300× (300 times).

Compound Microscopes

A ***compound microscope*** is a microscope that contains more than one magnifying lens. Although the first person to construct and use a compound microscope is not known with certainty, Hans Jansen and his son Zacharias are often given credit for being the first. (See the following Historical Note.) Compound light microscopes usually magnify objects about 1,000 times. Photographs taken through

TABLE 2-1

Relative Sizes of Microorganisms

ORGANISM(S)	DIMENSION(S)	APPROXIMATE SIZE (μM)
Viruses (most)	Diameter	0.01–0.3
Bacteria		
Cocci (spherical bacteria)	Diameter	average = 1
Bacilli (rod-shaped bacteria)	e.g., *Escherichia coli* (width × length)	average = 1 × 3
	Filaments (width)	1
Fungi		
Yeasts	e.g., *Candida albicans* (diameter)	3–5
Septate hyphae (hyphae with cross-walls)	Width	2–15
Aseptate hyphae (hyphae without cross-walls)	Width	10–30
Pond water protozoa		
Chlamydomonas	Length	5–12
Euglena	Length	35–55
Vorticella	Length	50–145
Paramecium	Length	180–300
Volvox[a]	Diameter	350–500
Stentor[a]	Length (extended)	1,000–2,000

[a]*These organisms are visible with the unaided human eye.*

the lens system of compound microscopes are called ***photomicrographs.***

Because visible light (from a built-in light bulb) is used as the source of illumination, the compound microscope is also referred to as a ***compound light microscope.*** It is the wavelength of visible light (approximately 0.45 μm) that limits the size of objects that can be seen using the compound light microscope. When using the compound light microscope, objects cannot be seen if they are smaller than half of the wavelength of visible light. A compound light microscope is shown in Figure 2-4, and the functions of its various components are described in Table 2-3.

The compound light microscopes used in today's laboratories contain two magnifying lens systems. Within the eyepiece or ocular is a lens called the ocular lens; it usually has a magnifying power of ×10. The second magnifying lens system is in the objective, which is positioned immediately above the object to be viewed. The four objectives used in most laboratory compound light microscopes are ×4, ×10, ×40, and ×100 objectives. As shown in Table 2-4, total magnification is calculated by multiplying the magnifying power of the ocular (×10) by the magnifying power of the objective that you are using.

The ×4 objective is rarely used in microbiology laboratories. Usually, specimens are first observed using the ×10 objective. Once the specimen is in focus, the high power or "high-dry" objective is then swung into position. This lens can be used to study algae, protozoa, and other large microorganisms. However, the oil-immersion objective (total magnification = 1,000×) must be used to study bacteria, because they are so tiny. To use the oil-immersion objective, a drop of immersion oil must first be placed between the specimen and the objective; the immersion oil reduces the scattering of light and ensures that the light will enter the oil-immersion lens.

For optimal observation of the specimen, the light must be properly adjusted and focused. The condenser, located beneath the stage, focuses light onto the specimen, adjusts the amount of light, and shapes the cone of light entering

TABLE 2-2

Characteristics of Various Types of Microscopes

TYPE	RESOLVING POWER	USEFUL MAGNIFICATION	CHARACTERISTICS
Brightfield	0.2000 μm	1,000×	Used to observe morphology of microorganisms such as bacteria, protozoa, fungi, and algae in living (unstained) and nonliving (stained) state Cannot observe organisms less than 0.2 μm in diameter or thickness, such as spirochetes and viruses
Darkfield	0.2000 μm	1,000×	Unstained organisms are observed against a dark background Useful for examining thin spirochetes Slightly more difficult to operate than brightfield
Phase-contrast	0.2000 μm	1,000×	Can be used to observe unstained living microorganisms
Fluorescence	0.2000 μm	1,000×	Fluorescent dye attached to organism Primarily an immunodiagnostic technique (immunofluorescence) Used to detect microorganisms in cells, tissues, and clinical specimens
Transmission electron microscope (TEM)	0.0002 mm (0.2 nm)	200,000×	Specimen is viewed on a screen Excellent resolution Allows examination of cellular and viral ultrastructure Specimen is nonliving Reveals internal features of thin specimens
Scanning electron microscope (SEM)	0.0200 mm (20 nm)	10,000×	Specimen is viewed on a screen Gives the illusion of depth (three-dimensions) Useful for examining surface features of cells and viruses Specimen is nonliving Resolution is less than that of TEM

the objective. Generally, the higher the magnification, the more light that is needed.

Magnification alone is of little value unless the enlarged image possesses increased detail and clarity. Image clarity depends on the microscope's *resolving power* (or *resolution*), which is the ability of the lens system to distinguish between two adjacent objects. If two objects are moved closer and closer together, there comes a point when the objects are so close together that the lens system can no longer resolve them as two separate objects (i.e., they are so close together that they appear to be one object). That distance between them, at which they cease to be seen as separate objects, is referred to as the resolving power of the optical instrument. Knowing the resolving power of an optical instrument also defines the smallest object that can be seen with that instrument. For example, the resolving power of the unaided human eye is approximately 0.2 mm. Thus, the unaided human eye is unable to see objects smaller than 0.2 mm in diameter.

The resolving power of the compound light microscope is approximately 1,000 times better than the resolving

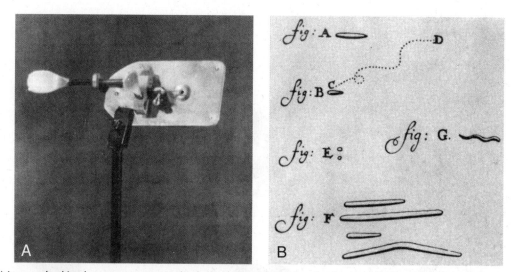

FIGURE 2-2. (*A*) Leeuwenhoek's microscopes were very simple devices. Each had a tiny glass lens, mounted in a brass plate. The specimen was placed on the sharp point of a brass pin, and two screws were used to adjust the position of the specimen. The entire instrument was about 3 to 4 inches long. It was held very close to the eye. (*B*) Although his microscopes had a magnifying capability of only around 200× to 300×, Leeuwenhoek was able to create remarkable drawings of different types of bacteria that he observed. (Volk WA, et al. Essentials of Medical Microbiology, 5th ed. Philadelphia: Lippincott-Raven, 1996.)

HISTORICAL NOTE

Early Compound Microscopes

Hans Jansen, an optician in Middleburg, Holland, is often given credit for developing the first compound microscope, sometime between 1590 and 1595. Although his son, Zacharias, was only a young boy at the time, Zacharias apparently later took over production of the Jansen microscopes. The Jansen microscopes contained two lenses and achieved magnifications of only 3× to 9×. Compound microscopes having a three-lens system were later used by Marcello Malpighi in Italy and Robert Hooke in England, both of whom published papers between 1660 and 1665 describing their microscopic findings. In his 1665 book entitled *Micrographia,* Hooke described a fossilized shell of a foraminiferan —a type of protozoan—and two species of microscopic fungi. Some scientists consider these to be the first written descriptions of microbes, and feel that Hooke should be given credit for discovering microorganisms. Some early compound microscopes are shown in Figure 2-3.

power of the unaided human eye. In practical terms, this means that objects can be examined with the compound microscope that are as much as 1,000 times smaller than the smallest objects that can be seen with the unaided human eye. Using a compound light microscope, we can see objects down to about 0.2 μm in diameter.

Additional magnifying lenses could be added to the compound light microscope, but this would not increase the resolving power. As stated earlier, as long as visible light is used as the source of illumination, objects smaller than half of the wavelength of visible light cannot be seen. Increasing magnification without increasing the resolving power is called ***empty magnification.*** It does no good to increase magnification without increasing resolving power.

Because objects are observed against a bright background (or "bright field") when using a compound light microscope, that microscope is sometimes referred to as a ***brightfield microscope.*** If the regularly used condenser is replaced with what is known as a darkfield condenser, illuminated objects are seen against a dark background (or "dark field"), and the microscope has been converted into a ***darkfield microscope.*** In the clinical microbiology laboratory, darkfield microscopy is routinely used to diagnose primary syphilis (the initial stage of syphilis). The etiologic (causative) agent of syphilis—a spiral-shaped bacterium, named *Treponema pallidum*—cannot be seen with a brightfield microscope because it is thinner than 0.2 mm and, therefore, is beneath the resolving power of the compound light microscope. *Treponema pallidum* can be seen

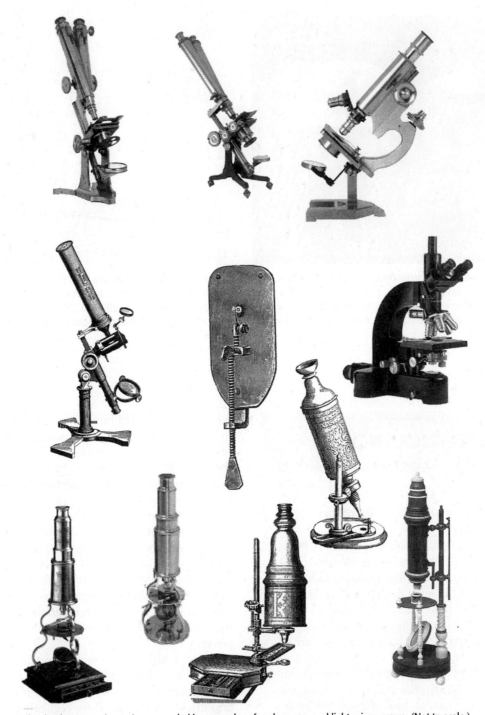

FIGURE 2-3. A Leeuwenhoek microscope (center), surrounded by examples of early compound light microscopes. (Not to scale.)

using a darkfield microscope, however, much in the same way that you can "see" dust particles in a beam of sunlight. Dust particles are actually beneath the resolving power of the unaided eye and, therefore, cannot really be seen. What you see in the beam is sunlight being reflected off the dust particles. With the darkfield microscope, laboratory technologists do not really see the treponemes—they see the light being reflected off the bacteria, and that light is easily seen against the dark background (Fig. 2-5).

Other types of compound microscopes include phase-contrast microscopes and fluorescence microscopes. ***Phase-contrast microscopes*** can be used to observe unstained living microorganisms. Because the light refracted by living cells is different from the light refracted by the surrounding medium, contrast is increased, and the organisms are more easily seen. ***Fluorescence microscopes*** contain a built-in ultraviolet (UV) light source. When UV light strikes certain dyes and pigments, these substances

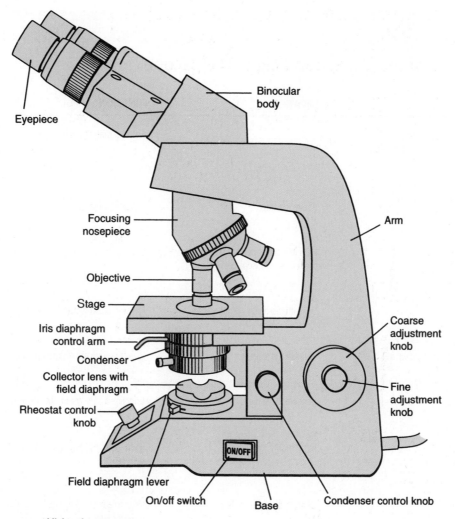

FIGURE 2-4. A modern compound light microscope.

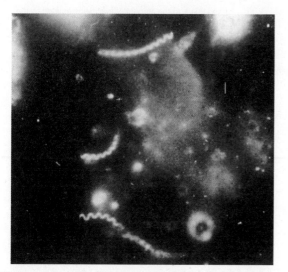

FIGURE 2-5. Spiral-shaped *Treponema pallidum,* the etiologic agent of syphilis, as seen by darkfield microscopy. (Koneman's Color Atlas and Textbook of Diagnostic Microbiology, 6th ed. Philadelphia: Lippincott-Raven, 2006. Courtesy of the Centers for Disease Control and Prevention.)

emit a longer wavelength light, causing them to glow against a dark background. Fluorescence microscopy is often used in immunology laboratories to demonstrate that antibodies stained with a fluorescent dye have combined with specific antigens; this is a type of immunodiagnostic procedure. (Immunodiagnostic procedures are described in Chapter 16.)

Electron Microscopes

Although extremely small infectious agents, such as rabies and smallpox viruses, were known to exist, they could not be seen until the electron microscope was developed. It should be noted that electron microscopes cannot be used to observe living organisms. Organisms are killed during the specimen-processing procedures. Even if they were not, they would be unable to survive in the vacuum created within the electron microscope.

Electron microscopes use an electron beam as a source of illumination and magnets to focus the beam. Because the wavelength of electrons traveling in a vacuum is much

TABLE 2-3

Components of the Compound Light Microscope

COMPONENT	LOCATION	FUNCTION
Ocular lens (also known as an eyepiece); a monocular microscope has one; a binocular microscope has two		An ×10 magnifying lens
Revolving nosepiece	Above the stage	Holds the objective lenses
Objective lenses	Held in place above the stage by the revolving nosepiece	Used to magnify objects placed on the stage
Stage	Beneath the revolving nosepiece	Flat surface on which the specimen is placed
Stage adjustment knobs (not shown in Fig. 2-4)	Beneath the stage	Used to move the microscope slide around on the stage
Condenser	Beneath the stage	Contains a lens system that focuses light onto the specimen
Iris diaphragm control arm	On the condenser	Used to adjust the amount of light coming through the condenser
Field diaphragm lever	Beneath the collector lens	Used to adjust the amount of light coming through the collector lens
Rheostat control knob	At the front of the base	Used to adjust the amount of light being emitted by the light bulb in the base
Condenser control knob	Beneath and behind the condenser	Used to adjust the height of the condenser
Coarse and fine adjustment knobs	On the arm of the microscope near the base	Used to focus the lenses

TABLE 2-4

Magnifications Achieved Using the Compound Light Microscope

OBJECTIVE	TOTAL MAGNIFICATION ACHIEVED WHEN THE OBJECTIVE IS USED IN CONJUNCTION WITH A 310 OCULAR LENS
×4 (scanning objective)	40×
×10 (low-power objective)	100×
×40 (high-dry objective)	400×
×100 (oil-immersion objective)	1,000×

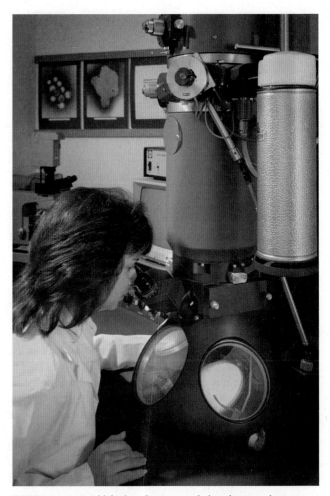

FIGURE 2-6. A CDC biologist using a transmission electron microscope. (Courtesy of James Gathany and the Centers for Disease Control and Prevention.)

shorter than the wavelength of visible light—about 100,000 times shorter—electron microscopes have a much greater resolving power than compound light microscopes. There are two types of electron microscopes: transmission electron microscopes and scanning electron microscopes.

A ***transmission electron microscope*** (Fig. 2-6) has a very tall column, at the top of which an electron gun fires a beam of electrons downward. When an extremely thin specimen (less than 1 μm thick) is placed into the electron beam, some of the electrons are transmitted through the specimen, and some are blocked. An image of the specimen is produced on a phosphor-coated screen at the bottom of the microscope's column. The object can be magnified up to approximately 1 million times. Thus, using a transmission electron microscope, a magnification is achieved that is about 1,000 times greater than the maximum magnification achieved using a compound light microscope. Even very tiny microbes (e.g., viruses) can be observed using a transmission electron microscope. Because thin sections of cells are examined, transmission electron microscopy enables scientists to study the internal structure of cells. Special staining procedures are used to increase contrast between different parts of the cell. The first transmission electron microscopes were developed during the late 1920s and early 1930s, but it was not until the early 1950s that electron microscopes began to be used routinely to study cells. A ***scanning electron microscope*** (Fig. 2-7) has a shorter column and instead of being placed into the electron beam, the specimen is placed at the bottom of the column. Electrons that bounce off the surface of the specimen are captured by detectors, and an image of the specimen

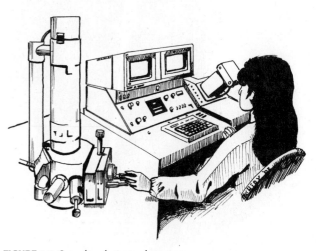

FIGURE 2-7. Scanning electron microscope.

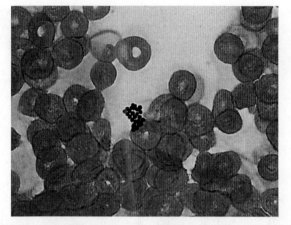

FIGURE 2-8. *Staphylococcus aureus* and red blood cells, as seen by light microscopy. (Marler LM, et al. Direct Smear Atlas. Philadelphia: Lippincott Williams & Wilkins, 2001.)

appears on a monitor. Scanning electron microscopes are used to observe the outer surfaces of specimens (i.e., surface detail). Although the resolving power of scanning electron microscopes (about 20 nm) is not quite as good as the resolving power of transmission electron microscopes (about 0.2 nm), it is still possible to observe extremely tiny objects using a scanning electron microscope. Scanning electron microscopes became available during the late 1960s.

Both types of electron microscopes have built-in camera systems. The photographs taken using transmission and scanning electron microscopes are called *transmission*

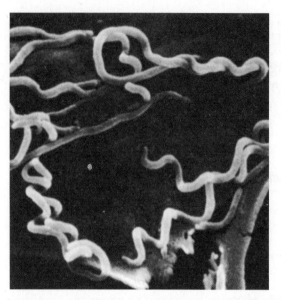

FIGURE 2-10. The illusion of depth when using scanning electron microscopy clearly reveals the corkscrew shape of cells of the syphilis-causing spirochete, *Treponema pallidum.* (Original magnification, 8,000×; Volk WA, et al. Essentials of Medical Microbiology, 5th ed. Philadelphia: Lippincott-Raven, 1996.)

electron micrographs (TEMs) and *scanning electron micrographs* (SEMs), respectively. They are black and white images. If you ever see **electron micrographs** in color, they have been artificially colorized. Figures 2-8, 2-9, and 2-10 show the differences in magnification and detail between electron micrographs and light photomicrographs. Refer to Table 2-2 for the characteristics of various types of microscopes.

◉ REVIEW OF KEY POINTS

- A meter (m) can be divided into 10 *deci*meters, 100 *centi*meters, 1,000 *milli*meters, 1 million *micro*meters, or 1 billion *nano*meters.

- The metric system is used to describe the sizes of microorganisms. The sizes of bacteria and protozoa are expressed in micrometers (μm), whereas the sizes of viruses are expressed in nanometers (nm).

- The development of simple and compound light microscopes enabled the discovery and visualization of microorganisms. Simple microscopes have only one magnifying lens, whereas compound microscopes have more than one magnifying lens.

- The limiting factor of compound light microscopes is the type of illumination being used. Because visible light is used as the source of illumination, objects that are smaller than half the wavelength of visible light cannot be seen. The resolving power (resolution) of the compound light microscope is 0.2 μm.

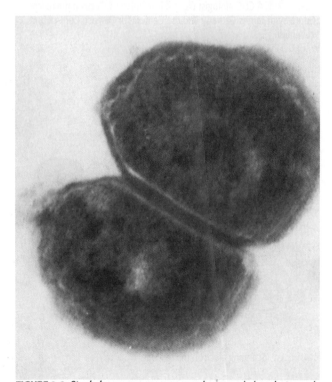

FIGURE 2-9. *Staphylococcus aureus,* as seen by transmission electron microscopy. (Original magnification, 40,000×; TEM courtesy of Ray Rupel.)

- Smaller objects can be seen using electron microscopes, because electrons are used as the source of illumination. The wavelength of electrons is shorter than that of visible light.

- Transmission electron microscopes enable scientists to see inside of cells (i.e., to see internal details). Using scanning electron microscopes, scientists are able to study surface details. The resolving power of the transmission electron microscope is 0.2 nm, whereas the resolving power of the scanning electron microscope is 20 nm.

- Because they are so tiny, most viruses can only be seen using electron microscopes.

- Photographs taken through the lens system of the compound light microscope are called photomicrographs, whereas those taken with electron microscopes are called transmission electron micrographs and scanning electron micrographs.

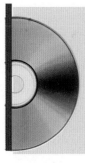

On the CD-ROM
- Critical Thinking
- Additional Self-Assessment Exercises

Self-Assessment Exercises

After studying this chapter, answer the following multiple-choice questions.

1. A millimeter is equivalent to how many nanometers?
   a. 1,000
   b. 10,000
   c. 100,000
   d. 1,000,000

2. Assume that a pinhead is 1 mm in diameter. How many spherical bacteria (cocci), lined up side-by-side, would fit across the pinhead? (Hint: Use information from Table 2-1.)
   a. 100
   b. 1,000
   c. 10,000
   d. 100,000

3. What is the length of an average rod-shaped bacterium (bacillus)?
   a. 3 μm
   b. 3 nm
   c. 0.3 mm
   d. 0.03 mm

4. What is the total magnification when using the high-power (high-dry) objective of a compound light microscope equipped with a ×10 ocular lens?
   a. 40
   b. 50
   c. 100
   d. 400

5. How many times better is the resolution of the transmission electron microscope than the resolution of the unaided human eye?
   a. 1,000
   b. 10,000
   c. 100,000
   d. 1,000,000

6. How many times better is the resolution of the transmission electron microscope than the resolution of the compound light microscope?
   a. 100
   b. 1,000
   c. 10,000
   d. 100,000

7. How many times better is the resolution of the transmission electron microscope than the resolution of the scanning electron microscope?
   a. 100
   b. 1,000
   c. 10,000
   d. 100,000

8. The limiting factor of any compound light microscope (i.e., the thing that limits its resolution to 0.2 μm) is the:
   a. number of condenser lenses it has.
   b. number of magnifying lenses it has.
   c. number of ocular lenses it has.
   d. wavelength of visible light.

9. Which of the following individuals is given credit for developing the first compound microscope?
   a. Anton van Leeuwenhoek
   b. Hans Jansen
   c. Louis Pasteur
   d. Robert Hooke

10. A compound light microscope differs from a simple microscope in that the compound light microscope contains more than one:
    a. condenser lens.
    b. magnifying lens.
    c. objective lens.
    d. ocular lens.

3

CELL STRUCTURE AND TAXONOMY

LEARNING OBJECTIVES

AFTER STUDYING THIS CHAPTER, YOU SHOULD BE
ABLE TO:

- Explain what is meant by the cell theory
- State the contributions of Hooke, Schleiden and Schwann, and Virchow to the study of cells
- Cite a function for each of the following parts of a eucaryotic cell: cell membrane, nucleus, ribosomes, Golgi complex, lysosomes, mitochondria, plastids, cytoskeleton, cell wall, flagella, and cilia
- Cite a function for each of the following parts of a bacterial cell: cell membrane, chromosome, cell wall, capsule, flagella, pili, and endospores
- Compare and contrast plant, animal, and bacterial cells
- Define the terms genus, specific epithet, and species
- Describe the Five-Kingdom and Three-Domain Systems of classification

INTRODUCTION

In this chapter, you will learn about the structure of microorganisms. Because they are so small, very little detail concerning their structure can be determined using the compound light microscope. Our knowledge of the fine structure of microbes has been gained through the use of electron microscopes. Such fine detail—detail that is beyond the resolving power of the compound light microscope—is referred to as the ultrastructure of the microorganisms. Also discussed in this chapter are the ways in which microorganisms and their cells reproduce and how microorganisms are classified.

In biology, a **cell** is defined as the fundamental living unit of any organism because, like the total organism, the cell exhibits the basic characteristics of life. A cell obtains food (nutrients) from the environment to produce energy for metabolism and other activities. *Metabolism* refers to

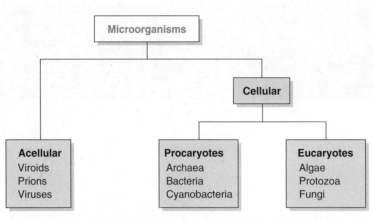

FIGURE 3-1. Acellular and cellular microbes. Acellular microbes include viroids, prions, and viruses. Cellular microbes include the less complex procaryotes (archaeans and bacteria) and the more complex eucaryotes (some algae, protozoa, and some fungi).

HISTORICAL NOTE

Cells

In 1665, an English physicist named Robert Hooke published a book, entitled *Micrographia,* containing descriptions of objects he had observed using a compound light microscope that he had made. These objects included molds, rusts, fleas, lice, fossilized plants and animals, and sections of cork. Hooke referred to the small empty chambers in the structure of cork as *cells,* probably because they reminded him of the bare rooms (called cells) in a monastery. Hooke was the first person to use the term "cells" in this manner. Around 1838–1839, a German botanist named Matthias Schleiden and a German zoologist named Theodor Schwann concluded that all plant and animal tissues were composed of cells; this later became known as the *cell theory.* Then in 1858, the German pathologist Rudolf Virchow proposed the theory of *biogenesis*—that life can only arise from preexisting life, and, therefore, that cells can only arise from preexisting cells. Biogenesis does not address the issue of the origin of life on earth, a complex topic about which much has been written.

all of the chemical reactions that occur within a cell (see Chapter 7 for a detailed discussion of metabolism and metabolic reactions). Because of its metabolism, a cell can grow and reproduce. It can respond to stimuli in its environment such as light, heat, cold, and the presence of

chemicals. A cell can mutate (change genetically) as a result of accidental changes in its genetic material—the *deoxyribonucleic acid* (**DNA**) that makes up the genes of its chromosomes—and, thus, can become better or less suited to its environment. As a result of these genetic changes, the mutant organism may be better adapted for survival and development into a new **species (pl. species)** of organism.

Considerable evidence exists to indicate that between 3.5 and 4 billion years ago, the first bit of life to appear on earth was a very primitive cell similar to the simple bacteria of today. Bacterial cells exhibit all the characteristics of life, although they do not have the complex system of membranes and *organelles* (tiny organlike structures) found in the more advanced single-celled organisms. These less complex cells, which include *Bacteria* and *Archaea,* are called *procaryotes* or **procaryotic cells.**[a] The more complex cells, containing a true nucleus and many membrane-bound organelles, are called *eucaryotes* or **eucaryotic cells.**[a] Eucaryotes include such organisms as algae, protozoa, fungi, plants, animals, and humans. Some microorganisms are procaryotic, some are eucaryotic, and some are not cells at all (Fig. 3-1).

Viruses appear to be the result of regressive or reverse evolution. They are composed of only a few genes protected by a protein coat, and sometimes may contain one or a few enzymes. Viruses depend on the energy and metabolic machinery of a host cell to reproduce. Because viruses are acellular (not composed of cells), they are placed in a completely separate category.

For those in the health professions, it is important to learn differences in the structure of various cells, not only for identification purposes, but also to understand differences in their metabolism. These factors must be known before one can determine or explain why antimicrobial

---

[a]Alternative spellings of procaryote and eucaryote are prokaryote and eukaryote.

agents (drugs) attack and destroy pathogens, but do not harm human cells.

Cytology, the study of the structure and function of cells, has developed during the past 75 years with the aid of the electron microscope and sophisticated biochemical research. Many books have been written about the details of these tiny functional factories—cells—but only a brief discussion of their structure and activities is presented here.

Eucaryotic Cell Structure

Eucaryotes (*eu* = true; *caryo* refers to a nut or nucleus) are so named because they have a true nucleus, in that their DNA is enclosed by a nuclear membrane. Most animal and plant cells are 10 to 30 μm in diameter, about 10 times larger than most procaryotic cells. Figure 3-2 illustrates a typical eucaryotic animal cell. This illustration is a composite of most of the structures that might be found in the various types of human body cells. Figure 3-3 is a transmission electron micrograph (TEM) of an actual yeast cell. A discussion of the functional parts of eucaryotic cells can be better understood by keeping the illustrated structures in mind.

Cell Membrane

The cell is enclosed and held intact by the **cell membrane,** which is also referred to as the plasma, cytoplasmic, or

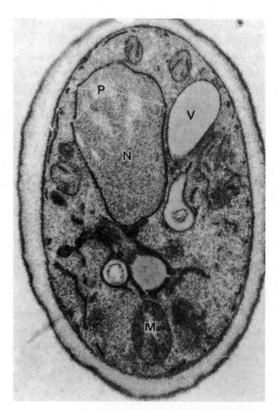

FIGURE 3-3. Cross-section through a yeast cell, showing the nucleus (N) with nuclear pores (P), mitochondrion (M), and vacuole (V). The cytoplasm is surrounded by the cell membrane. The thick outer portion is the cell wall. (Lechavalier HA, Pramer D. The Microbes. Philadelphia: JB Lippincott, 1970.)

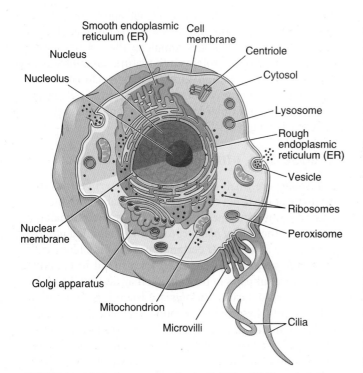

FIGURE 3-2. A typical eucaryotic animal cell. (Cohen BJ. Memmler's The Human Body in Health and Disease, 10th ed. Philadelphia: Lippincott Williams & Wilkins, 2005.)

cellular membrane. Structurally, it is a mosaic composed of large molecules of proteins and phospholipids (certain types of fats). The cell membrane is like a "skin" around the cell, separating the contents of the cell from the outside world. The cell membrane regulates the passage of nutrients, waste products, and secretions into and out of the cell. Because the cell membrane has the property of **selective permeability,** only certain substances may enter and leave the cell. The cell membrane is similar in structure and function to all of the other membranes that are found in eucaryotic cells.

Nucleus

As previously mentioned, the primary difference between procaryotic and eucaryotic cells is that eucaryotic cells possess a "true nucleus," whereas procaryotic cells do not. The **nucleus (pl. nuclei)** controls the functions of the entire cell and can be thought of as the "command center" of the cell. The nucleus has three components: nucleoplasm, chromosomes, and a nuclear membrane. **Nucleoplasm** (a type of **protoplasm**) is the gelatinous matrix or base material of the nucleus. The **chromosomes** are embedded or suspended in the nucleoplasm. The membrane that serves as a "skin" around the nucleus is called the **nuclear membrane;** it contains holes (nuclear pores) through which large molecules can enter and exit the nucleus.

Eucaryotic chromosomes consist of linear DNA molecules and proteins (histones and nonhistone proteins). **Genes** are located along the DNA molecules. Although genes are sometimes described as "beads on a string," each bead (gene) is actually a particular segment of the DNA molecule. Each gene contains the genetic information that enables the cell to produce a *gene product.* Most gene products are proteins, but some genes code for the production of two types of *ribonucleic acid* **(RNA):** ribosomal ribonucleic acid (rRNA) and transfer ribonucleic acid (tRNA) molecules (discussed in Chapter 6). The organism's complete collection of genes is referred to as that organism's *genotype* (or *genome*). To understand more about how genes control the activities of the entire organism, refer to Chapters 6 and 7.

The number and composition of chromosomes and the number of genes on each chromosome are characteristic of the particular species of organism. Different species have different numbers and sizes of chromosomes. Human diploid cells, for example, have 46 chromosomes (23 pairs), each consisting of thousands of genes. It has been estimated that the human genome consists of about 20,000 to 25,000 genes.

When observed using a transmission electron microscope, a dark (electron dense) area can be seen in the nucleus. This area is called the *nucleolus;* it is here that rRNA molecules are manufactured. The rRNA molecules then exit the nucleus and become part of the structure of ribosomes (discussed later).

Cytoplasm

Cytoplasm (a type of protoplasm) is a semifluid, gelatinous, nutrient matrix. Within the cytoplasm are found insoluble storage granules and a variety of cytoplasmic organelles, including endoplasmic reticulum, ribosomes, Golgi complexes, mitochondria, centrioles, microtubules, lysosomes, and other membrane-bound vacuoles. Each of these organelles has a highly specific function, and all of the functions are interrelated to maintain the cell and allow it to properly perform its activities. The cytoplasm is where most of the cell's metabolic reactions occur. The semifluid portion of the cytoplasm, excluding the granules and organelles, is sometimes referred to as the cytosol.

Endoplasmic Reticulum

The *endoplasmic reticulum* (ER) is a highly convoluted system of membranes that are interconnected and arranged to form a transport network of tubules and flattened sacs within the cytoplasm. Much of the ER has a rough, granular appearance when observed by transmission electron microscopy and is designated as *rough endoplasmic reticulum* **(RER).** This rough appearance is caused by the many *ribosomes* attached to the outer surface of the membranes. Endoplasmic reticulum to which ribosomes are not attached is called *smooth endoplasmic reticulum* **(SER).**

Ribosomes

Eucaryotic ribosomes are 18 to 22 nm in diameter. They consist mainly of rRNA and protein and play an important part in the synthesis (manufacture) of proteins. Clusters of ribosomes (called *polyribosomes* or *polysomes*), held together by a molecule of messenger RNA (mRNA), are sometimes observed by electron microscopy.

Each eucaryotic ribosome is composed of two subunits—a large subunit (the 60S subunit) and a small subunit (the 40S subunit)—that are produced in the nucleolus. The subunits are then transported to the cytoplasm where they remain separate until such time as they join together with an mRNA molecule to initiate protein synthesis (Chapter 6). When united, the 40S and 60S subunits form an 80S ribosome. (The "S" refers to Svedberg units, and 40S, 60S, and 80S are sedimentation coefficients. A sedimentation coefficient expresses the rate at which a particle or molecule moves in a centrifugal field; it is determined by the size and shape of the particle or molecule.)

Most of the proteins released from the ER are not mature. They must undergo further processing in an organelle known as a Golgi complex before they are able to perform their functions within or outside of the cell.

Golgi Complex

A *Golgi complex,* also known as a Golgi apparatus or Golgi body, connects or communicates with the ER. This stack of flattened, membranous sacs completes the transformation of newly synthesized proteins into mature, functional ones and packages them into small, membrane-enclosed vesicles for storage within the cell or export outside the cell (exocytosis or secretion). Golgi complexes are sometimes referred to as "packaging plants."

Lysosomes and Peroxisomes

Lysosomes are small (about 1 μm diameter) vesicles that originate at the Golgi complex. They contain lysozyme and other digestive enzymes that break down foreign material taken into the cell by *phagocytosis* (the engulfing of large particles by amebas and certain types of white blood cells called *phagocytes*). These enzymes also aid in breaking down worn out parts of the cell and may destroy the entire cell by a process called *autolysis* if the cell is damaged or deteriorating. Lysosomes are found in all eucaryotic cells.

Peroxisomes are membrane-bound vesicles in which hydrogen peroxide is both generated and broken down. Peroxisomes contain the enzyme catalase, which catalyzes (speeds up) the breakdown of hydrogen peroxide into water and oxygen. Peroxisomes are found in most eucaryotic cells, but are especially prominent in mammalian liver cells.

Mitochondria

The energy necessary for cellular function is provided by the formation of high-energy phosphate molecules such as adenosine triphosphate (ATP). ATP molecules are the major energy-carrying or energy-storing molecules within cells. *Mitochondria* **(sing., mitochondrion)** are referred to as the "power plants," "powerhouses," or "energy factories" of the eucaryotic cell, because this is where most of the ATP molecules are formed by cellular respiration. During this process, energy is released from glucose molecules and other nutrients to drive other cellular functions (see Chapter 7). The number of mitochondria in a cell varies greatly depending on the activities required of that cell. Mitochondria are about 0.5 to 1 μm in diameter and up to 7 μm in length. Many scientists believe that mitochondria and chloroplasts arose from bacteria living within eucaryotic cells (see "Insight: The Origin of Mitochondria and Chloroplasts" on the CD-ROM).

Plastids

Plant cells contain both mitochondria and another type of energy-producing organelle, called a plastid. *Plastids* are membrane-bound structures containing various photosynthetic pigments; they are the sites of photosynthesis. *Chloroplasts,* one type of plastid, contain a green, photosynthetic pigment called chlorophyll. Chloroplasts are found in plant cells and algae. *Photosynthesis* is the process by which light energy is used to convert carbon dioxide and water into carbohydrates and oxygen (Chapter 7). The chemical bonds in the carbohydrate molecules represent stored energy. Thus, photosynthesis is the conversion of light energy into chemical energy.

Cytoskeleton

Present throughout the cytoplasm is a system of fibers, collectively known as the *cytoskeleton.* The three types of cytoskeletal fibers are microtubules, microfilaments (actin filaments), and intermediate filaments. All three types serve to strengthen, support, and stiffen the cell, and give the cell its shape. In addition to their structural roles, microtubules and microfilaments are essential for a variety of activities, such as cell division, contraction, motility (see the section on flagella and cilia), and the movement of chromosomes within the cell. *Microtubules* are slender, hollow tubules composed of spherical protein subunits called tubulins.

Cell Wall

Some eucaryotic cells contain *cell walls*—external structures that provide rigidity, shape, and protection (Fig. 3-4). Eucaryotic cell walls, which are much simpler in structure than procaryotic cell walls, may contain cellulose, pectin, lignin, chitin, and some mineral salts (usually found in algae). The cell walls of algae contain a polysaccharide—

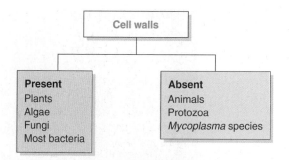

FIGURE 3-4. Presence or absence of cell wall in various types of cells.

cellulose—that is not found in the cell walls of any other microorganisms. Cellulose is also found in the cell walls of plants. The cell walls of fungi contain a polysaccharide—*chitin*—that is not found in the cell walls of any other microorganisms. Chitin, which is similar in structure to cellulose, is also found in the exoskeletons of beetles and crabs.

Flagella and Cilia

Some eucaryotic cells (e.g., spermatozoa and certain types of protozoa and algae) possess relatively long, thin structures called *flagella* **(sing., flagellum).** Such cells are said to be flagellated or motile; flagellated protozoa are called flagellates. The whipping motion of the flagella enables flagellated cells to "swim" through liquid environments; flagella are said to be whiplike. Flagella are referred to as organelles of locomotion (cell movement). Flagellated cells may possess one flagellum or two or more flagella. *Cilia* **(sing., cilium)** are also organelles of locomotion, but they tend to be shorter (more hairlike), thinner, and more numerous than flagella. Cilia can be found on some species of protozoa (called ciliates) and on certain types of cells in our bodies (e.g., the ciliated epithelial cells that line the respiratory tract). Unlike flagella, cilia tend to beat with a coordinated, rhythmic movement. Eucaryotic flagella and cilia, which contain an internal "9 + 2" arrangement of microtubules (Fig. 3-5), are structurally more complex than bacterial flagella.

Procaryotic Cell Structure

Procaryotic cells are about 10 times smaller than eucaryotic cells. A typical *Escherichia coli* cell is about 1 μm wide and 2 to 3 μm long. Structurally, *procaryotes* are very simple cells when compared with eucaryotic cells, and yet they are able to perform the necessary processes of life. Reproduction of procaryotic cells is by *binary fission*—the simple division of one cell into two cells, after DNA replication (Chapter 6) and the formation of a separating membrane and cell wall. All bacteria are procaryotes, as are the archaeans.

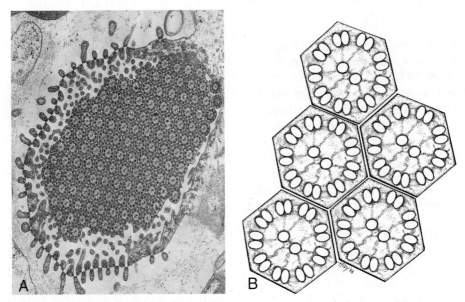

FIGURE 3-5. Cilia. (*A*) Transmission electron micrograph (TEM) showing the cross-section of a tapeworm flame cell (an excretory organ) containing numerous cilia. (TEM by P. Engelkirk.) (*B*) Diagrammatic representation of cilia in cross-section, illustrating the 9 + 2 arrangement of microtubules (see text). Individual cilia are round, but cilia within the flame cell are tightly squeezed together, resulting in their altered shape.

Embedded within the cytoplasm of procaryotic cells are a chromosome, ribosomes, and other cytoplasmic particles (Fig. 3-6). Unlike eucaryotic cells, the cytoplasm of procaryotic cells is not filled with internal membranes. The cytoplasm is surrounded by a cell membrane, a cell wall (usually), and sometimes a capsule or slime layer. These latter three structures make up the bacterial cell envelope. Depending on the particular species of bacterium, flagella or pili (description follows) or both may be observed outside the cell envelope, and a spore may sometimes be seen within the cell.

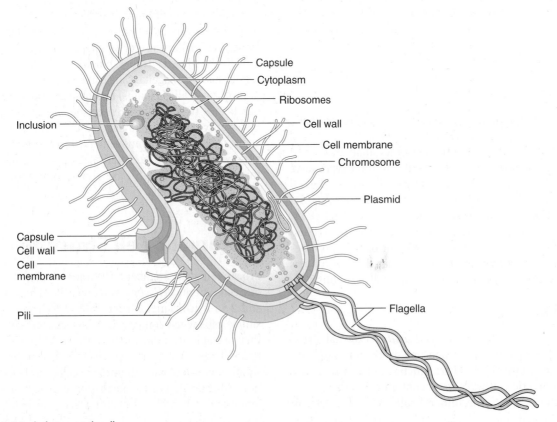

FIGURE 3-6. A typical procaryotic cell.

Cell Membrane

Enclosing the cytoplasm of a procaryotic cell is the cell membrane (or plasma, cytoplasmic, or cellular membrane). This membrane is similar in structure and function to the eucaryotic cell membrane. Chemically, the cell membrane consists of proteins and phospholipids, which are discussed further in Chapter 6. Being selectively permeable, the membrane controls which substances may enter or leave the cell. It is flexible and so thin that it cannot be seen with a compound light microscope. However, it is frequently observed in transmission electron micrographs of bacteria.

Many enzymes are attached to the cell membrane, and a variety of metabolic reactions take place there. Some scientists believe that inward foldings of the cell membranes—called mesosomes—are where cellular respiration takes place in bacteria. This process is similar to that which occurs in the mitochondria of eucaryotic cells, in which nutrients are broken down to produce energy in the form of ATP molecules. On the other hand, some scientists think that mesosomes are nothing more than artifacts created during the processing of bacterial cells for electron microscopy.

In cyanobacteria and other photosynthetic bacteria (bacteria that convert light energy into chemical energy), infoldings of the cell membrane contain chlorophyll and other pigments that serve to trap light energy for photosynthesis. However, procaryotic cells do not have complex internal membrane systems similar to the endoplasmic reticulum and Golgi complex of eucaryotic cells. Procaryotic cells do not contain any membrane-bound organelles or vesicles.

Chromosome

The procaryotic chromosome usually consists of a single, long, supercoiled, circular DNA molecule, which serves as the control center of the bacterial cell. It is capable of duplicating itself, guiding cell division, and directing cellular activities. A procaryotic cell contains neither nucleoplasm nor a nuclear membrane. The chromosome is suspended or embedded in the cytoplasm. The DNA-occupied space within a bacterial cell is sometimes referred to as the bacterial nucleoid.

The thin and tightly folded chromosome of *E. coli* is about 1.5 mm (1,500 μm) long and only 2 nm wide. Because a typical *E. coli* cell is about 2 to 3 μm long, its chromosome is approximately 500 to 750 times longer than the cell itself—quite a packaging feat! Bacterial chromosomes contain between 850 and 6,500 genes, depending on the species. Thus, a bacterial chromosome contains sufficient genetic information to code for between 850 to 6,500 gene products (enzymes, other proteins, and rRNA and tRNA molecules). In comparison, the chromosomes within a human cell contain about 25,000 genes, enough to code for approximately 25,000 gene products.

Small, circular molecules of double-stranded DNA that are not part of the chromosome (referred to as extrachromosomal DNA or *plasmids*) may also be present in the

cytoplasm of procaryotic cells. A **plasmid** may contain anywhere from fewer than 10 genes to several hundred genes. A bacterial cell may not contain any plasmids, or it may contain one plasmid, multiple copies of the same plasmid, or more than one type of plasmid (i.e., plasmids containing different genes). (Additional information about bacterial plasmids is found in Chapter 7.) Plasmids have also been found in yeast cells.

Cytoplasm

The semiliquid cytoplasm of procaryotic cells consists of water, enzymes, dissolved oxygen (in some bacteria), waste products, essential nutrients, proteins, carbohydrates, and lipids—a complex mixture of all the materials required by the cell for its metabolic functions.

Cytoplasmic Particles

Within the bacterial cytoplasm, many tiny particles have been observed. Most of these are ribosomes, often occurring in clusters called polyribosomes or polysomes (*poly* meaning many). Procaryotic ribosomes are smaller than eucaryotic ribosomes, but their function is the same—they are the sites of protein synthesis. A 70S procaryotic ribosome is composed of a 30S subunit and a 50S subunit. It has been estimated that there are about 15,000 ribosomes in the cytoplasm of an *E. coli* cell.

Cytoplasmic granules occur in certain species of bacteria. These may be stained by using a suitable stain, and then identified microscopically. The granules may consist of starch, lipids, sulfur, iron, or other stored substances.

Bacterial Cell Wall

The rigid exterior cell wall that defines the shape of bacterial cells is chemically complex. Thus, the structure of bacterial cell walls is quite different from the relatively simple structure of eucaryotic cell walls, although they serve the same functions—providing rigidity, strength, and protection. The main constituent of most bacterial cell walls is a complex

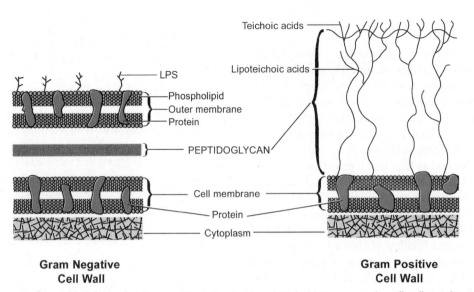

Teichoic acids
Lipoteichoic acids
LPS
Phospholipid
Outer membrane
Protein
PEPTIDOGLYCAN
Cell membrane
Protein
Cytoplasm

**Gram Negative
Cell Wall**

**Gram Positive
Cell Wall**

FIGURE 3-7. Differences between Gram-negative and Gram-positive cell walls. The relatively thin Gram-negative cell wall contains a thin layer of peptidoglycan, an outer membrane, and lipopolysaccharide (LPS). The thicker Gram-positive cell wall contains a thick layer of peptidoglycan and teichoic and lipoteichoic acids.

macromolecular polymer known as ***peptidoglycan*** (murein), consisting of many polysaccharide chains linked together by small peptide (protein) chains. Peptidoglycan is only found in bacteria. The thickness of the cell wall and its exact composition vary with the species of bacteria. The cell walls of certain bacteria, called "Gram-positive bacteria" (to be explained in Chapter 4), have a thick layer of peptidoglycan combined with teichoic acid and lipoteichoic acid molecules. The cell walls of "Gram-negative bacteria" (also explained in Chapter 4) have a much thinner layer of peptidoglycan, but this layer is covered with a complex layer of lipid macromolecules, usually referred to as the outer membrane, as shown

in Figures 3-7 and 3-8. These macromolecules are discussed in Chapter 6. Although most bacteria have cell walls, bacteria in the genus *Mycoplasma* do not. Archaeans (described later) have cell walls, but their cell walls do not contain peptidoglycan.

Glycocalyx (Slime Layers and Capsules)

Some bacteria have a thick layer of material (known as glycocalyx) located outside their cell wall. ***Glycocalyx*** is a slimy, gelatinous material produced by the cell membrane

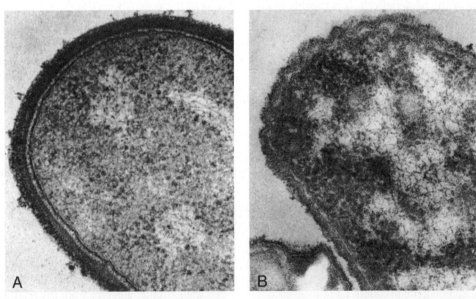

FIGURE 3-8. Bacterial cell walls. (*A*) A portion of the Gram-positive bacterium, *Bacillus fastidious;* note the cell wall's thick peptidoglycan layer, beneath which can be seen the cell membrane. (*B*) The Gram-negative bacterium, *Enterobacter aerogenes;* both the cell membrane and the outer membrane are visible along some sections of the cell wall. (Volk WA, et al. Essentials of Medical Microbiology, 5th ed. Philadelphia: Lippincott-Raven, 1996.)

and secreted outside of the cell wall. There are two types of glycocalyx. One type, called a **slime layer,** is not highly organized and is not firmly attached to the cell wall. It easily detaches from the cell wall and drifts away. Bacteria in the genus *Pseudomonas* produce a slime layer, which sometimes plays a role in diseases caused by *Pseudomonas* species. Slime layers enable certain bacteria to glide or slide along solid surfaces.

The other type of glycocalyx, called a **capsule,** is highly organized and firmly attached to the cell wall. Capsules usually consist of polysaccharides, which may be combined with lipids and proteins, depending on the bacterial species. Knowledge of the chemical composition of capsules is useful in differentiating among different types of bacteria within a particular species; for example, different strains of *Haemophilus influenzae,* a cause of meningitis and ear infections in children, are identified by their capsular types. A vaccine, called Hib vaccine, is available for protection against disease caused by *H. influenzae* capsular type b. Other examples of encapsulated bacteria are *Klebsiella pneumoniae, Neisseria meningitidis,* and *Streptococcus pneumoniae.*

Capsules can be detected using a capsule-staining procedure, which is a type of **negative stain.** The bacterial cell and background become stained, but the capsule remains unstained (Fig. 3-9). Thus, the capsule appears as an unstained halo around the bacterial cell. Antigen–antibody tests (described in Chapter 16) may be used to identify specific strains of bacteria possessing unique capsular molecules (antigens).

Encapsulated bacteria usually produce colonies on nutrient agar that are smooth, mucoid, and glistening; they are referred to as S-colonies. Nonencapsulated bacteria tend to grow as dry, rough colonies, called R-colonies. Capsules serve an antiphagocytic function, protecting the encapsulated bacteria from being phagocytized (ingested) by phagocytic white blood cells. Thus, encapsulated bacteria are able to survive longer in the human body than nonencapsulated bacteria.

Flagella

Flagella (sing., *flagellum*) are threadlike, protein appendages that enable bacteria to move. Flagellated bacteria are said to be motile, whereas nonflagellated bacteria are usually nonmotile. Bacterial flagella are about 10 to 20 nm thick; too thin to be seen with the compound light microscope. The number and arrangement of flagella possessed by a certain species of bacterium are characteristic of that species and can, thus, be used for classification and identification purposes (Fig. 3-10). Bacteria possessing flagella over their entire surface (perimeter) are called **peritrichous bacteria** (Fig. 3-11). Bacteria with a tuft of flagella at one end are described as being **lophotrichous bacteria,** whereas those having one or more flagella at each end are said to be **amphitrichous bacteria.** Bacteria possessing a single polar flagellum are described as **monotrichous bacteria.** In the laboratory, the number of flagella that a cell possesses and their locations on the cell can be determined using what is known as a flagella stain. The stain adheres to the flagella, making them thick enough to be seen under the microscope.

Bacterial flagella consist of three, four, or more threads of protein (called **flagellin**) twisted like a rope. Thus, the structures of bacterial flagella and eucaryotic flagella are quite different. You will recall that eucaryotic flagella (and cilia) contain a complex arrangement of internal microtubules, which run the length of the membrane-bound flagellum. Bacterial flagella do not contain microtubules, and their flagella are not membrane-bound. Bacterial flagella arise from a basal body in the cell membrane and project outward through the cell wall and capsule (if present), as shown in Figure 3-6.

Some **spirochetes** (spiral-shaped bacteria) have two flagella-like fibrils called **axial filaments,** one attached to each end of the bacterium. These axial filaments extend toward each other, wrap around the organism between the layers of the cell wall, and overlap in the midsection of the cell. As a result of its axial filaments, spirochetes can move in a spiral, helical, or inchworm manner.

Pili (Fimbriae)

Pili (sing., *pilus*) or *fimbriae* (sing., *fimbria*) are hairlike structures, most often observed on Gram-negative bacteria. They are composed of polymerized protein molecules called pilin. Pili are much thinner than flagella, have a rigid structure, and are not associated with motility. These tiny appendages arise from the cytoplasm and extend through

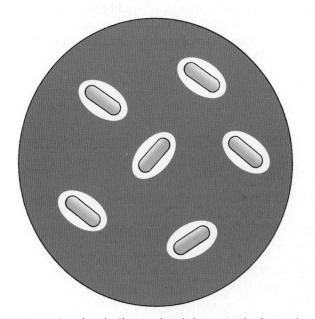

FIGURE 3-9. Capsule stain. The capsule stain is an example of a negative staining technique. The bacterial cells and the background stain, but the capsules do not. The capsules are seen as unstained "halos" around the bacterial cells.

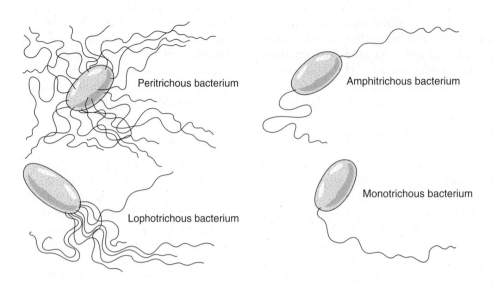

FIGURE 3-10. Flagellar arrangement. The four basic types of flagellar arrangement on bacteria: peritrichous, flagella all over the surface; lophotrichous, a tuft of flagella at one end; amphitrichous, one or more flagella at each end; monotrichous, one flagellum.

the plasma membrane, cell wall, and capsule (if present). There are two types of pili: one type enables bacteria to adhere or attach to surfaces; the other type (called a *sex pilus*) enables transfer of genetic material from one bacterial cell to another.

The pili that enable bacteria to anchor themselves to surfaces (e.g., tissues within the human body) are usually quite numerous (Fig. 3-12). In some species of bacteria, piliated strains (those possessing pili) are able to cause diseases like urethritis and cystitis, whereas nonpiliated

strains (those not possessing pili) of the same organisms are unable to cause these diseases.

A bacterial cell possessing a sex pilus (called a donor cell)—and the cell only possesses one sex pilus—is able to attach to another bacterial cell (called a recipient cell) by means of the sex pilus. Genetic material (usually in the form of a plasmid) is then transferred through the hollow sex pilus from the donor cell to the recipient cell—a process known as **conjugation** (described more fully in Chapter 7).

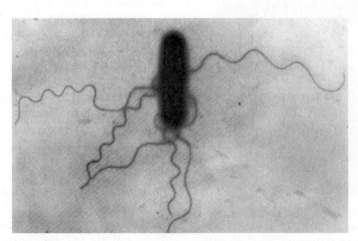

FIGURE 3-11. A peritrichous *Salmonella* cell. (Volk WA, et al. Essentials of Medical Microbiology, 5th ed. Philadelphia: Lippincott-Raven, 1996.)

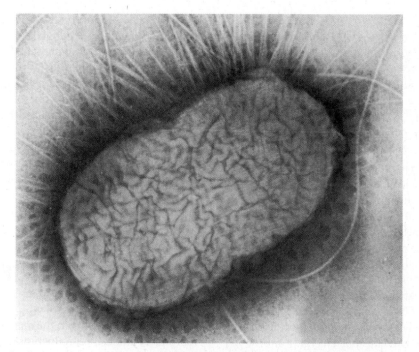

FIGURE 3-12. *Proteus vulgaris* cell, possessing numerous short, straight pili and several longer, curved flagella; the cell is undergoing binary fission. (Volk WA, et al. Essentials of Medical Microbiology, 5th ed. Philadelphia: Lippincott-Raven, 1996.)

Spores (Endospores)

A few genera of bacteria (e.g., *Bacillus* and *Clostridium*) are capable of forming thick-walled spores as a means of survival when their moisture or nutrient supply is low. Bacterial spores are referred to as **endospores,** and the process by which they are formed is called **sporulation.** During sporulation, a copy of the chromosome and some of the surrounding cytoplasm becomes enclosed in several thick protein coats. Spores are resistant to heat, cold, drying, and most chemicals. Spores have been shown to survive for many years in soil or dust, and some are quite resistant to disinfectants and boiling. When the dried spore lands on a moist, nutrient-rich surface, it germinates, and a new vegetative bacterial cell (a cell capable of growing and

dividing) emerges. Germination of a spore may be compared with germination of a seed. However, in bacteria, spore formation is related to the survival of the bacterial cell, not to reproduction. Usually, only one spore is produced in a bacterial cell and it germinates into only one vegetative bacterium (Fig. 3-13). In the laboratory, endospores can be stained using what is known as a spore stain. Once a particular bacterium's endospores are stained, the laboratory technologist can determine whether the organism is producing terminal or subterminal spores. A terminal spore is produced at the very end of the bacterial cell, whereas a subterminal spore is produced elsewhere in the cell. Where a spore is being produced within the cell and whether or not it causes a swelling of the cell serve as clues to the identity of the organism.

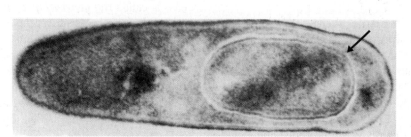

FIGURE 3-13. A bacillus with a well-defined endospore (arrow). (Lechavalier HA, Pramer D. The Microbes. Philadelphia: JB Lippincott, 1970.)

The Discovery of Endospores

While performing spontaneous generation experiments in 1876 and 1877, a British physicist named John Tyndall concluded that certain bacteria exist in two forms: a form which is readily killed by simple boiling (i.e., a heat-labile form), and a form that is not killed by simple boiling (i.e., a heat-stable form). He developed a fractional sterilization technique, known as *tyndallization*, which successfully killed both the heat labile and heat stable forms. Tyndallization involves boiling, followed by incubating, and then reboiling; these steps are repeated several times. The bacteria that emerge from the spores during the incubation steps are subsequently killed during the boiling steps. In 1877, Ferdinand Cohn, a German botanist, described the microscopic appearance of the two forms of the "hay bacillus," which Cohn named *Bacillus subtilis.* He referred to small refractile bodies within the bacterial cells as "spores" and observed the conversion of spores into actively growing cells. Cohn also concluded that when they were in the spore phase, the bacteria were heat resistant. Today, bacterial spores are known as endospores, whereas active, metabolizing, growing bacterial cells are referred to as vegetative cells. The experiments of Tyndall and Cohn supported Louis Pasteur's conclusions regarding spontaneous generation and dealt the final death blow to that theory.

Recap of Structural Differences Between Procaryotic and Eucaryotic Cells

Eucaryotic cells contain a true nucleus, whereas procaryotic cells do not. Eucaryotic cells are divided into plant and animal types. Animal cells do not have a cell wall, whereas plant cells have a simple cell wall, usually containing cellulose. Cellulose, a type of polysaccharide, is a rigid polymer of glucose (polymers and polysaccharides are described in Chapter 6). Procaryotic cells have complex cell walls consisting of proteins, lipids, and polysaccharides. Eucaryotic cells contain membranous structures (such as endoplasmic reticulum and Golgi complexes) and many membrane-bound organelles (such as mitochondria and plastids). Procaryotic cells possess no membranes other than the cell membrane that encloses the cytoplasm. Eucaryotic ribosomes (referred to as 80S ribosomes) are larger and denser than those found in procaryotes (70S ribosomes). The fact that 70S ribosomes are found in the mitochondria and chloroplasts of eucaryotes may indicate that these structures were derived from parasitic procaryotes during their evolutionary development. Other differences between procaryotic and eucaryotic cells are listed in Table 3-1.

Reproduction of Organisms and Their Cells

Reproduction (referring to the manner in which organisms reproduce) and cell reproduction (referring to the process by which individual cells reproduce) are complex topics, which can only be briefly discussed in a book of this size. It is hoped that students taking a microbiology course will have previously taken a biology course (in either high school or college) and will, therefore, have some prior knowledge of these topics. The following topics are discussed on the CD-ROM:

* asexual versus sexual reproduction
* life cycles
* eucaryotic cell reproduction (mitosis and meiosis)

Procaryotic Cell Reproduction

Procaryotic cell reproduction is quite simple when compared with eucaryotic cell division. Procaryotic cells reproduce by a process known as *binary fission,* in which one cell (the parent cell) splits in half to become two daughter cells. Before a procaryotic cell can divide in half, its chromosome must be duplicated (a process known as DNA replication; discussed in Chapter 6), so that each daughter cell will possess the same genetic information as the parent cell (Fig. 3-14).

The time it takes for binary fission to occur (i.e., the time it takes for one procaryotic cell to become two cells) is called the *generation time.* The generation time varies from one bacterial species to another and also depends on the growth conditions (e.g., pH, temperature, availability of nutrients). In the laboratory (in vitro), under ideal conditions, *E. coli* has a generation time of about 20 minutes—the number of cells will double every 20 minutes. Bacterial generation times range from as short as 10 minutes to as long as 24 hours, or even longer in some cases.

TABLE 3-1

Comparison Between Eucaryotic and Procaryotic Cells

| | EUCARYOTIC CELLS | | |
	PLANT TYPE	ANIMAL TYPE	PROCARYOTIC CELLS
Biologic distribution	All plants, fungi, and algae	All animals and protozoa	All bacteria
Nuclear membrane	Present	Present	Absent
Membranous structures other than cell membranes	Present	Present	Generally absent except for mesosomes and photosynthetic membranes
Microtubules	Present	Present	Absent
Cytoplasmic ribosomes (density)	80S	80S	70S
Chromosomes	Composed of DNA and proteins	Composed of DNA and proteins	Composed of DNA alone
Flagella or cilia	When present, have a complex structure	When present, have a complex structure	When present, flagella have a simple twisted protein structure; prokaryotic cells do not possess cilia
Cell wall	When present, of simple chemical constitution; usually contains cellulose	Absent	Of complex chemical constitution, containing peptidoglycan
Photosynthesis (chlorophyll)	Present	Absent	Present in cyanobacteria and some other bacteria

Taxonomy

According to *Bergey's Manual of Systematic Bacteriology* (described in Chapter 4 and on the CD-ROM), **taxonomy** (the science of classification of living organisms) consists of three separate but interrelated areas: classification, nomenclature, and identification. *Classification* is the arrangement of organisms into taxonomic groups (known as **taxa** [sing., **taxon**]) on the basis of similarities or relationships. Taxa include kingdoms or domains, divisions or phyla, classes, orders, families, genera, and species. Closely related organisms (i.e., organisms having similar characteristics) are placed into the same taxon. *Nomenclature* is the assignment of names to the various taxa according to international rules. *Identification* is the process of determining whether an isolate belongs to one of the established, named taxa or represents a previously unidentified species.

When attempting to identify an organism that has been isolated from a clinical specimen, laboratory technologists are very much like detectives. They gather "clues" (characteristics, attributes, properties, and traits) about the organism until they have sufficient clues to identify (speciate) the organism. In most cases, the clues that have been gathered will match the characteristics of an established species.

Parent cell

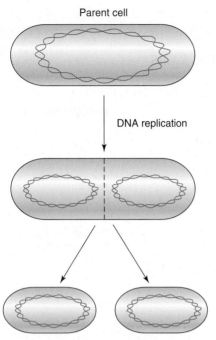

DNA replication

Two daughter cells

FIGURE 3-14. Binary fission. Note that DNA replication must occur before the actual splitting (fission) of the parent cell.

(Note: throughout this book, the term "to identify an organism" means to learn the organism's species name—i.e., to speciate it.)

Microbial Classification

Since Aristotle's time, naturalists have attempted to name and classify living organisms in a meaningful way, based on their appearance and behavior. Thus, the science of taxonomy was established, based on the binomial system of

---

nomenclature developed in the 18th century by the Swedish scientist, Carolus Linnaeus. In the binomial system, each organism is given two names (e.g., *Homo sapiens* for humans). The first name is the **genus (pl., genera)**, and the second name is the **specific epithet.** The first and second names together are referred to as the *species.*

Because written reference is often made to genera and species, biologists throughout the world have adopted a standard method of expressing these names. To express the genus, capitalize the first letter of the word and underline or italicize the whole word—for example, *Escherichia.* To express the species, capitalize the first letter of the genus name (the specific epithet is not capitalized) and then underline or italicize the entire species name—for example, *Escherichia coli.* Frequently, the genus is designated by a single letter abbreviation; in the example just given, *E. coli* indicates the species. In an essay or article about *Escherichia coli, Escherichia* would be spelled out the first time the organism is mentioned; thereafter, the abbreviated form, *E. coli,* could be used. The abbreviation "sp." is used to designate a single species, whereas the abbreviation "spp." is used to designate more than one species.

In addition to the proper scientific names for bacteria, acceptable terms like staphylococci (for *Staphylococcus* spp.), streptococci (for *Streptococcus* spp.), clostridia (for *Clostridium* spp.), pseudomonads (for *Pseudomonas* spp.), mycoplasmas (for *Mycoplasma* spp.), rickettsias (for *Rickettsia* spp.), and chlamydias (for *Chlamydia* spp.) are commonly used. Nicknames and slang terms frequently used within hospitals are GC and gonococci (for *Neisseria gonorrhoeae*), meningococci (for *Neisseria meningitidis*), pneumococci (for *Streptococcus pneumoniae*), staph (for *Staphylococcus* or staphylococcal), and strep (for *Streptococcus* or streptococcal). It is common to hear healthcare workers using terms like meningococcal meningitis, pneumococcal pneumonia, staph infection, and strep throat.

Quite often, bacteria are named for the disease that they cause (see Table 3-2 for examples). In a few cases, bacteria are misnamed. For example, *Haemophilus influenzae* does not cause influenza, which is a respiratory disease caused by influenza viruses.

Organisms are categorized into larger groups based on their similarities and differences. In 1969, Robert H. Whittaker proposed a Five-Kingdom System of Classification, in which all organisms are placed into five kingdoms:

- Bacteria and archaeans are in the Kingdom Procaryotae (or Monera)

- Algae and protozoa are in the Kingdom Protista (organisms in this kingdom are referred to as **protists**)

- Fungi are in the Kingdom Fungi

- Plants are in the Kingdom Plantae

- Animals are in the Kingdom Animalia (Although humans are in the Kingdom Animalia, in this book, the word "animals" refers to animals other than humans.)

○ STUDY AID

A Way to Remember the Sequence of Taxa From Kingdom to Species

Abbreviations and phrases are often helpful when trying to learn new material. A former student used the phrase "King David Came Over For Good Spaghetti" (KDCOFGS) to help her remember the sequence of taxa from Kingdom to Species. (K for Kingdom, D for Division, C for Class, O for Order, F for Family, G for Genus, and S for Species.) Or, if Phylum is preferred, rather than Division, King Philip can be substituted for King David. (KPCOFGS).

TABLE 3-2

Examples of Bacteria Named for the Diseases That They Cause[a]

BACTERIUM	DISEASE
Bacillus anthracis	Anthrax
Chlamydophila pneumoniae	Pneumonia
Chlamydophila psittaci	Psittacosis ("parrot fever")
Chlamydia trachomatis	Trachoma
Clostridium botulinum	Botulism
Clostridium tetani	Tetanus
Corynebacterium diphtheriae	Diphtheria
Francisella tularensis	Tularemia ("rabbit fever")
Klebsiella pneumoniae	Pneumonia
Mycobacterium leprae	Leprosy (Hansen's disease)
Mycobacterium tuberculosis	Tuberculosis
Mycoplasma pneumoniae	Pneumonia
Neisseria gonorrhoeae	Gonorrhea
Neisseria meningitidis	Meningitis
Streptococcus pneumoniae	Pneumonia
Vibrio cholerae	Cholera

[a]In some cases, these bacteria cause more than one disease.

HISTORICAL NOTE

What's in a Name?

Sometimes, bacteria and other microorganisms are named for the person who discovered the organism. An interesting example is the name of the plague bacillus. The bacterium that causes plague was discovered in 1894 by Alexandre Emile Jean Yersin (1863–1943), a French bacteriologist of Swiss descent, who worked for many years at various Pasteur Institutes in Vietnam. Yersin originally named the organism *Bacillus pestis,* but in 1896 the name was changed to *Pasteurella pestis,* to honor Louis Pasteur, with whom Yersin had studied. Then, many years later, taxonomists changed the name to *Yersinia pestis* to honor Yersin—the person who discovered the organism. Other genera named for bacteriologists include *Bordetella* (Jules Bordet), *Escherichia* (Theodore Escherich), *Neisseria* (Albert Ludwig Neisser), and *Salmonella* (Daniel Elmer Salmon).

Viruses are not included in the Five-Kingdom System of Classification because they are not living cells; they are acellular. Note that four of the five kingdoms consist of eucaryotic organisms. Each kingdom consists of divisions or phyla, which, in turn, are divided into classes, orders, families, genera, and species (Table 3-3). In some cases, species are subdivided into subspecies, their names consisting of a genus, a specific epithet, and a subspecific epithet (abbreviated "ssp."); an example would be *Haemophilus influenzae* ssp. *aegyptius,* the most common cause of "pink eye." Although Whittaker's Five-Kingdom System of Classification has been the most popular classification system for the past 30 or so years, not all scientists agree with it; other taxonomic classification schemes exist. For example, some scientists do not agree that algae and protozoa should be placed into the same kingdom, and in some classification schemes, protozoa are placed into a subkingdom of the Animal Kingdom.

In the late 1970s, Carl R. Woese (see Historical Note) devised a Three-Domain System of Classification, which is gaining in popularity among scientists. In this Three-Domain System, there are two domains of procaryotes (**Archaea** and **Bacteria**) and one domain (**Eucarya** or *Eukarya*), which includes all eucaryotic organisms. *Archaea* comes from *archae,* meaning "ancient." Although members of the Domain *Archaea* have been referred to in the past as

TABLE 3-3

Comparison of Human and Bacterial Classification

	HUMAN BEING	ESCHERICHIA COLI (A MEDICALLY IMPORTANT GRAM-NEGATIVE BACILLUS)[a]	STAPHYLOCOCCUS AUREUS (A MEDICALLY IMPORTANT GRAM-POSITIVE COCCUS)[a]
Kingdom (Domain)	Animalia (*Eucarya*)	Procaryotae (*Bacteria*)	Procaryotae (*Bacteria*)
Phylum	Chordata	Proteobacteria	Firmicutes
Class	Mammalia	Gammaproteobacteria	Bacilli
Order	Primates	Enterobacteriales	Bacillales
Family	*Hominidae*	*Enterobacteriaceae*	*Staphylococcaceae*
Genus	*Homo*	*Escherichia*	*Staphylococcus*
Species (a species has two names; the first name is the genus, and the second name is the specific epithet)	*Homo sapiens*	*Escherichia coli*	*Staphylococcus aureus*

[a]Based on Bergey's Manual of Systematic Bacteriology, vol. 1, 2nd ed. New York: Springer-Verlag, 2001. A bacillus is a rod-shaped bacterium. A coccus is a spherical-shaped bacterium.

archaebacteria and archaeobacteria (meaning "ancient" bacteria), these names have fallen out of favor because the **archaeans** are so different from bacteria. Similarly, organisms in the Domain *Bacteria* have, at times, been referred to as eubacteria, meaning "true" bacteria, but are now usually referred to simply as **bacteria.** Note that the domain names are italicized. Domain *Archaea* contains 2 phyla and Domain *Bacteria* contains 23. The Three-Domain System of Classification is based on differences in the structure of certain rRNA molecules among organisms in the three domains.

Determining Relatedness Among Organisms

How do scientists determine how closely related one organism is to another? The most widely used technique for gauging diversity or relatedness is called rRNA sequencing. Ribosomes are made up of two subunits: a small subunit and a large subunit. The small subunit contains only one RNA molecule, which is referred to as the "small subunit rRNA" or SSUrRNA. The SSUrRNA in procaryotic ribosomes is a 16S rRNA molecule, whereas the SSUrRNA in eucaryotes is an 18S rRNA molecule. (The "S" in 16S and 18S refers to Svedberg units, which were discussed earlier.) The gene that codes for the 16S rRNA molecule contains about 1,500 DNA nucleotides, whereas the gene that codes for the 18S rRNA molecule contains about 2,000 nucleotides. The sequence of nucleotides in the gene that codes for the 16S rRNA molecule is called the 16s rDNA sequence. To determine "relatedness," researchers compare the sequence of nucleotide base pairs in the gene, rather than comparing the actual SSUrRNA molecules. If the 16S rDNA sequence of one procaryotic organism is quite similar to the 16S rDNA sequence of another procaryotic organism, then the organisms are closely related. The less similar the 16S rDNA sequences in procaryotes (or the 18S rDNA sequences in eucaryotes), the less related are the organisms. For example, the 18S rDNA sequence of a human is much more similar to the 18S rDNA sequence of a chimpanzee than to the 18S rDNA sequence of a fungus.

HISTORICAL NOTE

Carl R. Woese

During the 1970s, a molecular biologist named Carl Woese and his colleagues at the University of Illinois shook up the scientific community by developing a system of classifying organisms that was based on the sequences of nucleotide bases in their ribosomal RNA molecules. They demonstrated that procaryotic organisms can be divided into two major groups (referred to as domains), based on differences in their rRNA sequences, and that the rRNA from these two groups differed from the rRNA of eucaryotic organisms. Although this system of classification was not widely accepted at first, Woese's Three-Domain System of Classification has become the classification system most favored by microbiologists.

Perhaps taxonomists will some day combine the Three-Domain System and the Five-Kingdom System, producing either a Six-Kingdom System (Bacteria, Archaea, Protista, Fungi, Plantae, and Animalia) or a Seven-Kingdom System (Bacteria, Archaea, Algae, Protozoa, Fungi, Plantae, and Animalia).

⊙ REVIEW OF KEY POINTS

- The cell is the fundamental unit of any living organism; it exhibits the basic characteristics of life. All living organisms are composed of one or more cells.

- Complex eucaryotic cells contain membrane-bound organelles and a true nucleus, containing DNA. Procaryotic cells (archaeans and bacteria) exhibit all the characteristics of life, but do not have a true nucleus or a complex system of membranes and membrane-bound organelles.

- Some eucaryotic cells have cell walls to provide rigidity, shape, and protection; these simple cell walls may contain cellulose, pectin, lignin, chitin, or mineral salts. Procaryotic bacterial cell walls are more complex, containing peptidoglycan and, in some cases, lipopolysaccharides.

- In eucaryotic cells, energy is produced within mitochondria ("energy factories"). Energy-producing reactions occur at the cell membranes of procaryotic cells.

- External to the cell wall, some bacteria have either a capsule or a slime layer. Capsules serve an antiphagocytic function and have been used in the production of certain vaccines. Determining whether a bacterium possesses a capsule is valuable when attempting to identify the organism.

- Many bacteria have flagella that enable motility, and some produce spores for survival. Determining whether a bacterium possesses flagella is valuable when attempting to identify the organism, as are the number and location of the flagella. Likewise, the presence or absence of spores and their location within cells are of value when identifying bacteria.

- Eucaryotic cells reproduce either by mitosis or meiosis, whereas procaryotic cells reproduce by binary fission.

- In the binomial system of nomenclature, the first name is the genus, the second name is the specific epithet, and the two names together represent the species.

- Taxonomic classification of organisms separates them into kingdoms, divisions, classes, orders, families, genera, and species, based on their characteristics, attributes, properties, and traits.

- In the Five-Kingdom System of Classification, microorganisms are found in the first three kingdoms—Procaryotae (bacteria), Protista (algae and protozoa), and Fungi. In the Three-Domain System of Classification, microorganisms are found in all three domains—*Archaea, Bacteria,* and *Eucarya.*

- The most widely used technique for determining how closely one procaryotic organism is related to another involves the gene that codes for the 16S rRNA molecule of ribosomes. The more similar the 16S sequences, the more closely related are the organisms. The less similar the 16S sequences, the less related are the organisms. For eucaryotes, the 18s rRNA gene is used.

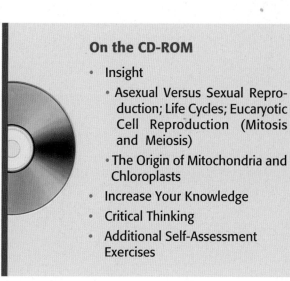

On the CD-ROM

- Insight
  - Asexual Versus Sexual Reproduction; Life Cycles; Eucaryotic Cell Reproduction (Mitosis and Meiosis)
  - The Origin of Mitochondria and Chloroplasts
- Increase Your Knowledge
- Critical Thinking
- Additional Self-Assessment Exercises

Self-Assessment Exercises

After studying this chapter, answer the following multiple-choice questions.

1. Molecules of extrachromosomal DNA are also known as:
   a. Golgi bodies.
   b. lysosomes.
   c. plasmids.
   d. plastids.

2. A bacterium possessing a tuft of flagella at one end of its cell would be called what kind of bacterium?
   a. amphitrichous
   b. lophotrichous
   c. monotrichous
   d. peritrichous

3. One way in which an archaean would differ from a bacterium is that the archaean would possess no:
   a. DNA in its chromosome.
   b. peptidoglycan in its cell walls.
   c. ribosomes in its cytoplasm.
   d. RNA in its ribosomes.

4. Some bacteria stain Gram-positive and others stain Gram-negative as a result of differences in the structure of their:
   a. capsule.
   b. cell membrane.
   c. cell wall.
   d. ribosomes.

5. Of the following, which one is *not* found in procaryotic cells?
   a. cell membrane
   b. chromosome
   c. mitochondria
   d. plasmids

6. The Three-Domain System of Classification is based on differences in which of the following molecules?
   a. mRNA
   b. peptidoglycan
   c. rRNA
   d. tRNA

7. Which of the following is in the correct sequence?
   a. Kingdom, Class, Division, Order, Family, Genus
   b. Kingdom, Division, Class, Order, Family, Genus
   c. Kingdom, Division, Order, Class, Family, Genus
   d. Kingdom, Order, Division, Class, Family, Genus

8. Which one of the following is *never* found in procaryotic cells?
   a. flagella
   b. capsule
   c. cilia
   d. ribosomes

9. The semipermeable structure controlling the transport of materials between the cell and its external environment is the:
   a. cell membrane.
   b. cell wall.
   c. cytoplasm.
   d. nuclear membrane.

10. In eucaryotic cells, what are the sites of photosynthesis?
    a. mitochondria
    b. plasmids
    c. plastids
    d. ribosomes

4

DIVERSITY OF MICROORGANISMS
PART 1 Acellular and Procaryotic Microbes

LEARNING OBJECTIVES

AFTER STUDYING THIS CHAPTER, YOU SHOULD BE ABLE TO:

- Describe the characteristics used to classify or categorize viruses
- Compare and contrast viruses and bacteria
- List several important viral diseases of humans
- Discuss differences between viroids and virions, and the diseases they cause
- List various ways in which bacteria can be classified or categorized
- Define the terms diplococci, streptococci, staphylococci, tetrad, octad, coccobacilli, diplobacilli, streptobacilli, and pleomorphism
- Define the terms obligate aerobe, microaerophile, facultative anaerobe, aerotolerant anaerobe, obligate anaerobe, and capnophile
- State key differences among rickettsias, chlamydias, and mycoplasmas
- Identify several important bacterial diseases of humans
- State several ways in which archaeans differ from bacteria

INTRODUCTION

Imagine the excitement that Anton van Leeuwenhoek experienced as he gazed through his tiny glass lenses and became the first person to see live microorganisms. In the years that have followed his eloquently written late 17th–early 18th century accounts of the bacteria and protozoa that he observed, tens of thousands of microorganisms have been discovered, described, and classified. In this chapter and the next, you will be introduced to the diversity of form and function that exists in the microbial world.

As you will recall, microbiology is the study of microorganisms—organisms too small to be seen by the naked eye. Microorganisms can be divided into those that are truly cellular (bacteria, archaeans, algae, protozoa, and fungi) and those that are acellular (viruses, viroids, and prions). The cellular microorganisms can be subdivided into those that are procaryotic (bacteria and archaeans) and those that are eucaryotic (algae, protozoa, and fungi). For a variety of reasons, acellular microorganisms are not considered by most scientists to be living organisms. Thus, rather than using the term microorganisms to describe them, viruses, viroids, and prions are often referred to as infectious agents or infectious particles.

Acellular Infectious Agents

Viruses

Complete virus particles, called *virions,* are very small and simple in structure. Most viruses range in size from 10 to 300 nm in diameter, although some—like Ebola virus—can be up to 1 μm in length. The smallest virus is about the size of the large hemoglobin molecule of a red blood cell. Viruses could not be seen until electron microscopes were invented in the 1930s. The first photographs of viruses were obtained in 1940. The negative staining procedure, developed in 1959, revolutionized the study of viruses, making it possible to observe unstained viruses against an electron-dense, dark background.

No type of organism is safe from viral infections; viruses infect humans, animals, plants, fungi, protozoa, algae, and bacterial cells (Table 4-1). Many human diseases are caused by viruses (refer back to Table 1-1). Some viruses—called oncogenic viruses or oncoviruses—cause specific types of cancer, including human cancers such as lymphomas, carcinomas, and some types of leukemia.

Viruses are said to have five specific properties that distinguish them from living cells:

- They possess *either* DNA or RNA, unlike living cells, which possess both.

- They are unable to replicate (multiply) on their own; their replication is directed by the viral nucleic acid once it has been introduced into a host cell.

- Unlike cells, they do not divide by binary fission, mitosis, or meiosis.

- They lack the genes and enzymes necessary for energy production.

- They depend on the ribosomes, enzymes, and metabolites ("building blocks") of the host cell for protein and nucleic acid production.

A typical virion consists of a genome of either DNA or RNA, surrounded by a *capsid* (protein coat), which is composed of many small protein units called *capsomeres* (Fig.

TABLE 4-1

Relative Sizes and Shapes of Some Viruses

VIRUSES	NUCLEIC ACID TYPE	SHAPE	SIZE RANGE (nm)
Animal Viruses			
Vaccinia	DNA	Complex	200 × 300
Mumps	RNA	Helical	150–250
Herpes simplex	DNA	Polyhedral	100–150
Influenza	RNA	Helical	80–120
Retroviruses	RNA	Helical	100–120
Adenoviruses	DNA	Polyhedral	60–90
Retroviruses	RNA	Polyhedral	60–80
Papovaviruses	DNA	Polyhedral	40–60
Polioviruses	RNA	Polyhedral	28
Plant Viruses			
Turnip yellow mosaic	RNA	Polyhedral	28
Wound tumor	RNA	Polyhedral	55–60
Alfalfa mosaic	RNA	Polyhedral	18 × 36–40
Tobacco mosaic	RNA	Helical	18 × 300
Bacteriophages			
T2	DNA	Complex	65 × 210
L	DNA	Complex	54 × 194
F_x-174	DNA	Complex	25

4-1). Some viruses (called enveloped viruses) have an outer envelope composed of lipids and polysaccharides. Bacterial viruses may also have a tail, sheath, and tail fibers. There are no ribosomes for protein synthesis or sites of energy production; hence, the virus must invade and take over a functioning cell to produce new virions.

Viruses are classified by the following characteristics: (1) type of genetic material (either DNA or RNA), (2) shape of the capsid, (3) number of capsomeres, (4) size of the capsid, (5) presence or absence of an envelope, (6) type of host that it infects, (7) type of disease it produces, (8) target cell, and (9) immunologic or antigenic properties.

There are four categories of viruses, based on the type of nucleic acid they possess. The genetic material of most viruses is either double-stranded DNA or single-stranded RNA, but a few viruses possess single-stranded DNA or double-stranded RNA. Viral genomes are usually circular

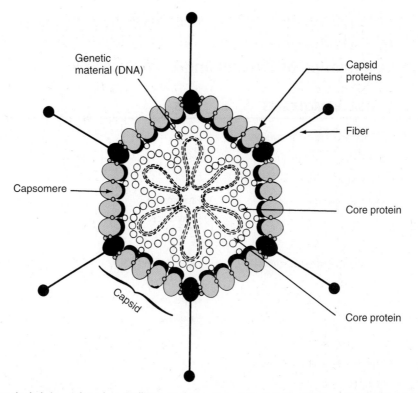

FIGURE 4-1. Model of an icosahedral virus: adenovirus. (Volk WA, et al. Essentials of Medical Microbiology, 4th ed. Philadelphia: JB Lippincott, 1991.)

molecules, but some are linear (having two ends). Capsids of viruses have various shapes and symmetry. They may be polyhedral (many sided), helical (coiled tubes), bullet shaped, spherical, or a complex combination of these shapes. Polyhedral capsids have 20 sides or facets; geometrically, they are referred to as icosahedrons. Each facet consists of several capsomeres; thus, the size of the virus is determined by the size of each facet and the number of capsomeres in each. Frequently, the envelope around the capsid makes the virus appear spherical or irregular in shape in electron micrographs. The envelope is acquired by certain animal viruses as they escape from the nucleus or cytoplasm of the host cell by budding (Fig. 4-2). In other words, the envelope is derived from either the host

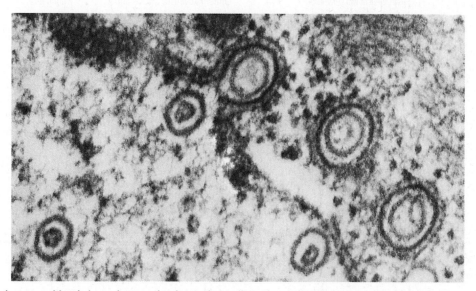

FIGURE 4-2. Herpesviruses acquiring their envelopes as they leave a host cell's nucleus by budding. From left to right: three viruses within the nucleus; one virus in the process of leaving the nucleus by budding; two viruses that have already acquired their envelopes. (Original magnification, 100,000×.) (Volk WA, et al. Essentials of Medical Microbiology, 5th ed. Philadelphia: Lippincott-Raven, 1996.)

TABLE 4-2

Selected Important Groups of Viruses and Viral Diseases

VIRUS TYPE	VIRAL CHARACTERISTICS	VIRUS	DISEASE
Poxviruses	Large, brick shape with envelope, dsDNA	Variola Vaccinia	Smallpox Cowpox
Polyoma-papilloma	dsDNA, polyhedral	Papillomavirus Polyomavirus	Warts Some tumors, some cancer
Herpesvirus	Polyhedral with envelope, dsDNA	Herpes simplex I Herpes simplex II Herpes zoster Varicella	Cold sores or fever blisters Genital herpes Shingles Chickenpox
Adenovirus	dsDNA, icosahedral, with envelope		Respiratory infections, pneumonia, conjunctivitis, some tumors
Picornaviruses (the name means small RNA viruses)	ssRNA, tiny icosahedral, with envelope	Rhinovirus Poliovirus Hepatitis types A and B Coxsackievirus	Colds Poliomyelitis Hepatitis Respiratory infections, meningitis
Reoviruses	dsRNA, icosahedral with envelope	Enterovirus	Intestinal infections
Myxoviruses	RNA, helical with envelope	Orthomyxoviruses types A and B Myxovirus parotidis Paramyxovirus Rhabdovirus	Influenza Mumps Measles (rubeola) Rabies
Arbovirus	Arthropodborne RNA, cubic	Mosquitoborne type B Mosquitoborne types A and B Tickborne, coronavirus	Yellow fever Encephalitis (many types) Colorado tick fever
Retrovirus	dsRNA, helical with envelope	RNA tumor virus HTLV virus HIV	Tumors Leukemia AIDS

ds, double-stranded; ss, single-stranded.

cell's nuclear membrane or cell membrane. Apparently, viruses are then able to alter these membranes by adding protein fibers, spikes, and knobs that enable the virus to recognize the next host cell to be invaded. A list of some viruses, their characteristics, and diseases they cause is presented in Table 4-2. Sizes of viruses are depicted in Figure 4-3.

Origin of Viruses

Where did viruses come from? Two main theories have been proposed to explain the origin of viruses. One theory states that viruses existed before cells, but this seems unlikely in view of the fact that viruses require cells for their replication. The other theory states that cells came first and that viruses represent ancient derivatives of degenerate cells or cell fragments. The question of whether viruses are alive depends on one's definition of life and, thus, is not an easy question to answer. However, most scientists agree that viruses lack most of the basic features of cells; thus, they consider viruses to be nonliving entities.

Bacteriophages

The viruses that infect bacteria are known as ***bacteriophages*** (or simply, *phages*). Like all viruses, they are obligate intracellular pathogens, in that they must enter a bacterial cell to replicate. There are three categories of bacteriophages, based on their shape:

* Icosahedron bacteriophages: an almost spherical shape, with 20 triangular facets; the smallest icosahedron phages are about 25 nm in diameter.

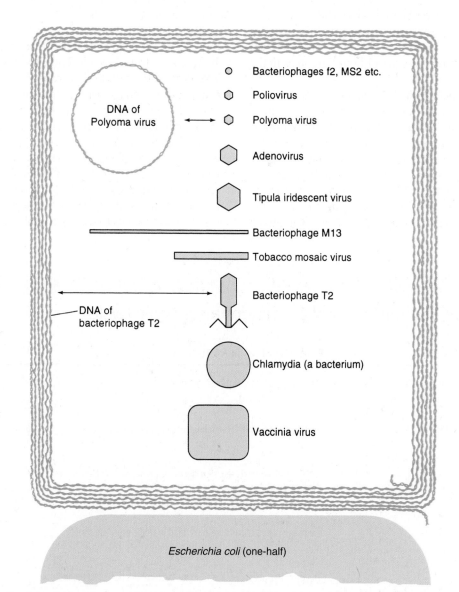

FIGURE 4-3. Comparative sizes of virions, their nucleic acids, and bacteria. (Davis BD, et al. Microbiology, 4th ed. Philadelphia: JB Lippincott, 1990.)

- Filamentous bacteriophages: long tubes formed by capsid proteins assembled into a helical structure; they can be up to about 900 nm long.

- Complex bacteriophages: icosahedral heads attached to helical tails; may also possess base plates and tail fibers.

In addition to shape, bacteriophages can be categorized by the type of nucleic acid that they possess; there are single-stranded DNA phages, double-stranded DNA phages, single-stranded RNA phages, and double-stranded RNA phages. From this point, only DNA phages will be discussed.

Bacteriophages can be categorized by the events that occur after invasion of the bacterial cell: some are virulent phages, whereas others are temperate phages. Phages in either category do not actually enter the bacterial cell—rather, they inject their nucleic acid into the cell. It is what happens next that distinguishes virulent phages from temperate phages.

Virulent bacteriophages always cause what is known as the **lytic cycle,** which ends with the destruction (lysis) of the bacterial cell. For most phages, the whole process (from attachment to lysis) takes less than 1 hour. The steps in the lytic cycle are shown in Table 4-3.

The first step in the lytic cycle is *attachment* (adsorption) of the phage to the surface of the bacterial cell. The phage can only attach to bacterial cells that possess the appropriate receptor—a protein or polysaccharide molecule on the surface of the cell that is recognized by a molecule on the surface of the phage. Most bacteriophages are species- and strain-specific, meaning that they only infect a particular species or strain of bacteria. Those that infect *Escherichia coli* are called coliphages. Some bacteriophages can attach to more than one species of bacterium. Figure 4-4 shows a number of bacteriophages attached to the surface of a *Vibrio cholerae* cell.

The second step in the lytic cycle is called *penetration*. In this step, the phage injects its DNA into the bacterial cell, acting much like a hypodermic needle (Fig. 4-5). From this point on, the phage DNA "dictates" what occurs within the bacterial cell. This is sometimes described as the phage DNA taking over the host cell's "machinery."

The third step in the lytic cycle is called *biosynthesis*. It is during this step that the phage genes are expressed, resulting in the production (biosynthesis) of viral pieces. It is also during this step that the host cell's enzymes (e.g., DNA polymerase and RNA polymerase), nucleotides, amino acids, and ribosomes are used to make viral DNA and viral proteins. In the fourth step of the lytic cycle, called *assembly,* the viral pieces are assembled to produce complete viral particles (virions). It is during this step that viral DNA is packaged up into capsids.

The final step in the lytic cycle, called *release,* is when the host cell bursts open and all of the new virions (about 50 to 1000) escape from the cell. Thus, the lytic cycle ends with lysis of the host cell. Lysis is caused by an enzyme that is coded for by a phage gene. At the appropriate time—after assembly—the appropriate viral gene is expressed, the enzyme is produced, and the bacterial cell wall is destroyed. With certain bacteriophages, a phage gene codes for an enzyme that interferes with cell wall synthesis, leading to weakness and, finally, collapse of the cell wall. Bacteriophage enzymes that destroy cell walls or prevent their synthesis are currently being studied for possible use as therapeutic agents (i.e., for use as drugs to treat bacterial infections).

TABLE 4-3

Steps in the Multiplication of Bacteriophages (Lytic Cycle)

STEP	NAME OF STEP	WHAT OCCURS DURING THIS STEP
1	Attachment (adsorption)	The phage attaches to a protein or polysaccharide molecule (receptor) on the surface of the bacterial cell
2	Penetration	The phage injects its DNA into the bacterial cell; the capsid remains on the outer surface of the cell
3	Biosynthesis	Phage genes are expressed, resulting in the production of phage pieces or parts (i.e., phage DNA and phage proteins)
4	Assembly	The phage pieces or parts are assembled to create complete phages
5	Release	The complete phages escape from the bacterial cell by lysis of the cell

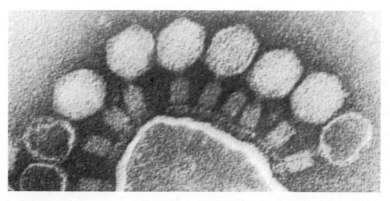

FIGURE 4-4. A partially lysed cell of *Vibrio cholerae* with attached virions of phage CP-T1. Note the empty capsids, full capsids, contracted tail sheaths, base plates, and spikes. (Original magnification, 257,000×.) (Courtesy of R.W. Taylor and J.E. Ogg, Colorado State University, Fort Collins, CO.)

The other category of bacteriophages—*temperate phages* (also known as *lysogenic phages*)—do not immediately initiate the lytic cycle, but rather, their DNA remains integrated into the bacterial cell chromosome, generation after generation. **Temperate bacteriophages** are discussed in Chapter 7.

Bacteriophages are involved in two of the four major ways in which bacteria acquire new genetic information. These processes—called lysogenic conversion and transduction—are discussed in Chapter 7.

Animal Viruses

Viruses that infect humans and animals are collectively referred to as "animal viruses." Some animal viruses are DNA viruses; others are RNA viruses. Animal viruses may consist solely of nucleic acid surrounded by a protein coat (capsid), or they may be more complex. For example, they may be enveloped or they may contain enzymes that play a role in viral multiplication within host cells. The steps in the multiplication of animal viruses are shown in Table 4-4.

The first step in the multiplication of animal viruses is *attachment* (or adsorption) of the virus to the cell. Like bacteriophages, animal viruses can only attach to cells bearing the appropriate protein or polysaccharide receptors on their surface. Did you ever wonder why certain viruses cause infections in dogs, but not humans, or vice versa? Did you ever wonder why certain viruses cause respiratory infections, whereas others cause gastrointestinal infections? It all boils down to receptors. Viruses can only attach to and invade cells that bear a receptor that they can recognize and attach to.

The second step in the multiplication of animal viruses is *penetration,* but, unlike bacteriophages, the entire virion usually enters the host cell, sometimes because the cell phagocytizes the virus (Fig. 4-6). This necessitates a third step that was not required for bacteriophages—*uncoating*—whereby the viral nucleic acid escapes from the capsid.

As with bacteriophages, from this point on, the viral nucleic acid "dictates" what occurs within the host cell. The fourth step is *biosynthesis,* whereby many viral pieces (viral nucleic acid and viral proteins) are produced. This step can be quite complicated, depending on what type of virus infected the cell (i.e., whether it was a single-stranded DNA virus, a double-stranded DNA virus, a single-stranded RNA virus, or a double-stranded RNA virus). Some animal viruses do not initiate biosynthesis right

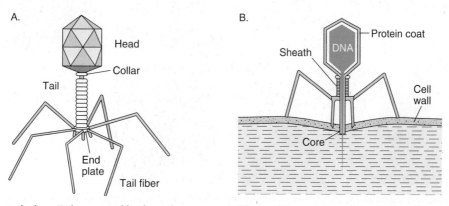

FIGURE 4-5. (*A*) The bacteriophage T4 is an assembly of protein components. The head is a protein membrane with 20 facets, filled with DNA. It is attached to a tail consisting of a hollow core surrounded by a sheath and based on a spiked end plate to which six fibers are attached. (*B*) The sheath contracts, driving the core through the cell wall, and viral DNA enters the cell.

TABLE 4-4

Steps in the Multiplication of Animal Viruses

STEP	NAME OF STEP	WHAT OCCURS DURING THIS STEP
1	Attachment (adsorption)	The virus attaches to a protein or polysaccharide molecule (receptor) on the surface of a host cell
2	Penetration	The entire virus enters the host cell, in some cases because it was phagocytized by the cell
3	Uncoating	The viral nucleic acid escapes from the capsid
4	Biosynthesis	Viral genes are expressed, resulting in the production of pieces or parts of viruses (i.e., viral DNA and viral proteins)
5	Assembly	The viral pieces or parts are assembled to create complete virions
6	Release	The complete virions escape from the host cell by lysis or budding

away, but rather, remain latent within the host cell for variable periods. Latent viral infections are discussed in more detail in a subsequent section.

The fifth step—*assembly*—involves fitting the virus pieces together to produce complete virions. After the virus particles are assembled, they must escape from the cell—a sixth step called *release*. How they escape from the cell depends on the type of virus that it is. Some animal viruses escape by destroying the host cell, leading to cell destruction and some of the symptoms associated with infection with that particular virus. Other viruses escape the cell by a process known as budding. Viruses that escape from the

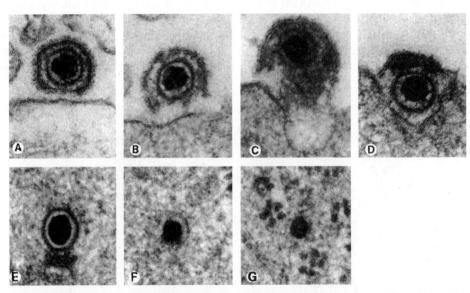

FIGURE 4-6. Adsorption (*A*), penetration (*B–D*), and uncoating and digestion of the capsid (*E–G*) of herpes simplex on HeLa cells, as deduced from electron micrographs of infected cell sections. Penetration involves local digestion of the viral and cellular membranes (*B, C*), resulting in fusion of the two membranes and release of the nucleocapsid into the cytoplasmic matrix (*D*). The naked nucleocapsid is intact in *E,* is partially digested in *F,* and has disappeared in *G,* leaving a core containing DNA and protein. (Morgan C, et al. J Virol 1968;2:507.)

host cell cytoplasm by budding become surrounded with pieces of the cell membrane, thus becoming enveloped viruses. If it is an enveloped virus, you know that it escaped from its host cell by budding.

Remnants or collections of viruses, called **inclusion bodies,** are often seen in infected cells and are used as a diagnostic tool to identify certain viral diseases. Inclusion bodies may be found in the cytoplasm (cytoplasmic inclusion bodies) or within the nucleus (intranuclear inclusion bodies), depending on the particular disease. In rabies, the cytoplasmic inclusion bodies in nerve cells are called Negri bodies. The inclusion bodies of AIDS and the Guarnieri bodies of smallpox are also cytoplasmic. Herpes and poliomyelitis viruses cause intranuclear inclusion bodies. In each case, inclusion bodies may represent aggregates or collections of viruses. Some important human viral diseases include AIDS, chickenpox, cold sores, the common cold, Ebola virus infections, genital herpes infections, German measles, Hantavirus pulmonary syndrome, infectious mononucleosis, influenza, measles, mumps, poliomyelitis, rabies, severe acute respiratory syndrome (SARS), and viral encephalitis. In addition, all human warts are caused by viruses.

Latent Virus Infections

Herpes virus infections, such as cold sores (fever blisters), are good examples of latent virus infections. Although the infected person is always harboring the virus in nerve cells, the cold sores come and go. A fever, stress, or excessive sunlight can trigger the viral genes to take over the cells and produce more viruses; in the process, cells are destroyed and a cold sore develops. Latent viral infections are usually limited by the defense systems of the human body—phagocytes and antiviral proteins called interferons that are produced by virus-infected cells (discussed in Chapter 15). Shingles, a painful nerve disease that is also caused by a herpesvirus, is another example of a latent viral infection. After a chickenpox infection, the virus can remain latent in the human body for many years. Then, when the body's immune defenses become weakened by old age or disease, the latent chickenpox virus resurfaces to cause shingles.

Antiviral Agents

It is important for healthcare professionals to understand that antibiotics are not effective against viral infections. Antibiotics function by inhibiting certain metabolic activities within cellular pathogens, and viruses are not cells. However, for certain patients with colds and influenza, antibiotics may be prescribed in an attempt to prevent secondary bacterial infections that might follow the virus infection. In recent years, a few chemicals—called antiviral agents—have been developed. They interfere with virus-specific enzymes and virus production by either disrupting critical phases in viral

cycles or inhibiting the synthesis of viral DNA, RNA, or proteins. Antiviral agents are discussed further in Chapter 9.

Oncogenic Viruses

Viruses that cause cancer are called **oncogenic viruses** or *oncoviruses.* The first evidence that viruses cause cancers came from experiments with chickens. Subsequently, viruses were shown to be the cause of various types of cancers in rodents, frogs, and cats. Although the cause of many (perhaps most) types of human cancers remains unknown, it is known that *some* human cancers are caused by viruses. Epstein-Barr virus (a type of herpesvirus) is the cause of infectious mononucleosis (not a type of cancer), but it also causes three types of human cancers: nasopharyngeal cancer, Burkitt's lymphoma, and B-cell lymphoma. Kaposi sarcoma, a type of cancer that is common in AIDS patients, is caused by human herpesvirus 8. Associations between hepatitis B and C viruses and hepatocellular (liver) carcinoma have been established. Human papillomaviruses (HPV; wart viruses) can cause different types of cancer, including cervical cancer and other types of cancer of the genital tract. A retrovirus that is closely related to human immunodeficiency virus (HIV; discussed in the next section), called HTLV-1, causes a rare type of adult T-cell leukemia. All the above-mentioned viruses, except HTLV-1, are DNA viruses. HTLV-1 is an RNA virus.

Human Immunodeficiency Virus

Human immunodeficiency virus (HIV), the cause of acquired immune deficiency syndrome (AIDS), is an enveloped, double-stranded RNA virus (Fig. 4-7). It is a member of a genus of viruses called lentiviruses, in a family of viruses called Retroviridae (retroviruses). HIV is able to attach to and invade cells bearing receptors that the virus recognizes. The most important of these receptors is designated CD4, and cells possessing that receptor are called CD4$^+$ cells. The most important of the CD4$^+$ cells is the helper T cell (discussed in Chapter 16); HIV infections destroy these important cells of the immune system. Macrophages also possess CD4 receptors and can, thus, be invaded by HIV. In addition, HIV is able to invade certain cells that do not possess CD4 receptors, but do possess other receptors that HIV is able to recognize.

Plant Viruses

More than 1,000 different viruses cause plant diseases, including diseases of citrus trees, cocoa trees, rice, barley, tobacco, turnips, cauliflower, potatoes, tomatoes, and many other fruits, vegetables, trees, and grains. These diseases result in huge economic losses, estimated to be in excess of $70 billion per year worldwide. Plant viruses are usually transmitted via insects (e.g., aphids, leaf hoppers, whiteflies); mites; nematodes (round worms); infected seeds, cuttings, and tubers; and contaminated tools (e.g., hoes, clippers, and saws).

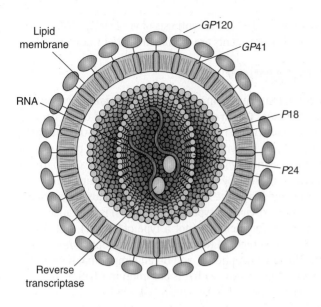

FIGURE 4-7. Human immunodeficiency virus (HIV). HIV is an enveloped virus, containing two identical RNA strands. Each of its 72 surface knobs contains a glycoprotein (designated *gp*120) capable of binding to a CD4 receptor on the surface of certain host cells (e.g., T-helper cells). The "stalk" that supports the knob is a transmembrane glycoprotein (designated *gp*41), which may also play a role in attachment to host cells. Reverse transcriptase is an RNA-dependent DNA polymerase. (Porth CM. Pathophysiology: Concepts of Altered Health States, 5th Ed. Philadelphia: Lippincott Williams & Wilkins, 1998.)

Viroids and Prions

Although viruses are extremely small nonliving infectious agents, viroids and prions are even smaller and less complex infectious agents. *Viroids* consist of short, naked fragments of single-stranded RNA (about 300 to 400 nucleotides in length) that can interfere with the metabolism of plant cells and stunt the growth of plants, sometimes killing the plants in the process. They are transmitted between plants in the same manner as viruses. Plant diseases thought or known to be caused by viroids include potato spindle tuber (producing small, cracked, spindle-shaped potatoes), citrus exocortis (stunting of citrus trees), and diseases of chrysanthemums, coconut palms, and tomatoes. Thus far, no animal diseases have been discovered that are caused by viroids.

Prions (pronounced "pree-ons") are small infectious proteins that apparently cause fatal neurologic diseases in animals, such as scrapie (pronounced "scrape-ee") in sheep and goats; bovine spongiform encephalopathy (BSE; "mad cow disease;" see "Insight: Microbes in the News: 'Mad Cow Disease' " on the CD-ROM); and kuru, Creutzfeldt-Jakob (C-J) disease, Gerstmann-Sträussler-Scheinker (GSS) disease, and fatal familial insomnia in humans. Similar diseases in mink, mule deer, Western white-tailed deer, elk, and cats may also be caused by prions. The name "scrapie" comes from the observation that infected animals scrape

themselves against fence posts and other objects in an effort to relieve the intense pruritus (itching) associated with the disease. The disease in deer and elk is called "chronic wasting disease," in reference to the irreversible weight loss that the animals experience.

Kuru is a disease that was once common among natives in Papua, New Guinea, where women and children ate human brains as part of a traditional burial custom (ritualistic cannibalism). If the brain of the deceased person contained prions, then persons who ate that brain developed kuru. Kuru, C-J disease, and GSS disease involve loss of coordination and dementia. Dementia, a general mental deterioration, is characterized by disorientation and impaired memory, judgment, and intellect. In fatal familial insomnia, insomnia and dementia follow difficulty sleeping. All these diseases are fatal spongiform encephalopathies, in which the brain becomes riddled with holes (spongelike).

Scientists have been investigating the link between "mad cow disease" and a form of C-J disease (called variant CJD or vCJD) in humans. As of March 2006, 190 cases of vCJD had been diagnosed worldwide, including 160 in the United Kingdom; these cases probably resulted from eating prion-infected beef. The cattle may have acquired the disease through ingestion of cattle feed that contained ground-up parts of prion-infected sheep.

The 1997 Nobel Prize for Physiology or Medicine was awarded to Stanley B. Prusiner, the scientist who coined the term prion and studied the role of these proteinaceous infectious particles in disease. Of all pathogens, prions are believed to be the most resistant to disinfectants. The mechanism by which prions cause disease remains a mystery, although it is thought that prions convert normal protein molecules into nonfunctional ones by causing the normal molecules to change their shape. Many scientists remain unconvinced that proteins alone can cause disease.

The Domain *Bacteria*

Characteristics

Chapter 3 explained that there are two domains of procaryotic organisms: Domain *Bacteria* and Domain *Archaea*. The bacteriologist's most important reference (sometimes referred to as the bacteriologist's "bible") is a five-volume set of books entitled *Bergey's Manual of Systematic Bacteriology,* which is currently being rewritten. (An outline of these volumes can be found on CD-ROM Appendix 2: "Phyla and Medically Significant Genera Within the Domain *Bacteria*.") When all five volumes have been completed, they will contain descriptions of more than 5,000 validly named species of bacteria. Some authorities believe that this number represents only from less than 1% to a few percent of the total number of bacteria that exist in nature.

The Domain *Bacteria* contains 23 phyla, 32 classes, 5 subclasses, 77 orders, 14 suborders, 182 families, 871 genera, and 5,007 species. Organisms in this domain are broadly divided into three phenotypic categories (i.e., categories based on their physical characteristics): (1) those that are Gram-negative and have a cell wall, (2) those that are Gram-positive and have a cell wall, and (3) those that lack a cell wall. (The terms Gram-positive and Gram-negative are explained in a subsequent section of this chapter.) Using computers, microbiologists have established numerical taxonomy systems that not only help to identify bacteria by their physical characteristics, but also can help establish how closely related these organisms are by comparing the composition of their genetic material and other cellular characteristics. (Note: as previously mentioned, throughout this book, the term "to identify an organism" means to learn the organism's species name—i.e., to speciate it.)

Many characteristics of bacteria are examined to provide data for identification and classification. These characteristics include cell morphology (shape), staining reactions, motility, colony morphology, atmospheric requirements, nutritional requirements, biochemical and metabolic activities, specific enzymes that the organism produces, pathogenicity (the ability to cause disease), and genetic composition.

Cell Morphology

With the compound light microscope, the size, shape, and morphologic arrangement of various bacteria are easily observed. Bacteria vary greatly in size, usually ranging from spheres measuring about 0.2 μm in diameter to 10.0 μm-long spiral-shaped bacteria, to even longer filamentous bacteria. As previously mentioned, the average coccus is about 1 μm in diameter, and the average bacillus is about 1 μm wide × 3 μm long. Some unusually large bacteria and unusually small bacteria have also been discovered (discussed later).

There are three basic shapes of bacteria (Fig. 4-8): (1) round or spherical bacteria—the *cocci* (sing., *coccus*); (2) rectangular or rod-shaped bacteria—the *bacilli* (sing., *bacillus*); and (3) curved and spiral-shaped bacteria (sometimes referred to as spirilla). Recall from Chapter 3 that bacteria divide by binary fission—one cell splits in half to become two daughter cells. After binary fission, the

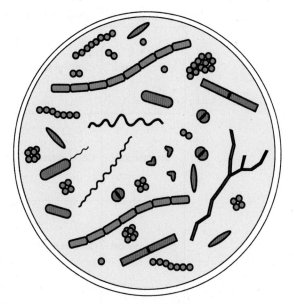

FIGURE 4-8. Various forms of bacteria, including single cocci, diplococci, tetrads, octads, streptococci, staphylococci, single bacilli, diplobacilli, streptobacilli, branching bacilli, loosely coiled spirochetes, and tightly coiled spirochetes. (See text for explanation of terms.)

daughter cells may separate completely from each other or may remain connected, forming various morphologic arrangements.

Cocci may be seen singly or in pairs (**diplococci**), chains (**streptococci**), clusters (**staphylococci**), packets of four (**tetrads**), or packets of eight (**octads**), depending on the particular species and the manner in which the cells divide (Figs. 4-9 and 4-10). Examples of medically important cocci

⊙ STUDY AID

Bacterial Names Sometimes Provide a Clue to Their Shape

If "coccus" appears in the name of a bacterium, you automatically know the shape of the organism—spherical. Examples include genera such as *Enterococcus, Peptococcus, Peptostreptococcus, Staphylococcus,* and *Streptococcus.* However, not all cocci have "coccus" in their names (e.g., *Neisseria* spp.). If "bacillus" appears in the name of a bacterium, you automatically know the shape of the organism—rod-shaped or rectangular. Examples include genera such as *Actinobacillus, Bacillus, Lactobacillus,* and *Streptobacillus.* However, not all bacilli have "bacillus" in their names (e.g., *E. coli*).

Arrangement	Description	Appearance	Example	Disease
Diplococci	Cocci in pairs	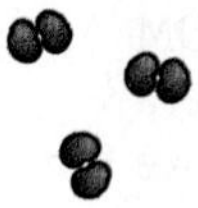	*Neisseria gonorrhoeae*	Gonorrhea
Streptococci	Cocci in chains	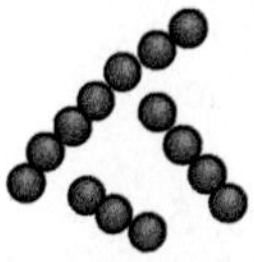	*Streptococcus pyogenes*	Strep throat
Staphylococci	Cocci in clusters	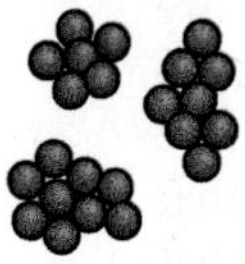	*Staphylococcus aureus*	Boils
Tetrad	A packet of 4 cocci	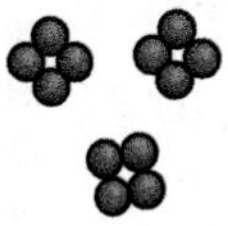	*Micrococcus luteus*	Rarely pathogenic
Octad	A packet of 8 cocci	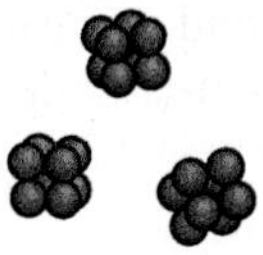	*Sarcina ventriculi*	Rarely pathogenic

FIGURE 4-9. Morphologic arrangements of cocci.

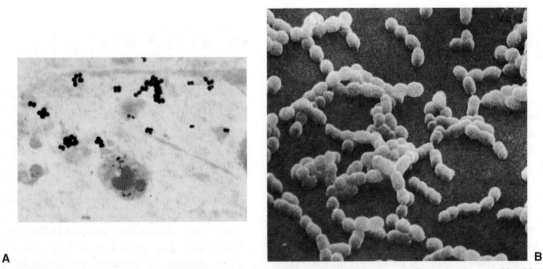

A   **B**

FIGURE 4-10. Morphologic arrangements of cocci. (*A*) Photomicrograph of Gram-stained *Staphylococcus aureus* illustrating Gram-positive (blue) cocci in grapelike clusters. A pink-stained white blood cell can also be seen in the lower portion of the photomicrograph. (*B*) scanning electron micrograph of *Streptococcus mutans* illustrating cocci in chains. (Original magnification, 5,000×.) (*A:* Koneman's Color Atlas and Textbook of Diagnostic Microbiology, 6th ed. Philadelphia: Lippincott Williams & Wilkins, 2006. *B:* Volk WA, et al. Essentials of Medical Microbiology, 5th ed. Philadelphia: Lippincott-Raven, 1996.)

Beware the Word "Bacillus"

Whenever you see the word *Bacillus,* capitalized and underlined or italicized, it is a particular genus of rod-shaped bacteria. However, if you see the word bacillus, and it is not capitalized, underlined, or italicized, it refers to any rod-shaped bacterium.

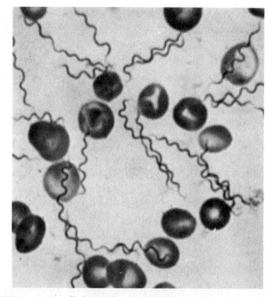

FIGURE 4-11. *Borrelia hermsii,* a cause of relapsing fever, in a stained blood smear. (Original magnification, 2,700×.) (Volk WA, et al. Essentials of Medical Microbiology, 5th ed. Philadelphia: Lippincott-Raven, 1996.)

include *Enterococcus* spp., *Neisseria* spp., *Staphylococcus* spp., and *Streptococcus* spp.

Bacilli (often referred to as rods) may be short or long, thick or thin, and pointed or with curved or blunt ends. They may occur singly, in pairs (**diplobacilli**), in chains (**streptobacilli**), in long filaments, or branched. Some rods are quite short, resembling elongated cocci; they are called *coccobacilli. Listeria monocytogenes* and *Haemophilus influenzae* are examples of **coccobacilli.** Some bacilli stack up next to each other, side-by-side in a palisade arrangement, which is characteristic of *Corynebacterium diphtheriae* (the cause of diphtheria) and organisms that resemble it in appearance (called diphtheroids). Examples of medically important bacilli include members of the family *Enterobacteriaceae* (e.g., *Enterobacter, Escherichia, Klebsiella, Proteus, Salmonella,* and *Shigella* spp.), *Pseudomonas aeruginosa, Bacillus* spp., and *Clostridium* spp.

Curved and spiral-shaped bacilli are placed into a third morphologic grouping. For example, *Vibrio* spp., such as *Vibrio cholerae* (the cause of cholera) and *Vibrio parahaemolyticus* (a cause of diarrhea), are curved (comma-shaped) bacilli. Curved bacteria usually occur singly, but some species may form pairs. A pair of curved bacilli resembles a bird and is described as having a gull-wing morphology. *Campylobacter* spp. (a common cause of diarrhea) have a gull-wing morphology. Spiral-shaped bacteria are referred to as spirochetes. Different species of spirochetes vary in size, length, rigidity, and the number and amplitude of their coils. Some are tightly coiled, such as *Treponema pallidum,* the cause of syphilis, with a flexible cell wall that enables them to move readily through tissues (refer back to Fig. 2-5). Its morphology and characteristic motility—spinning around its long axis—make *T. pallidum* easy to recognize in wet preparations of clinical specimens obtained from patients with primary syphilis. *Borrelia* spp., the causative agents of Lyme disease and relapsing fever, are examples of less tightly coiled spirochetes (Fig. 4-11).

Some bacteria may lose their characteristic shape because adverse growth conditions (e.g., the presence of certain antibiotics) prevent the production of normal cell walls.

They are referred to as cell-wall–deficient (CWD) bacteria. Some CWD bacteria revert to their original shape when placed in favorable growth conditions, whereas others do not. Bacteria in the genus *Mycoplasma* do not have cell walls; thus, when examined microscopically, they appear in various shapes. Bacteria that exist in a variety of shapes are described as being *pleomorphic;* the ability to exist in a variety of shapes is known as **pleomorphism.** Because they have no cell walls, mycoplasmas are resistant to antibiotics that inhibit cell wall synthesis.

Staining Procedures

As they exist in nature, bacteria are colorless, transparent, and difficult to see. Therefore, various staining methods have been devised to enable scientists to examine bacteria. In preparation for staining, the bacteria are smeared onto a glass microscope slide (resulting in what is known as a "smear"), air-dried, and then "fixed." (Methods for preparing and fixing smears are further described in CD-ROM Appendix 5: "Clinical Microbiology Laboratory Procedures.") The two most common methods of fixation are heat-fixation and methanol-fixation. Heat-fixation is usually accomplished by passing the smear through a Bunsen burner flame. If not performed properly, excess heat can distort the morphology of the cells. Methanol fixation, which is accomplished by flooding the smear with absolute methanol for 30 seconds, is a more satisfactory fixation technique. Fixation serves three purposes:

- it kills the organisms
- it preserves their morphology (shape)
- it anchors the smear to the slide

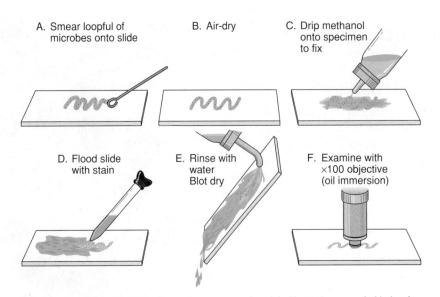

A. Smear loopful of microbes onto slide

B. Air-dry

C. Drip methanol onto specimen to fix

D. Flood slide with stain

E. Rinse with water Blot dry

F. Examine with ×100 objective (oil immersion)

FIGURE 4-12. Simple bacterial staining technique. (*A*) With a flamed loop, smear a loopful of bacteria suspended in broth or water onto a slide. (*B*) Allow slide to air-dry. (*C*) Fix the smear with absolute (100%) methanol. (*D*) Flood the slide with the stain. (*E*) Rinse with water and blot dry with bibulous paper or paper towel. (*F*) Examine the slide with the ×100 microscope objective, using a drop of immersion oil directly on the smear.

Specific stains and staining techniques are used to observe bacterial cell morphology (e.g., size, shape, morphologic arrangement, composition of cell wall, capsules, flagella, and endospores).

A *simple stain* is sufficient to determine bacterial shape and morphologic arrangement (e.g., pairs, chains, clusters).

HISTORICAL NOTE

The Origin of the Gram Stain

While working in a laboratory in the morgue of a Berlin hospital in the 1880s, a Danish physician named **Hans Christian Gram** developed what was to become the most important of all bacterial staining procedures. He was developing a staining technique that would enable him to see bacteria in the lung tissues of patients who had died of pneumonia. The procedure he developed—now called the **Gram stain**—demonstrated that two general categories of bacteria cause pneumonia: some of them stained blue and some of them stained red. The blue ones came to be known as Gram-positive bacteria, and the red ones came to be known as Gram-negative bacteria. It was not until 1963 that the mechanism of Gram differentiation was explained by M.R.J. Salton.

For this method, shown in Figure 4-12, a dye (such as methylene blue) is applied to the fixed smear, rinsed, dried, and examined using the oil immersion lens of the microscope. The procedures used to observe bacterial capsules, spores, and flagella are collectively referred to as *structural staining procedures.*

In 1883, Dr. Hans Christian Gram developed a staining technique that bears his name—the *Gram stain* or Gram staining procedure. (The details of this staining procedure are found in CD-ROM Appendix 5: "Clinical Microbiology Laboratory Procedures.") The Gram stain has become the most important staining procedure in the bacteriology laboratory, because it differentiates between "Gram-positive" and "Gram-negative" bacteria (these terms will be explained shortly). The organism's Gram reaction serves as an extremely important "clue" when attempting to learn the identity (species) of a particular bacterium. There are nine steps in the Gram staining procedure, as described in CD-ROM Appendix 5: "Clinical Microbiology Laboratory Procedures."

The color of the bacteria at the end of the Gram staining procedure depends on the chemical composition of their cell wall (Table 4-5). If the bacteria were not decolorized during the decolorization step, they will be blue-to-purple at the conclusion of the Gram staining procedure; such bacteria are said to be "Gram-positive." The thick layer of peptidoglycan in the cell walls of Gram-positive bacteria makes it difficult to remove the crystal violet–iodine complex during the decolorization step. Figures 4-13 through 4-17 depict various Gram-positive bacteria.

If, on the other hand, the crystal violet was removed from the cells during the decolorization step, and the cells were subsequently stained by the safranin (a red dye), they

TABLE 4-5

Differences Between Gram-Positive and Gram-Negative Bacteria

	GRAM-POSITIVE BACTERIA	GRAM-NEGATIVE BACTERIA
Color at the end of the Gram staining procedure	Blue-to-purple	Pink-to-red
Peptidoglycan in cell walls	Thick layer	Thin layer
Teichoic acids and lipoteichoic acids in cell walls	Present	Absent
Lipopolysaccharide in cell walls	Absent	Present

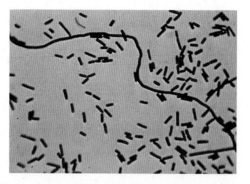

FIGURE 4-15. Gram-positive bacilli (*Clostridium perfringens*) in a Gram-stained smear prepared from a broth culture. Individual bacilli and chains of bacilli (streptobacilli) can be seen. (Koneman's Color Atlas and Textbook of Diagnostic Microbiology, 6th ed. Philadelphia: Lippincott Williams & Wilkins, 2006.)

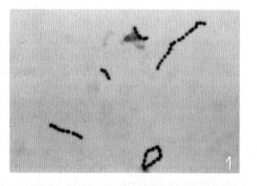

FIGURE 4-13. Chains of Gram-positive streptococci in a Gram-stained smear from a broth culture. (Koneman's Color Atlas and Textbook of Diagnostic Microbiology, 6th ed. Philadelphia: Lippincott Williams & Wilkins, 2006.)

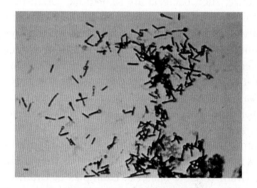

FIGURE 4-16. Gram-positive bacilli (*Clostridium tetani)* in a Gram-stained smear from a broth culture. Terminal spores can be seen on some of the cells. (Koneman's Color Atlas and Textbook of Diagnostic Microbiology, 6th ed. Philadelphia: Lippincott Williams & Wilkins, 2006.)

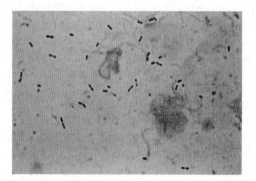

FIGURE 4-14. Gram-positive *Streptococcus pneumoniae* in a Gram-stained smear of a blood culture. Note the pairs of cocci (known as diplo-cocci). (Koneman's Color Atlas and Textbook of Diagnostic Microbiology, 6th ed. Philadelphia: Lippincott Williams & Wilkins, 2006.)

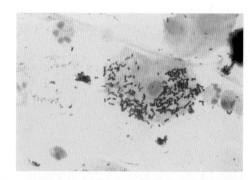

FIGURE 4-17. Many Gram-positive bacteria can be seen on the surface of a pink-stained epithelial cell in this Gram-stained sputum specimen. Several smaller pink-staining polymorphonuclear leukocytes can also be seen. (Koneman's Color Atlas and Textbook of Diagnostic Microbiology, 6th ed. Philadelphia: Lippincott Williams & Wilkins, 2006.)

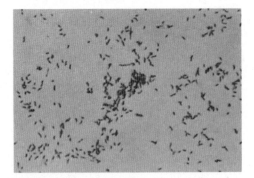

FIGURE 4-18. Gram-negative bacilli in a Gram-stained smear prepared from a bacterial colony. Individual bacilli and a few short chains of bacilli can be seen. (Koneman et al. Color Atlas and Textbook of Diagnostic Microbiology, 5th ed. Philadelphia: Lippincott Williams & Wilkins, 1997.)

will be pink-to-red at the conclusion of the Gram staining procedure; such bacteria are said to be "Gram-negative." The thin layer of peptidoglycan in the cell walls of Gram-negative bacteria makes it easier to remove the crystal violet–iodine complex during decolorization. In addition, the decolorizer dissolves the lipid in the cell walls of Gram-negative bacteria; this destroys the integrity of the cell wall and makes it much easier to remove the crystal violet–iodine complex. Figures 4-18 and 4-19 depict various Gram-negative bacteria.

Some strains of bacteria are neither consistently blue-to-purple nor pink-to-red after Gram staining; they are referred to as Gram-variable bacteria. Examples of Gram-variable bacteria are members of the genus *Mycobacterium,* such as *M. tuberculosis* and *M. leprae.* Refer to Table 4-6 and Figures 4-13 through 4-19 for the staining characteristics of certain pathogens.

Mycobacterium species are more often identified using a staining procedure called the *acid-fast stain.* In this proce-

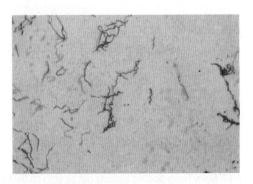

FIGURE 4-19. Loosely, coiled Gram-negative spirochetes. *Borrelia burgdorferi* is the etiologic agent (cause) of Lyme disease. (Koneman's Color Atlas and Textbook of Diagnostic Microbiology, 6th ed. Philadelphia: Lippincott Williams & Wilkins, 2006.)

dure, carbol fuchsin (a bright red dye) is first driven into the bacterial cell using heat (usually by flooding the smear with carbol fuchsin, and then holding a Bunsen burner flame under the slide until steaming of the carbol fuchsin occurs). The heat is necessary because the cell walls of mycobacteria contain waxes, which prevent the stain from penetrating the cells. The heat softens the waxes, enabling the stain to penetrate. A decolorizing agent (a mixture of acid and alcohol) is then used in an attempt to remove the red color from the cells. Because mycobacteria are not decolorized by the acid–alcohol mixture (again owing to the waxes in their cell walls), they are said to be acid-fast. Most other bacteria are decolorized by the acid–alcohol treatment; they are said to be non–acid-fast. The acid-fast stain is especially useful in the tuberculosis laboratory ("TB lab") where the acid-fast mycobacteria are readily seen as red bacilli (referred to as acid-fast bacilli or AFB) against a blue or green background in a sputum specimen from a tuberculosis patient. Figures 4-20 and 4-21 depict the appearance of mycobacteria after the acid-fast staining procedure. The acid-fast staining procedure was developed in 1882 by Paul Ehrlich—a German chemist (see *Microbiology—Hollywood Style* on the CD-ROM that accompanies this book).

The Gram and acid-fast staining procedures are referred to as ***differential staining procedures*** because they enable microbiologists to differentiate one group of bacteria from another (i.e., Gram-positive bacteria from Gram-negative bacteria, and acid-fast bacteria from non–acid-fast bacteria). Table 4-7 summarizes the various types of bacterial staining procedures.

TABLE 4-6

Characteristics of Some Important Pathogenic Bacteria

BACTERIUM	DISEASES	TYPE	GRAM-STAIN REACTION[a]
Bacillus anthracis	Anthrax	Spore-forming rod	+
Bordetella pertussis	Whooping cough	Rod	−
Brucella abortus and B. melitensis	Brucellosis, undulant fever	Rod	−
Chlamydia trachomatis	Lymphogranuloma venereum, trachoma	Pleomorphic	−
Clostridium botulinum	Botulism (food poisoning)	Spore-forming rod	+
Clostridium perfringens	Gas gangrene, wound infections	Spore-forming rod	+
Clostridium tetani	Tetanus (lockjaw)	Spore-forming rod	+
Corynebacterium diphtheriae	Diphtheria	Rod	+
Escherichia coli	Urinary tract infections	Rod	−
Francisella tularensis	Tularemia	Rod	−
Haemophilus ducreyi	Chancroid	Rod	−
Haemophilus influenzae	Meningitis, pneumonia	Rod	−
Klebsiella pneumoniae	Pneumonia	Rod	−
Mycobacterium leprae	Leprosy	Rod	+/−
Mycobacterium tuberculosis	Tuberculosis	Rod	+/−
Neisseria gonorrhoeae	Gonorrhea	Diplococcus	−

(continues)

TABLE 4-6

Characteristics of Some Important Pathogenic Bacteria *(continued)*

BACTERIUM	DISEASES	TYPE	GRAM-STAIN REACTION[a]
Neisseria meningitidis	Nasopharyngitis, meningitis	Diplococcus	−
Proteus vulgaris	Gastroenteritis, urinary tract infections	Rod	−
Pseudomonas aeruginosa	Respiratory, urogenital, and wound infections	Rod	−
Rickettsia rickettsii	Rocky Mountain spotted fever	Rod	−
Salmonella typhi	Typhoid fever	Rod	−
Salmonella species	Gastroenteritis	Rod	−
Shigella species	Shigellosis (bacillary dysentery)	Rod	−
Staphylococcus aureus	Boils, carbuncles, pneumonia, septicemia	Cocci in clusters	+
Streptococcus pyogenes	Strep throat, scarlet fever, rheumatic fever, septicemia	Cocci in chains	+
Streptococcus pneumoniae	Pneumonia, meningitis	Diplococcus	+
Treponema pallidum	Syphilis	Spirochete	−
Vibrio cholerae	Cholera	Curved rod	−
Yersinia pestis	Plague	Rod	−

[a]+, Gram-positive; −, Gram-negative; +/−, Gram-variable.

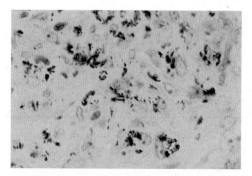

FIGURE 4-20. Many red acid-fast mycobacteria can be seen in this acid-fast stained liver biopsy specimen. (Koneman's Color Atlas and Textbook of Diagnostic Microbiology, 6th ed. Philadelphia: Lippincott Williams & Wilkins, 2006.)

Motility

If a bacterium is able to "swim," it is said to be motile. Bacteria unable to swim are said to be nonmotile. Bacterial motility is most often associated with the presence of flagella or axial filaments, although some bacteria exhibit a type of gliding motility on secreted slime. Most spiral-shaped bacteria and about one half of the bacilli are motile by means of flagella, but cocci are generally nonmotile. A flagella stain can be used to demonstrate the presence, number, and location of flagella on bacterial cells. Various terms (e.g., monotrichous, amphitrichous, lophotrichous, peritrichous) are used to describe the number and location of flagella on bacterial cells (see Chapter 3).

Motility can be demonstrated by stabbing the bacteria into a tube of semisolid medium or by using the hanging-drop technique. Growth (multiplication) of bacteria in semisolid medium produces turbidity (cloudiness). Nonmotile organisms will grow only along the stab line (thus, turbidity will be seen only along the stab line), but motile organisms will spread away from the stab line (thus, producing turbidity throughout the medium; see Fig. 4-22). In the hanging-drop

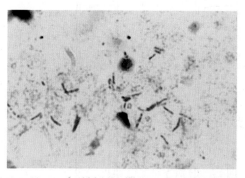

FIGURE 4-21. Many red acid-fast bacilli (*Mycobacterium tuberculosis*) can be seen in this acid-fast stained concentrate from a digested sputum specimen. (Koneman et al. Color Atlas and Textbook of Diagnostic Microbiology, 5th ed. Philadelphia: Lippincott Williams & Wilkins, 1997.)

method (Fig. 4-23), a drop of a bacterial suspension is placed onto a glass coverslip. The coverslip is then inverted over a depression slide. When the preparation is examined microscopically, motile bacteria within the "hanging drop" will be seen darting around in every direction.

Colony Morphology

After a bacterial cell lands on the surface of a solid culture medium, it divides over and over again, ultimately producing a mound or pile of bacteria, known as a bacterial colony (Fig. 4-24). A colony contains millions of organisms. The colony morphology (appearance of the colonies) of bacteria varies from one species to another. Colony morphology includes the size, color, overall shape, elevation, and the appearance of the edge or margin of the colony. As is true for cell morphology and staining characteristics, colony features serve as important "clues" in the identification of bacteria. Size of colonies is determined by the organism's rate of growth (generation time), and is an important characteristic of a particular bacterial species. Colony morphology also includes the results of enzymatic activity on various types of culture media, such as those shown in Figures 8-3 through 8-5 in Chapter 8.

Atmospheric Requirements

In the microbiology laboratory, it is useful to classify bacteria on the basis of their relationship to oxygen (O_2) and carbon dioxide (CO_2). With respect to oxygen, a bacterial isolate can be classified into one of five major groups: obligate aerobes, microaerophilic aerobes (microaerophiles), facultative anaerobes, aerotolerant anaerobes, and obligate anaerobes. In a liquid medium such as thioglycollate broth, the region of the medium in which the organism grows depends on the oxygen needs of that particular species.

To grow and multiply, **obligate aerobes** require an atmosphere containing molecular oxygen in concentrations comparable to that found in room air (i.e., 20 to 21% O_2). Mycobacteria and certain fungi are examples of microorganisms that are obligate aerobes. **Microaerophiles** (microaerophilic aerobes) also require oxygen for multiplication, but in concentrations lower than that found in room air. *Neisseria gonorrhoeae* (the causative agent of gonorrhea) and *Campylobacter* spp. (which are major causes of bacterial diarrhea) are examples of microaerophilic bacteria that prefer an atmosphere containing about 5% oxygen.

Anaerobes can be defined as organisms that do not require oxygen for life and reproduction. However, they vary in their sensitivity to oxygen. The terms obligate anaerobe, aerotolerant anaerobe, and facultative anaerobe are used to describe the organism's relationship to molecular oxygen. An **obligate anaerobe** is an anaerobe that can only grow in an anaerobic environment (i.e., an environment containing no oxygen). (See "Insight: Life in the Absence of Oxygen" on the CD-ROM.)

An **aerotolerant anaerobe** does not require oxygen, grows better in the absence of oxygen, but can survive in at-

TABLE 4-7

Types of Bacterial Staining Procedures

CATEGORY	EXAMPLE(S)	PURPOSE
Simple staining procedure	Staining with methylene blue	Merely to stain the cells so that their size, shape, and morphologic arrangement can be determined
Structural staining procedures	Capsule stains	To determine whether the organism is encapsulated
	Flagella stains	To determine whether the organism possesses flagella and, if so, their number and location on the cell
	Endospore stains	To determine whether the organism is a spore-former and, if so, to determine whether the spores are terminal or subterminal spores
Differential staining procedures	Gram stain	To differentiate between Gram-positive and Gram-negative bacteria
	Acid-fast stain	To differentiate between acid-fast and non–acid-fast bacteria

mospheres containing molecular oxygen (such as air and a CO_2 incubator). The concentration of oxygen that an aerotolerant anaerobe can tolerate varies from one species to another. **Facultative anaerobes** are capable of surviving in either the presence or absence of oxygen; anywhere from 0% O_2 to 20 to 21% O_2. Many of the bacteria routinely isolated from clinical specimens are facultative anaerobes (e.g., members of the family *Enterobacteriaceae*, most streptococci, most staphylococci).

Room air contains less than 1% CO_2. Some bacteria, referred to as **capnophiles** (capnophilic organisms), grow better in the laboratory in the presence of increased

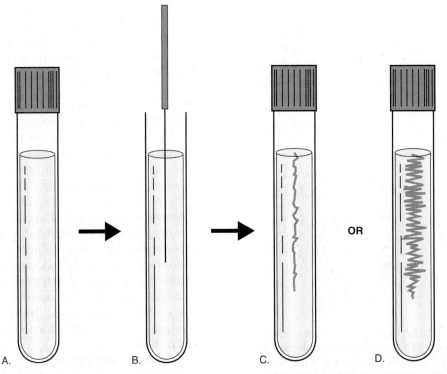

FIGURE 4-22. Semisolid agar method for determining motility. (*A*) Uninoculated tube of semisolid agar. (*B*) Same tube being inoculated by stabbing the inoculating wire into the medium. (*C*) Pattern of growth of a nonmotile organism, after incubation. (*D*) Pattern of growth of a motile organism, after incubation.

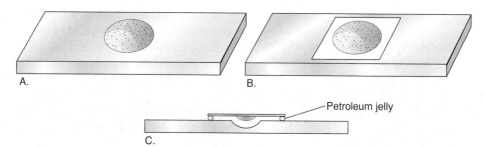

FIGURE 4-23. Hanging-drop preparation for study of living bacteria. (*A*) Depression slide. (*B*) Depression slide with coverglass over the depression area. (*C*) Side view of hanging-drop preparation showing the drop of liquid culture medium hanging from the center of the coverglass above the depression.

concentrations of CO_2. Some anaerobes (e.g., *Bacteroides* and *Fusobacterium* species) are capnophiles, as are some aerobes (e.g., certain *Neisseria*, *Campylobacter*, and *Haemophilus* species). In the clinical microbiology laboratory, CO_2 incubators are routinely calibrated to contain between 5% and 10% CO_2.

Nutritional Requirements

All bacteria need some form of the elements carbon, hydrogen, oxygen, sulfur, phosphorus, and nitrogen for growth. Special elements, such as potassium, calcium, iron, manganese, magnesium, cobalt, copper, zinc, and uranium, are required by some bacteria. Certain microbes have specific vitamin requirements and some need organic substances secreted by other living microorganisms during their growth. Organisms with especially demanding nutritional requirements are said to be fastidious; think of them as being "fussy." Special enriched media must be used to grow fastidious organisms in the laboratory. The nutritional needs of a particular organism are usually characteristic for that species of bacteria and sometimes serve as important clues when attempting to identify the organism. Nutritional requirements are discussed further in Chapters 7 and 8.

Biochemical and Metabolic Activities

As bacteria grow, they produce many waste products and secretions, some of which are enzymes that enable them to invade their host and cause disease. The pathogenic strains of many bacteria, such as staphylococci and streptococci, can be tentatively identified by the enzymes they secrete. Also, in particular environments, some bacteria are characterized by the production of certain gases, such as carbon dioxide, hydrogen sulfide, oxygen, or methane. To aid in the identification of certain types of bacteria in the laboratory, they are inoculated into various substrates (e.g., carbohydrates and amino acids) to determine whether they possess the enzymes necessary to break down those substrates. Learning whether a particular organism is able to break down a certain substrate serves as a clue to the identity of that organism. Different types of culture media are also used in the laboratory to learn information about an organism's metabolic activities (to be discussed in Chapter 8).

Pathogenicity

The characteristics that enable bacteria to cause disease are discussed in Chapter 14. Many pathogens are able to cause disease because they possess capsules, pili, or endotoxins (part of the cell wall of Gram-negative bacteria), or because they secrete exotoxins and exoenzymes that damage cells and tissues. Frequently, pathogenicity (the ability to cause disease) is tested by injecting the organism into mice or cell cultures. Some common pathogenic bacteria are listed in Table 4-6.

Genetic Composition

Most modern laboratories are moving toward the identification of bacteria using some type of test procedure that analyzes the organism's deoxyribonucleic acid (DNA) or ribonucleic acid (RNA). These test procedures are collectively referred to as molecular diagnostic procedures. The composition of the genetic material (DNA) of an organism is unique to each species. DNA probes make it possible to identify an isolate without relying on phenotypic characteristics. A DNA probe is a single-stranded DNA sequence that can be used to identify an organism by hybridizing with a unique complimentary sequence on the DNA or rRNA of that organism. Also, through the use of 16S rRNA sequencing (see Chapter 3), a researcher can determine the degree of relatedness between two different bacteria.

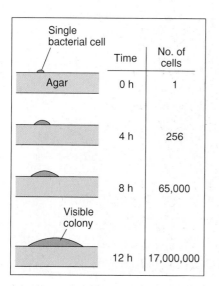

Single bacterial cell	Time	No. of cells
Agar	0 h	1
	4 h	256
	8 h	65,000
Visible colony	12 h	17,000,000

FIGURE 4-24. Formation of a bacterial colony on solid growth medium. In this illustration, the generation time is assumed to be 30 minutes.

Unique Bacteria

Rickettsias, chlamydias, and mycoplasmas are bacteria, but they do not possess all the attributes of typical bacterial cells. Thus, they are often referred to as "unique" or "rudimentary" bacteria. Because they are so small and difficult to isolate, they were formerly thought to be viruses.

Rickettsias, Chlamydias, and Closely Related Bacteria

Rickettsias and chlamydias are bacteria with a Gram-negative-type cell wall. They are obligate intracellular pathogens that cause diseases in humans and other animals. As the name implies, an obligate intracellular pathogen is a pathogen that *must* live within a host cell. To grow such organisms in the laboratory, they must be inoculated into embryonated chicken eggs, laboratory animals, or cell cultures. They will not grow on artificial (synthetic) culture media.

The genus *Rickettsia* was named for Howard T. Ricketts, a U.S. pathologist; these organisms have no connection to the disease called rickets, which is the result of vitamin D deficiency. Because they appear to have leaky cell membranes, most rickettsias must live inside another cell to retain all necessary cellular substances (Fig. 4-25). All diseases caused by *Rickettsia* species are arthropodborne, meaning that they are transmitted by arthropod **vectors** (carriers); see Table 4-8.

Arthropods such as lice, fleas, and ticks transmit the rickettsias from one host to another by their bites or waste products. Diseases caused by *Rickettsia* spp. include typhus and typhuslike diseases (e.g., Rocky Mountain spotted fever). All these diseases involve production of a rash. Medically important bacteria that are closely related to rickettsias include *Coxiella burnetii, Bartonella quintana* (formerly *Rochalimaea quintana*), and *Ehrlichia* spp. *Coxiella burnetii* (the cause of Q fever) is transmitted primarily by aerosols, but can be transmitted to animals by ticks. *Bartonella quintana* is associated with trench fever (a louseborne disease), cat scratch disease, bacteremia, and endocarditis. *Ehrlichia* and *Anaplasma* spp. cause human tickborne diseases such as human monocytic ehrlichiosis (HME) and human granulocytic ehrlichiosis (HGE). *Ehrlichia* and *Anaplasma* spp. are intraleukocytic pathogens, meaning that they live within certain types of white blood cells.

The term "chlamydias" refers to *Chlamydia* spp. and closely related organisms (such as *Chlamydophila* spp.). Chlamydias are referred to as "energy parasites." Although they can produce adenosine triphosphate (ATP) molecules, they preferentially use ATP molecules produced by their host cells. ATP molecules are the major energy-storing or energy-carrying molecules of cells (see Chapter 7). Chlamydias are obligate intracellular pathogens that are transferred by inhalation of aerosols or by direct contact between hosts—*not* by arthropods. Medically important

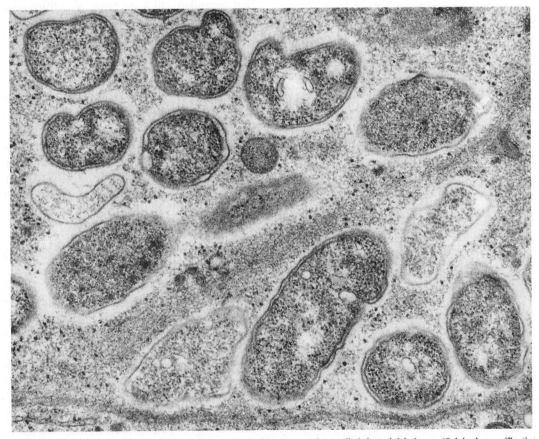

FIGURE 4-25. *Rickettsia prowazekii,* the cause of epidemic louseborne typhus, in experimentally infected tick tissue. (Original magnification, 45,000×.) (Volk WA, et al. Essentials of Medical Microbiology, 5th ed. Philadelphia: Lippincott-Raven, 1996.)

TABLE 4-8

Human Diseases Caused by Unique Bacteria

GENUS	SPECIES	HUMAN DISEASE(S)
Rickettsia	R. akari R. prowazekii R. rickettsii R. typhi	Rickettsialpox (a miteborne disease) Epidemic typhus (a louseborne disease) Rocky Mountain spotted fever (a tickborne disease) Endemic or murine typhus (a fleaborne disease)
Ehrlichia spp.	E. chaffeensis	Human monocytic ehrlichiosis
Anaplasma spp.	Anaplasma phagocytophilum (formerly E. phagocytophilum)	Human granulocytic ehrlichiosis
Chlamydia (and Chlamydia–like bacteria)	Chlamydophila pneumoniae	Pneumonia
	Chlamydophila psittaci Chlamydia trachomatis	Psittacosis (a respiratory disease; a zoonosis; sometimes called "parrot fever") Different serotypes cause different diseases, including trachoma (an eye disease) inclusion conjunctivitis (an eye disease), nongonococcal urethritis (NGU; a sexually transmitted disease), lymphogranuloma venereum (LGV; a sexually transmitted disease)
Mycoplasma	M. pneumoniae M. genitalium	Atypical pneumonia Nongonococcal urethritis (NGU)
Orientia	O. tsutsugamushi	Scrub typhus (a miteborne disease)
Ureaplasma	U. urealyticum	Nongonococcal urethritis (NGU)

chlamydias include *Chlamydia trachomatis, Chlamy-dophila pneumoniae,* and *Chlamydophila psittaci.* Different serotypes of *C. trachomatis* cause different diseases, including trachoma (the leading cause of blindness in the world), inclusion conjunctivitis (another type of eye disease), and nongonococcal urethritis (NGU; a term given to urethritis that is not caused by *Neisseria gonorrhoeae*). *C. pneumoniae* causes a type of pneumonia, and *C. psittaci* causes a respiratory disease called psittacosis. Chlamydial diseases are listed in Table 4-8.

Mycoplasmas

Mycoplasmas are the smallest of the cellular microbes (Fig. 4-26). Because they lack cell walls, they assume many shapes, from coccoid to filamentous; thus, they appear pleomorphic when examined microscopically. Sometimes they are confused with CWD bacteria, described earlier; however, even in the most favorable growth media, mycoplasmas are not able to produce cell walls, which is not

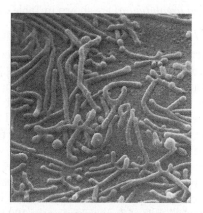

FIGURE 4-26. Scanning electron micrograph of *Mycoplasma pneumoniae.* (Strohl WA, et al. Lippincott's Illustrated Reviews: Microbiology. Philadelphia: Lippincott Williams & Wilkins, 2001.)

true for CWD. Mycoplasmas were formerly called pleuropneumonia-like organisms (PPLO), first isolated from cattle with lung infections. They may be free-living or parasitic and are pathogenic to many animals and some plants. In humans, pathogenic mycoplasmas cause primary atypical pneumonia and genitourinary infections; some species can grow intracellularly. Because they have no cell wall, they are resistant to treatment with penicillin and other antibiotics that work by inhibiting cell wall synthesis. Mycoplasmas can be cultured on artificial media in the laboratory, where they produce tiny colonies (called "fried egg colonies") that resemble sunny-side-up fried eggs in appearance. The absence of a cell wall prevents mycoplasmas from staining with the Gram stain procedure. Diseases caused by mycoplasmas and a closely related organism (*Ureaplasma urealyticum*) are shown in Table 4-8.

Especially Large and Especially Small Bacteria

The size of a typical coccus (e.g., a *Staphylococcus aureus* cell) is 1 μm in diameter. A typical bacillus (e.g., an *E. coli* cell) is about 1.0 μm wide × 3.0 μm long, although some bacilli are long thin filaments—up to about 12 μm in length or even longer—but still only about 1 μm wide. Thus, most bacteria are microscopic, requiring the use of a microscope to be seen.

Perhaps the largest of all bacteria—large enough to be seen with the unaided human eye—is *Thiomargarita namibiensis,* a colorless, marine, sulfide-oxidizing bacterium. Single spherical cells of *T. namibiensis* are 100 to 300 μm, but may be as large as 750 μm (0.75 mm). In terms of size, comparing a *T. namibiensis* cell to an *E. coli* cell would be like comparing a blue whale to a newly born mouse. Other marine sulfide-oxidizing bacteria in the genera *Beggiatoa* and *Thioploca* are also especially large, having diameters from 10 μm to more than 100 μm. Although *Beggiatoa* and *Thioploca* form filaments, *Thiomargarita* cells do not.

Another enormous bacterium, named *Epulopiscium fishelsonii,* has been isolated from the intestines of the reef surgeonfish; this bacillus is about 80 μm wide × 600 μm (0.6 mm) long. *Epulopiscium* cells are about five times longer than eucaryotic *Paramecium* cells. The volume of an *Epulopiscium* cell is about a million times greater than the volume of a typical bacterial cell. Spore-forming bacteria called metabacteria, found in the intestines of herbivorous rodents, are closely related to *Epulopiscium,* but they reach lengths of only 20 to 30 μm. Although shorter than *Epulopiscium,* metabacteria are much longer than most bacteria.

At the other end of the spectrum, there are especially tiny bacteria called **nanobacteria.** Their sizes are expressed in nanometers because these bacteria are less than 1 μm in diameter; hence the name, nanobacteria. In some cases, they are as small as 20 nm in diameter. Nanobacteria have been found in soil, minerals, ocean water, human and animal blood, human dental calculus (plaque), arterial plaque, and even rocks (meteorites) of extraterrestrial origin.

Photosynthetic Bacteria

Photosynthetic bacteria include purple bacteria, green bacteria, and cyanobacteria (erroneously referred to in the past as blue-green algae). Although all three groups use light as an energy source, they do not all carry out photosynthesis in the same way. For example, purple and green bacteria (which, in some cases, are not actually those colors) do not produce oxygen, whereas cyanobacteria do. Photosynthesis that produces oxygen is called **oxygenic photosynthesis,** whereas photosynthesis that does not produce oxygen is called **anoxygenic photosynthesis.**

In photosynthetic eucaryotes (algae and plants), photosynthesis takes place in plastids, which were discussed in Chapter 3. In cyanobacteria, photosynthesis takes place on intracellular membranes known as thylakoids. Thylakoids are attached to the cell membrane at various points and are thought to represent invaginations of the cell membrane. Attached to the thylakoids, in orderly rows, are numerous phycobilisomes—complex protein pigment aggregates where light harvesting occurs.

Many scientists believe that cyanobacteria were the first organisms capable of carrying out oxygenic photosynthesis and, thus, played a major part in the oxygenation of the atmosphere (see "Insight: The Oxygen Holocaust" on the CD-ROM). Fossil records reveal that cyanobacteria were already in existence 3.3 to 3.5 billion years ago. Photosynthesis is discussed further in Chapter 7. Cyanobacteria vary widely in shape; some are cocci, some are bacilli, and others form long filaments.

When appropriate conditions exist, cyanobacteria in pond or lake water will overgrow, creating a water bloom— a "pond scum" that resembles a thick layer of bluish-green (turquoise) oil paint. The conditions include a mild or no wind, a balmy water temperature ($15°$ to $30°C$), a water pH of 6 to 9, and an abundance of the nutrients nitrogen and phosphorous in the water. Many cyanobacteria are able to convert nitrogen gas (N_2) from the air into ammonium ions (NH_4^+) in the soil or water; this process is known as ***nitrogen fixation*** (Chapter 10).

Some cyanobacteria produce toxins (poisons), such as neurotoxins (which affect the central nervous system), hepatotoxins (which affect the liver), and cytotoxins (which affect other types of cells). Additional information about these toxins can be found in the CD-ROM Appendix 1, entitled "Microbial Intoxications."

The Domain *Archaea*

Procaryotic organisms thus far described in this chapter are all members of the Domain *Bacteria*. Procaryotic organisms in the Domain *Archaea* were discovered in 1977. Although they were once referred to as archaebacteria (or archaeobacteria), most scientists now feel that there are sufficient differences between archaeans (or archaeons) and bacteria to stop referring to archaeans as bacteria. "Archae" means "ancient," and the name *archaea* was originally assigned when it was thought that these procaryotes evolved earlier than bacteria. Now, there is considerable debate as to whether bacteria or archaeans came first. Genetically, archaeans are more closely related to eucaryotes than they are to bacteria; some possess genes otherwise found only in eucaryotes. Many scientists believe that bacteria and archaeans diverged from a common ancestor relatively soon after life began on this planet. Later, the eucaryotes split off from the archaeans (refer back to Fig. 1-1). According to *Bergey's Manual of Systematic Bacteriology,* the Domain *Archaea* contains 2 phyla, 8 classes, 12 orders, 21 families, 69 genera, and 217 species. Archaeans vary widely in shape; some are cocci, some are bacilli, and others

form long filaments. Many, but not all, archaeans are "extremophiles," in the sense that they live in extreme environments, such as extremely acidic, extremely hot, and extremely salty environments. Some live at the bottom of the ocean in and near thermal vents, where, in addition to heat and salinity, there is extreme pressure. Other archaeans, called methanogens, produce methane, which is a flammable gas. Although virtually all archaeans possess cell walls, their cell walls contain no peptidoglycan. In contrast, all bacterial cell walls contain peptidoglycan. The 16S rRNA sequences of archaeans are quite different from the 16S rRNA sequences of bacteria. The 16S rRNA sequence data suggest that archaeans are more closely related to eucaryotes than they are to bacteria. You will recall from Chapter 3 that differences in rRNA structure form the basis of the Three-Domain System of Classification.

REVIEW OF KEY POINTS

- Microbes can be divided into those that are cellular (bacteria, algae, protozoa, and fungi) and those that are acellular (viruses, viroids, and prions). The cellular microorganisms can be divided into those that are procaryotic and those that are eucaryotic.

- Complete virus particles, called virions, may be distinguished from living cells because they possess *either* DNA or RNA—never both. Most viruses consist merely of nucleic acid surrounded by a protein coat. Viruses must invade host cells to replicate; they lack the enzymes necessary for the production of energy, proteins, and nucleic acid.

- Viruses are classified by type of nucleic acid, shape of the capsid, size of the capsid, number of capsomeres, presence or absence of an envelope, type of host(s) and host cell(s) they infect, type of disease they cause, and antigenic properties.

- Bacteriophages are viruses that infect bacteria. There are two categories of bacteriophages: virulent bacteriophages, which cause destruction (lysis) of the host cell, and temperate bacteriophages, which change the host cell genetically.

- Viroids are infectious RNA molecules that interfere with the metabolism of plant cells. Prions are infectious protein molecules that cause certain diseases in animals. The highly publicized "mad cow disease" is an example of a prion-caused disease.

- Characteristics used for identification and classification of bacteria include cell morphology, staining reactions, motility, colony morphology, atmospheric requirements, nutritional needs, biochemical and metabolic activities, pathogenicity, amino acid sequencing of proteins, and genetic composition.

- The three basic shapes of bacteria are cocci, bacilli, and curved and spiral-shaped bacteria. Cocci occur singly or in pairs (diplococci), chains (streptococci), clusters (staphylococci), or packets of four (tetrads) or eight (octads). Bacilli occur singly, in pairs (diplobacilli), or in chains (streptobacilli), or they may be branched or filamentous. Very short bacilli are called coccobacilli. Curved bacteria may occur singly, or in pairs or chains. Spiral-shaped bacteria usually occur singly.

- Bacterial smears must be fixed before staining. The two most common types of fixation are heat-fixation and methanol-fixation; the latter technique is preferred. The fixation process serves to kill the organisms, preserve their morphology, and anchor the smear to the slide.

- Most motile bacteria possess whiplike structures called flagella. The terms monotrichous, amphitrichous, lophotrichous, and peritrichous are used to describe the number and location of flagella on the bacterial cell.

- A pile or mound of bacteria on the surface of a solid culture medium is referred to as a colony; it contains millions of bacterial cells. Bacterial colony morphology includes size, color, overall shape, elevation, consistency, and the appearance of the margin of the colony.

- On the basis of its oxygen requirements, a bacterial isolate can be classified as an obligate aerobe, a microaerophile, a facultative anaerobe, an aerotolerant anaerobe, or an obligate anaerobe. Bacteria requiring increased concentrations of carbon dioxide are called capnophiles.

- All bacteria need some form of the elements carbon, hydrogen, oxygen, sulfur, phosphorus, and nitrogen. In addition, certain bacteria require potassium, calcium, iron, manganese, magnesium, cobalt, copper, zinc, and uranium. Fastidious (nutritionally demanding) microbes may require additional vitamins, amino acids, and other organic compounds.

- Pathogenic bacteria may produce pili, capsules, endotoxin, exotoxins, and exoenzymes that enable them to cause disease.

- Rickettsias, chlamydias, and mycoplasmas are rudimentary Gram-negative bacteria. Mycoplasmas differ from other bacteria because they have no cell walls. Rickettsias and chlamydias are unique because they are obligate intracellular pathogens.

- Extremely tiny bacteria (less than 1 μm in diameter), called nanobacteria, have been found in soil, minerals, ocean water, human and animal blood, human dental calculus (plaque), arterial plaque, and even rocks (meteorites) of extraterrestrial origin.

- Certain bacteria, including a group of bacteria referred to as cyanobacteria, are photosynthetic. Some photosynthetic bacteria, including cyanobacteria, produce oxygen as a byproduct of photosynthesis; this type of photosynthesis is known as oxygenic photosynthesis.

- Genetically, archaeans are more closely related to eucaryotic organisms than to bacteria, although both archaeans and bacteria are procaryotic. Archaeans differ from bacteria in several ways: they possess a different type of rRNA; their cell walls contain no peptidoglycan; many of them live in extreme environments; and some (called methanogens) produce methane.

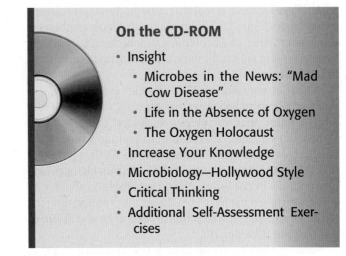

On the CD-ROM
- Insight
  - Microbes in the News: "Mad Cow Disease"
  - Life in the Absence of Oxygen
  - The Oxygen Holocaust
- Increase Your Knowledge
- Microbiology—Hollywood Style
- Critical Thinking
- Additional Self-Assessment Exercises

Self-Assessment Exercises

After studying this chapter, answer the following multiple-choice questions.

1. Which one of the following steps occurs during the multiplication of animal viruses, but not during the multiplication of bacteriophages?
   a. assembly
   b. biosynthesis
   c. penetration
   d. uncoating

2. Which one of the following diseases or groups of diseases is not caused by prions?
   a. certain plant diseases
   b. chronic wasting disease of deer and elk
   c. Creutzfeldt-Jacob disease of humans
   d. "mad cow disease"

3. Most procaryotic cells reproduce by:
   a. binary fission.
   b. budding.
   c. gamete production.
   d. spore formation.

4. The group of bacteria that lack rigid cell walls and take on irregular shapes is:
   a. chlamydias.
   b. mycobacteria.
   c. mycoplasmas.
   d. rickettsias.

5. At the end of the Gram staining procedure, Gram-positive bacteria will be:
   a. blue-to-purple.
   b. green.
   c. orange.
   d. pink-to-red.

6. Which one of the following statements about rickettias is false?
   a. Diseases caused by rickettsias are arthropodborne.
   b. Rickets is caused by a *Rickettsia* species.
   c. *Rickettsia* species cause typhus and typhuslike diseases.
   d. Rickettsias have leaky membranes.

7. Which one of the following statements about *Chlamydia* and *Chlamydophila* spp. is false?
   a. They are obligate intracellular pathogens.
   b. They are considered to be "energy parasites."
   c. The diseases they cause are all arthropodborne.
   d. They are considered to be Gram-negative bacteria.

8. Which one of the following statements about cyanobacteria is false?
   a. Although cyanobacteria are photosynthetic, they do not produce oxygen as a result of photosynthesis.
   b. At one time, cyanobacteria were called blue-green algae.
   c. Some cyanobacteria are capable of nitrogen fixation.
   d. Some cyanobacteria are important medically because they produce toxins.

9. Which one of the following statements about archaeans is false?
   a. Archaeans are more closely related to eucaryotes than they are to bacteria.
   b. Both archaeans and bacteria are procaryotic organisms.
   c. Some archaeans live in extremely hot environments.
   d. The cell walls of archaeans contain a thicker layer of peptidoglycan than the cell walls of bacteria.

10. An organism that does not require oxygen, grows better in the absence of oxygen, but can survive in atmospheres containing some molecular oxygen is known as a(n):
    a. aerotolerant anaerobe.
    b. capnophile.
    c. facultative anaerobe.
    d. microaerophile.

DIVERSITY OF MICROORGANISMS
PART 2 Eucaryotic Microbes

LEARNING OBJECTIVES

AFTER STUDYING THIS CHAPTER, YOU SHOULD BE ABLE TO:

- Compare and contrast the differences among algae, protozoa, and fungi
- Explain what is meant by a "red tide" (i.e., what causes it) and its medical significance
- List the four major categories of protozoa and their most important differentiating characteristics
- Define the terms pellicle, cytostome, and stigma
- List five infectious diseases of humans that are caused by protozoa and five that are caused by fungi
- State the importance of phycotoxins and mycotoxins
- Explain the differences between aerial and vegetative hyphae, septate and aseptate hyphae, sexual and asexual spores
- Explain the major difference between a lichen and a slime mold

INTRODUCTION

Acellular and procaryotic microbes were described in Chapter 4. This chapter describes the eucaryotic microbes, which include some algae, all protozoa, some fungi, all lichens, and all slime molds. Scientists have not yet determined when the first eucaryotic organisms appeared on earth. The best guesses are between 2 and 3.5 billion years ago.

Algae

Characteristics and Classification

Algae (sing., *alga*) are photosynthetic, eucaryotic organisms that, together with protozoa, are classified in the second kingdom (Protista) of the Five-Kingdom System of Classification. Not all taxonomists agree, however, that algae and protozoa should be combined in the same kingdom. The study of algae is called phycology (or algology), and a person who studies algae is called a phycologist (or algologist).

All algal cells consist of cytoplasm, a cell wall (usually), cell membrane, a nucleus, plastids, ribosomes, mitochondria, and Golgi bodies. In addition, some algal cells have a **pellicle** (a thickened cell membrane), a **stigma** (a light-sensing organelle, also known as an eyespot), and flagella. Although they are not plants, algae are more plantlike than protozoa. (See Table 5-1 for similarities and differences between algae and plants.) Algae lack true roots, stems, and leaves.

Algae range in size from tiny, unicellular, microscopic organisms (e.g., diatoms, dinoflagellates, desmids) to large, multicellular, plantlike seaweeds (e.g., kelp; Table 5-2). Thus, not all algae are microorganisms. Algae may be arranged in colonies or strands and are found in freshwater and salt water, in wet soil, and on wet rocks. Algae produce their energy by photosynthesis, using energy from the sun, carbon dioxide, water, and inorganic nutrients from the soil to build cellular material. However, a few species use organic nutrients, and others survive with very little sunlight. Most algal cell walls contain cellulose, a polysaccharide not found in the cell walls of any other microorganisms. Depending on the types of photosynthetic pigments they possess, algae are classified as green, golden (or golden brown), brown, or red.

Diatoms are tiny, usually unicellular algae that live in both freshwater and seawater. They are important members of the phytoplankton. Diatoms have silicon dioxide in their cell walls; thus, they have cell walls made of glass. Deposits of diatoms are used to make diatomaceous earth, which is used in filtration systems, insulation, and abrasives. Because of their attractive, geometric, and varied appearance, diatoms are quite interesting to observe microscopically.

Dinoflagellates are microscopic, unicellular, flagellated, often photosynthetic algae. Like diatoms, they are important members of the phytoplankton, producing much of the oxygen in our atmosphere and serving as

TABLE 5-1

Similarities and Differences Between Algae and Plants

	ALGAE	PLANTS
Eucaryotic	Yes	Yes
Photosynthetic	Yes	Yes
Cells contain chlorophyll	Yes	Yes
Use carbon dioxide as an energy source	Yes	Yes
Store energy in the form of starch	Yes	Yes
Composed of roots, stems, and leaves	No	Most (bryophytes, such as mosses, are the exception)
Cell walls contain cellulose	Most (exceptions include diatoms and dinoflagellates; *Euglena* and *Volvox* do not have cell walls)	Yes
Method of reproduction	Both asexual and sexual	Sexual
Contain a vascular system to transport internal fluids	No	Most (mosses and other bryophytes are avascular)

TABLE 5-2

Characteristics of Algae

PHYLUM (AND COMMON NAME)	STRUCTURAL ARRANGEMENT	PREDOMINANT COLOR	PHOTOSYNTHETIC PIGMENTS[a]	HABITAT
Bacillariophyta (diatoms)	Unicellular	Olive brown	Chlorophyll c, carotenoids, xanthophylls	Freshwater and seawater
Chlorophyta (green algae)	Unicellular and multicellular	Green	Chlorophyll b, carotenoids	Freshwater (predominantly) and seawater
Chrysophyta (golden algae)	Unicellular	Golden olive	Chlorophyll c, carotenoids, xanthophylls	Freshwater
Dinoflagellata (dinoflagellates)	Unicellular	Brown	Chlorophyll c, carotenoids, xanthophylls	Freshwater and seawater
Euglenophyta (*Euglena* spp. and closely related organisms)	Unicellular	Green	Chlorophyll b, carotenoids, xanthophylls	Freshwater
Phaeophyta (brown algae)	Multicellular seaweeds	Olive brown	Chlorophyll c, carotenoids, xanthophylls	Seawater; most commonly, cold environments
Rhodophyta (red algae)	Multicellular seaweeds	Red to black	Chlorophyll d (in some), carotenoids, phycobilins	Seawater (predominantly) and freshwater; most commonly, tropical environments

[a]In addition to chlorophyll a, which is possessed by all algae. Carotenoids are yellow-orange; chlorophylls are greenish; phycobilins are red and blue; and xanthophylls are brownish.

important links in food chains. Some dinoflagellates produce light and, for this reason, are sometimes referred to as fire algae. Dinoflagellates are responsible for what are known as "red tides" (discussed in CD-ROM Appendix 1: "Microbial Intoxications").

Green algae include desmids, *Spirogyra, Chlamydomonas, Volvox,* and *Euglena,* all of which can be found in pond water. Desmids are unicellular algae, some of which resemble a microscopic banana. *Spirogyra* is an example of a filamentous alga, often producing long green strands in pond water. *Chlamydomonas* is a unicellular, biflagellated alga, containing one chloroplast and a stigma.

Volvox is a multicellular alga (sometimes referred to as a colonial alga or colony), consisting of as many as 60,000 interconnected, biflagellated cells, arranged to form a hollow sphere. The flagella beat in a coordinated manner,

causing the *Volvox* colony to move through the water in a rolling motion. Sometimes, daughter colonies can be seen within a *Volvox* colony.

Euglena is a rather interesting alga, in that it possesses features possessed by both algae and protozoa. Like algae, *Euglena* contains chloroplasts, is photosynthetic, and stores energy in the form of starch. Protozoan features include the presence of a primitive mouth (called a **cytostome**) and the absence of a cell wall (hence, no cellulose). *Euglena* possesses a photosensing organelle called a stigma and a single flagellum. With its stigma, it can sense light; with its flagellum, it can swim into the light. When there is no light, *Euglena* can continue to obtain nutrients by ingesting food through its cytostome. Although it has no cell wall, *Euglena* does possess a pellicle, which serves the same function as a cell wall—protection.

Algae are easy to find. They include large seaweeds of various colors, brown kelp (up to 10 meters in length) found along ocean shores, the green scum floating on ponds, and the slippery green material on wet rocks. There are also many microscopic forms in pond water that differ from the colorless, nonphotosynthetic protozoa in that they are pigmented and photosynthetic. Some algae (e.g., *Chlamydomonas, Euglena,* and *Volvox*) have characteristics (e.g., cytostome, pellicle, flagella) that cause them to be classified as protozoa by some taxonomists. (Although there is some disagreement among taxonomists as to where *Chlamydomonas, Volvox,* and *Euglena* should be classified, they are referred to as algae in this book, primarily because they are photosynthetic. In this book, photosynthetic protists are considered to be algae, and nonphotosynthetic protists are considered to be protozoa.)

Algae are an important source of food, iodine and other minerals, fertilizers, emulsifiers for pudding, and stabilizers for ice cream and salad dressings; they are also used as a gelling agent for jams and nutrient media for bacterial growth. The agar used as a solidifying agent in laboratory culture media is a complex polysaccharide derived from a red marine alga. Damage to water systems is frequently caused by algae clogging filters and pipes if many nutrients are present. Some typical algae are shown in Figure 5-1.

Medical Significance

One genus of algae (*Prototheca*) is a very rare cause of human infections (causing a disease known as protothecosis). *Prototheca* lives in soil and can enter wounds, especially those located on the feet. It produces a small subcutaneous lesion that can progress to a crusty, warty-looking lesion. If the organism enters the lymphatic system, it may cause a debilitating, sometimes fatal infection, especially in immunosuppressed individuals. Algae in several other genera secrete substances (**phycotoxins**) that are poisonous to humans, fish, and other animals. For additional information on these toxins, see CD-ROM Appendix 1: "Microbial Intoxications."

Protozoa

Characteristics

Protozoa (sing., **protozoan**) are eucaryotic organisms that, together with algae, are classified in the second kingdom (Protista) of the Five-Kingdom System of Classification. As previously stated, not all taxonomists agree that algae and protozoa should be combined in the same kingdom. The study of protozoa is called protozoology, and a person who studies protozoa is called a protozoologist.

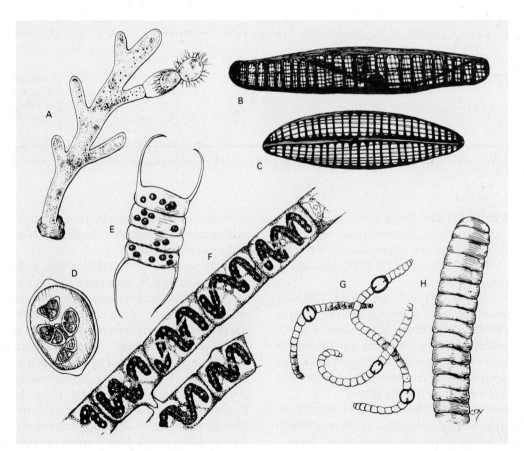

FIGURE 5-1. Typical algae. (*A*) *Vaucheria*. (*B*) Diatom. (*C*) *Navicula*. (*D*) *Oocystis*. (*E*) *Scenedesmus*. (*F*) *Spirogyra*. (*G*) *Nostoc*. (*H*) *Oscillatoria*.

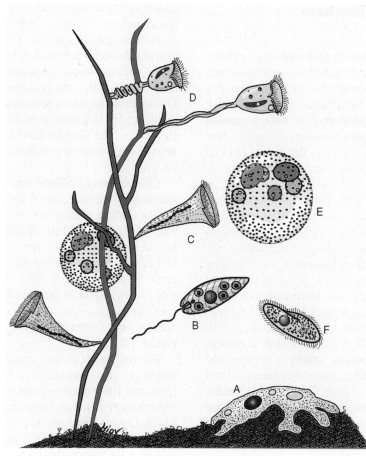

FIGURE 5-2. Typical pond water algae and protozoa. (*A*) *Amoeba* sp. (*B*) *Euglena* sp. (*C*) *Stentor* sp. (*D*) *Vorticella* sp. in extended and contracted positions. (*E*) *Volvox* sp. (*F*) *Paramecium* sp.

Most protozoa are unicellular (single-celled), ranging in length from 3 to 2,000 μm. Most of them are free-living organisms, found in soil and water (Fig. 5-2). Protozoal cells are more animal-like than plantlike. All protozoal cells possess a variety of eucaryotic structures and organelles, including cell membranes, nuclei, endoplasmic reticulum, mitochondria, Golgi bodies, lysosomes, centrioles, and food vacuoles. In addition, some protozoa possess pellicles, cytostomes, contractile vacuoles, pseudopodia, cilia, and flagella. Protozoa have no chlorophyll and, therefore, cannot make their own food by photosynthesis. Some ingest whole algae, yeasts, bacteria, and other smaller protozoans as their source of nutrients; others live on dead and decaying organic matter.

Protozoa do not have cell walls, but some, including some flagellates and some ciliates, possess a pellicle, which serves the same purpose as a cell wall—protection. Some flagellates and some ciliates ingest food through a primitive mouth or opening, called a cytostome. *Paramecium* spp. (common pond water ciliates) possess both a pellicle and a cytostome. Some pond water protozoa (such as amebae and *Paramecium*) contain an organelle called a **contractile vacuole,** which pumps water out of the cell.

Vorticella spp. (pond water ciliates) have a contractile stalk (Fig. 5-2). Within the stalk is a primitive muscle fiber called a myoneme.

A typical protozoan life cycle consists of two stages: the trophozoite stage and the cyst stage. The **trophozoite** is the motile, feeding, dividing stage in a protozoan's life cycle, whereas the **cyst** is the dormant, survival stage. In some ways (e.g., a thick outer wall), cysts are like bacterial spores.

Some protozoa are parasites. Parasitic protozoa break down and absorb nutrients from the body of the host in which they live. Many parasitic protozoa are pathogens, such as those that cause malaria, giardiasis, African sleeping sickness, and amebic dysentery (see Chapter 18). Other protozoa coexist with the host animal in a type of mutualistic symbiotic relationship—a relationship in which both organisms benefit. A typical example of such a symbiotic relationship is the termite and its intestinal protozoa. The protozoa digest the wood eaten by the termite, enabling both organisms to absorb the nutrients necessary for life. Without the intestinal protozoa, the termite would be unable to digest the wood that it eats and would starve to death. Symbiotic relationships are discussed in greater detail in Chapter 10.

Classification and Medical Significance

Protozoa are divided into groups (referred to in various classification schemes as phyla, subphyla, or classes) according to their method of locomotion (Table 5-3). *Amebae* (amebas) move by means of cytoplasmic extensions called *pseudopodia* (sing., *pseudopodium*; false feet). An **ameba (pl., amebae)** first extends a pseudopodium in the direction the ameba intends to move, and then the rest of the cell slowly flows into it; this process is called ameboid movement. An ameba ingests a food particle (e.g., a yeast or bacterial cell) by surrounding the particle with pseudopodia, which then fuse together; this process is known as phagocytosis. The ingested particle, surrounded by a membrane, is referred to as a food vacuole (or phagosome). Digestive enzymes, released from lysosomes, then digest or break down the food into nutrients. Some of the white blood cells in our bodies ingest and digest materials in the same manner as amebae. (Phagocytosis by white blood cells is discussed further in Chapter 15.) When fluids are ingested in a similar manner, the process is known as *pinocytosis*. One medically important ameba is *Entamoeba histolytica*, which causes amebic dysentery (amebiasis) and extraintestinal (meaning away from the intestine) amebic abscesses. Other amebae of medical significance, described in Chapter 18, include *Naegleria fowleri* (the cause of primary amebic meningoencephalitis) and *Acanthamoeba* spp. (which cause eye infections).

Flagellated protozoa or *flagellates* (sing., *flagellate*) move by means of whiplike flagella. A basal body (also called a kinetosome or kinetoplast) anchors each flagellum within the cytoplasm. Flagella exhibit a wavelike motion. Some flagellates are pathogenic. For example, *Trypanosoma brucei* subspecies *gambiense*, transmitted by the tsetse fly, causes African sleeping sickness in humans; *Trypanosoma cruzi* causes American trypanosomiasis (Chagas' disease); *Trichomonas vaginalis* causes persistent sexually transmitted infections (trichomoniasis) of the male and female genital tracts; and *Giardia lamblia* (also known as *Giardia intestinalis*) causes a persistent diarrheal disease (giardiasis; Fig. 5-3).

Ciliates (sing., *ciliate*) move about by means of large numbers of hairlike cilia on their surfaces. Cilia exhibit an oarlike motion. Ciliates are the most complex of all protozoa. A pathogenic ciliate, *Balantidium coli,* causes dysentery in underdeveloped countries. It is usually transmitted to humans from drinking water that has been contaminated by swine feces. *B. coli* is the only ciliated protozoan that causes disease in humans. Examples of pond water ciliates are *Blepharisma, Didinium, Euplotes, Paramecium, Stentor,* and *Vorticella* spp., some of which are shown in Figure 5-2.

Nonmotile protozoa—protozoa lacking pseudopodia, flagella, or cilia—are classified together in a category called sporozoa. The most important sporozoan pathogens are the *Plasmodium* spp. that cause malaria in many areas of the world. One of these species, *Plasmodium vivax*, causes a few cases of malaria annually in the United States. Malarial parasites are transmitted by female *Anopheles* mosquitoes, which become infected when they take a blood meal from a person with malaria. Another sporozoan, *Cryptosporidium*

TABLE 5-3

Characteristics of Major Protozoa

CATEGORY	MEANS OF MOVEMENT	METHOD OF ASEXUAL REPRODUCTION	METHOD OF SEXUAL REPRODUCTION	REPRESENTATIVES
Ciliates	Cilia	Transverse fission	Conjugation	*Balantidium coli, Paramecium, Stentor, Tetrahymena, Vorticella*
Amebae (amebas)	Pseudopodia (false feet)	Binary fission	When present, involves flagellated sex cells	*Amoeba, Naegleria, Entamoeba histolytica*
Flagellates	Flagella	Binary fission	None	*Chlamydomonas, Giardia lamblia, Trichomonas, Trypanosoma*
Sporozoa	Generally nonmotile except for certain sex cells	Multiple fission	Involves flagellated sex cells	*Plasmodium, Toxoplasma gondii, Cryptosporidium*

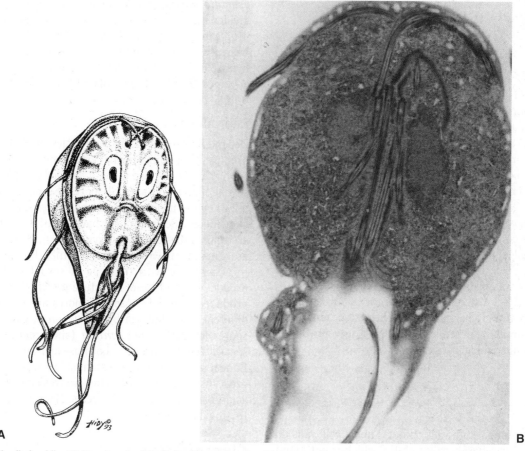

FIGURE 5-3. *Giardia lamblia*. (*A*) Drawing of a *Giardia lamblia* trophozoite. (*B*) Transmission electron micrograph (TEM) showing a longitudinal section of a *Giardia lamblia* trophozoite. (TEM by S. Koester and P. Engelkirk.)

parvum, causes severe diarrheal disease (cryptosporidiosis) in immunosuppressed patients, especially those with acquired immunodeficiency syndrome (AIDS). A 1993 epidemic in Milwaukee, Wisconsin, caused by *Cryptosporidium* oocysts in drinking water, resulted in more than 400,000 cases of cryptosporidiosis, including some fatal cases. Other pathogenic sporozoans include *Babesia* spp. (the cause of babesiosis), *Cyclospora cayetanensis* (the cause of a diarrheal disease called cyclosporiasis), and *Toxoplasma gondii* (the cause of toxoplasmosis). Pathogenic protozoa are described in Chapter 18.

Fungi

Characteristics

In the Five-Kingdom System of Classification, fungi (sing., fungus) are in a kingdom all by themselves—the Kingdom Fungi. The study of fungi is called mycology, and a person who studies fungi is called a mycologist.

Fungi are found almost everywhere on earth; some (the saprophytic fungi) living on organic matter in water and soil, and others (the parasitic fungi) living on and within animals and plants. Some are harmful, whereas others are beneficial. Fungi also live on many unlikely materials, causing deterioration of leather and plastics and spoilage of jams, pickles, and many other foods. Beneficial fungi are important in the production of cheeses, beer, wine, and other foods, as well as certain drugs (e.g., the immunosuppressant drug cyclosporine) and antibiotics (e.g., penicillin).

Fungi are a diverse group of eucaryotic organisms that include yeasts, molds, and mushrooms. As saprophytes, their main source of food is dead and decaying organic matter. Fungi are the "garbage disposers" of nature—the "vultures" of the microbial world. By secreting digestive enzymes into dead plant and animal matter, they decompose this material into absorbable nutrients for themselves and other living organisms; thus, they are the original "recyclers." Imagine living in a world without saprophytes, stumbling through endless piles of dead plants and animals and animal waste products. Not a pleasant thought!

Fungi are sometimes incorrectly referred to as plants. They are not plants. One way that fungi differ from plants and algae is that they are not photosynthetic; they have no chlorophyll or other photosynthetic pigments. The cell walls of algal and plant cells contain cellulose (a polysac-

Decomposer Versus Saprophyte

The term **decomposer** relates to what an organism "does for a living," so to speak—decomposers break materials down. The term **saprophyte** (or saprobe) relates to how an organism obtains nutrients; saprophytes absorb nutrients from dead and decaying organic matter. Sometimes the terms decomposer and saprophyte are used to describe the same organism. For example, all saprophytes are decomposers—they decompose organic materials, such as corpses, dead plants, and feces. However, not all decomposers are saprophytes. Some decomposers decompose materials such as minerals, rocks, inorganic industrial wastes, rubber, plastic, and textiles. Also note the difference between a saprophyte and a parasite. A parasite obtains nutrients from living organisms, whereas a saprophyte obtains nutrients from dead ones.

charide), but fungal cell walls do not. Fungal cell walls do contain a polysaccharide called chitin, which is not found in the cell walls of any other microorganisms. Chitin is also found in the exoskeletons of arthropods. Although many fungi are unicellular (e.g., yeasts), others grow as filaments called *hyphae* (**sing., *hypha***), which intertwine to form a mass called a *mycelium* (**pl., *mycelia***) or thallus; thus, they are quite different from bacteria, which are always unicellular. Also remember that bacteria are procaryotic, whereas fungi are eucaryotic. Some fungi have *septate hyphae* (meaning that the cytoplasm within the hypha is divided into cells by cross-walls or septa), whereas others have

aseptate hyphae (the cytoplasm within the hypha is not divided into cells; no septa). Aseptate hyphae contain mult-inucleated cytoplasm (described as being coenocytic). Learning whether the fungus possesses septate or aseptate hyphae is an important "clue" when attempting to identify a fungus that has been isolated from a clinical specimen (Fig. 5-4).

Reproduction

Depending on the particular species, fungal cells can reproduce by budding, hyphal extension, or the formation of spores. There are two general categories of fungal spores: sexual spores and asexual spores. Sexual spores are produced by the fusion of two gametes (thus, by the fusion of two nuclei). Sexual spores have a variety of names (e.g., ascospores, basidiospores, zygospores), depending on the exact manner in which they are formed. Fungi are classified in accordance with the type of sexual spore that they produce or the type of structure on which the spores are produced (Fig. 5-5). Asexual spores are formed in many different ways, but not by the fusion of gametes. Asexual spores are also called **conidia (sing., conidium)**. Some species of fungi produce both asexual and sexual spores. Fungal spores are very resistant structures that are carried great distances by wind. They are resistant to heat, cold, acids, bases, and other chemicals. Many people are allergic to fungal spores.

Classification

The classification of fungi changes periodically. Currently, the Kingdom Fungi is divided into five phyla. Classification of fungi into these phyla is based primarily on their mode of sexual reproduction. The two phyla known as "lower fungi" are the Zygomycotina (or Zygomycetes) and the Chytridiomycotina (or Chytridiomycetes). Zygomycotina include the common bread molds and other fungi that cause food spoilage. Chytridiomycotina, which are not considered to be true fungi by some taxonomists, live in water ("water

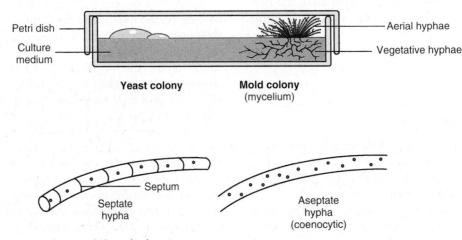

FIGURE 5-4. Fungal colonies and terms relating to hyphae.

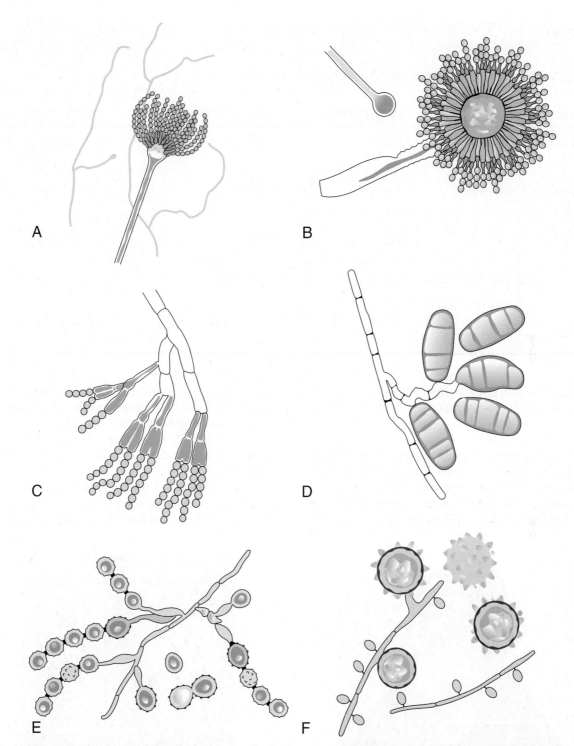

FIGURE 5-5. Microscopic appearance of various fungi. (*A*) *Aspergillus fumigatus.* (*B*) *Aspergillus flavus.* (*C*) *Penicillium* sp. (*D*) *Curvularia* sp. (*E*) *Scopulariopsis* sp. (*F*) *Histoplasma capsulatum.* (Koneman's Color Atlas and Textbook of Diagnostic Microbiology, 6th ed. Philadelphia: Lippincott Williams & Wilkins, 2006.)

molds") and soil. The two phyla known as "higher fungi" are the Ascomycotina (or Ascomycetes) and the Basidiomycotina (or Basidiomycetes). Ascomycotina include certain yeasts and some fungi that cause plant diseases (e.g., Dutch Elm disease). Basidiomycotina include some yeasts, some fungi that cause plant diseases, and the large "fleshy fungi"

that live in the woods (e.g., mushrooms, toadstools, bracket fungi, puffballs). The fifth phylum—Deuteromycotina (or Deuteromycetes)—contains fungi having no mode of sexual reproduction, or in which the mode of sexual reproduction is not known. This phylum is sometimes referred to as Fungi Imperfecti. Deuteromycetes include certain medically

TABLE 5-4

Selected Characteristics of the Phyla of Fungi

PHYLUM	TYPE OF HYPHAE	TYPE OF SEXUAL SPORE	TYPE OF ASEXUAL SPORE
Zygomycotina (Zygomycetes)	Aseptate	Zygospore	Nonmotile sporangiospores
Chytridiomycotina (Chytridiomycetes)	Aseptate	Oospore	Motile zoospores
Ascomycotina (Ascomycetes)	Septate	Ascospore	Conidiospores
Basidiomycotina (Basidiomycetes)	Septate	Basidiospore	Rare
Deuteromycotina (Deuteromycetes)	Septate	None observed	Conidiospores

important molds such as *Aspergillus* and *Penicillium*. Characteristics of each of these phyla are shown in Table 5-4.

Yeasts

Yeasts are microscopic, eucaryotic, single-celled (unicellular) organisms that lack mycelia. Individual yeast cells, sometimes referred to as blastospores or blastoconidia, can only be observed using a microscope. They usually reproduce by budding (Fig. 5-6), but occasionally do so by a type of spore formation. Sometimes a string of elongated buds is formed; this string of elongated buds is called a ***pseudohypha*** (pl., ***pseudohyphae***). It resembles a hypha, but it is *not* a hypha (Fig. 5-7). Some yeasts produce thick-walled, sporelike structures called chlamydospores (or chlamydoconidia; Fig. 5-7).

Yeasts are found in soil and water and on the skins of many fruits and vegetables. Wine, beer, and alcoholic beverages had been produced for centuries before Louis

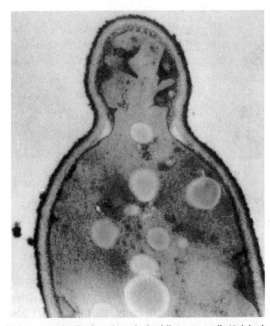

FIGURE 5-6. Longitudinal section of a budding yeast cell. (Original magnification, 15,500×.) (Lechavalier HA, Pramer D. The Microbes. Philadelphia: JB Lippincott, 1970.)

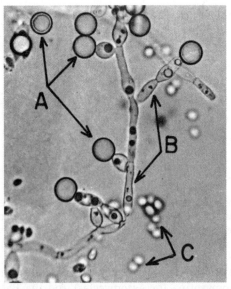

FIGURE 5-7. Microscopic examination of a culture of *Candida albicans* showing (*A*) chlamydospores, (*B*) pseudohyphae (elongated yeast cells, linked end to end), and (*C*) budding yeast cells (blastospores). (Original magnification, 450×.) (Davis BD, et al. Microbiology, 4th ed. Philadelphia: Harper & Row, 1987.)

Pasteur discovered that naturally occurring yeasts on the skin of grapes and other fruits and grains were responsible for these fermentation processes. The common yeast *Saccharomyces cerevisiae* ("baker's yeast") ferments sugar to alcohol under anaerobic conditions. Under aerobic conditions, this yeast breaks down simple sugars to carbon dioxide and water; for this reason, it has long been used to leaven light bread. Yeasts are also a good source of nutrients for humans because they produce many vitamins and proteins. Some yeasts (e.g., *Candida albicans* and *Cryptococcus neoformans*) are human pathogens. *Candida albicans* is the yeast most frequently isolated from human clinical specimens, and is also the fungus most frequently isolated from human clinical specimens.

In the laboratory, yeasts produce colonies that are quite similar in appearance to bacterial colonies (Figs. 5-4 and 5-8). To distinguish between a yeast colony and a bacterial colony, a wet mount can be performed. A small portion of the colony is mixed with a drop of water or saline on a microscope slide, a coverslip is added, and the preparation is examined under the microscope. Yeasts are usually larger than bacteria (ranging from 3 to 8 μm in diameter) and are usually oval-shaped; some may be observed in the process of budding. Bacteria do not produce buds.

Molds

Molds (also spelled moulds) are the fungi often seen in water and soil and on food. They grow in the form of cytoplasmic filaments or hyphae that make up the mycelium of the mold. Some of the hyphae (called **aerial hyphae**) extend above the surface of whatever the mold is growing on, and some (called **vegetative hyphae**) are beneath the surface (Fig. 5-4). Reproduction is by spore formation, either sexually or asexually, on the aerial hyphae; for this reason, aerial hyphae are sometimes referred to as reproductive hyphae. Various species of molds are found in each of the classes of fungi except Basidiomycotina. An interesting mold in class Chytridiomycotina is *Phytophthora infestans,* the potato blight mold that caused a famine in Ireland in the mid-19th century (see the following Historical Note).

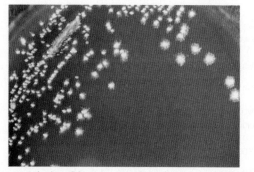

FIGURE 5-8. Colonies of the yeast, *Candida albicans,* on a blood agar plate. The footlike extensions from the margins of the colonies are typical of this species. (Koneman's Color Atlas and Textbook of Diagnostic Microbiology, 6th ed. Philadelphia: Lippincott Williams & Wilkins, 2006.)

HISTORICAL NOTE

The Great Potato Famine

Although St. Patrick may have driven the snakes out of Ireland, it was a mold named *Phytophthora infestans* that drove away many of the Irish people. The mold killed off Ireland's potato crops in 1845, 1846, and 1848, causing more than 1 million people to die of starvation and illnesses resulting from malnutrition. When their crops failed, many people could not pay their rent; about 800,000 were forced out of their homes. Nearly 2 million Irish abandoned their homeland to start new lives in America and other countries; many died aboard ship while en route. Ireland lost about one third of its population between 1847 and 1860. Some blamed the "little people" for the potato disease; others blamed the Devil. It was not until 1861 that Antoine De Bary proved that it was a fungus that had caused the blight. Late blight of potato was the first disease known with certainty to be caused by a microorganism.

Molds have great commercial importance. For example, within the Ascomycotina and the Basidiomycotina classes are found many antibiotic-producing molds, such as *Penicillium* and *Cephalosporium*. Penicillin, the first antibiotic to be discovered by a scientist, was actually discovered by accident (discussed in Chapter 9). Many additional antibiotics were later developed by culturing soil samples in laboratories and isolating any molds that inhibited growth of bacteria. Today, to increase their spectrum of activity, antibiotics can be chemically altered in pharmaceutical company laboratories, as has been done with the various semi-synthetic penicillins (e.g., ampicillin, amoxicillin, and carbenicillin).

Some molds are also used to produce large quantities of enzymes (such as amylase, which converts starch to glucose), citric acid, and other organic acids that are used commercially. The flavor of cheeses such as bleu cheese, Roquefort, camembert, and limburger are the result of molds that grow in them.

Fleshy Fungi

The large fungi that are encountered in forests, such as mushrooms, toadstools, puffballs, and bracket fungi, are collectively referred to as fleshy fungi. Obviously, they are not microorganisms. Mushrooms are a class of true fungi that consist of a network of filaments or strands (the mycelium) that grow in the soil or in a rotting log, and a fruiting body (the mushroom that rises above the ground) that forms and releases spores. Each spore, much like the seed of a plant, germinates into a new organism. Many mushrooms are delicious to eat, but others, including some that resemble edible fungi, are extremely toxic and may cause permanent liver and brain damage or death if ingested.

Medical Significance

A variety of fungi (including yeasts, molds, and some fleshy fungi) are of medical, veterinary, and agricultural importance because of the diseases they cause in humans, animals, and plants. Many diseases of crop plants, grains, corn, and potatoes, are caused by molds. Some of these plant diseases are referred to as blights and rusts. Not only do these fungi destroy crops, but some produce toxins (**mycotoxins**) that cause disease in humans and animals (discussed in CD-ROM Appendix 1: "Microbial Intoxications"). Molds and yeasts also cause a variety of infectious diseases of humans and animals—collectively referred to as *mycoses* (discussed below and in Chapter 17). Considering the large number of fungal species, very few are pathogenic for humans.

Fungal Infections of Humans

Fungal infections are known as **mycoses (sing., *mycosis*)**, and are categorized as superficial, cutaneous, subcutaneous, or systemic mycoses. In some cases the infection may progress through all these stages. Representative mycoses are listed in Table 5-5.

Superficial and Cutaneous Mycoses. Superficial mycoses are fungal infections of the outermost areas of the human body: hair, fingernails, toenails, and the dead, outermost layers of the skin (the epidermis). Cutaneous mycoses are fungal infections of the living layers of skin (the dermis). A group of molds, collectively referred to as dermatophytes, cause tinea infections, which are often referred to as "ringworm" infections. (Please note that "ringworm" infections have absolutely nothing to do with worms.) Tinea infections are named in accordance with the part of the anatomy that is infected; examples include tinea pedis (athlete's foot), tinea unguium (fingernails and toenails), tinea capitis (scalp), tinea barbae (face and neck), tinea corporis (trunk of the body), and tinea cruris (groin area).

Candida albicans is an opportunistic yeast that lives harmlessly on the skin and mucous membranes of the mouth, gastrointestinal tract, and genitourinary tract. However, when conditions cause a reduction in the number of indigenous bacteria at these anatomic locations, *Candida albicans* flourishes, leading to yeast infections of the mouth (thrush), skin, and vagina (yeast vaginitis). This type of local infection may become a focal site from which the organisms invade the bloodstream to become a generalized or systemic infection in many internal areas of the body.

Subcutaneous and Systemic Mycoses. Subcutaneous and systemic mycoses are the more severe types of mycoses. Subcutaneous mycoses are fungal infections of the dermis

---

TABLE 5-5

Selected Fungal Diseases of Humans

CATEGORY	GENUS/SPECIES	DISEASES
Yeasts	*Candida albicans*	Thrush; yeast vaginitis; nail infections; systemic infection
	Cryptococcus neoformans	Cryptococcosis (lung infection; meningitis, etc.)
Molds	*Aspergillus* spp.	Aspergillosis (lung infection; systemic infection)
	Mucor and *Rhizopus* spp. and other species of bread molds	Mucormycosis or zygomycosis (lung infection; systemic infection)
	Various dermatophytes	Tinea ("ringworm") infections
Dimorphic fungi	*Blastomyces dermatitidis*	Blastomycosis (primarily a disease of lungs and skin)
	Coccidioides immitis	Coccidioidomycosis (lung infection; systemic infection)
	Histoplasma capsulatum	Histoplasmosis (lung infection; systemic infection)
	Sporothrix schenckii	Sporotrichosis (a skin disease)
Other	*Pneumocystis jiroveci*	*Pneumocystis* pneumonia (PCP)

and underlying tissues. These conditions can be quite grotesque in appearance. An example is Madura foot (a type of eucaryotic mycetoma), in which the patient's foot becomes covered with large, unsightly, fungus-containing bumps.

Systemic or generalized mycoses are fungal infections of internal organs of the body, sometimes affecting two or more different organ systems simultaneously (e.g., simultaneous infection of the respiratory system and the bloodstream, or simultaneous infection of the respiratory tract and the central nervous system).

Spores of some pathogenic fungi may be inhaled with dust from contaminated soil or dried bird and bat feces (guano), or they may enter through wounds of the hands and feet. If the spores are inhaled into the lungs, they may germinate there to cause a respiratory infection similar to tuberculosis. Examples of deep-seated pulmonary infections are blastomycosis, coccidioidomycosis, cryptococcosis, and histoplasmosis. In each case, the pathogens may invade further to cause widespread systemic infections, especially in immunosuppressed individuals [see Insight: Microbes in the News: "Sick Building Syndrome" (Black Mold in Buildings) on the CD-ROM].

Did you know that common bread molds can cause human disease—even death? Inhalation of spores of bread molds like *Rhizopus* and *Mucor* spp. by an immunosuppressed patient can lead to a respiratory disease called zygomycosis or mucormycosis. The mold can then become disseminated throughout the patient's body and can lead to death. *Rhizopus, Mucor,* and other bread molds are primitive molds with aseptate hyphae. As previously mentioned, the cytoplasm of aseptate hyphae is not divided into individual cells by cross-walls (septa).

To diagnose mycoses, clinical specimens are submitted to the Mycology Section of the Clinical Microbiology Laboratory (discussed in Chapter 13). When isolated from clinical specimens, yeasts are identified by inoculating them into a series of biochemical tests. In this way, the laboratory technologist can determine which substrates (usually carbohydrates) the yeast is able to use as nutrients; this depends on what enzymes the yeast possesses. Minisystems (miniaturized biochemical test systems) are commercially available for the identification of clinically important yeasts.

Biochemical tests are rarely used, however, for identification of molds isolated from clinical specimens. Rather, molds are identified by a combination of macroscopic and microscopic observations. Macroscopic observations include the color, texture, and topography of the mold colony (mycelium). Microscopic examination of the mold reveals the types of structures on which or within which spores are produced; the method of spore production varies from one species of mold to another. Immunodiagnostic procedures, including skin tests, are also available for diagnosing certain types of mycoses.

Mycoses are most effectively treated with antifungal agents like nystatin, amphotericin B, or 5-fluorocytosine (discussed in Chapter 9). Because these chemotherapeutic agents may be toxic to humans, they are prescribed with due consideration and caution.

Dimorphic Fungi. A few fungi, including some human pathogens, can live either as yeasts or as molds, depending on growth conditions. This phenomenon is called **dimorphism,** and the organisms are referred to as *dimorphic fungi* (Fig. 5-9). When grown in vitro at body temperature (37°C), dimorphic fungi exist as unicellular yeasts and produce yeast colonies. Within the human body (in vivo), dimorphic fungi exist as yeasts. However, when grown in vitro at room temperature (25°C), dimorphic fungi exist as molds, producing mold colonies (mycelia). Dimorphic fungi that cause human diseases include *Histoplasma capsulatum* (which causes histoplasmosis), *Sporothrix schenckii* (which causes sporotrichosis), *Coccidioides immitis* (which causes coccidioidomycosis), and *Blastomyces dermatitidis* (which causes blastomycosis).

Lichens

Nearly everyone has seen lichens, usually while hiking in the woods. They appear as colored, often circular patches on tree trunks and rocks. A *lichen* is actually a combination of two organisms—an alga (or a cyanobacterium) and a fungus—living together in such a close relationship that they appear to be one organism. Close relationships of this type are referred to as symbiotic relationships. A lichen represents a particular type of symbiotic relationship known as mutualism—a relationship in which both parties benefit (discussed further in Chapter 10). There are about 20,000 different species of lichens. Lichens may be brown, black, orange, various shades of green, and other colors, depending on the specific combination of alga and fungus. Lichens are classified as protists.

Slime Molds

Slime molds, which are found in soil and on rotting logs, have both fungal and protozoal characteristics and very interesting life cycles. Some slime molds (known as cellular slime molds) start out in life as independent amebae, ingesting bacteria and fungi by phagocytosis. When they run out of food, they fuse together to form a motile, multicellular form known as a slug, which is only about 0.5 mm long. The slug then becomes a fruiting body, consisting of a stalk and a spore cap. Spores produced within the spore cap become disseminated, and from each spore emerges an ameba. Cellular slime molds represent cell differentiation at the lowest level, and scientists are studying them in an attempt to determine how some of the cells in the slug know that they are to become part of the stalk, how others know that they are to become part of the spore cap, and still

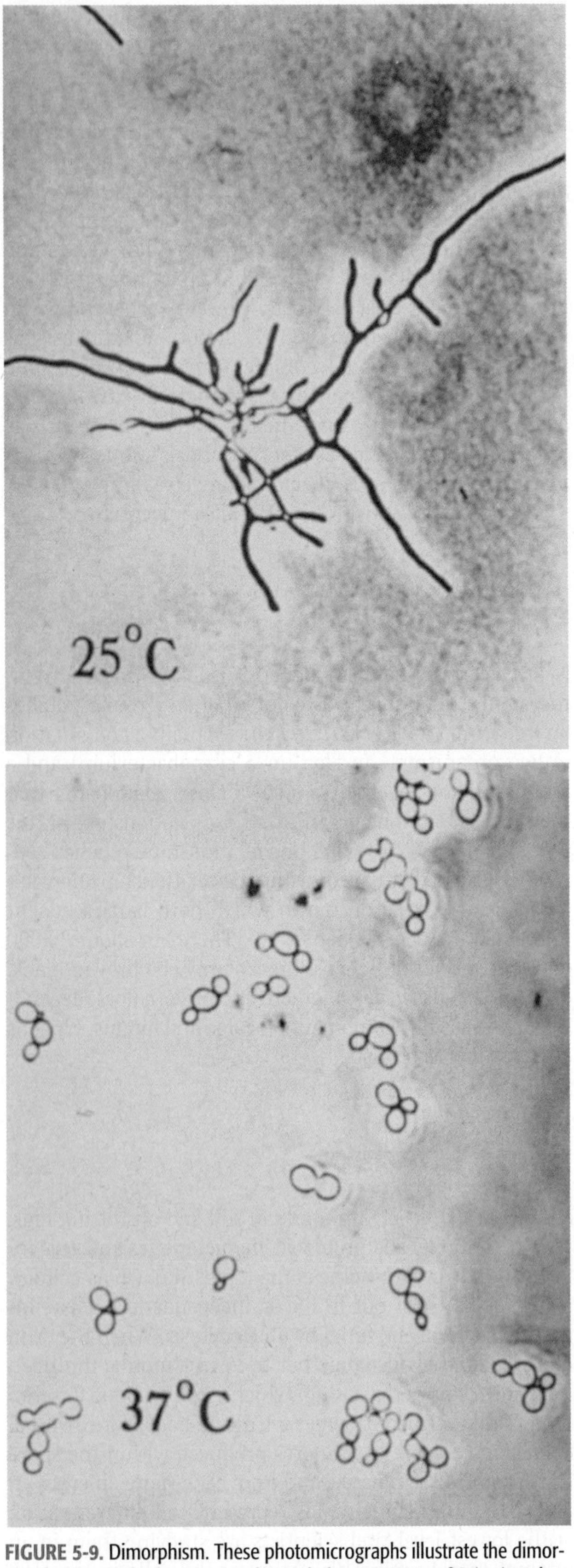

FIGURE 5-9. Dimorphism. These photomicrographs illustrate the dimorphic fungus, *Histoplasma capsulatum,* being grown at 25°C (*top*) and at 37°C (*bottom*). (Schaeter M, et al., eds. Mechanisms of Microbial Disease, 3rd ed. Philadelphia: Lippincott Williams & Wilkins, 1999.)

others know that they are to differentiate into spores within the spore cap. Other slime molds, known as plasmodial (or acellular) slime molds, also produce stalks and spores, but their life cycles differ somewhat from those of cellular slime molds. In the life cycle of a plasmodial slime mold, haploid cells fuse to become diploid cells, which develop into very large masses of motile, multinucleated protoplasm, each such mass being known as a plasmodium. Slime molds are classified as protists.

REVIEW OF KEY POINTS

- Algae are eucaryotic, photosynthetic organisms that range in size from tiny, unicellular, microscopic cells to large, multicellular, plantlike seaweeds. Algal cells are more plantlike than animal-like. In the Five-Kingdom System of Classification, algae are classified in the Kingdom Protista. Algae are an important source of food, iodine and other minerals, fertilizers, emulsifiers, stabilizers, and gelling agents. Some algae produce toxins (called phycotoxins), but infections caused by algae are extremely rare.

- Protozoa are eucaryotic, usually single-celled and nonphotosynthetic microbes, composed of cells that are more animal-like than plantlike. In the Five-Kingdom System of Classification, protozoa are classified in the Kingdom Protista. Protozoa are placed in categories based on their mode of locomotion. Amebae move by means of pseudopodia, flagellates by means of flagella, and ciliates by means of cilia. Protozoa that lacks pseudopodia, flagella, and cilia are called sporozoans. Many protozoa are free-living, but others are parasitic. Some parasitic protozoa are human parasites.

- Fungi are eucaryotic, nonphotosynthetic organisms that include mushrooms, toadstools, bracket fungi, puffballs, molds, and yeasts. Many fungi are saprophytic decomposers in nature, and many others are parasitic on animals or plants. Fungi cause a wide variety of plant diseases, including rusts and smuts. Some molds and fleshy fungi produce toxins (mycotoxins) that cause disease in humans and animals. The human infectious diseases caused by fungi (specifically, yeasts and molds) are classified as superficial, cutaneous, subcutaneous, and systemic mycoses.

- A lichen represents a symbiotic relationship between an alga (or a cyanobacterium) and a fungus. It is an example of a mutualistic relationship (mutualism), because both parties benefit from the association. Lichens are classified as protists.

- Slime molds are classified as protists. They have complex life cycles. At various stages in their life cycles, they have protozoan and fungal characteristics.

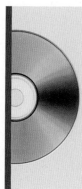

On the CD-ROM

- Insight: Microbes in the News: "Sick Building Syndrome" (Black Mold in Buildings)
- Increase Your Knowledge
- Critical Thinking
- Additional Self-Assessment Exercises

Self-Assessment Exercises

After studying this chapter, answer the following multiple-choice questions.

1. Which of the following statements about algae and fungi is (are) true?
   a. Algae are photosynthetic, whereas fungi are not.
   b. Algal cell walls contain cellulose, whereas fungal cell walls do not.
   c. Fungal cell walls contain chitin, whereas algal cell walls do not.
   d. all of the above

2. All of the following are algae except:
   a. desmids.
   b. diatoms.
   c. dinoflagellates.
   d. sporozoa.

3. All of the following are fungi except:
   a. molds.
   b. *Paramecium.*
   c. *Penicillium.*
   d. yeasts.

4. A protozoan may possess any of the following except:
   a. cilia.
   b. flagella.
   c. hyphae.
   d. pseudopodia.

5. Which one of the following terms is not associated with fungi?
   a. conidia
   b. hyphae
   c. mycelium
   d. pellicle

6. All of the following terms can be used to describe hyphae except:
   a. aerial and reproductive.
   b. septate and aseptate.
   c. sexual and asexual.
   d. vegetative.

7. A lichen usually represents a symbiotic relationship between which of the following pairs?
   a. a fungus and an ameba
   b. a yeast and an ameba
   c. an alga and a cyanobacterium
   d. an alga and a fungus

8. A stigma is a:
   a. light-sensing organelle.
   b. primitive mouth.
   c. thickened membrane.
   d. type of plastid.

9. If a dimorphic fungus is causing a respiratory infection, which of the following might be seen in a sputum specimen from that patient?
   a. amebae
   b. conidia
   c. hyphae
   d. yeasts

10. Which one of the following is not a fungus?
    a. *Aspergillus*
    b. *Candida*
    c. *Penicillium*
    d. *Prototheca*

6

BIOCHEMISTRY: THE CHEMISTRY OF LIFE

LEARNING OBJECTIVES

AFTER STUDYING THIS CHAPTER, YOU SHOULD BE ABLE TO:
- Name the four main categories of biochemical molecules discussed in this chapter
- Differentiate among trioses, tetroses, pentoses, hexoses, and heptoses
- Differentiate among monosaccharides, disaccharides, and polysaccharides and cite two examples of each
- Differentiate between a dehydration synthesis reaction and a hydrolysis reaction and cite an example of each
- Differentiate among covalent, glycosidic, and peptide bonds
- Describe the role of enzymes in metabolism
- Define the following terms: apoenzyme, cofactor, coenzyme, holoenzyme, substrate
- Cite important differences between the structures of DNA and RNA
- Differentiate between a DNA nucleotide and an RNA nucleotide
- Define what is meant by "the central dogma"
- Describe the processes of DNA replication, transcription, and translation

INTRODUCTION

Some students are surprised to learn that they must study chemistry as part of a microbiology course. The reason why chemistry is an important component of a microbiology course is the answer to the question, "What exactly is a microorganism?" A microbe can be thought of as a "bag" of chemicals that interact with each other in a variety of ways. Even the bag itself is composed of chemicals. Everything a microorganism is and does relates to chemistry. The various ways microorganisms function and survive in their environment depend on their chemical makeup. The same things are true about the cells that make up any living organisms—including human beings; these cells, too, can be thought of as bags of chemicals.

To understand microbial cells and how they function, one must have a basic knowledge of the chemistry of atoms, molecules, and compounds. CD-ROM Appendix 3: "Basic Chemistry Concepts" contains such information. Students having little or no background in chemistry should study the material in CD-ROM Appendix 3 before attempting to learn the material in this chapter. CD-ROM Appendix 3 can serve as a review for students who have already studied basic chemistry, either in a biology course or an introductory chemistry course. Your instructor will inform you as to whether the material in CD-ROM Appendix 3 is "testable."

Even the most simple procaryotic cells consist of very large molecules (macromolecules), such as deoxyribonucleic acid (DNA), ribonucleic acid (RNA), proteins, lipids, and polysaccharides, as well as many combinations of these macromolecules that combine to make up structures like capsules, cell walls, cell membranes, and flagella. These macromolecules can be broken down into smaller units or "building blocks," such as monosaccharides (simple sugars), fatty acids, amino acids, and nucleotides. Each of these molecules, in turn, may be broken down into even smaller molecules of water, carbon dioxide, ammonia, sulfides, and phosphates, which, in turn, can be broken down into atoms of carbon (C), hydrogen (H), oxygen (O), nitrogen (N), sulfur (S), phosphorus (P), etc. *Organic chemistry* is the study of compounds that contain carbon; *inorganic chemistry* involves all other chemical reactions; *biochemistry* is the chemistry of living cells. Basic inorganic chemistry is introduced in CD-ROM Appendix 3: "Basic Chemistry Concepts"; organic chemistry and biochemistry are discussed in this chapter.

Only when all these molecules and compounds are in place and working together properly can the cell function like a well-managed factory. As in industry, a cell must have the appropriate machinery, regulatory molecules (enzymes) to control its activities, fuel (nutrients or light) to provide energy, and raw materials (nutrients) for manufacturing essential end products.

Everything that a microorganism is and does involves biochemistry. Biochemicals make up the structure of a microorganism, and a multitude of biochemical reactions take place within the microorganism. What is true for microbes is also true for every other living organism. The characteristics that distinguish living organisms from inanimate objects—(1) their complex and highly organized structure; (2) their ability to extract, transform, and use energy from their environment; and (3) their capacity for precise self-replication and self-assembly—all result from the nature, function, and interaction of biomolecules. Because biochemistry is a branch of organic chemistry, a brief introduction to organic chemistry will be presented first.

Organic Chemistry

Organic compounds are compounds that contain carbon, and *organic chemistry* is that branch of the science of chemistry that specializes in the study of organic compounds. The term "organic" is somewhat misleading, as it implies that all these compounds are produced by or are in some way related to living organisms. This is not true! Although some organic compounds are associated with living organisms, many are not. A typical *Escherichia coli* cell contains more than 6,000 different kinds of organic compounds, including about 3,000 different proteins and approximately the same number of different molecules of nucleic acid. Proteins make up about 15% of the total weight of an *E. coli* cell, whereas nucleic acids, polysaccharides, and lipids make up about 7%, 3%, and 2%, respectively.

Organic chemistry is a broad and important branch of chemistry, involving the chemistry of fossil fuels (petroleum and coal), dyes, drugs, paper, ink, paints, plastics, gasoline, rubber tires, food, and clothing. The number of compounds that contain carbon far exceeds the number of compounds that do not contain carbon. Some carbon-containing compounds are very large and complex, some containing thousands of atoms.

Carbon Bonds

In our current understanding of life, carbon is the primary requisite for all living systems. The element carbon exists in three forms: diamond, graphite, and carbon or carbon black. These three forms have dramatically different physical properties, and it is difficult to believe that they are truly the same element. Carbon atoms have a valence of four, meaning that a carbon atom can bond to four other atoms. For convenience, the carbon atom is illustrated in this text with the symbol C and four bonds.

$$-\overset{|}{\underset{|}{C}}-$$

The uniqueness of carbon lies in the ability of its atoms to bond to each other to form a multitude of compounds. The variety of carbon compounds increases still more when atoms of other elements also attach in different ways to the carbon atom.

There are three ways in which carbon atoms can bond to each other: *single bond, double bond,* and *triple bond.* In the following illustrations, each line between the carbon atoms represents a pair of shared electrons (known as a *covalent bond*). In a carbon–carbon single bond, the two carbon atoms share one pair of electrons; in a carbon–carbon double bond, two pairs of electrons; and in a carbon–carbon triple bond, three pairs of electrons. Covalent bonds are typical of the compounds of carbon and are the bonds of primary importance in organic chemistry. Organic chemistry is sometimes defined as the chemistry of carbon and its covalent bonds.

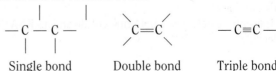

Single bond   Double bond   Triple bond

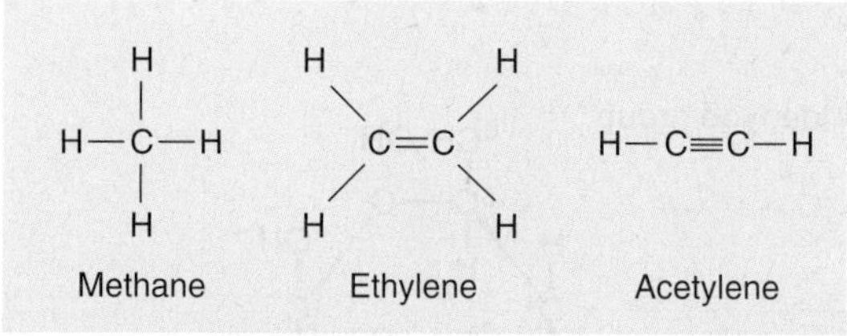

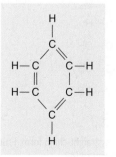

FIGURE 6-1. Simple hydrocarbons.

When atoms of other elements attach to available bonds of carbon atoms, compounds are formed. For example, if only hydrogen atoms are bonded to the available bonds, compounds called hydrocarbons are formed. In other words, a **hydrocarbon** is an organic molecule that contains only carbon and hydrogen atoms. Just a few of the many hydrocarbon compounds are shown in Figure 6-1.

When more than two carbons are linked together, longer molecules are formed. A series of many carbon atoms bonded together is referred to as a *chain*. Long-chain carbon compounds are usually liquids or solids, whereas short-chain carbon compounds, such as the hydrocarbons shown in Figure 6-1, are gases.

Cyclic Compounds

Carbon atoms may link to carbon atoms to close the chain, forming *rings* or cyclic compounds. An example is benzene, which has six carbons and six hydrogens, as shown in Figure 6-2. Although benzene contains six carbon atoms, other ring structures contain fewer or more carbon atoms, and some compounds contain fused rings (e.g., double- or triple-ringed compounds).

Biochemistry

Biochemistry is the study of biology at the molecular level and can, thus, be thought of as the chemistry of life or the chemistry of living organisms. Not only is biochemistry a branch of biology, but it is also a branch of organic chemistry. Biochemistry involves the study of the biomolecules that are present within living organisms. These biomolecules are usually large molecules (called macromolecules)

FIGURE 6-2. The benzene ring.

and include carbohydrates, lipids, proteins, and nucleic acids. Other examples of biomolecules are vitamins, enzymes, hormones, and energy-carrying molecules, such as adenosine triphosphate (ATP).

Humans obtain their nutrients from the foods they eat. The carbohydrates, fats, nucleic acids, and proteins contained in these foods are digested, and their components are absorbed into the blood and carried to every cell in the body. Within cells, these components are then broken down and rearranged. In this way, the compounds necessary for cell structure and function are synthesized. Microorganisms also absorb their essential nutrients into the cell by various means, to be described in Chapter 7. These nutrients are then used in metabolic reactions as sources of energy and as "building blocks" for enzymes, structural macromolecules, and genetic materials.

Carbohydrates

Carbohydrates are biomolecules composed of carbon, hydrogen, and oxygen, in the ratio of 1:2:1, or simply CH_2O. Glucose, fructose, sucrose, lactose, maltose, starch, cellulose, and glycogen are all examples of carbohydrates.

Monosaccharides

The simplest carbohydrates are sugars, and the smallest sugars (or simple sugars) are called **monosaccharides** (Greek *mono* meaning "one"; *sakcharon* meaning "sugar"). The "one" refers to the number of rings; in other words, monosaccharides are sugars composed of only one ring. The most important monosaccharide in nature is **glucose** ($C_6H_{12}O_6$), which may occur as a chain or in alpha or beta ring configurations, as shown in Figure 6-3. Monosaccharides may contain from three to nine carbon atoms (Table 6-1), although most of them contain five or six. A three-carbon monosaccharide is called a **triose**; one containing four carbons is called a **tetrose;** five, a **pentose;** six, a **hexose;** seven, a **heptose;** eight, an *octose;* and nine, a *nonose*. Ribose and deoxyribose are pentoses that are found in RNA and DNA, respectively. Glucose (also called dextrose) is a hexose. Octoses and nonoses are quite rare.

The main source of energy for body cells, glucose, is found in most sweet fruits and in blood. The glucose carried in the blood to the cells is oxidized to produce the energy-carrying molecule ATP, with its high-energy phosphate bonds. ATP molecules are the main source of the energy that is used to drive most metabolic reactions. Other monosaccharides are galactose and fructose, both of which are hexoses. Fructose (Fig. 6-4), the sweetest of the monosaccharides, is found in fruits and honey.

Disaccharides

Disaccharides (*di* meaning "two") are double-ringed sugars that result from the combination of two monosaccharides. The synthesis of a disaccharide from two monosaccharides by removal of a water molecule is called a

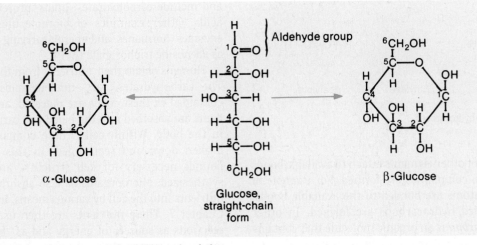

FIGURE 6-3. Glucose. All three forms may exist in equilibrium in solution.

dehydration synthesis reaction (Fig. 6-5). The bond holding the two monosaccharides together is called a *glycosidic bond;* it is a type of covalent bond. Glucose is the major constituent of disaccharides. Sucrose (table sugar) is a sweet disaccharide made by joining together a glucose molecule and a fructose molecule. Sucrose comes from sugar cane, sugar beets, and maple sugar. Lactose (milk sugar) and maltose (malt sugar) are also disaccharides. Lactose is made by joining together a molecule of glucose and a molecule of galactose. People who lack the digestive enzyme lactase, needed to split lactose into its monosaccharide components, are said to be lactose intolerant. Maltose is made by combining two molecules of glucose.

Disaccharides react with water in a process called a *hydrolysis reaction,* which causes them to break down into two monosaccharides:

disaccharide + H_2O → two monosaccharides
sucrose + H_2O → glucose + fructose
lactose + H_2O → glucose + galactose
maltose + H_2O → glucose + glucose

Peptidoglycan (mentioned in Chapter 3) is a complex macromolecular network found in the cell walls of all members of the Domain *Bacteria.* Peptidoglycan consists of a repeating disaccharide, attached by polypeptides (proteins) to form a lattice that surrounds and protects the entire bacterial cell. A number of antibiotics (including penicillin) prevent the final cross-linking of the rows of disaccharides, thus weakening the cell wall and leading to

TABLE 6-1

Monosaccharides

NUMBER OF CARBON ATOMS	GENERAL NAME	EXAMPLES
3	Triose	Glyceraldehyde (glycerose), dihydroxyacetone
4	Tetrose	Erythrose
5	Pentose	Ribose, deoxyribose, arabinose, xylose, ribulose
6	Hexose	Glucose, fructose, galactose, mannose
7	Heptose	Sedoheptulose, mannoheptulose
8	Octose	Octoses have been synthetically prepared; they do not occur in nature
9	Nonose	Neuraminic acid

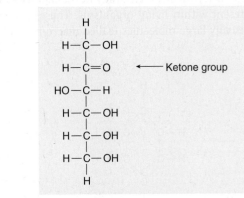

FIGURE 6-4. Fructose in straight-chain form. Fructose may also exist in the ring form shown in Figure 6-5.

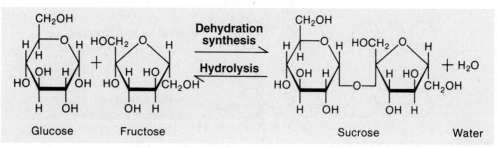

FIGURE 6-5. The dehydration synthesis and hydrolysis of sucrose.

lysis (bursting) of the bacterial cell. Although most members of the Domain *Archaea* have cell walls, their cell walls do not contain peptidoglycan.

Carbohydrates composed of three monosaccharides are called trisaccharides; those composed of four are called tetrasaccharides; those composed of five are called pentasaccharides; and so on, until one comes to polysaccharides.

Polysaccharides

The definition of a **polysaccharide** varies from one reference book to another, with some stating that a polysaccharide consists of more than six monosaccharides, others stating more than eight, and others stating more than ten. Poly means "many," and in reality, most polysaccharides contain many monosaccharides—up to hundreds or even thousands of monosaccharides. Thus, in this book, polysaccharides are defined as carbohydrate polymers containing many monosaccharides. Examples include starch and glycogen, which are composed of hundreds of repetitive glucose units held together by different types of covalent bonds, known as glycosidic bonds (or glycosidic linkages). Glucose is the major constituent of polysaccharides. Polysaccharides are examples of **polymers**—molecules consisting of many similar subunits. Some of these molecules are so large that they are insoluble in water. In the presence of the proper enzymes or acids, polysaccharides may be hydrolyzed or broken down into disaccharides, and then finally into monosaccharides (Fig. 6-6).

Polysaccharides serve two main functions. One is to store energy that can be used when the external food supply is low. The common storage molecule in animals is **glycogen,** which is found in the liver and in muscles. In plants, glucose is stored as **starch** and is found in potatoes and other vegetables and seeds. Some algae store starch, whereas bacteria contain glycogen granules as a reserve nutrient supply. The other function of polysaccharides is to provide a "tough" molecule for structural support and protection. Many bacteria produce polysaccharide capsules, which protect the bacteria from being phagocytized (eaten) by white blood cells.

Cellulose is another example of a polysaccharide. Plant and algal cells have cellulose cell walls to provide support and shape as well as protection against the environment. Cellulose is insoluble in water and indigestible for humans and most animals. Some protozoa, fungi, and bacteria have enzymes that will break the β-glycosidic bonds linking the glucose units in cellulose. Some of these microorganisms (saprophytes) are able to disintegrate dead plants in the soil, and others (parasites) live in the digestive organs of herbivores (plant eaters). Protozoa in the gut of termites digest the cellulose in the wood that the termites eat. Fibers of cellulose extracted from certain plants are used to make paper, cotton, linen, and rope. These fibers are relatively rigid, strong, and insoluble because they consist of 100 to 200 parallel strands of cellulose. Starch and glycogen are easily digested by animals because they possess the

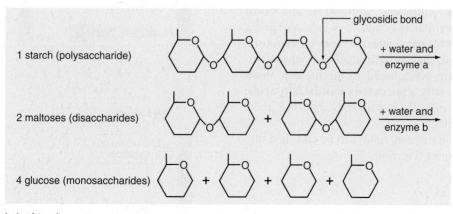

FIGURE 6-6. The hydrolysis of starch.

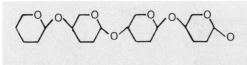

FIGURE 6-7. The difference between cellulose and starch.

digestive enzyme that hydrolyzes the α-glycosidic bonds that link the glucose units into long, helical, or branched polymers (Fig. 6-7).

When polysaccharides combine with other chemical groups (amines, lipids, and amino acids), extremely complex macromolecules are formed that serve specific purposes. Glucosamine and galactosamine (amine derivatives of glucose and galactose, respectively) are important constituents of the supporting polysaccharides in connective tissue fibers, cartilage, and chitin. Chitin is the main component of the hard outer covering of insects, spiders, and crabs, and is also found in the cell walls of fungi. The main portion of the rigid cell wall of bacteria consists of amino sugars and short polypeptide chains that combine to form the peptidoglycan layer.

Lipids

Lipids constitute an important class of biomolecules. Most lipids are insoluble in water but soluble in fat solvents, such as ether, chloroform, and benzene. Lipids are essential constituents of almost all living cells.

Fatty Acids

Fatty acids can be thought of as the building blocks of lipids. Fatty acids are long-chain carboxylic acids that are insoluble in water. **Saturated fatty acids** contain only single bonds between the carbon atoms. Fats containing saturated fatty acids are usually solids at room temperature. **Monounsaturated fatty acids** (such as those found in butter, olives, and peanuts) have one double bond in the carbon chain. **Polyunsaturated fatty acids** (such as those found in soybeans, safflowers, sunflowers, and corn) contain two or more double bonds. Most fats containing unsaturated fatty acids are liquids at room temperature. The terms saturated, monounsaturated, and polyunsaturated fatty acids are often heard in discussions about human diet. Certain fatty acids, called **essential fatty acids,** cannot be synthesized in the human body and, thus, must be provided in the diet.

For purposes of discussion, lipids can be classified into the following categories (Fig. 6-8):

- Waxes
- Fats and oils
- Phospholipids
- Glycolipids
- Steroids
- Prostaglandins and leukotrienes

Waxes

A **wax** consists of a saturated fatty acid and a long-chain alcohol. Wax coatings on the fruits, leaves, and stems of plants help to prevent loss of water and damage from pests. Waxes on the skin, fur, and feathers of animals and birds provide a waterproof coating. Lanolin, a mixture of waxes obtained from wool, is used in hand and body lotions to aid in retention of water, thus softening the skin. The waxes that are present in the cell walls of *Mycobacterium tuberculosis* (the

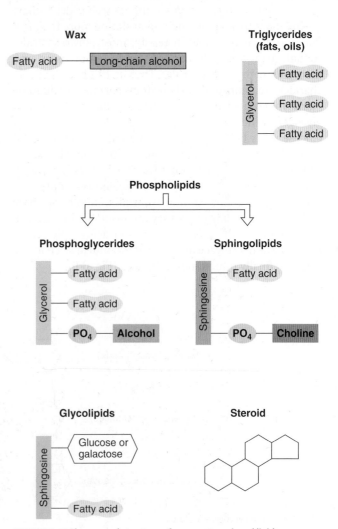

FIGURE 6-8. The general structure of some categories of lipids.

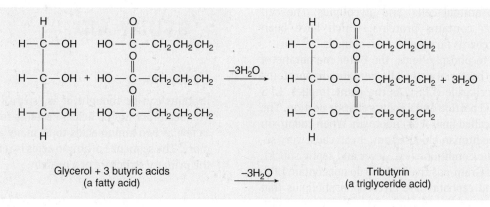

FIGURE 6-9. The synthesis of a fat.

causative agent of tuberculosis) are responsible for several interesting characteristics of this bacterium. For example, should a *M. tuberculosis* cell be phagocytized by a phagocytic white blood cell (a phagocyte), the waxes protect the cell from being digested. This enables the bacterial cell to survive and multiply within the phagocyte. Also, the waxes in the cell walls of *M. tuberculosis* make the organism difficult to stain, and, once stained, the waxes make it difficult to remove the stain from the cell. In the acid-fast staining procedure, for example, it is necessary to heat the carbolfuchsin dye to drive it into the cell; once the cell has been stained, the waxes prevent decolorization of the cell when a mixture of acid and alcohol is applied. Because the cell does not decolorize in the presence of acid, the organism is described as being acid-fast.

Fats and Oils

Fats and oils are the most common types of lipids. Fats and oils are also known as **triglycerides,** because they are composed of glycerol (a three-carbon alcohol) and three fatty acids (Fig. 6-9). Fats are triglycerides that are solid at room temperature. Most fats come from animal sources;

examples include the fats found in meat, whole milk, butter, and cheese. Most oils are triglycerides that are liquid at room temperature. The most commonly used oils come from plant sources. Olive oil and peanut oil are monounsaturated oils, whereas oils from corn, cottonseed, safflower, and sunflower are polyunsaturated.

Phospholipids

Phospholipids contain glycerol, fatty acids, a phosphate group, and an alcohol. There are two types: *glycerophospholipids* (also called *phosphoglycerides*) and *sphingolipids.* Glycerophospholipids are the most abundant lipids in cell membranes. The basic structure of a cell membrane is a lipid bilayer, consisting of two rows of phospholipids, arranged tail-to-tail (Fig. 6-10). The hydrophobic tails, lacking an affinity for water molecules, point toward each other, enabling them to get as far away from water as possible. The hydrophilic heads, being able to associate with water molecules, project to the inner and outer surfaces of the membrane. Two other types of lipids are also found in eucaryotic cell membranes: steroids (primarily

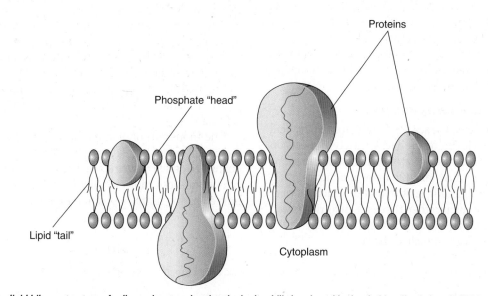

FIGURE 6-10. The lipid bilayer structure of cell membranes, showing the hydrophilic heads and hydrophobic tails of phospholipid molecules. Cell membranes also contain protein molecules, which resemble "icebergs floating in a sea of lipids."

cholesterol, in animal cells) and glycolipids. The cell membrane also contains proteins, which have been described as "icebergs floating in a sea of lipids."

In addition to phospholipids, the outer membrane of Gram-negative bacterial cell walls contains lipoproteins and lipopolysaccharide (LPS). As the name implies, LPS consists of a lipid portion and a polysaccharide portion. The lipid portion is called lipid-A or endotoxin. When endotoxin is present in the human bloodstream, it can cause very serious physiologic conditions (e.g., fever and septic shock). The cell walls of Gram-positive bacteria do not contain LPS.

Lecithins and cephalins are glycerophospholipids that are found in brain and nerve tissues as well as in egg yolks, wheat germ, and yeast.

Sphingolipids are phospholipids that contain an 18-carbon alcohol called sphingosine rather than glycerol. Sphingolipids are found in brain and nerve tissues. One of the most abundant sphingolipids is sphingomyelin, which makes up the white matter of the myelin sheath that coats nerve cells.

Glycolipids

Glycolipids are abundant in the brain and in the myelin sheaths of nerves. Some glycolipids contain glycerol plus two fatty acids and a monosaccharide. Cerebrosides and gangliosides are examples of glycolipids; both are found in the human nervous system. A person's blood group (A, B, AB, or O) is determined by the particular glycolipids that are present on the surface of that person's red blood cells.

Steroids

Steroids are rather complex, four-ringed structures. Steroids include cholesterol, bile salts, fat-soluble vitamins, and steroid hormones. Cholesterol is a component of cell membranes, myelin sheath, and brain and nerve tissue. Bile salts are synthesized in the liver from cholesterol and stored in the gallbladder. The fat-soluble vitamins are vitamins A, D, E, and K. Steroid hormones include male sex hormones (testosterone and androsterone) and female sex hormones (estrogens such as estradiol and progesterone). The adrenal corticosteroids (aldosterone and cortisone) are steroid hormones produced by the adrenal glands, one of which is located at the top of each kidney.

Prostaglandins and Leukotrienes

Prostaglandins and leukotrienes are derived from a fatty acid called arachidonic acid. Both have a wide variety of effects on body chemistry. They act as mediators of hormones, lower or raise blood pressure, cause inflammation, and induce fever. Leukotrienes are produced in leukocytes (for which they are named), but also occur in other tissues. Leukotrienes can produce long-lasting muscle contractions, especially in the lungs, where they cause asthmalike attacks.

Proteins

Proteins are among the most essential chemicals in all living cells, referred to by some scientists as "the substance

---

of life." Some proteins are the structural components of membranes, cells, and tissues, whereas others are enzymes and hormones that chemically control the metabolic balance within both the cell and the entire organism. All proteins are polymers of amino acids; however, they vary widely in the number of amino acids present and in the sequence of amino acids as well as their size, configuration, and functions. Proteins contain carbon, hydrogen, oxygen, nitrogen, and sometimes sulfur.

Amino Acid Structure

A total of 23 different *amino acids* have been found in proteins, 20 primary or naturally occurring amino acids plus 3 secondary amino acids (derived from primary amino acids). Each amino acid is composed of carbon, hydrogen, oxygen, and nitrogen; 3 of the amino acids also have sulfur atoms in the molecule. Humans can synthesize certain amino acids, but not others. Those that cannot be synthesized (called *essential amino acids*) must be ingested as part of our diets. The term *essential amino acids* is somewhat misleading, however, in view of the fact that *all* of the amino acids are necessary for protein synthesis. Because we cannot manufacture the essential amino acids, it is *essential* that they be included in our diets.

The general formula for amino acids is shown in Figure 6-11. In this figure, the "R" group represents any of the 23 groups that may be substituted into that position to build the various amino acids. For instance, "H" in place of the "R" represents the amino acid glycine, and "CH$_3$" in that position results in the structural formula for the amino acid alanine.

The thousands of different proteins in the human body are composed of a great variety of amino acids in various quantities and arrangements. The number of proteins that can be synthesized is virtually unlimited. Proteins are not limited by the number of different amino acids, just as the

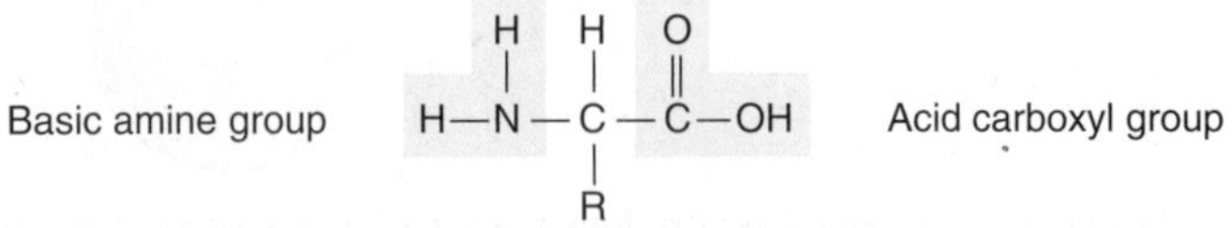

Basic amine group   H—N—C—C—OH   Acid carboxyl group

FIGURE 6-11. The basic structure of an amino acid.

Names of Amino Acids

Alanine (1°)	Glutamic acid (1°)	Isoleucine (1°, E)	Serine (1°)
Arginine (1°, E*)	Glutamine (1°)	Leucine (1°, E)	Threonine (1°, E)
Asparagine (1°)	Glycine (1°)	Lysine (1°, E)	Tryptophan (1°, E)
Aspartic acid (1°)	Histidine (1°, E*)	Methionine (1°, E)	Tyrosine (1°)
Cysteine (1°)	Hydroxylysine (2°)	Phenylalanine (1°, E)	Valine (1°, E)
Cystine (2°)	Hydroxyproline (2°)	Proline (1°)	

Key: 1°, a primary amino acid; 2°, a secondary amino acid; E, an essential amino acid; E, additional essential amino acid in infants*

number of words in a written language is not limited by the number of letters in the alphabet. The actual number of proteins produced by an organism and the amino acid sequence of those proteins are determined by the particular genes present on the organism's chromosome(s).

Protein Structure

When water is removed, by dehydration synthesis, amino acids become linked together by a covalent bond, referred to as a **peptide bond** (as shown in Fig. 6-12). A **dipeptide** is formed by bonding two amino acids, whereas the bonding of three amino acids forms a **tripeptide.** A chain (polymer) consisting of more than three amino acids is referred to as a **polypeptide.** Polypeptides are said to have *primary protein structure*—a linear sequence of amino acids in a chain (Fig. 6-13).

Most polypeptide chains naturally twist into helices or sheets as a result of the charged side chains protruding from the carbon–nitrogen backbone of the molecule. This helical or sheetlike configuration is referred to as *secondary protein structure* and is found in fibrous proteins. Fibrous proteins are long, threadlike molecules that are insoluble in water. They make up keratin (found in hair, nails, wool, horns, feathers), collagen (in tendons), myosin (in muscles), and the microtubules and microfilaments of cells.

Because a long coil can become entwined by folding back on itself, a polypeptide helix may become globular (Fig. 6-13). In some areas the helix is retained, but other areas curve randomly. This globular, *tertiary protein structure* is stabilized not only by hydrogen bonding but also by disulfide bond cross-links between two sulfur groups (S–S). This three-dimensional configuration is characteristic of enzymes, which work by fitting on and into specific molecules (see the next section). Other examples of globular proteins include many hormones (e.g., insulin), albumin in eggs, and hemoglobin and fibrinogen in blood. Globular proteins are soluble in water.

When two or more polypeptide chains are bonded together by hydrogen and disulfide bonds, the resulting structure is referred to as *quaternary protein structure* (Fig. 6-13). For instance, hemoglobin consists of four globular myoglobins. The size, shape, and configuration of a protein are specific for the function it must perform. If the amino acid sequence and, thus, the configuration of hemoglobin in red blood cells is not perfect, the red blood cells may become distorted and assume a sickle shape (as in sickle cell anemia). In this state, they are unable to carry the oxygen that is necessary for cellular metabolism. Myoglobin, the oxygen-binding protein found in skeletal muscles, was the first protein to have its primary, secondary, and tertiary structure defined by scientists.

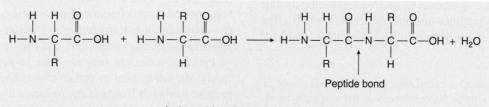

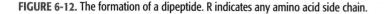

Amino acid$_1$ + Amino acid$_2$ ⟶ Dipeptide

FIGURE 6-12. The formation of a dipeptide. R indicates any amino acid side chain.

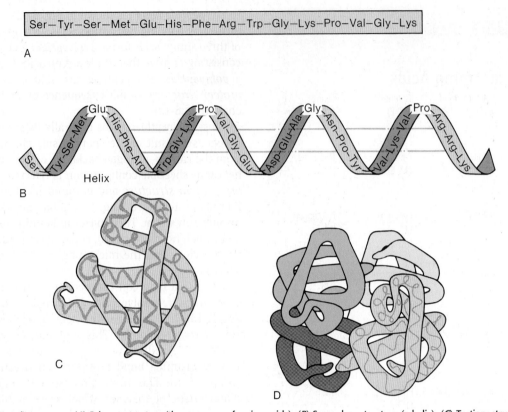

Ser—Tyr—Ser—Met—Glu—His—Phe—Arg—Trp—Gly—Lys—Pro—Val—Gly—Lys

A

Helix

B

C

D

FIGURE 6-13. Protein structure. (*A*) Primary structure (the sequence of amino acids). (*B*) Secondary structure (a helix). (*C*) Tertiary structure (globular). (*D*) Quaternary structure (four polypeptide chains).

Enzymes

Enzymes are protein molecules[a] produced by living cells as "instructed" by genes on the chromosomes. Enzymes are referred to as **biological catalysts**—biologic molecules that **catalyze** metabolic reactions. A ***catalyst*** is defined as an agent that speeds up a chemical reaction without being consumed in the process. In some cases, a particular metabolic reaction will not occur at all in the absence of an enzyme catalyst. Almost every reaction in the cell requires the presence of a specific enzyme. Although enzymes influence the direction of the reaction and increase its rate of reaction, they do not provide the energy needed to activate the reaction.

Some protein molecules function as enzymes all by themselves. Other proteins (called ***apoenzymes***) can only function as enzymes (i.e., can only catalyze a chemical reaction) after they link up with a nonprotein ***cofactor.*** Some apoenzymes require metal ions (e.g., Ca^{2+}, Fe^{2+}, Mg^{2+}, Cu^{2+}) as cofactors, whereas others require vitamin-type compounds (called ***coenzymes***), such as vitamin C, flavin-adenine dinucleotide (FAD), and nicotinamide-adenine dinucleotide (NAD). The combination of the apoenzyme plus the cofactor is called a ***holoenzyme*** (a "whole" enzyme); the holoenzyme can function as an enzyme.

apoenzyme + cofactor = holoenzyme (a functional enzyme)

Enzymes are usually named by adding the ending "-ase" to the word, indicating the compound or types of compounds on which an enzyme acts or exerts its effect. For example, proteases, carbohydrases, and lipases are enzymes that exert their effects on proteins, carbohydrates, and lipids, respectively. The specific molecule on which an enzyme acts is referred to as that enzyme's ***substrate.*** Each enzyme has a particular substrate on which it exerts its effect; thus, enzymes are said to be very specific. Although most enzymes end in "ase," some do not; lysozyme and hemolysins are examples.

Some toxins and other poisonous substances cause damage to the human body by interfering with the action of certain necessary enzymes. For example, cyanide poison binds to the iron and copper ions in the cytochrome systems of the mitochondria of eucaryotic cells. As a result, the cells cannot use oxygen to synthesize ATP, which is essential for energy production, and they soon die.

Proteins, including enzymes, may be denatured (structurally altered) by heat or certain chemicals. In a denatured protein, the bonds that hold the molecule in a tertiary structure are broken. With these bonds broken, the protein is no longer functional. Enzymes are discussed further in Chapter 7.

[a]Certain RNA molecules, called ribozymes, have been shown to have enzymatic activity. However, because the vast majority of enzymes are proteins, enzymes are discussed in this book as if all of them are proteins.

Examples of Enzymes

Catalase	Lysozyme
Coagulase	Oxidase
DNA polymerase	Peptidases
DNAse	Proteases
Hemolysins	RNA polymerase
Lipases	RNase

Nucleic Acids

Function

Nucleic acids—DNA and RNA—comprise the fourth major group of biomolecules in living cells. Nucleic acids play extremely important roles in a cell; they are critical to the proper functioning of a cell. DNA is the "hereditary molecule"—the molecule that contains the genes and genetic code. DNA makes up the major portion of chromosomes. The information in DNA must flow to the rest of the cell for the cell to function properly; this flow of information is accomplished by RNA molecules. RNA molecules participate in the conversion of the genetic code into proteins and other gene products.

Structure

In addition to the elements C, H, O, and N, DNA and RNA also contain P (phosphorus). The building blocks of these nucleic acid polymers are called *nucleotides.* These are more complex monomers (single molecular units that can be repeated to form a polymer) than amino acids, which are the building blocks of proteins. Nucleotides consist of three subunits: a nitrogen-containing (nitrogenous) base, a five-carbon sugar (pentose), and a phosphate group, joined together, as shown in Figure 6-14. The building blocks of DNA are called *DNA nucleotides;* they contain a nitrogenous base, deoxyribose, and a phosphate group. The building blocks of RNA are called *RNA nucleotides;* they contain a nitrogenous base, ribose, and a phosphate group.

HISTORICAL NOTE

The Discovery of the "Hereditary Molecule"

In 1944, **Oswald T. Avery** and his colleagues at the Rockefeller Institute wrote one of the most important papers ever published in biology. In that paper, they announced their discovery that DNA, not proteins as had earlier been suspected, is the molecule that contains genetic information (i.e., that DNA is the hereditary molecule). They made this discovery while repeating Frederick Griffith's 1928 transformation experiments (see Chapter 7). Whereas Griffith's experiments involved mice, Avery's group conducted in vitro experiments. The importance of this discovery was not fully appreciated at the time, and Avery and his colleagues did not receive a Nobel Prize. Additional evidence that DNA is the molecule that contains genetic information was provided by Alfred Hershey and Martha Chase in 1952. Their work involved a bacteriophage that infects *Escherichia coli.* In 1969, Hershey shared a Nobel Prize with Max Delbrück and Salvador Luria for their discoveries involving the genetic structure and replication of bacteriophages.

As previously stated, there are two kinds of nucleic acids in cells: DNA and RNA. DNA contains deoxyribose as its pentose, whereas RNA contains ribose as its pentose. There are three types of RNA, which are named for the function they serve: *messenger RNA (mRNA), ribosomal RNA (rRNA),* and *transfer RNA (tRNA).* The five nitrogenous bases in nucleic acids are adenine (A), guanine (G), thymine (T), cytosine (C), and uracil (U). Thymine is found in DNA, but not in RNA. Uracil is found in RNA, but not in DNA. The other three bases (A, G, C) are present in both DNA and RNA. Both A and G are *purines* (double-ring structures), whereas T, C, and U are *pyrimidines* (single-ring structures; Fig. 6-15).

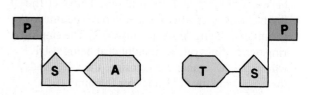

FIGURE 6-14. Two nucleotides, each consisting of a nitrogenous base (A or T), a five-carbon sugar (S), and a phosphate group (P).

Nucleotides

THREE PARTS TO EVERY NUCLEOTIDE	FOUR DNA NUCLEOTIDES (DEOXYRIBONU-CLEOTIDES)	FOUR RNA NUCLEOTIDES (RIBONU-CLEOTIDES)
1. Nitrogenous base	Adenine (a purine) Guanine (a purine) Cytosine (a pyrimidine) Thymine (a pyrimidine)	Adenine (a purine) Guanine (a purine) Cytosine (a pyrimidine) Uracil (a pyrimidine)
2. Pentose	Deoxyribose	Ribose
3. Phosphate group	Phosphate group	Phosphate group

The nucleotides join together (via covalent bonds) between their sugar and phosphate groups to form very long polymers—100,000 or more monomers long—as shown in Figure 6-16.

DNA Structure

For a double-stranded DNA molecule to form, the nitrogenous bases on the two separate strands must bond together.

Purines and Pyrimidines

Here is one way to remember the difference between purines and pyrimidines. Think of the double-ring structure of a purine (adenine or guanine) as being "pure and un-CUT." The single-ring pyrimidines can be thought of as being "CUT," where the "C" stands for cytosine, the "U" stands for uracil, and the "T" stands for thymine.

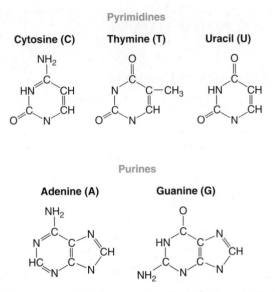

FIGURE 6-15. The pyrimidines and purines found in DNA and RNA. Note that pyrimidines are single-ring structures, whereas purines are double-ring structures.

It was found that because of the size and bonding attraction between the molecules, A (a purine) always bonds with T (a pyrimidine) via two hydrogen bonds, and G (a purine) always bonds with C (a pyrimidine) via three hydrogen bonds (Fig. 6-17). (A–T and G–C are known as "base pairs.") The bonding forces of the double-stranded polymer cause it to assume the shape of a double α-helix, which is similar to a right-handed spiral staircase (Fig. 6-18).

DNA Replication

When a cell is preparing to divide, all the DNA molecules in the chromosomes of that cell must duplicate, thereby ensuring that the same genetic information is passed on to both daughter cells. This process is called *DNA replication.*

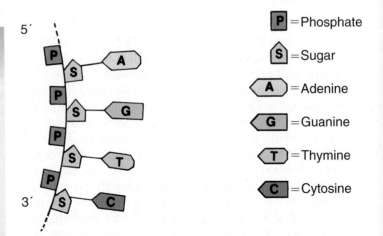

P	=Phosphate
S	=Sugar
A	=Adenine
G	=Guanine
T	=Thymine
C	=Cytosine

FIGURE 6-16. One small section of a nucleic acid polymer.

HISTORICAL NOTE

The Discovery of the Structure of DNA

In the early 1950s, an American named **James Watson** and an Englishman named **Francis Crick** published two extremely important papers. The first (published in 1953) proposed a double-stranded, helical structure for DNA (a "double helix"), and the second (published in 1954) proposed a method by which a DNA molecule could copy (replicate) itself exactly, so that identical genetic information could be passed on to each daughter cell. The idea for the double-helical structure was based on an x-ray diffraction photograph of crystallized DNA that Watson had seen in the London laboratory of Maurice Wilkins. The now famous photograph had been produced by Rosalind Franklin, an x-ray crystallographer who worked in Wilkins's lab. Watson, Crick, and Wilkins received a Nobel Prize in Chemistry in 1962 for their contributions to our understanding of DNA. Franklin had died before 1962; the Nobel Prize is not awarded posthumously.

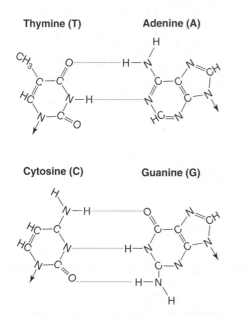

FIGURE 6-17. Base pairs that occur in double-stranded DNA molecules. Note that A and T are connected by two hydrogen bonds, whereas G and C are connected by three hydrogen bonds. The arrows represent the points at which the bases are bonded to deoxyribose molecules.

STUDY AID

Major Differences Between DNA and RNA

DNA is double-stranded, whereas RNA is single-stranded.
DNA contains deoxyribose, whereas RNA contains ribose.
DNA contains thymine, whereas RNA contains uracil.

It occurs by separation of the DNA strands and the building of complementary strands by the addition of the correct DNA nucleotides, as indicated in Figure 6-19. The point on the molecule where DNA replication starts is called the *replication fork*. The most important enzyme required for DNA replication is ***DNA polymerase*** (also known as DNA-dependent DNA polymerase). Other enzymes are also required, including DNA helicase and DNA topoisomerase (which initiate the separation of the two strands of the DNA molecule), primase (which synthesizes a short RNA primer), and DNA ligase (which connects fragments of newly synthesized DNA).

The duplicated DNA of the chromosomes can then be separated during cell division, so that each daughter cell contains the same number of chromosomes, the same genes, and the same amount of DNA as in the parent cell (except during meiosis, the reduction division by which ova and sperm cells are produced in eucaryotes). There are subtle differences between DNA replication in procaryotes and eucaryotes.

Gene Expression

As you learned in Chapter 3, a gene is a particular segment of a DNA molecule or chromosome. A gene contains the instructions (the "recipe" or "blueprint") that will enable a cell to make what is known as a *gene product*. The ***genetic code*** contains four "letters" (the letters that stand for the four nitrogenous bases found in DNA): "A" for adenine, "G" for guanine, "C" for cytosine, and "T" for thymine. It is the sequence of these four bases that spell out the instructions for a particular gene product.

Although most genes code for proteins (meaning that each gene contains the instructions for the production of a particular protein), some code for rRNA and tRNA molecules. However, because the vast majority of gene products are proteins, gene products are discussed in this chapter as if all of them are proteins.

The Central Dogma. It was Francis Crick who, in 1957, proposed what is referred to as the ***central dogma*** to explain the flow of genetic information within a cell:

$$\text{DNA} \rightarrow \text{mRNA} \rightarrow \text{protein}$$

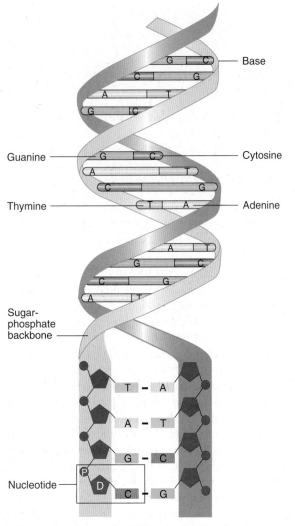

FIGURE 6-18. Double-stranded DNA molecule, also referred to as a double helix.

The central dogma (also known as the "one gene–one protein hypothesis") states that:

1. The genetic information contained in one gene of a DNA molecule is used to make one molecule of mRNA by a process known as transcription.

2. The genetic information in that mRNA molecule is then used to make one protein by a process known as translation.

When the information in a gene has been used by the cell to make a gene product, the gene that codes for that particular gene product is said to have been *expressed*. All the genes on the chromosome are not being expressed at any given time. That would be a terrible waste of energy! For example, it would not be logical for a cell to produce a particular enzyme if that enzyme was not actually needed. Genes that are expressed at all times are called **constitutive genes.** Those that are expressed only when the gene products are needed are called **inducible genes.**

Transcription. When a cell is stimulated (by need) to produce a particular protein, the DNA of the appropriate gene is activated to unwind temporarily from its helical configuration. This unwinding exposes the bases, which then attract the bases of free RNA nucleotides, and an mRNA molecule begins to be assembled alongside one of the strands of the unwound DNA. Thus, one of the DNA strands has served as a template, or pattern (it is referred to as the *DNA template*), and has coded for a complementary mirror image of its structure in the mRNA molecule. On the growing mRNA molecule, an A will be introduced opposite a T on the DNA molecule, a G opposite a C, a C opposite a G, and a U opposite an A (see the study aid on page 103). Remember that there is no T in RNA molecules. This process is called **transcription** because the genetic code from the DNA molecule is transcribed to produce an mRNA molecule. After the mRNA has been synthesized over the length of the gene, it is released from the DNA strand to carry the message to the cytoplasm and direct the synthesis of a particular protein. The primary enzyme involved in

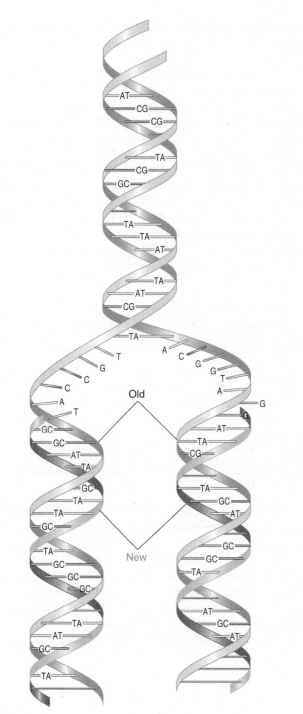

FIGURE 6-19. DNA replication. (See text for details.)

STUDY AID

Transcription

SEQUENCE OF BASES IN THE DNA TEMPLATE	SEQUENCE OF BASES IN THE MRNA MOLECULE
A	U
T	A
G	C
C	G
C	G
G	C
A	U
A	U
T	A

transcription is called **RNA polymerase** (also known as DNA-dependent RNA polymerase). Located along the DNA template are various nucleotide sequences known as "traffic signals" that let the RNA polymerase know where to start and stop the transcription process (i.e., the "traffic signals" are the starting and stopping points for each gene). Each mRNA molecule contains the same genetic information that was contained in the gene on the DNA template. Note, however, that the genetic code in the mRNA molecule is made up of RNA nucleotides, whereas the genetic code in the DNA template is made up of DNA nucleotides. The information in the mRNA molecule will then be used to synthesize one protein.

In eucaryotes, transcription occurs within the nucleus. The newly formed mRNA molecules then travel through the pores of the nuclear membrane, out into the cytoplasm, where they take up positions on the protein "assembly line." Ribosomes, which are composed of proteins and ribosomal RNA (rRNA), attract the mRNA molecules. In eucaryotic cells, ribosomes are usually attached to endoplasmic reticulum membranes.

In procaryotes, transcription occurs in the cytoplasm. Ribosomes attach to the mRNA molecules as they are being transcribed at the DNA; thus, transcription and translation (protein synthesis) may occur simultaneously.

Translation (Protein Synthesis). The base sequence of the mRNA molecule is read or interpreted in groups of three bases, called **codons.** The sequence of a codon's three bases is the code that determines which amino acid is inserted in that position in the protein being synthesized. Also located on the mRNA molecule are various codons that act as start and stop signals.

Before they can be used to build a protein molecule, amino acids must first be "activated." Each amino acid is activated by attaching to an appropriate *transfer RNA (tRNA)* molecule, which then carries (transfers) the amino acid from the cytoplasmic matrix to the site of protein

assembly. The enzyme responsible for attaching amino acids to their corresponding tRNA molecules is amino acyl-tRNA synthetase.

The three-base sequence of the codon determines which tRNA brings its specific amino acid to the ribosome, because the tRNA molecule contains an **anticodon**: a three-base sequence that is complementary to, or attracted to, the codon of the mRNA. For example, the tRNA with the anticodon base sequence UUU carries the amino acid lysine to the mRNA codon AAA. Similarly, the mRNA codon CCG codes for the tRNA anticodon GGC, which carries the amino acid proline. The following chart illustrates the sequence of three bases (GGC) in the DNA template that codes for a particular codon (CCG) in mRNA, which, in turn, attracts a particular anticodon (GGC) on the tRNA carrying a specific amino acid (proline):

DNA TEMPLATE	mRNA (CODON)	tRNA (ANTICODON)	AMINO ACID
G	C	G	
G	C	G	Proline
C	G	C	

The process of translating the message carried by the mRNA, whereby particular tRNAs bring amino acids to be bound together in the proper sequence to make a specific protein, is called **translation** (summarized in Fig. 6-20). It should be noted that a eucaryotic cell is constantly producing mRNAs in its nucleus, which direct the synthesis of all the proteins, including metabolic enzymes necessary for the normal functions of that specific type of cell. Also, mRNA and tRNA are short-lived nucleic acids that may be

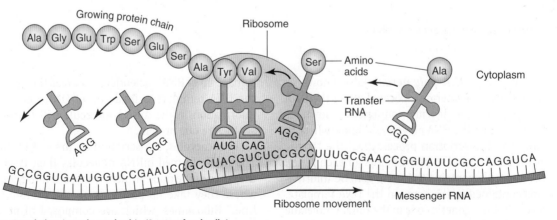

FIGURE 6-20. Translation (protein synthesis). (See text for details.)

reused many times and then destroyed and resynthesized. The rRNA molecules are made in the dense portion of the nucleus called the nucleolus. Ribosomes last longer in the cell than do mRNA molecules.

As tRNA molecules attach to mRNA while it is sliding over the ribosome, they bring the correct activated amino acids into contact with each other so that peptide bonds are formed and a polypeptide is synthesized. Recent evidence suggests a role for rRNA (a structural component of the ribosome) in the formation of the peptide bonds. As the polypeptide grows and becomes a protein, it folds into the unique shape determined by the amino acid sequence. This characteristic shape allows the protein to perform its specific function. If one of the bases of a DNA gene is incorrect or out of sequence (known as a *mutation*), the amino acid sequence of the gene product will be incorrect and the altered protein configuration may not allow the protein to function properly. For example, some diabetics may not produce a functional insulin molecule because a mutation in one of their chromosomes caused a rearrangement of the bases in the gene that codes for insulin. Such errors are the basis for most genetic and inherited diseases, such as phenylketonuria (PKU), sickle cell anemia, cerebral palsy, cystic fibrosis, cleft lip, clubfoot, extra fingers, albinism, and many other birth defects. Likewise, nonpathogenic microbes may mutate to become pathogens, and pathogens may lose the ability to cause disease by mutation. Mutations are discussed further in Chapter 7.

The relatively new sciences of genetic engineering and gene therapy attempt to repair the genetic damage in some diseases. As yet, the morality of manipulation of human genes has not been resolved by society. However, many genetically engineered microbes are able to produce substances, such as human insulin, interferon, growth hormones, new pharmaceutical agents, and vaccines, that will have a substantial effect on the medical treatment of humans (see Chapter 7).

REVIEW OF KEY POINTS

- Organic compounds contain carbon atoms that are connected to each other by single, double, or triple bonds. A single bond represents one covalent bond (*i.e.*, the sharing of a pair of electrons). A double bond represents two covalent bonds, or four shared electrons. A triple bond represents three covalent bonds, or six electons.

- Organic compounds may be small molecules, cyclic molecules, short chain molecules, or long chain molecules.

- Organic compounds containing only carbon and hydrogen are called hydrocarbons.

- Biochemistry is both a branch of biology and a branch of organic chemistry; it involves the study of biomolecules, including macromolecules such as carbohydrates, lipids, proteins, and nucleic acids.

- Carbohydrates are organic molecules containing C, H, and O. Carbohydrates include monosaccharides, disaccharides, trisaccharides, and polysaccharides.

- The "building blocks" of carbohydrates are monosaccharides, which contain between three and nine carbon atoms. If the monosaccharide contains three carbon atoms it is called a triose; a four-carbon monosaccharide is called a tetrose; five carbons, a pentose; six carbons, a hexose; and seven carbons, a heptose.

- Disaccharides consist of two monosaccharides, held together by covalent bonds called glycosidic bonds. Sucrose, lactose, and maltose are examples of disaccharides. Trisaccharides consist of three monosaccharides. Polysaccharides consist of many monosaccharides. Starch, glycogen, and cellulose are examples of polysaccharides.

- Lipids are essential constituents of most living cells. Lipids include waxes, fats, oils, phospholipids, glycolipids, and steroids. Phospholipids are important components of cell membranes.

- The thousands of different proteins in an organism are composed of various numbers and arrangements of amino acids (*i.e.*, amino acids are the "building blocks" of proteins). The simplest protein is a dipeptide, containing two amino acids, held together by covalent bonds called peptide bonds. A tripeptide contains three amino acis. A polypeptide contains more than three amino acids.

- Nucleic acids are polymers, composed of nucleotides (*i.e.*, nucleotides are the "building blocks" of nucleic acids). The nucleotides in a single-stranded nucleic acid molecule are held together by covalent bonds.

- The two categories of nucleic acids are deoxyribonucleic acid (DNA; the hereditary molecule) and ribonucleic acid (RNA). The three types of RNA are messenger RNA (mRNA), transfer RNA (tRNA), and ribosomal RNA (rRNA).

- In a double-stranded DNA molecule, the nucleotides in one strand are connected to nucleotides in the other strand by hydrogen bonds.

- DNA is the primary component of chromosomes. Genes are located along the DNA molecule. DNA molecules are used as templates to produce other DNA molecules by the process known as DNA replication. The most important enzyme in DNA replication is DNA polymerase.

- The flow of genetic information within a cell follows the sequence DNA → mRNA → protein. This is known as the central dogma.

- The information (genetic code) in one gene of a DNA molecule is used to produce a mRNA molecule. This process is known as transcription. The most important enzyme in transcription is RNA polymerase.

- Information in one mRNA molecule is used to produce a protein. This process is known as translation (protein synthesis) and occurs at a ribosome.

- Transfer RNA (tRNA) molecules activate amino acids and transfer them to the growing protein chain. Specific amino acids are added at the correct locations because three-nucleotide sequences (anticodons) on the tRNA molecules recognize three-nucleotide sequence (codons) on the mRNA molecule.

- The newly formed protein (polypeptide) molecule twists into secondary spirals that can be used as fibrous structural cell proteins, or the spirals may fold back on themselves to become tertiary globular structures. Quaternary globular proteins, like hemoglobin, consist of more than one globular protein.

- The size, shape, and configuration of a protein is specific for the function it must perform and is determined by the genes on the chromosome.

SELF-ASSESSMENT EXERCISES

After studying this chapter, answer the following multiple-choice questions.

On the CD-ROM
- Increase Your Knowledge
- Microbiology—Hollywood Style
- Critical Thinking
- Additional Self-Assessment Exercises

1. Which of the following are the building blocks of proteins?
   a. amino acids
   b. monosaccharides
   c. nucleotides
   d. peptides

2. Glucose, sucrose, and cellulose are examples of:
   a. carbohydrates.
   b. disaccharides.
   c. monosaccharides.
   d. polysaccharides.

3. Which of the following nitrogenous bases is *not* found in an RNA molecule?
   a. adenine
   b. guanine
   c. thymine
   d. uracil

4. Which of the following are purines?
   a. adenine and guanine
   b. adenine and thymine
   c. guanine and uracil
   d. guanine and cytosine

5. Which one of the following is *not* found at the site of protein synthesis?
   a. DNA
   b. mRNA
   c. rRNA
   d. tRNA

6. Which of the following statements about DNA is (are) true?
   a. DNA contains thymine but not uracil.
   b. DNA molecules contain deoxyribose.
   c. In a double-stranded DNA molecule, adenine on one strand will be connected to thymine on the complementary strand by two hydrogen bonds.
   d. All of the above statements are true.

7. The amino acids in a polypeptide chain are connected by:
   a. covalent bonds.
   b. glycosidic bonds.
   c. peptide bonds.
   d. both a and c.

8. Which of the following statements about nucleotides is (are) true?
   a. A nucleotide contains a nitrogenous base.
   b. A nucleotide contains a pentose.
   c. A nucleotide contains a phosphate group.
   d. All of the above statements are true.

9. A heptose contains how many carbon atoms?
   a. 4
   b. 5
   c. 6
   d. 7

10. Virtually all enzymes are:
   a. carbohydrates.
   b. nucleic acids.
   c. proteins.
   d. substrates.

MICROBIAL PHYSIOLOGY AND GENETICS

LEARNING OBJECTIVES

AFTER STUDYING THIS CHAPTER, YOU SHOULD BE
ABLE TO:

- Define phototroph, chemotroph, autotroph, heterotroph, photoautotroph, chemoheterotroph, endoenzyme, exoenzyme, plasmid, R-factor, "superbug," mutation, mutant, and mutagen
- Discuss the relationships among apoenzymes, coenzymes, and holoenzymes
- Differentiate between catabolism and anabolism
- Explain the role of ATP molecules in metabolism
- Briefly describe each of the following: biochemical pathway, aerobic respiration, glycolysis, the Krebs cycle, the electron transport chain, oxidation–reduction reactions, photosynthesis
- Differentiate among beneficial, harmful, and silent mutations
- Briefly describe each of the following ways in which bacteria acquire genetic information: lysogenic conversion, transduction, transformation, conjugation

Microbial Physiology

Introduction

Physiology is the study of the vital life processes of organisms, especially how these processes normally function in living organisms. ***Microbial physiology*** concerns the vital life processes of microorganisms. Microorganisms, especially bacteria, are ideally suited for use in studies of the basic metabolic reactions that occur within cells. Bacteria are inexpensive to maintain in the laboratory, take up little space, and reproduce quickly. Their morphology, nutritional needs, and metabolic reactions are easily observable.

Of special importance is the fact that species of bacteria can be found that represent each of the nutritional types of organisms on earth. Scientists can learn a great deal about cells—including human cells—by studying the nutritional needs of bacteria, their metabolic pathways, and why they live, grow, multiply, or die under certain conditions.

Each tiny single-celled bacterium strives to produce more cells like itself, and, as long as water and an adequate nutrient supply are available, it often does so at an alarming rate. Under favorable conditions, in 24 hours, the offspring (progeny) of a single *Escherichia coli* cell would outnumber the entire human population on the earth! Because some bacteria, fungi, and viruses produce generation after generation so rapidly, they have been used extensively in genetic studies. In fact, most of today's genetic knowledge was and still is being obtained by studying these microorganisms.

Nutritional Requirements

Studies of bacterial nutrition and other aspects of microbial physiology enable scientists to understand the vital chemical processes that occur within every living cell, including those of the human body. All living protoplasm contains six major chemical elements: carbon, hydrogen, oxygen, nitrogen, phosphorus, and sulfur. Other elements, usually required in lesser amounts, include sodium, potassium, chlorine, magnesium, calcium, iron, iodine, and some trace elements. Combinations of all these elements make up the vital macromolecules of life, including carbohydrates, lipids, proteins, and nucleic acids.

To build necessary cellular materials, every organism requires a source (or sources) of energy, a source (or sources) of carbon, and additional nutrients. Those materials that organisms are unable to synthesize, but are required for the building of macromolecules and sustaining life, are termed **essential nutrients.** Essential nutrients (e.g., essential amino acids and essential fatty acids) must be continually supplied to an organism for it to survive. Essential nutrients vary from species to species.

Categorizing Microorganisms According to Their Energy and Carbon Sources

Since the beginning of life on earth, microorganisms have been evolving, some in different directions than others. Today, there are microbes representing each of the four major nutritional categories (photoautotrophs, photoheterotrophs, chemoautotrophs, chemoheterotrophs; terms defined later in this chapter). Various terms are used to indicate an organism's energy source and carbon source. As you will see, these terms can be used in combination (Table 7-1).

Terms Relating to an Organism's Energy Source

The terms phototroph and chemotroph pertain to what an organism uses as an energy source. **Phototrophs** use light as an energy source. The process by which organisms convert light energy into chemical energy is called *photosynthesis.* **Chemotrophs** use either inorganic or organic chemicals as an energy source. Chemotrophs can be subdivided into two categories: chemolithotrophs and chemoorganotrophs. **Chemolithotrophs** (or simply lithotrophs) are organisms that use inorganic chemicals as an energy source. **Chemoorganotrophs** (or simply organotrophs) are organisms that use organic chemicals as an energy source.

Terms Relating to an Organism's Carbon Source

The terms autotroph and heterotroph pertain to what an organism uses as a carbon source. **Autotrophs** use carbon dioxide (CO_2) as their sole source of carbon. Photosynthetic organisms such as plants, algae, and cyanobacteria are examples of autotrophs. **Heterotrophs** are organisms that use organic compounds other than CO_2 as their carbon source. (Recall that all organic compounds contain carbon.) Humans, animals, fungi, and protozoa are examples of heterotrophs. Both saprophytic fungi, which live on dead and decaying organic matter, and parasitic fungi are heterotrophs. Most bacteria are also heterotrophs.

The terms relating to energy source can be combined with the terms relating to carbon source, yielding terms that indicate both an organism's energy source and carbon source. For example, **photoautotrophs** are organisms (such as plants, algae, cyanobacteria, purple and green sulfur bacteria) that use light as an energy source and CO_2 as a carbon source. **Photoheterotrophs,** like purple nonsulfur and green nonsulfur bacteria, use light as an energy source and organic compounds other than CO_2 as a carbon source. **Chemoautotrophs** (such as nitrifying, hydrogen, iron, and sulfur bacteria) use chemicals as an energy source and CO_2 as a carbon source. **Chemoheterotrophs** use chemicals as an energy source and organic compounds other than CO_2 as a carbon source. All animals, all protozoa, all fungi, and most bacteria are chemo-

---

⊙ STUDY AID

Nutrients

The term "nutrients" refers to the various chemical compounds that organisms (including microorganisms) use to sustain life. Many nutrients are energy sources; organisms will obtain energy from these chemicals by breaking chemical bonds. Whenever a chemical bond is broken, energy is released. As nutrients are broken down by enzymatic action, smaller molecules are produced, which are then used by cells as building blocks. Nutrients also serve as sources of carbon, nitrogen, and other elements.

TABLE 7-1

Terms Relating to Energy and Carbon Sources

TERMS RELATING TO ENERGY SOURCE		TERMS RELATING TO CARBON SOURCE
	Autotrophs (organisms that use CO_2 as a carbon source)	Heterotrophs (organisms that use organic compounds other than CO_2 as a carbon source)
Phototrophs (organisms that use light as an energy source)	Photoautotrophs (e.g., algae, plants, some photosynthetic bacteria, including cyanobacteria)	Photoheterotrophs (e.g., some photosynthetic bacteria)
Chemotrophs[a] (organisms that use chemicals as an energy source)	Chemoautotrophs (e.g., some bacteria)	Chemoheterotrophs (e.g., protozoa, fungi, animals, most bacteria)

[a]Chemotrophs can be divided into two categories: (1) chemolithotrophs (or simply lithotrophs) are organisms that use inorganic chemicals as an energy source, and (2) chemoorganotrophs (or simply organotrophs) are organisms that use organic chemicals as an energy source.

heterotrophs. All medically important bacteria are chemoheterotrophs.

Ecology is the study of the interactions between organisms and the world around them. The term **ecosystem** refers to the interactions between living organisms and their nonliving environment. Interrelationships among the different nutritional types are of prime importance in the functioning of the ecosystem. Phototrophs (like algae and plants) are the producers of food and oxygen for chemoheterotrophs (such as animals). Dead plants and animals would clutter the earth if chemoheterotrophic, saprophytic decomposers (certain fungi and bacteria) did not break down the dead organic matter into small inorganic and organic compounds (carbon dioxide, nitrates, phosphates) in soil, water, and air—compounds that are then used and recycled by chemotrophs. Photoautotrophs contribute energy to the ecosystem by trapping energy from the sun and using it to build organic compounds (carbohydrates, lipids, proteins, and nucleic acids) from inorganic materials in the soil, water, and air. In oxygenic photosynthesis (described later), oxygen is released for use by aerobic organisms, such as animals and humans.

Metabolic Enzymes

The term *metabolism* refers to all the chemical reactions that occur within any cell. These chemical reactions are referred to as **metabolic reactions.** The metabolic processes that occur in microbes are similar to those that occur in cells of the human body. Metabolic reactions are enhanced and regulated by enzymes, known as *metabolic enzymes.* A cell can only perform a certain metabolic reaction if it possesses the appropriate metabolic enzyme, and it can only possess that enzyme if the genome of the cell contains the gene that codes for production of that enzyme.

Biologic Catalysts

As you learned in Chapter 6, enzymes are known as *biologic catalysts.* Enzymes are proteins that catalyze (speed up or accelerate) the rate of biochemical reactions. In some cases, the reaction will not occur at all in the absence of the enzyme. Thus, a complete definition of a biologic catalyst would be a protein that either causes a particular chemical reaction to occur or accelerates it.

Recall that enzymes are very specific. A particular enzyme can only catalyze one particular chemical reaction. In most cases, a particular enzyme can only exert its effect or act on one particular substance—known as the *substrate* for that enzyme. The unique three-dimensional shape of the enzyme enables it to fit the combining site of the substrate, much like a key fits into a lock (Fig. 7-1).

An enzyme does not become altered during the chemical reaction that it catalyzes. At the conclusion of the reaction, the enzyme is unchanged and is available to drive that reaction over and over. The enzyme moves from substrate molecule to substrate molecule at a rate of several hundred each second, producing a supply of the end product for as long as this particular end product is needed by the cell. However, enzymes do not last indefinitely; they finally degenerate and lose their activity. Therefore, the cell must synthesize and replace these important proteins. Because there are thousands of metabolic reactions continually occurring in the cell, there are thousands of enzymes avail-

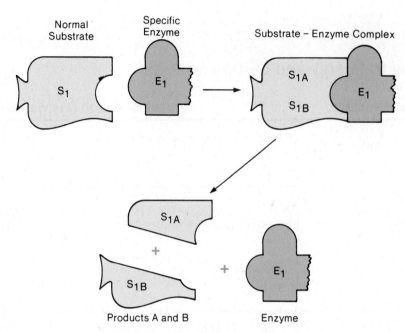

FIGURE 7-1. Action of a specific enzyme (E) breaking down a substrate (S) molecule.

able to control and direct the essential metabolic pathways. At any particular time, all the required enzymes need not be present; this situation is controlled by genes on the chromosomes and the needs of the cell, which are determined by the internal and external environments. For example, if no lactose is present in the organism's external environment, the organism does not need the enzyme required to break down lactose.

Enzymes produced within a cell that remain within the cell—to catalyze reactions within the cell—are called ***endoenzymes.*** The digestive enzymes within phagocytes are good examples of endoenzymes; they are used to digest materials that the phagocytes have ingested. Enzymes produced within a cell that are then released from the cell—to catalyze extracellular reactions—are called ***exoenzymes.*** Examples of exoenzymes are cellulase and pectinase, which are secreted by saprophytic fungi to digest cellulose and pectin in the external environment (e.g., in rotting leaves on the forest floor). Cellulose and pectin molecules are too large to be absorbed into fungal cells. The exoenzymes cellulase and pectinase break down these large molecules into smaller molecules, which can then be absorbed into the cells.

Hydrolases and polymerases are additional examples of metabolic enzymes. Hydrolases break down macromolecules by the addition of water, in a process called hydrolysis or a hydrolysis reaction. These hydrolytic processes enable saprophytes to break apart such complex materials as leather, wax, cork, wood, rubber, hair, and some plastics. Some of the enzymes involved in the formation of large polymers like DNA and RNA are called polymerases. As was discussed in Chapter 6, DNA polymerase is active each time the DNA of a cell is replicated, and RNA polymerase is required for the synthesis of mRNA molecules.

As was discussed in Chapter 6, some proteins (called apoenzymes) cannot, on their own, catalyze a chemical reaction. An apoenzyme must link up with a cofactor to catalyze a chemical reaction. Cofactors are either mineral ions (e.g., magnesium, calcium, or iron cations) or coenzymes. Coenzymes are small organic, vitamin-type molecules such as flavin-adenine dinucleotide (FAD) and nicotinamide-adenine dinucleotide (NAD). These particular coenzymes participate in the Krebs cycle, which is discussed later in this chapter. Like enzymes, coenzymes do not have to be present in large amounts because they are not altered during the chemical reaction that they catalyze; thus, they are available for use over and over. However, a lack of certain vitamins from which the coenzymes are synthesized will halt all reactions involving that particular coenzyme.

Factors That Affect the Efficiency of Enzymes

Many factors affect the efficiency or effectiveness of enzymes. Certain physical or chemical changes can diminish or completely stop enzyme activity, because enzymes function properly only under optimum conditions. Optimum conditions for enzyme activity include a relatively limited range of pH and temperature as well as the appropriate concentration of enzyme and substrate. Extremes in heat and acidity can denature (or alter) enzymes by breaking the bonds responsible for their three-dimensional shape, resulting in the loss of enzymatic activity.

An enzyme will function at peak efficiency over a particular pH range. If the pH is too high or too low, the enzyme will not function at peak efficiency, and the reaction that the enzyme catalyzes will not proceed at its maximum rate.

Likewise, an enzyme will function at peak efficiency over a particular temperature range. If the temperature is too high or too low, the enzyme will not function at peak efficiency, and the reaction that the enzyme catalyzes will not proceed at its maximum rate.

This explains why a particular bacterium grows best at a certain temperature and pH; these are the optimal conditions for the enzymes possessed by that bacterium. The optimal pH and temperature for growth vary from one species to another.

Substrate concentration is another factor that influences the efficiency of an enzyme. If the substrate concentration is too high or too low, the enzyme will not function at peak efficiency, and the reaction that the enzyme catalyzes will not proceed at its maximum rate.

Although certain mineral ions (e.g., calcium, magnesium, and iron) enhance the activity of enzymes by serving as cofactors, other heavy metal ions (e.g., lead, zinc, mercury, and arsenic) usually act as poisons to the cell. These toxic ions inhibit enzyme activity by replacing the cofactors at the combining site of the enzyme, thus inhibiting normal metabolic processes. Some disinfectants containing mineral ions are effective in inhibiting the growth of bacteria in this manner.

Sometimes, a molecule that is similar in structure to the substrate can be used as an inhibitor to deliberately interfere with a particular metabolic pathway. The enzyme binds to the molecule having a similar structure to the substrate, thus, tying the enzyme up, so that it cannot attach to the substrate and cannot catalyze the chemical reaction. If that reaction is essential for the life of the cell, the cell will stop growing and may die. For example, a chemotherapeutic agent, such as a sulfonamide drug, can bind to certain bacterial enzymes, blocking attachment of the enzymes to their substrates and preventing essential metabolites from being formed. This could lead to the death of the bacteria.

Metabolism

As previously mentioned, the term metabolism refers to all the chemical reactions occurring within a cell. The reactions are referred to as metabolic reactions. A *metabolite* is any molecule that is a nutrient, an intermediary product, or an end product in a metabolic reaction. Within a cell, many metabolic reactions proceed simultaneously, breaking down some compounds and synthesizing (building) others. Most metabolic reactions fall into two categories: catabolism and anabolism.

The term *catabolism* refers to all the catabolic reactions that are occurring in a cell. *Catabolic reactions,* which are described in greater detail in a subsequent section, involve the breaking down of larger molecules into smaller molecules, requiring the breaking of bonds. Any time that chemical bonds are broken, energy is released. Catabolic reactions are a cell's major source of energy. Catabolic reactions in bacteria are quite diverse, because energy sources range from inorganic compounds (e.g., sulfide, ferrous ion, hydrogen) to organic compounds (e.g., carbohydrates, lipids, amino acids).

Anabolism refers to all the anabolic reactions that are occurring in a cell. *Anabolic reactions,* which are described in greater detail in a subsequent section, involve the assembly of smaller molecules into larger molecules, requiring the formation of bonds. Energy is required for bond formation. Once formed, the bonds represent stored energy. Anabolic reactions tend to be quite similar for all types of cells; the pathways for the biosynthesis of macromolecules do not differ much among organisms. Table 7-2 illustrates the key differences between catabolism and anabolism.

The energy that is released during catabolic reactions is used to drive anabolic reactions. A kind of energy balancing act occurs within a cell, with some metabolic reactions releasing energy and other metabolic reactions requiring energy. The energy required by a cell may be trapped from the rays of the sun (as in photosynthesis), or it may be produced by certain catabolic reactions. Then the energy can be temporarily stored within high-energy bonds in special molecules, usually *adenosine triphosphate* (ATP) molecules. Although ATP molecules are not the only high-

TABLE 7-2

Differences Between Catabolism and Anabolism

CATABOLISM	ANABOLISM
All the catabolic reactions in a cell	All the anabolic reactions in a cell
Catabolic reactions release energy	Anabolic reactions require energy
Catabolic reactions involve the breaking of bonds; whenever chemical bonds are broken, energy is released	Anabolic reactions involve the creation of bonds; it takes energy to create chemical bonds
Larger molecules are broken down into smaller molecules (sometimes referred to as degradative reactions)	Smaller molecules are bonded together to create larger molecules (sometimes referred to as biosynthetic reactions)

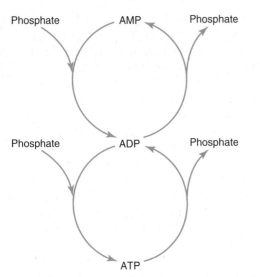

FIGURE 7-2. Interrelationships among ATP, ADP, and AMP molecules.

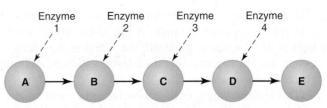

FIGURE 7-3. A biochemical pathway. There are four steps in this hypothetical biochemical pathway, in which compound A is ultimately converted to compound E. Compound A is first converted to compound B, which in turn is converted to compound C, which in turn is converted to compound D, which in turn is converted to compound E. Compound A is referred to as the starting material; compounds B, C, and D are referred to as intermediate (or intermediary) products; and compound E is referred to as the end product. A total of four enzymes are required in this pathway. The substrate for enzyme 1 is compound A; the substrate for enzyme 2 is compound B, and so on.

energy compounds found within a cell, they are the most important ones. <u>ATP molecules are the major energy-storing or energy-carrying molecules in a cell.</u>

ATP molecules are found in all cells because they are used to transfer energy from energy-yielding molecules, like glucose, to an energy-requiring reaction. Thus, ATP is a temporary, intermediate molecule. If ATP is not used shortly after it is formed, it is soon hydrolyzed to adenosine diphosphate (ADP), a more stable molecule; the hydrolysis of ATP is an example of a catabolic reaction. If a cell runs out of ATP molecules, ADP molecules can be used as an emergency energy source by the removal of another phosphate group to produce adenosine monophosphate (AMP); the hydrolysis of ADP is also a catabolic reaction. Figure 7-2 illustrates the interrelationships between ATP, ADP, and AMP molecules.

In addition to the energy required for metabolic pathways, energy is also required by the organism for growth, reproduction, sporulation, movement, and the active transport of substances across membranes. Some organisms (e.g., certain planktonic dinoflagellates) even use energy for bioluminescence. They cause a glowing that can sometimes be seen at the surface of an ocean, in a ship's wake, or as waves break on a beach. The value of bioluminescence to these organisms is unclear.

Chemical reactions are essentially energy transformation processes during which the energy that is stored in chemical bonds is transferred to produce new chemical bonds. The cellular mechanisms that release small amounts of energy as the cell needs it usually involve a sequence of catabolic and anabolic reactions.

Catabolism

As previously stated, the term catabolism refers to all the catabolic reactions that occur within a cell. <u>The key thing about catabolic reactions is that they release energy.</u>

Catabolic reactions are a cell's major source of energy. Catabolic reactions involve the breaking of chemical bonds. Any time chemical bonds are broken, energy is released. The energy produced by catabolic reactions can be used to wiggle flagella and actively transport substances through membranes, but most of the energy produced by catabolic reactions is used to drive anabolic reactions. Unfortunately, some of the energy is lost as heat. Catabolic reactions are often referred to as degradative reactions; they degrade larger molecules down into smaller molecules. For example, breaking a disaccharide down into its two original monosaccharides—a hydrolysis reaction—is an example of a catabolic reaction.

Biochemical Pathways

A biochemical pathway is a series of linked biochemical reactions that occur in a stepwise manner, leading from a starting material to an end product (Fig. 7-3).

Glucose is the favorite "food" or nutrient of cells, including microorganisms. <u>Nutrients should be thought of as energy sources, and chemical bonds should be thought of as stored energy.</u> Whenever the chemical bonds within the nutrients are broken, energy is released.

○ STUDY AID

A Biochemical Pathway

Think of a biochemical pathway as a journey by car. To drive from City A to City E, you must pass through Cities B, C, and D. City A is the starting point. City E is the destination or end point. Cities B, C, and D are intermediate points along the journey.

There are many chemical processes by which glucose is catabolized within cells. Two common processes are the biochemical pathways known as aerobic respiration and fermentation reactions, which will be discussed in this chapter. Additional pathways for catabolizing glucose, such as the Entner-Doudoroff pathway, the pentose phosphate pathway, and anaerobic respiration, will not be described because they are beyond the scope of this book.

Aerobic Respiration of Glucose

The complete catabolism of glucose by the process known as aerobic respiration (or cellular respiration) occurs in three phases, each of which is a biochemical pathway: (1) glycolysis, (2) the Krebs cycle, and (3) the electron-transport chain. Although the first phase—glycolysis—is an anaerobic process, the other two phases require aerobic conditions; hence the name, *aerobic* respiration.

Glycolysis. Glycolysis, also known as the glycolytic pathway, the Embden-Meyerhof pathway, and the Embden-Meyerhof-Parnas pathway, is a nine-step biochemical pathway, involving nine separate biochemical reactions, each of which requires a specific enzyme (Fig. 7-4).

In glycolysis, a six-carbon molecule of glucose is ultimately broken down into two three-carbon molecules of pyruvic acid (also called pyruvate). Glycolysis can take place in either the presence or absence of oxygen; oxygen does not participate in this phase of aerobic respiration. Glycolysis produces very little energy—a net yield of only two molecules of ATP. Glycolysis takes place in the cytoplasm of both procaryotic and eucaryotic cells.

Krebs Cycle. The pyruvic acid molecules produced during glycolysis are converted into acetyl-CoA molecules, which then enter the Krebs cycle (Fig. 7-5).

The Krebs cycle is a biochemical pathway consisting of eight separate reactions, each of which is controlled by a different enzyme. In the first step of the Krebs cycle, acetyl-CoA combines with oxaloacetate to produce citric acid (a tricarboxylic acid); hence, the other names for the Krebs cycle—the citric acid cycle, the tricarboxylic acid cycle, and the TCA cycle. It is referred to as a cycle because at the end of the eight reactions, the biochemical pathway ends up back at its starting point—oxaloacetate. Only two ATP molecules are produced during the Krebs cycle, but a number of products (e.g., NADH, $FADH_2$, and hydrogen ions) that are formed during the Krebs cycle enter the electron transport chain. (NADH is the reduced form of nicotinamide-adenine dinucleotide or NAD, and $FADH_2$ is the reduced form of flavin-adenine dinucleotide or FAD.) In eucaryotic cells, the Krebs cycle and the electron transport chain are located within mitochondria. (Recall that mitochondria are referred to as "energy factories" or "power houses.") In procaryotic cells, both the Krebs cycle and the electron transport chain occur at the inner surface of the cell membrane.

Electron Transport Chain. As previously mentioned, certain of the products produced during the Krebs cycle enter the **electron transport chain** (also called the electron

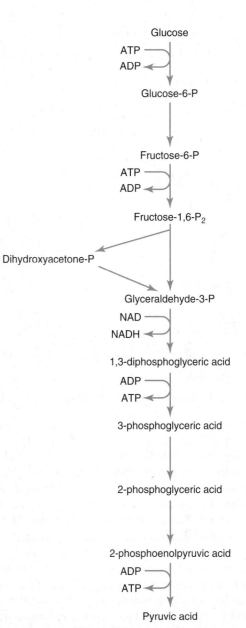

FIGURE 7-4. Glycolysis. Each of the compounds from glucose to fructose-1,6-P_2 contains six carbon atoms. Fructose-1,6-P_2 is broken into two three-carbon compounds: dihydroxyacetone-P and glyceraldehyde-3-P, each of which is ultimately transformed into a molecule of pyruvic acid. Thus, in glycolysis, one six-carbon molecule of glucose is converted to two three-carbon molecules of pyruvic acid. (See text for additional details.) (Volk WA, et al. Essentials of Medical Microbiology, 5th ed. Philadelphia: Lippincott-Raven, 1996.)

transport system or respiratory chain). The electron transport chain consists of a series of oxidation–reduction reactions (described in a subsequent section), whereby energy is released as electrons are transferred from one compound to another. These compounds include flavoproteins, quinones, nonheme iron proteins, and cytochromes. Oxygen is at the end of the chain; it is referred to as the final or terminal electron acceptor.

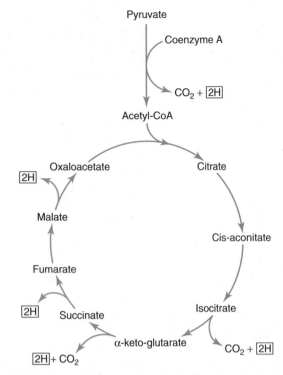

Pyruvate

Coenzyme A

CO_2 + $\boxed{2H}$

Acetyl-CoA

Oxaloacetate

$\boxed{2H}$

Citrate

Malate

Cis-aconitate

Fumarate

$\boxed{2H}$

Succinate

Isocitrate

α-keto-glutarate

$\boxed{2H}$ + CO_2

CO_2 + $\boxed{2H}$

FIGURE 7-5. The Krebs cycle. (See text for details.)

TABLE 7-3

Recap of the Number of ATP Molecules Produced From One Molecule of Glucose by Aerobic Respiration

	PROCARYOTIC CELLS	EUCARYOTIC CELLS
Glycolysis	2	2
Krebs cycle	2	2
Electron transport chain	32	34
Total ATP molecules	36	38

Many different enzymes are involved in the electron transport chain, including cytochrome oxidase (also called cytochrome *c*, or merely oxidase), the enzyme responsible for transferring electrons to oxygen, the final electron acceptor. In the clinical microbiology laboratory, the oxidase test is useful in the identification (speciation) of a Gram-negative bacillus that has been isolated from a clinical specimen. Whether or not the organism possesses oxidase is an important clue to the organism's identity.

During the electron transport chain, a large number of ATP molecules (32 in procaryotic cells and 34 in eucaryotic cells) are produced by a process known as oxidative phosphorylation. The net yield of ATP molecules from the catabolism of one glucose molecule by aerobic respiration is 36 (in procaryotic cells) or 38 (in eucaryotic cells; Table 7-3). That is a great deal of energy from one molecule of glucose! Aerobic respiration is a very efficient system. Aerobic respiration of glucose produces 18 times (procaryotic cells) or 19 times (eucaryotic cells) as much energy than does fermentation of glucose (discussed in a subsequent section).

The chemical equation representing aerobic respiration is:

$$C_6H_{12}O_6 + 6\,O_2 + 38\,ADP + 38\,\textcircled{P} \rightarrow 6\,H_2O + 6\,CO_2 + 38\,ATP$$

where $\textcircled{P}$ indicates an activated phosphate group.

The catabolism of glucose by aerobic respiration is just one of many ways in which cells can catabolize glucose molecules. How glucose is utilized by a cell depends on the individual organism, its available nutrient and energy resources, and the enzymes it is able to produce. Some bacteria degrade glucose to pyruvic acid by other metabolic pathways. Also, glycerol, fatty acids from lipids, and amino acids from protein digestion may enter the Krebs cycle to produce energy for the cell when necessary (i.e., when there are insufficient carbohydrates available).

Fermentation of Glucose

The first thing to note about **fermentation** reactions is that they do not involve oxygen; therefore, fermentations usually take place in anaerobic environments. The first step in the fermentation of glucose is glycolysis, which occurs exactly as previously described. Remember that glycolysis does not involve oxygen, and very little energy (two ATP molecules) is produced by glycolysis.

The next step in fermentation reactions is the conversion of pyruvic acid into an end product. The particular end product that is produced depends on the specific organism involved. The various end products of fermentation have many industrial applications. For example, certain yeasts (*Saccharomyces* spp.) and bacteria (*Zymomonas* spp.) convert pyruvic acid into ethyl alcohol (ethanol) and CO_2. Such yeasts are used to make wine, beer, other alcoholic beverages, and bread.

A group of Gram-positive bacteria, called lactic acid bacteria, convert pyruvic acid to lactic acid. These bacteria are used to make a variety of food products, including cheeses, yogurt, pickles, and cured sausages. In human muscle cells, the lack of oxygen during extreme exertion results in pyruvic acid being converted to lactic acid. The presence of lactic acid in muscle tissue is the cause of soreness that develops in exhausted muscles. Some oral bacteria (e.g., various *Streptococcus* spp.) convert glucose into lactic acid, which then eats away the enamel on our teeth, leading to tooth decay. The presence of lactic acid bacteria in milk causes the souring of milk into curd and whey.

Some bacteria convert pyruvic acid into propionic acid. *Propionibacterium* spp. are used in the production of Swiss cheese. The propionic acid they produce gives the cheese its characteristic flavor, and the CO_2 that is produced creates the holes. Other end products of fermentation include acetic acid, acetone, butanol, butyric acid, isopropanol, and succinic acid.

Fermentation reactions produce very little energy (approximately two ATP molecules); therefore, they are very inefficient ways to catabolize glucose. Aerobes and facultative anaerobes are much more efficient in energy production than obligate anaerobes because they are able to catabolize glucose via aerobic respiration.

Oxidation–Reduction (Redox) Reactions

Oxidation–reduction reactions are paired reactions in which electrons are transferred from one compound to another (Fig. 7-6). Whenever an atom, ion, or molecule loses one or more electrons (e^2) in a reaction, the process is called *oxidation,* and the molecule is said to be *oxidized.* The electrons that are lost do not float about at random but, because they are very reactive, attach immediately to another molecule. The resulting gain of one or more electrons by a molecule is called *reduction,* and the molecule is said to be *reduced.* Within the cell, an oxidation reaction is always paired (or coupled) with a reduction reaction, thus the term oxidation–reduction or "redox" reactions. In a redox reaction, the electron donor is referred to as the reducing agent and the electron acceptor is referred to as the oxidizing agent. Thus, in Figure 7-6, compound A is the reducing agent and compound B is the oxidizing agent.

As stated earlier, the electron transport chain consists of a series of oxidation–reduction reactions, whereby energy is released as electrons are transferred from one compound to another. Many biologic oxidations are referred to as *dehydrogenation reactions* because hydrogen ions (H^+) as well as electrons are removed. Concurrently, those hydrogen ions must be picked up in a reduction reaction. Many good illustrations are found in the aerobic respiration of glucose, in which the hydrogen ions released during the Krebs cycle enter the electron transport chain. (See "Insight: Why Anaerobes Die in the Presence of Oxygen" on the CD-ROM).

Anabolism

As previously stated, anabolism refers to all the *anabolic reactions* that are occurring in a cell. Anabolic reactions require energy because chemical bonds are being formed. It takes energy to create a chemical bond. Most of the energy required for anabolic reactions is provided by the catabolic reactions that are occurring simultaneously in the cell. Anabolic reactions are often referred to as biosynthetic reactions. Examples of anabolic reactions include creating a disaccharide from two monosaccharides by dehydration synthesis, the biosynthesis of polypeptides by linking amino acids molecules together, and the biosynthesis of nucleic acid molecules by linking nucleotides together.

Biosynthesis of Organic Compounds

The biosynthesis of organic compounds requires energy and may occur either through photosynthesis (biosynthesis using light energy) or **chemosynthesis** (biosynthesis using chemical energy).

Photosynthesis. In photosynthesis, light energy is converted to chemical energy in the form of chemical bonds. Phototrophs that use CO_2 as their carbon source are called photoautotrophs; examples are algae, plants, cyanobacteria, and certain other photosynthetic bacteria. Phototrophs that use small organic molecules, such as acids and alcohols, to build organic molecules are called photoheterotrophs; some types of bacteria are photoheterotrophs.

The goal of photosynthetic processes is to trap the radiant energy of light and convert it into chemical bond energy in ATP molecules and carbohydrates, particularly glucose, which can then be converted into more ATP molecules at a later time through aerobic respiration. Bacteria that produce oxygen by photosynthesis are called *oxygenic photosynthetic bacteria,* and the process is known as *oxygenic photosynthesis.* The oxygenic photosynthesis reaction is

$$6\,CO_2 + 12\,H_2O \xrightarrow[ATP]{light} C_6H_{12}O_6$$
$$+ 6\,O_2 + 6\,H_2O + ADP + \textcircled{P}$$

Note that this reaction is almost the reverse of the aerobic respiration reaction; it is nature's way of balancing substrates in the environment. In aerobic respiration, glucose and oxygen are ultimately converted into water and carbon dioxide. In oxygenic photosynthesis, water and carbon dioxide are converted into glucose and oxygen.

Photosynthetic reactions do not always produce oxygen. Purple sulfur bacteria and green sulfur bacteria (which are obligately anaerobic photoautotrophs) are referred to as *anoxygenic photosynthetic bacteria* because their photosynthetic processes do not produce oxygen (*anoxygenic photosynthesis*). These bacteria use sulfur, sulfur

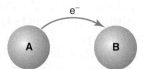

FIGURE 7-6. An oxidation–reduction reaction. In this illustration, an electron has been transferred from compound A to compound B. Two reactions have occurred simultaneously. Compound A has lost an electron (an oxidation reaction), and compound B has gained an electron (a reduction reaction). Oxidation is the loss of an electron. Reduction is the gain of an electron. Compound A has been oxidized, and compound B has been reduced. The term *reduction* relates to the fact that an electron has a negative charge. When compound B receives an electron, its electrical charge is reduced.

compounds (e.g., H_2S gas), or hydrogen gas to reduce CO_2, rather than H_2O.

Bacterial photosynthetic pigments use shorter wavelengths of light, which penetrate deep within a body of water or into mud where it appears to be dark. In the absence of light, some phototrophic organisms may survive anaerobically by the fermentation process alone. Other phototrophic bacteria also have a limited ability to use simple organic molecules in photosynthetic reactions; thus, they become photoheterotrophic organisms under certain conditions.

Chemosynthesis. The chemosynthetic process involves a chemical source of energy and raw materials for synthesis of the metabolites and macromolecules required for growth and function of the organisms. Chemotrophs that use CO_2 as their carbon source are called chemoautotrophs. Examples of chemoautotrophs are a few primitive types of bacteria. You will recall that some archaeans are methanogens; they are chemoautotrophs also. Methanogens produce methane in the following manner:

$$4\,H_2 + CO_2 \rightarrow CH_4 + 2\,H_2O$$

Chemotrophs that use organic molecules other than CO_2 as their carbon source are called chemoheterotrophs. Most bacteria, as well as all protozoa, fungi, animals, and humans, are chemoheterotrophs.

Bacterial Genetics

It would be impossible to discuss the genetics of all types of microorganisms in a book of this size. (Recall that some microbes are procaryotic and others are eucaryotic.) Therefore, the following discussion of bacterial genetics will serve as an introduction to the subject of microbial genetics.

Genetics—the study of heredity—involves many topics, some of which (e.g., DNA, genes, the genetic code, chromosomes, DNA replication, transcription, translation) have already been addressed in this book. The topics thus far discussed all relate to molecular genetics—genetics at the molecular level.

An organism's *genotype* (or genome) is its complete collection of genes, whereas an organism's **phenotype** is all the organism's physical traits, attributes, or characteristics. Phenotypic characteristics of humans include hair, eye, and skin color. Phenotypic characteristics of bacteria include the presence or absence of certain enzymes and such structures as capsules, flagella, and pili. An organism's phenotype is dictated by that organism's genotype. Phenotype is the manifestation of genotype. For example, an organism cannot produce a particular enzyme unless it possesses the gene that codes for that enzyme. It cannot produce flagella unless it possesses the genes necessary for flagella production.

Most bacteria possess one chromosome, which usually consists of a long, continuous (circular), double-stranded DNA molecule, with no protein on the outside (as is found in eucaryotic chromosomes). A particular segment of the chromosome constitutes a gene. The chromosome can be thought of as a circular strand of genes, all linked together—somewhat like a string of beads. Genes are the fundamental units of heredity that carry the information needed for the special characteristics of each different species of bacteria. Genes direct all functions of the cell, providing it with its own particular traits and individuality.

As you learned in Chapter 6, the information in a gene is used by the cell to make a mRNA molecule (via the process known as transcription). Then, the information in the mRNA molecule is used to make a *gene product* (via the process known as translation). Most gene products are proteins, but rRNA and tRNA molecules are also coded for by genes and, therefore, represent other types of gene products. When the information in a gene has been used by the cell to make a gene product, the gene coding for that particular gene product is said to have been *expressed*. All the genes on the chromosome are not being expressed at any given time. That would be a terrible waste of energy! For example, it would be pointless for a cell to produce a particular enzyme if that enzyme was not needed. Genes that are expressed at all times are called *constitutive genes*. Those that are expressed only when the gene products are needed are called *inducible genes*.

Because there is only one chromosome that replicates just before cell division, identical traits of a species are passed from the parent bacterium to the daughter cells after binary fission has occurred. DNA replication must precede binary fission to ensure that each daughter cell has exactly the same genetic composition as the parent cell.

Mutations

The DNA of any gene on the chromosome is subject to accidental alteration (e.g., the deletion of a base pair), which alters the gene product and perhaps also alters the trait that is controlled by that gene. If the change in the gene alters or eliminates a trait in such a way that the cell does not die or become incapable of division, the altered trait is transmitted to the daughter cells of each succeeding generation. A change in the characteristics of a cell caused by a change in the DNA molecule (genetic alteration) that is transmissible to the offspring is called a **mutation.** There are three categories of mutations: beneficial mutations, harmful (and sometimes lethal) mutations, and silent mutations.

Beneficial mutations, as the name implies, are of benefit to the organism. An example would be a mutation that enables the organism to survive in an environment where organisms without that mutation would die. Perhaps the mutation enables the organism to be resistant to a particular antibiotic.

An example of a **harmful mutation** would be a mutation that leads to the production of a nonfunctional enzyme. A nonfunctional enzyme is unable to catalyze the chemical reaction that it would normally catalyze if it were functional. If it happens to be an enzyme that catalyzes a metabolic reaction essential to the life of the cell, the cell will die. Thus, this is an example of a ***lethal mutation.*** Not all harmful mutations are lethal.

In all likelihood, most mutations are ***silent mutations*** (or neutral mutations), meaning that they have no effect on the cell. For example, if the mutation causes an incorrect amino acid to be placed near the center of a large, highly convoluted enzyme, composed of hundreds of amino acids, it is doubtful that the mutation would cause any change in the structure or function of that enzyme. If the mutation causes no change in function, it is considered silent.

Most likely, spontaneous mutations (random mutations that occur naturally) occur more or less constantly throughout a bacterial genome. However, some genes are more prone to spontaneous mutations than others. The rate at which spontaneous mutations occur is usually expressed in terms of the frequency at which a mutation will occur in a particular gene. This rate varies from one mutation every 10^4 (10,000) rounds of DNA replication to one mutation every 10^{12} (1 trillion) rounds of DNA replication. The average spontaneous mutation rate is about one mutation every 10^6 (1 million) rounds of DNA replication. In other words, the odds that a spontaneous mutation will occur in a particular gene are about 1 mutation per million cell divisions.

The mutation rate can be increased by exposing cells to physical or chemical agents that affect the chromosome. Such agents are called ***mutagens.*** In research laboratories, x-rays, ultraviolet light, and radioactive substances, as well as certain chemical agents, are used to increase the mutation rate of bacteria, thus causing more mutations to occur. The organism containing the mutation is called a ***mutant.*** Bacterial mutants are used in genetic and medical research and in the development of vaccines. The types of mutagenic changes frequently observed in bacteria involve cell shape, biochemical activities, nutritional needs, antigenic sites, colony characteristics, virulence, and drug resistance. Nonpathogenic "live" virus vaccines, such as the Sabin vaccine for polio, are examples of laboratory-induced mutations of pathogenic microorganisms.

STUDY AID

Ways in Which Bacteria Acquire New Genetic Information

Mutations (involve changes in the base sequences of genes)

Lysogenic conversion (involves bacteriophages and the acquisition of new viral genes)

Transduction (involves bacteriophages and the acquisition of new bacterial genes)

Transformation (involves the uptake of "naked" DNA)

Conjugation (involves the transfer of genetic information from one cell to another through a hollow sex pilus)

In a test procedure called the ***Ames test*** (developed by Bruce Ames in the 1960s), a mutant strain of *Salmonella* is used to learn whether a particular chemical (e.g., a food additive or a chemical used in some type of cosmetic product) is a mutagen. If exposure to the chemical causes a reversal of the organism's mutation (known as a back mutation), then the chemical has been shown to be mutagenic. If the chemical is mutagenic, then it might also be carcinogenic (cancer-causing) and should be tested using laboratory animals or cell cultures. Many substances found to be mutagenic by the Ames test have been shown to be carcinogenic in laboratory animals. Substances that are carcinogenic in laboratory animals might also be carcinogenic in humans.

Ways in Which Bacteria Acquire New Genetic Information

There are at least four additional ways that the genetic composition of bacteria can be changed: lysogenic conversion,

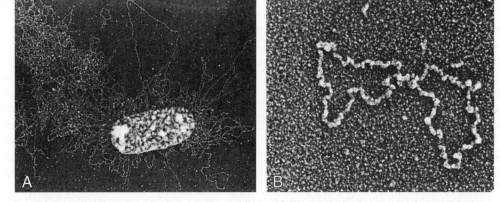

FIGURE 7-7. Plasmids. (*A*) Disrupted *Escherichia coli* cell. The DNA has spilled out and a plasmid can be seen slightly to the left of top center. (*B*) Enlargement of a plasmid, which is about 1 μm from side to side. (Volk WA, et al. Essentials of Medical Microbiology, 4th ed. Philadelphia: JB Lippincott, 1991.)

transduction, transformation, and conjugation. These are ways in which bacteria acquire new genetic information (i.e., acquire new genes). If the new genes remain in the cytoplasm of the cell, the DNA molecule on which they are located is called a *plasmid* (Fig. 7-7). Because they are not part of the chromosome, plasmids are referred to as extrachromosomal DNA. Many different types of plasmids have been discovered, and information about them all would fill many books. Some plasmids contain many genes, others only a few, but, in all cases, the cell is changed by the acquisition of these genes. Some plasmids replicate simultaneously with chromosomal DNA replication; others replicate independently at various other times. A plasmid that can exist either autonomously (by itself) or can integrate into the chromosome is referred to as an **episome.** Some plasmid genes can be expressed as extrachromosomal genes, but others must integrate into the chromosome before the genes become functional.

Lysogenic Conversion

As mentioned in Chapter 4, there are two categories of bacteriophages (phages): virulent phages and temperate phages. Virulent phages always cause the lytic cycle to occur, ending with the destruction (lysis) of the bacterial cell. Virulent phages are described in Chapter 4.

After *temperate phages* (also known as lysogenic phages) inject their DNA into the bacterial cell, the phage DNA integrates into (becomes part of) the bacterial chromosome but does not cause the lytic cycle to occur. This situation—in which the phage genome is present in the cell but is not causing the lytic cycle to occur—is known as **lysogeny.** During lysogeny, all that remains of the phage is its DNA; in this form, the phage is referred to as a **prophage.** The bacterial cell containing the prophage is referred to as a **lysogenic cell** or *lysogenic bacterium.* Each time a lysogenic cell undergoes binary fission, the phage DNA is replicated along with the bacterial DNA and is passed on to each of the daughter cells. Thus, the daughter cells are also lysogenic cells.

Although the prophage does not usually cause the lytic cycle to occur, certain events (e.g., exposure of the bacterial cell to ultraviolet light or certain chemicals) can trigger it to do so. While the prophage is integrated into the bacterial chromosome, the bacterial cell can produce gene products that are coded for by the prophage genes. The bacterial cell will exhibit new properties—a phenomenon known as **lysogenic conversion** (or *phage conversion*). In other words, the bacterial cell has been converted as a result of lysogeny and is now able to produce one or more gene products that it previously was unable to produce.

A medically related example of lysogenic conversion involves the disease diphtheria. Diphtheria is caused by a toxin—called diphtheria toxin—that is produced by a Gram-positive bacillus named *Corynebacterium diphtheriae.* Interestingly, the *C. diphtheriae* genome does not normally contain the gene that codes for diphtheria toxin. Only cells of *C. diphtheriae* that contain a prophage can produce

diphtheria toxin, because it is actually a phage gene (called the tox gene) that codes for the toxin. Strains of *C. diphtheriae* capable of producing diphtheria toxin are called *toxigenic strains,* and those unable to produce the toxin are called *nontoxigenic strains.* A nontoxigenic *C. diphtheriae* cell can be converted to a toxigenic cell as a result of lysogeny. As previously mentioned, conversion as a result of lysogeny is referred to as lysogenic conversion. The phage that infects *C. diphtheriae*—the phage having the tox gene in its genome—is called a corynebacteriophage.

Other medically related examples of lysogenic conversion involve *Streptococcus pyogenes, Clostridium botulinum,* and *Vibrio cholerae.* Only strains of *S. pyogenes* that carry a prophage are capable of producing erythrogenic toxin—the toxin that causes scarlet fever. Only strains of *C. botulinum* that carry a prophage can produce botulinal toxin, and only strains of *V. cholerae* that carry a prophage can produce cholera toxin. Thus, without being infected by bacteriophages, these bacteria could not cause scarlet fever, botulism, and cholera, respectively. A recap of bacteriophage terminology can be found in Table 7-4.

Transduction

Transduction also involves bacteriophages. Transduction means "to carry across." Some bacterial genetic material may be carried across from one bacterial cell to another by a bacterial virus. This phenomenon may occur after infection of a bacterial cell by a temperate bacteriophage. The viral DNA combines with the bacterial chromosome, becoming a prophage. If a stimulating chemical, heat, or ultraviolet light activates the prophage, it begins to produce new viruses via the production of phage DNA and proteins. As the chromosome disintegrates, small pieces of bacterial DNA may remain attached to the maturing phage DNA. During the assembly of the virus particles, one or more bacterial genes may be incorporated into some of the mature bacteriophages. When all the phages are released by cell lysis, they proceed to infect other cells, some injecting bacterial genes as well as viral genes. Thus, bacterial genes that are attached to the phage DNA are carried to new cells by the virus. Check this book's CD-ROM for "A Closer Look at Transduction."

Only small segments of DNA are transferred from cell to cell by transduction compared with the amount that can be transferred by transformation and conjugation.

Transformation

In **transformation,** a bacterial cell becomes genetically transformed after the uptake of DNA fragments ("naked DNA") from the environment. Transformation experiments, performed by Oswald Avery and his colleagues, proved that DNA is indeed the genetic material (see Historical Note on page 120). In those experiments, a DNA extract from encapsulated, pathogenic *Streptococcus pneumoniae* (referred to as *S. pneumoniae* type 1) was added to a broth culture of nonencapsulated, nonpathogenic *S. pneumoniae* (referred to as *S. pneumoniae* type 2). Thus, at the beginning of the

TABLE 7-4

Recap of Bacteriophage Terminology

TERM	MEANING
Bacteriophage (or phage)	A virus that infects bacteria
Lysogenic cell (or lysogenic bacterium)	A bacterial cell with bacteriophage DNA integrated into its chromosome
Lysogenic conversion	When a bacterial cell has acquired new phenotypic characteristics as a result of lysogeny
Lysogeny	When the bacteriophage DNA is integrated into the bacterial chromosome; the bacteriophage DNA replicates along with the chromosome
Lytic cycle	The sequence of events in the multiplication of a virulent bacteriophage; ends with lysis of the bacterial cell
Prophage	The name given to the bacteriophage when all that remains of it is its DNA, integrated into the bacterial chromosome
Temperate bacteriophage (or lysogenic bacteriophage)	A bacteriophage whose DNA integrates into the bacterial chromosome but does not cause the lytic cycle to occur
Virulent bacteriophage	A bacteriophage that always causes the lytic cycle to occur

experiment, there were no live encapsulated bacteria in the culture. After incubation, however, live type 1 (encapsulated) bacteria were recovered from the culture. How was that possible? The only possible explanation was that some of the live type 2 bacteria must have taken up (absorbed) some of the type 1 DNA from the broth. Type 2 bacteria that absorbed pieces of type 1 DNA containing the gene(s) for capsule production were now able to produce capsules. In other words, type 2 (nonencapsulated) bacteria were converted to type 1 (encapsulated) bacteria as a result of the uptake of the genes that code for capsule production.

Transformation is probably not widespread in nature. In the laboratory, it has been demonstrated to occur in several genera including *Bacillus, Escherichia, Haemophilus, Pseudomonas,* and *Neisseria.* Transformations have even been shown to occur between two different species (e.g., between *Staphylococcus* and *Streptococcus*). Extracellular pieces of DNA molecules can only penetrate the cell wall and cell membrane of certain bacteria. The ability to absorb naked DNA into the cell is referred to as **competence,** and bacteria capable of taking up naked DNA molecules are said to be **competent bacteria.**

Some competent bacterial cells have incorporated DNA fragments from certain animal viruses (e.g., cowpox), retaining the latent virus genes for long periods. This knowledge may have some importance in the study of viruses that remain latent in humans for many years before they finally cause disease, as may be the case in Parkinson's disease. These human virus genes may hide in the bacteria of the indigenous microflora until they are released to cause disease.

Conjugation

The transfer of genetic material by the process known as conjugation was discovered by Joshua Lederberg and Edward Tatum in 1946, while experimenting with *E. coli.* Conjugation involves a specialized type of pilus called a sex pilus (sometimes referred to as an F pilus). A bacterial cell (called the donor cell) possessing a sex pilus attaches by means of the sex pilus to another bacterial cell (called the recipient cell). Some genetic material (usually in the form of a plasmid) is then transferred through the hollow sex pilus from

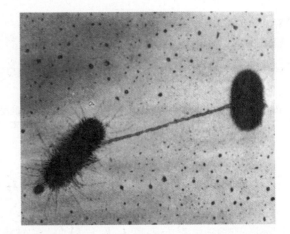

FIGURE 7-8. Conjugation in *Escherichia coli.* The donor cell (having numerous short pili) is connected to the recipient cell by a sex pilus. (Original magnification, 3,000×.) (Volk WA, et al. Essentials of Medical Microbiology, 5th ed. Philadelphia: Lippincott-Raven, 1996.)

of enteric, Gram-negative bacilli, but has been reported within species of *Pseudomonas* and *Streptococcus* as well. In electron micrographs, microbiologists have observed that sex pili are thicker and longer than other pili.

Although many different genes may be transferred by conjugation, the ones most frequently noted include those coding for antibiotic resistance, colicin (a protein produced by *E. coli* that kills certain other bacteria), and fertility factors (F^+ and Hfr^+), where F stands for fertility and Hfr stands for high frequency of recombination. Check this book's CD-ROM for "A Closer Look at Fertility Factors."

If a plasmid contains multiple genes for antibiotic resistance, the plasmid is referred to as a resistance factor or ***R-factor.*** A recipient cell that receives an R-factor becomes a multiply drug-resistant organism (referred to by the press as a "superbug"). Superbugs are discussed in detail in Chapter 9.

Transduction, transformation, and conjugation are excellent tools for mapping bacterial chromosomes and for studying bacterial and viral genetics. Although all these methods are frequently used in the laboratory, it is believed that they also occur in natural environments under certain circumstances.

the donor cell to the recipient cell (Fig. 7-8). Although conjugation has nothing to do with reproduction, the process is sometimes referred to as "bacterial mating," and the terms "male" and "female" cells are sometimes used in reference to the donor and recipient cells, respectively. This type of genetic recombination occurs mostly among species

Genetic Engineering

An array of techniques has been developed to transfer eucaryotic genes, particularly human genes, into other easily cultured cells to facilitate the large-scale production of important gene products (proteins, in most cases). This process is known as ***genetic engineering*** or recombinant DNA technology. Plasmids are frequently used as vectors or vehicles for inserting genes into cells. Bacteria, yeasts, human leukocytes, macrophages, and fibroblasts have been used as genetically engineered "manufacturing plants" for proteins such as human growth hormone (somatotropin), somatostatin (which inhibits the release of somatotropin), plasminogen-activating factor, insulin, and interferon. Somatostatin and insulin were first produced by recombinant DNA technology in 1978.

Many industrial and medical benefits may be derived from genetic engineering research. In agriculture, there is a potential for incorporating nitrogen-fixing capabilities into additional soil microorganisms; to make plants that are resistant to insects, as well as to bacterial and fungal diseases; and to increase the size and nutritional value of foods.

Genetically engineered microorganisms can also be used to clean up the environment (e.g., to get rid of toxic wastes). Consider this hypothetical example. A soil bacterium contains a gene that enables the organism to break oil down into harmless byproducts, but, because the organism cannot survive in salt water, it cannot be used to clean up oil spills at sea. Remove the gene from the soil bacterium, and, using a plasmid vector, insert it into a marine bacterium. Now the marine bacterium has the ability to break down oil and, in large numbers, can be used to clean up oil spills at sea.

In medicine, there is potential for making engineered antibodies, antibiotics, and drugs; for synthesizing important enzymes and hormones for treatment of inherited diseases; and for making vaccines. Such vaccines would contain only part of the pathogen (e.g., the capsid proteins of a virus) to which the person would form protective antibodies (see "Insight: Genetically Engineered Bacteria and Yeasts" on the CD-ROM).

Gene Therapy

Gene therapy of human diseases involves the insertion of a normal gene into cells to correct a specific genetic or acquired disorder that is being caused by a defective gene. The first gene therapy trials were conducted in the United States in 1990. Viral delivery is currently the most common method for inserting genes into cells, in which specific viruses are selected to target the DNA of specific cells. For example, a virus capable of infecting liver cells would be used to insert a therapeutic gene or genes into the DNA of liver cells. Viruses currently being used or considered for use as vectors include adenoviruses, retroviruses, adeno-associated virus, and herpesviruses. It is likely that genes will someday be regularly prescribed as "drugs" in the treatment of certain diseases (e.g., autoimmune diseases, sickle cell anemia, cancer, certain liver and lung diseases, cystic fibrosis, heart disease, hemoglobin defects, hemophilia, muscular dystrophy, and various immune deficiencies). In the future, synthetic vectors, rather than viruses, may be used to insert genes into cells.

REVIEW OF KEY POINTS

- Scientists have learned a great deal about cells—including human cells—by studying the nutritional needs of bacteria, their metabolic pathways, and why they live, grow, multiply, or die under certain conditions.

- All living organisms require sources of energy and carbon so that they can build the molecules necessary for life. In addition, organisms must be provided with certain materials (called essential nutrients) that they themselves are unable to synthesize but are required for survival; these essential nutrients vary from species to species.

- The energy source for certain organisms (called phototrophs) is light and for other organisms (called chemotrophs) is organic or inorganic chemicals. Chemolithotrophs (or simply lithotrophs) use inorganic chemicals as an energy source, whereas chemoorganotrophs (or simply organotrophs) use organic chemicals as an energy source.

- An organism's carbon source may be CO_2 (in which case the organism is called an autotroph) or other organic compounds (in which case the organism is called a heterotroph). Humans, animals, protozoa, and fungi are heterotrophs, as are most bacteria.

- Interrelationships among the different nutritional types are of prime importance in the functioning of the ecosystem. Phototrophs (plants, algae, and certain bacteria) are the producers of food and oxygen for the chemoheterotrophs (animals). Dead plants and animals are recycled by the chemoheterotrophic saprophytic decomposers (certain fungi and bacteria) into nutrients for phototrophs and chemotrophs.

- Metabolism refers to all the chemical reactions that occur within any cell, including the production of energy and the synthesis of new molecules; such reactions are regulated by enzymes.

- Metabolic reactions include catabolic reactions and anabolic reactions. Catabolic reactions (also called degradative reactions) involve the breaking of chemical bonds and the release of energy. Anabolic reactions (also called biosynthetic reactions) require energy because they involve the formation of chemical bonds.

- Enzymes are biologic molecules (proteins) that serve as catalysts to control the rate of metabolic reactions. The enzymes produced by any particular cell are governed by the genotype of that cell, and the presence or absence of any particular enzyme is part of the phenotype of that cell. All the enzymes that a cell is capable of producing need not be present in the cell at a given moment in time; they are produced to meet the metabolic needs of the cell as determined by the internal and external environments.

- An enzyme operates at peak efficiency within a particular pH and temperature range and when an appropriate concentration of the substrate for that enzyme exists. If the environment is too acidic, basic, hot, or cold, or contains too much or too little substrate, the enzyme will not operate at peak efficiency and the reaction will not proceed at its maximum rate.

- Adenosine triphosphate (ATP) is the principal energy-storing or energy-carrying molecule in the cell. Should a cell require energy, one of the high-energy bonds in an ATP molecule can be broken, producing energy, an ADP molecule, and a free phosphate. The energy can then be used for growth, reproduction, active transport of substances across membranes, sporulation, movement, anabolic reactions, and other energy-requiring activities.

- A common pathway by which bacteria catabolize glucose is aerobic respiration, which consists of three phases: glycolysis, the Krebs cycle, and the electron transport chain. Most of the energy that is produced by aerobic respiration is produced by the electron transport chain. The breakdown of one molecule of glucose by aerobic respiration yields either 36 ATP molecules (procaryotic cells) or 38 ATP molecules (eucaryotic cells).

- Aerobes and facultative anaerobes are able to produce more energy than anaerobes, because they can catabolize glucose molecules via aerobic pathways. Anaerobes must catabolize glucose by fermentation, a relatively inefficient method, that yields only two ATP molecules from a molecule of glucose.

- Phototrophic organisms (algae, plants, and photosynthetic bacteria) derive their energy from the sun by photosynthesis. Chemosynthetic organisms use a chemical source of energy and raw materials to synthesize metabolites and macromolecules for growth and function of the organisms.

- As with humans, animals, and plants, the genetics of microbes involves DNA, genes, the genetic code, chromosomes, DNA replication, transcription, and translation—all part of molecular genetics.

- The base sequence of any gene on a chromosome may be altered accidentally in many ways, resulting in a mutation. Mutations are expressed not only in the cell in which the mutation occurred, but in subsequent generations as well. The altered genetic code will result in an altered protein, which could affect any of a number of different phenotypic characteristics (e.g., changes in colony characteristics, cell shape, biochemical activities, nutritional needs, antigenic sites, virulence, pathogenicity, drug resistance). Mutant bacteria are used in genetic and medical research and the production of vaccines.

- Mutations may be beneficial, harmful, or of no consequence to the cell or organism containing the mutation. Those of no consequence are called silent or neutral mutations.

- In addition to mutations, genetic changes in a bacterial cell may be the result of lysogenic conversion, transduction, transformation, or conjugation, all of which occur in nature as well as in the laboratory.

- Lysogenic conversion and transduction involve bacteriophages. Transformation involves the uptake of naked DNA from the environment. Conjugation involves the transfer of genetic material (usually a plasmid) from a donor cell to a recipient cell through a hollow sex pilus.

- The field of genetic engineering involves the introduction of new genes into cells. When a cell receives a new gene, it can produce the gene product that is coded for by that gene. Genetically engineered bacteria are used to produce products such as insulin, interferon, human growth hormone, and materials for use as vaccines. Gene therapy involves the use of viruses and plasmids to introduce normal genes into cells that contain abnormal genes.

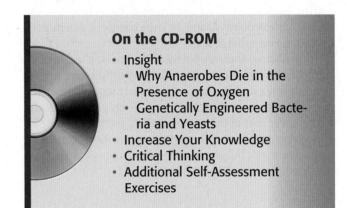

On the CD-ROM
- Insight
  - Why Anaerobes Die in the Presence of Oxygen
  - Genetically Engineered Bacteria and Yeasts
- Increase Your Knowledge
- Critical Thinking
- Additional Self-Assessment Exercises

SELF-ASSESSMENT EXERCISES

After studying this chapter, answer the following multiple-choice questions.

1. Which of the following characteristics do animals, fungi, and protozoa have in common?
   a. They obtain their carbon from carbon dioxide.
   b. They obtain their carbon from inorganic compounds.
   c. They obtain their energy and carbon atoms from chemicals.
   d. They obtain their energy from light.

2. Most ATP molecules are produced during which phase of aerobic respiration?
   a. electron transport chain
   b. fermentation
   c. glycolysis
   d. Krebs cycle

3. Which of the following processes does not involve bacteriophages?
   a. lysogenic conversion
   b. lytic cycle
   c. transduction
   d. transformation

4. In transduction, bacteria acquire new genetic information in the form of:
   a. bacterial genes.
   b. naked DNA.
   c. R-factors.
   d. viral genes.

5. The process whereby naked DNA is absorbed into a bacterial cell is known as:
   a. transcription.
   b. transduction.
   c. transformation.
   d. translation.

6. In lysogenic conversion, bacteria acquire new genetic information in the form of:
   a. bacterial genes.
   b. naked DNA.
   c. R-factors.
   d. viral genes.

7. Saprophytic fungi are able to digest organic molecules outside of the organism by means of:
   a. apoenzymes.
   b. coenzymes.
   c. endoenzymes.
   d. exoenzymes.

8. The process by which a nontoxigenic *Corynebacterium diphtheriae* cell is changed into a toxigenic cell is called:
   a. conjugation.
   b. lysogenic conversion.
   c. transduction.
   d. transformation.

9. Which of the following does (do) not occur in anaerobes?
   a. anabolic reactions
   b. catabolic reactions
   c. electron transport chain
   d. fermentation reactions

10. Proteins that must link up with a cofactor to function as an enzyme are called:
    a. apoenzymes.
    b. coenzymes.
    c. endoenzymes.
    d. holoenzymes.

8

CONTROLLING MICROBIAL GROWTH IN VITRO

LEARNING OBJECTIVES

AFTER STUDYING THIS CHAPTER, YOU SHOULD BE ABLE TO:

- List several factors that affect the growth of microorganisms
- Describe the following types of microorganisms: psychrophilic, mesophilic, thermophilic, halophilic, haloduric, alkaliphilic, acidophilic, and barophilic
- List three in vitro sites where microbial growth is encouraged
- Differentiate among enriched, selective, and differential media and cite two examples of each

- Explain the importance of using "sterile technique" in the microbiology laboratory
- Describe the three types of incubators that are used in the microbiology laboratory
- Draw a bacterial growth curve and label its four phases
- Cite two reasons why bacteria die during the death phase
- Name three ways in which obligate intracellular pathogens can be cultured in the laboratory
- List three in vitro sites where microbial growth must be inhibited
- Differentiate among sterilization, disinfection, and sanitization

- Differentiate between bactericidal and bacteriostatic agents
- Explain the processes of pasteurization and lyophilization
- List several physical methods used to inhibit the growth of microorganisms
- Cite three ways in which disinfectants kill microorganisms
- Identify several factors that can influence the effectiveness of disinfectants
- Explain briefly why the use of antibiotics in animal feed and household products is controversial

INTRODUCTION

In certain locations—such as within microbiology laboratories—the growth of microorganisms is encouraged; in other words, scientists *want* them to grow. In other locations—such as on hospital wards, in intensive care units, and in operating rooms—it is necessary to *inhibit* the growth of microorganisms. Both concepts—encouraging and inhibiting the in vitro growth of microorganisms—are discussed in this chapter. (Recall that in vitro refers to events outside the body, whereas in vivo refers to events inside the body.) Before discussing these concepts, however, various factors that affect the growth of microorganisms are examined.

Factors That Affect Microbial Growth

Microbial growth is affected by many different environmental factors, including the availability of nutrients and moisture, temperature, pH, osmotic pressure, barometric pressure, and composition of the atmosphere. These environmental factors affect microorganisms in our daily lives and play important roles in the control of microorganisms in laboratory, industrial, and hospital settings. Whether scientists wish to encourage or inhibit the growth of microorganisms, they must first understand the fundamental needs of microbes.

Availability of Nutrients

As discussed in Chapter 7, all living organisms require nutrients—the various chemical compounds that organisms use to sustain life. Therefore, to survive in a particular environment, appropriate nutrients must be available. Many nutrients are energy sources; organisms will obtain energy from these chemicals by breaking chemical bonds. Nutrients also serve as sources of carbon, oxygen, hydrogen, nitrogen, phosphorus, and sulfur as well as other elements (e.g., sodium, potassium, chlorine, magnesium, calcium, and trace elements such as iron, iodine, and zinc) that are

usually required in lesser amounts. About 25 of the 92 naturally occurring elements are essential to life.

Moisture

On earth, water is essential for life. Cells consist of anywhere between 70 and 95% water. All living organisms require water to carry out their normal metabolic processes, and most will die in environments containing too little moisture. There are certain microbial stages (e.g., bacterial endospores and protozoan cysts), however, that can survive the complete drying process (***desiccation***). The organisms contained within the spores and cysts are in a dormant or resting state; if they are placed in a moist, nutrient-rich environment, they will grow and reproduce normally.

Temperature

Every microorganism has an optimum growth temperature—the temperature at which the organism grows best. Every microorganism also has a minimum growth temperature, below which it ceases to grow, and a maximum growth temperature, above which it dies. The temperature range (i.e., the range of temperatures from the minimum growth temperature to the maximum growth temperature) at which an organism grows can differ greatly from one microbe to another. To a large extent, the temperature and pH ranges over which an organism grows best are determined by the enzymes present within the organism. As discussed in Chapter 7, enzymes have optimum temperature and pH ranges at which they operate at peak efficiency. If an organism's enzymes are operating at peak efficiency, the organism will be metabolizing and growing at its maximum rate.

Microorganisms that grow best at high temperatures are called ***thermophiles*** (meaning organisms that love heat). Thermophiles can be found in hot springs, compost pits, and silage as well as in and near hydrothermal vents at the bottom of the ocean (check this book's CD-ROM for "A Closer Look at Hydrothermal Vents"). Thermophilic cyanobacteria, certain other types of bacteria, and algae cause many of the colors observed in the near-boiling hot springs found in Yellowstone National Park. Organisms that favor temperatures above 100°C are referred to as hyperthermophiles (or extreme thermophiles). The highest temperature at which a bacterium has been found living is around 113°C; it was an archaean named *Pyrolobus fumarii.*

Microbes that grow best at moderate temperatures are called ***mesophiles.*** This group includes most of the species that grow on plants and animals and in warm soil and water. Most pathogens and members of the indigenous microflora are mesophilic, because they grow best at normal body temperature (37°C).

Psychrophiles prefer cold temperatures. They thrive in cold ocean water. At high altitudes, algae (often pink) can be seen living on snow. Ironically, the optimum growth temperature of one group of psychrophiles (called **psychrotrophs**) is refrigerator temperature (4°C); perhaps you encountered some of these microbes (bread molds, for example) the last time you cleaned out your refrigerator. Microorganisms that prefer warmer temperatures, but can tolerate or endure very cold temperatures and can be preserved in the frozen state, are known as **psychroduric organisms**. Fecal material left by early Arctic explorers contained psychroduric *Escherichia coli* that survived the Arctic temperatures. Refer to Table 8-1 for the temperature ranges of psychrophilic, mesophilic, and thermophilic bacteria.

pH

The term "pH" refers to the acidity or alkalinity of a solution (see CD-ROM Appendix 3: "Basic Chemistry Concepts"). Most microorganisms prefer a neutral or slightly alkaline growth medium (pH 7.0 to 7.4), but *acidophilic* microbes (**acidophiles**), such as those that can live in the stomach and in pickled foods, prefer a pH of 2 to 5. Fungi prefer acidic environments. Acidophiles thrive in highly acidic environments, such as those created by the production of sulfurous gases in hydrothermal vents and hot springs as well as in the debris produced from coal mining. **Alkaliphiles** prefer an alkaline environment (pH greater than 8.5), such as is found inside the intestine (pH of approximately 9.0), in soils laden with carbonate, and in so-called soda lakes. *Vibrio cholerae*—the causative agent of cholera—is the only human pathogen that grows well above pH 8.

Osmotic Pressure and Salinity

Osmotic pressure is the pressure that is exerted on a cell membrane by solutions both inside and outside the cell. When cells are suspended in a solution, the ideal situation is that the pressure inside the cell is equal to the pressure of the solution outside the cell. Substances dissolved in liquids are referred to as solutes. When the concentration of solutes in the environment outside of a cell is greater than the concentration of solutes inside the cell, the solution in which the cell is suspended is said to be **hypertonic.** In such a situation, whenever possible, water leaves the cell by osmosis in an attempt to equalize the two concentrations. **Osmosis** is defined as the movement of a solvent (e.g., water), through a permeable membrane, from a solution having a lower concentration of solute to a solution having a higher concentration of solute. If the cell is a human cell, such as a red blood cell (erythrocyte), the loss of water causes the cell to shrink; this shrinkage is called **crenation** and the cell is said to be **crenated.** If the cell is a bacterial cell, having a rigid cell wall, the cell does not shrink. Instead, the cell membrane and cytoplasm shrink away from the cell wall. This condition, known as **plasmolysis,** inhibits bacterial cell growth and multiplication. Salts and sugars are added to certain foods as a way of preserving them. Bacteria that enter such hypertonic environments will die as a result of desiccation.

When the concentration of solutes outside a cell is less than the concentration of solutes inside the cell, the solution in which the cell is suspended is said to be **hypotonic.** In such a situation, whenever possible, water enters the cell in an attempt to equalize the two concentrations. If the cell is a human cell, such as an erythrocyte, the increased water within the cell causes the cell to swell. If sufficient water enters, the cell will burst (lyse). In the case of erythrocytes, this bursting is called **hemolysis.** If a bacterial cell is placed in a hypotonic solution (such as distilled water), the cell may not burst (because of the rigid cell wall), but the fluid pressure within the cell increases greatly. This increased pressure occurs in cells having rigid cell walls such as plant cells and bacteria. If the pressure becomes so great that the cell ruptures, the escape of cytoplasm from the cell is referred to as **plasmoptysis.**

When the concentration of solutes outside a cell equals the concentration of solutes inside the cell, the solution is said to be **isotonic.** In an isotonic environment, excess

TABLE 8-1

Categories of Bacteria on the Basis of Growth Temperature

CATEGORY	MINIMUM GROWTH TEMPERATURE	OPTIMUM GROWTH TEMPERATURE	MAXIMUM GROWTH TEMPERATURE
Thermophiles	25°C	50°–60°C	113°C
Mesophiles	10°C	20°–40°C	45°C
Psychrophiles	–5°C	10°–20°C	30°C

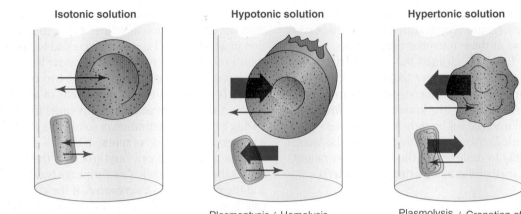

Isotonic solution	Hypotonic solution	Hypertonic solution
	Plasmoptysis / Hemolysis of bacteria / (red blood cell)	Plasmolysis / Crenation of of bacteria / red blood cell

FIGURE 8-1. Changes in osmotic pressure. No change in pressure occurs inside the cell in an isotonic solution. Internal pressure is increased in a hypotonic solution, resulting in swelling of the cell. Internal pressure is decreased in a hypertonic solution, resulting in shrinking of the cell. (Arrows indicate the direction of water flow. The larger the arrow, the greater the amount of water flowing in that direction.)

water neither leaves nor enters the cell and, thus, no plasmolysis or plasmoptysis occurs; the cell has normal turgor (fullness). Refer to Figure 8-1 for a comparison of the effects of various solution concentrations on bacteria and red blood cells.

Sugar solutions for jellies and pickling brines (salt solutions) for meats preserve these foods by inhibiting the growth of most microorganisms. However, some types of molds and bacteria can survive and even grow in a salty environment.

Those microbes that actually prefer salty environments (such as the concentrated salt water found in the Great Salt Lake and solar salt evaporation ponds) are called *halophilic,* *halo* referring to "salt" and *philic* meaning "to love." Microbes that live in the ocean, such as *V. cholerae* (mentioned earlier) and other *Vibrio* species, are halophilic. Organisms that do not prefer to live in salty environments but are capable of surviving there (such as *Staphylococcus aureus*) are referred to as **haloduric organisms.**

Barometric Pressure

Most bacteria are not affected by minor changes in barometric pressure. Some thrive at normal atmospheric pressure (about 14.7 pounds per square inch or psi). Others, known as **barophiles** (*baro,* referring to "pressure"), thrive deep in the ocean and in oil wells, where the atmospheric pressure is very high. Some archaeans, for example, are barophiles, capable of living in the deepest parts of the ocean. Check this book's CD-ROM for "A Closer Look at Barometric Pressure."

Gaseous Atmosphere

As discussed in Chapter 4, microorganisms vary with respect to the type of gaseous atmosphere that they require. For example, some microbes (obligate aerobes) prefer the same at-

mosphere that humans do (i.e., about 20 to 21% O_2 and 78 to 79% N_2, with all other atmospheric gases combined representing less than 1%). Although microaerophiles also require oxygen, they require reduced concentrations of oxygen (around 5% O_2). Obligate anaerobes are killed by the presence of oxygen. Thus, in nature, the types and concentrations of gases present in a particular environment determine which species of microbes are able to live there. To grow a particular microorganism in the laboratory, it is necessary to provide the atmosphere that it requires. For example, to obtain maximum growth in the laboratory, capnophiles require increased concentrations of carbon dioxide (usually from 5 to 10% CO_2).

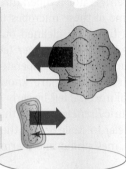

⊙ STUDY AID

-Phile

The suffix *-phile* means to love something. For example, acidophiles are organisms that love acidic conditions; therefore, they live in acidic environments. Alkaliphiles live in alkaline environments. Halophiles live in salty environments. Barophiles live in environments where there is high barometric pressure, such as at the bottom of the ocean. Thermophiles prefer hot temperatures. Mesophiles prefer moderate temperatures. Psychrophiles prefer cold temperatures. Microaerophiles live in environments containing reduced concentrations of oxygen (around 5% O_2). Capnophiles grow best in environments rich in carbon dioxide.

Encouraging the Growth of Microorganisms In Vitro

Introduction

There are many reasons why the growth of microorganisms is encouraged in microbiology laboratories. For example, technologists and technicians who work in clinical microbiology laboratories must be able to isolate microorganisms from clinical specimens and grow them on culture media so they can then gather information that will enable identification of any pathogens that are present. In microbiology research laboratories, scientists must culture microbes so that they can learn more about them, harvest antibiotics and other microbial products, test new antimicrobial agents, and produce vaccines. Microbes must also be cultured in genetic engineering laboratories and in the laboratories of certain food and beverage companies, as well as other industries.

Many different types of microorganisms can be cultured (grown) in vitro, including viruses, bacteria, fungi, and protozoa. In this chapter, emphasis is placed on culturing bacteria. Culturing other types of microorganisms will be mentioned only briefly.

Culturing Bacteria in the Laboratory

In many ways, modern microbiology laboratories resemble those of 50, 100, or even 150 years ago. Today's laboratories still use many of the same basic tools that were used in the past. For example, microbiologists still use compound light microscopes, Petri dishes containing solid culture media, tubes containing liquid culture media, Bunsen burners, wire inoculating loops, bottles of staining reagents, and incubators. However, a closer inspection will reveal many modern, commercially available products and instruments that would have been inconceivable in the days of Louis Pasteur and Robert Koch.

Bacterial Growth

"Human growth" refers to an increase in size; going from a tiny newborn baby to a large adult. Although bacteria do increase in size before cell division, "bacterial growth" refers to an increase in the number of organisms rather than an increase in their size. When each bacterial cell reaches its optimum size, it divides by binary fission (bi meaning "two") into two daughter cells (i.e., each bacterium simply splits in half to become two identical cells). (Recall from Chapter 3 that DNA replication must occur before binary fission occurs, so that each daughter cell has exactly the same genetic makeup as the parent cell.) On solid medium, binary fission continues through many generations until a colony is produced. A bacterial colony is a mound or pile of bacteria containing millions of cells. Binary fission continues for as long as the nutrient supply, water, and space allow and ends when the nutrients are depleted or the concentration of cellular waste products reaches a toxic level. The division of staphylococci by binary fission is shown in Figure 8-2.

The time it takes for one cell to become two cells by binary fission is called the *generation time.* The generation time varies from one bacterial species to another. In the laboratory, under ideal growth conditions, *E. coli, V. cholerae, Staphylococcus,* and *Streptococcus* all have a generation time of about 20 minutes, whereas some *Pseudomonas* and *Clostridium* species may divide every 10 minutes, and *Mycobacterium tuberculosis* may divide only every 18 to 24 hours. Bacteria with short generation times are referred to as rapid growers, whereas those with long generation times are referred to as slow growers.

The growth of microorganisms in the body, in nature, or in the laboratory is greatly influenced by temperature, pH, moisture content, available nutrients, and the characteristics of other organisms present. Therefore, the number of bacteria in nature fluctuates unpredictably because these factors vary with the seasons, rainfall, temperature, and time of day.

In the laboratory, however, a pure culture of a single species of bacteria can usually be maintained if the appropriate growth medium and environmental conditions are provided. The temperature, pH, and proper atmosphere are quite easily controlled to provide optimum conditions for growth. Appropriate nutrients must be provided in the growth medium, including an appropriate energy and carbon source. Some bacteria, described as being *fastidious,* have complex nutritional requirements. Often, special mixtures of vitamins and amino acids must be added to the medium to culture these fastidious organisms. Some organisms will not grow at all on artificial culture; these include obligate intracellular pathogens, such as viruses, rickettsias, and chlamydias. To propagate obligate intracellular pathogens in the laboratory, they must be inoculated into live animals, embryonated chicken eggs, or cell cultures. Other microorganisms that will not grow on artificial media include *Treponema pallidum* (the causative agent of syphilis) and *Mycobacterium leprae* (the causative agent of leprosy).

Culture Media

The media (sing., medium) that are used in microbiology laboratories to culture bacteria are referred to as **artificial media** or *synthetic media,* because they do not occur naturally; rather, they are prepared in the laboratory. There are a number of ways of categorizing the media that are used to culture bacteria.

One way to classify culture media is based on whether the exact contents of the media are known. A **chemically defined medium** is one in which all the ingredients are known; this is because the medium was prepared in the laboratory by adding a certain number of grams of each of the components (e.g., carbohydrates, amino acids, salts). A **complex medium** is one in which the exact contents are not

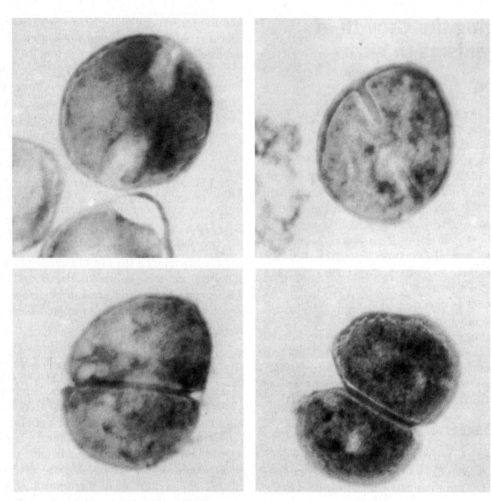

FIGURE 8-2. Binary fission of staphylococci. (Original magnification, 30,000×; photograph courtesy of Ray Rupel.)

known. Complex media contain ground up or digested extracts from animal organs (e.g., hearts, livers, brains), fish, yeasts, and plants, which provide the necessary nutrients, vitamins, and minerals.

Culture media can also be categorized as liquid or solid. Liquid media (also known as broths) are contained in tubes and are thus often referred to as tubed media. Solid media are prepared by adding agar to liquid media and then pouring the media into tubes or Petri dishes, where the media solidifies. Bacteria are then grown on the surface of the agar-containing solid media. Agar is a complex polysaccharide that is obtained from a red marine alga; it is used as a solidifying agent, much like gelatin is used as a solidifying agent in the kitchen.

An **enriched medium** is a broth or solid medium containing a rich supply of special nutrients that promotes the growth of fastidious organisms. It is usually prepared by adding extra nutrients to a medium called nutrient agar. Blood agar (nutrient agar plus 5% sheep red blood cells) and chocolate agar (nutrient agar plus powdered hemoglobin) are examples of solid enriched media that are used routinely in the clinical bacteriology laboratory. Blood agar is bright red, whereas chocolate agar is brown (the color of

chocolate). Although both of these media contain hemoglobin, chocolate agar is considered to be more enriched than blood agar because the hemoglobin is more readily accessible in chocolate agar. Chocolate agar is used to culture important, fastidious, bacterial pathogens, like *Neisseria gonorrhoeae* and *Haemophilus influenzae,* that will not grow on blood agar.

A **selective medium** has added inhibitors that discourage the growth of certain organisms without inhibiting growth of the organism being sought. For example, MacConkey agar inhibits growth of Gram-positive bacteria and thus is selective for Gram-negative bacteria. Phenylethyl alcohol (PEA) agar and colistin-nalidixic acid (CNA) agar inhibit growth of Gram-negative bacteria and thus are selective for Gram-positive bacteria. Thayer-Martin agar and Martin-Lewis agar (chocolate agars containing extra nutrients plus several antimicrobial agents) are selective for *Neisseria gonorrhoeae.* Only salt-tolerant (haloduric) bacteria can grow on mannitol salt agar (MSA).

A **differential medium** permits the differentiation of organisms that grow on the medium. For example, MacConkey agar is frequently used to differentiate among various Gram-negative bacilli that are isolated from fecal

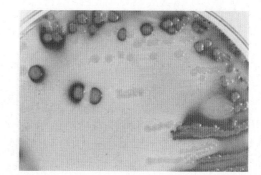

HISTORICAL NOTE

Culturing Bacteria in the Laboratory

The earliest successful attempts to culture microorganisms in a laboratory setting were made by Ferdinand Cohn (1872), Joseph Schroeter (1875), and Oscar Brefeld (1875). Robert Koch described his culture techniques in 1881. Initially, Koch used slices of boiled potatoes on which to culture bacteria, but he later developed both liquid and solid forms of artificial media. Gelatin was initially used as a solidifying agent in Koch's culture media, but in 1882, Fanny Hesse, the wife of Dr. Walther Hesse—one of Koch's assistants—suggested the use of agar. Frau Hesse (as she is most commonly called) had been using agar in her kitchen for many years as a solidifying agent in fruit and vegetable jellies. Another of Koch's assistants, Richard Julius Petri, invented glass Petri dishes in 1887 for use as containers for solid culture media and bacterial cultures. The Petri dishes in use today are virtually unchanged from the original design, except that most of today's laboratories use plastic, presterilized, disposable Petri dishes. In 1878, Joseph Lister became the first person to obtain a pure culture of a bacterium (*Streptococcus lactis*) in a liquid medium. As a result of their ability to obtain pure cultures of bacteria in their laboratories, Louis Pasteur and Robert Koch made significant contributions to the germ theory of disease.

FIGURE 8-3. Bacterial colonies on MacConkey agar, which is a selective and differential medium. It is selective for Gram-negative bacteria, meaning that only Gram-negative bacteria will grow on this medium. Colonies of lactose-fermenters (pink colonies) and nonlactose-fermenters (clear colonies) can be seen. (Koneman's Color Atlas and Textbook of Diagnostic Microbiology, 6th ed. Philadelphia: Lippincott Williams & Wilkins, 2006.)

seen, blood agar is enriched and differential. MacConkey agar and MSA are selective and differential. PEA and CNA are enriched and selective: they are blood agars to which selective inhibitory substances have been added. Thayer-Martin and Martin-Lewis agars are highly enriched and highly selective.

Thioglycollate broth (THIO) is a very popular liquid medium for use in the bacteriology laboratory. THIO supports the growth of all categories of bacteria from obligate aerobes to obligate anaerobes. How is this possible? Within the tube of THIO there is a concentration gradient of dissolved oxygen. The concentration of oxygen decreases with depth. The concentration of oxygen in the broth at the top of the tube is about 20 to 21%. At the bottom of the tube, there is no oxygen in the broth. Organisms will grow only in that part of the broth where the oxygen concentration meets their needs (Fig. 8-6). For example, microaerophiles will grow where there is around 5% oxygen, and obligate

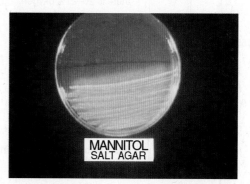

FIGURE 8-4. Mannitol-salt-agar, a selective and differential medium, is used to screen for *Staphylococcus aureus*. Any bacteria capable of growing in a 7.5% sodium chloride concentration will grow on this medium, but *S. aureus* will turn the medium yellow because of its ability to ferment the mannitol in the medium. The organism growing on the upper section of the plate is unable to ferment mannitol, but the organism growing on the lower section is a mannitol fermenter. (Koneman, et al. Color Atlas and Textbook of Diagnostic Microbiology, 5th ed. Philadelphia: Lippincott Williams & Wilkins, 1997.)

specimens. Gram-negative bacteria able to ferment lactose (an ingredient of MacConkey agar) produce pink colonies, whereas those unable to ferment lactose produce colorless colonies (Fig. 8-3). Thus, MacConkey agar differentiates between lactose-fermenting (LF) and nonlactose-fermenting (NLF) Gram-negative bacteria. Mannitol salt agar is used to screen for *Staphylococcus aureus;* not only will *S. aureus* grow on MSA, but it turns the originally pink medium to yellow because of its ability to ferment mannitol (Fig. 8-4). In a sense, blood agar is also a differential medium because it is used to determine the type of hemolysis (alteration or destruction of red blood cells) that the bacterial isolate produces (Fig. 8-5).

The various categories of media (enriched, selective, differential) are not mutually exclusive. For example, as just

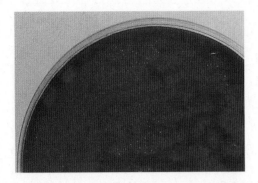

FIGURE 8-5. Colonies of a β-hemolytic *Streptococcus* species on a blood agar plate. The clear zones (β hemolysis) around the pinpoint, shiny colonies are caused by enzymes (hemolysins) that lyse the red blood cells in the agar. (Koneman's Color Atlas and Textbook of Diagnostic Microbiology, 6th ed. Philadelphia: Lippincott Williams & Wilkins, 2006.)

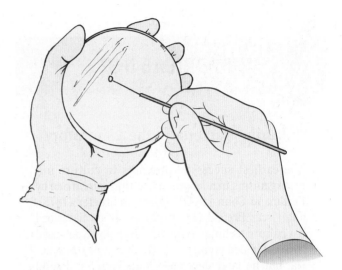

FIGURE 8-7. The proper method of inoculating an agar plate. The plate is held in the palm of one hand. The other hand is used to lightly drag the inoculating loop over the surface of the solid culture medium. The inoculating loop is held in much the same manner as a small camelhair paint brush is held by an artist when applying paint to the surface of a canvas.

anaerobes will only grow at the very bottom of the tube where there is no oxygen. Facultative anaerobes can grow anywhere in the tube. (Recall that facultative anaerobes can live in the presence or absence of oxygen.)

Inoculation of Culture Media

In clinical microbiology laboratories, culture media are routinely inoculated with clinical specimens (i.e., specimens that have been collected from patients suspected of having infectious diseases). **Inoculation** of a liquid medium involves adding a portion of the specimen to the medium.

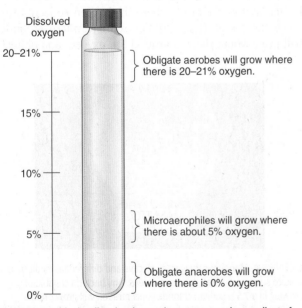

FIGURE 8-6. Thioglycollate broth contains a concentration gradient of dissolved oxygen, ranging from 20 to 21% O_2 at the top of the tube to 0% O_2 at the bottom of the tube. A particular bacterium will grow only in that part of the broth containing the concentration of oxygen that it requires.

Inoculation of a solid or plated medium involves the use of a sterile inoculating loop to apply a portion of the specimen to the surface of the medium; a process commonly referred to as "streaking" (Fig. 8-7). The proper method of inoculating plated media to obtain well-isolated colonies is described in CD-ROM Appendix 5: "Clinical Microbiology Laboratory Procedures."

Importance of Using "Sterile Technique"

Individuals working in a microbiology laboratory must practice what is known as **sterile technique,** and must understand its importance. Sterile technique is practiced when it is necessary to exclude <u>all</u> microorganisms from a particular area, so that the area will be sterile. For example, when inoculating plated media, it is important to keep the Petri dish lid in place at all times, except for the few seconds that it takes to inoculate the specimen to the surface of the culture medium. Every additional second that the lid is off provides an opportunity for airborne organisms (e.g., bacterial and fungal spores) to land on the surface of the medium, where they will then grow. Such unwanted organisms are referred to as **contaminants,** and the plate is said to be *contaminated*. Of equal importance is to maintain the sterility of the media before inoculation and to avoid touching the agar surface with fingertips or other nonsterile objects. Inoculating media within a biologic safety cabinet (BSC) minimizes the possibility of contamination and protects the laboratory worker from becoming infected with the organism(s) that he or she is working with. BSCs are further discussed in CD-ROM Appendix 4: "Responsibilities of the Clinical Microbiology Laboratory."

Incubation

After media are inoculated, they must be incubated (i.e., they must be placed into a chamber [called an *incubator*] that contains the appropriate atmosphere and moisture level and is set to maintain the appropriate temperature). This is called **incubation.** To culture most human pathogens, the incubator is set at 35° to 37°C. Three types of incubators are used in a clinical microbiology laboratory:

- A CO_2 (carbon dioxide) incubator is an incubator to which a cylinder of CO_2 is attached. CO_2 is periodically introduced into the incubator to maintain a CO_2 concentration of about 5 to 10%. Such an incubator is used to isolate capnophiles (organisms that grow best in atmospheres containing increased CO_2). It is important to keep in mind that a CO_2 incubator contains oxygen (about 15 to 20%) in addition to CO_2. Thus, a CO_2 incubator is *not* an anaerobic incubator.

- A non-CO_2 incubator is an incubator containing room air; thus, it contains about 20 to 21% O_2.

- An anaerobic incubator is an incubator containing an atmosphere devoid of oxygen.

Once a particular species of bacteria has been isolated from a clinical specimen, it can be separated from any other organisms that were present in the specimen and can be grown as a pure culture. The term *pure culture* refers to the fact that there is only one bacterial species present. The changes in a bacterial population over an extended period follow a definite predictable pattern that can be shown by plotting the population growth curve on a graph (discussed later in this chapter).

Bacterial Population Counts

Microbiologists sometimes need to know how many bacteria are present in a particular liquid at any given time (e.g., to determine the degree of bacterial contamination in drinking water, milk, and other foods). The microbiologist may (1) determine the total number of bacterial cells in the liquid (the total number would include both viable and dead cells) or (2) determine the number of viable (living) cells.

Various types of instruments are available to determine the total number of cells (e.g., a spectrophotometer could be used). In a spectrophotometer, a beam of light is passed through the liquid. When no bacteria are present in the liquid, the liquid is clear, and a large amount of light passes through. As bacteria increase in number, the liquid becomes turbid (cloudy), and less light passes through. Turbidity increases (i.e., the solution becomes more cloudy) as the number of organisms increases; therefore, the amount of transmitted light decreases as the bacteria increase in number. Formulas are available to equate the amount of transmitted light to the concentration of organisms in the liquid, which is usually expressed as the number of organisms per milliliter (mL) of suspension.

The *viable plate count* is used to determine the number of viable bacteria in a liquid sample, such as milk, water, ground food diluted in water, or a broth culture. In this procedure, serial dilutions of the sample are prepared, and then 0.1-mL or 1.0-mL aliquots (portions) are inoculated onto plates of nutrient agar. After overnight incubation, the number of colonies are counted. (Usually, a plate containing 30 to 300 colonies is used.) To determine the concentration of bacteria in the original sample, the number of colonies must be multiplied by the dilution factor(s). For example, if 220 colonies were counted on an agar plate that had been inoculated with a 1.0-mL sample of a 1:10,000 dilution, there were $220 \times 10,000 = 2,200,000$ bacteria/mL of the original material at the time the dilutions were made and cultured. If, however, 220 colonies were counted on an agar plate that had been inoculated with a 0.1-mL sample of a 1:10,000 dilution, there were $220 \times 10 \times 10,000 = 22,000,000$ bacteria/mL of the original material at the time the dilutions were made and cultured.

In the clinical microbiology laboratory, a viable cell count is an important part of a urine culture. (The technique is described in Chapter 13.) The number of viable bacteria per milliliter of a urine specimen is used as an indicator of a urinary tract infection (UTI). As explained in Chapter 13, high colony counts may also be caused by contamination of the urine specimen with indigenous microflora during specimen collection or failure to refrigerate the specimen between collection and transport to the laboratory.

Bacterial Population Growth Curve

A *population growth curve* for any particular species of bacterium may be determined by growing a pure culture of the organism in a liquid medium at a constant temperature. Samples of the culture are collected at fixed intervals (e.g., every 30 minutes), and the number of viable organisms in each sample is determined. The data are then plotted on logarithmic graph paper. The graph in Figure 8-8 was obtained by plotting the logarithm ($\log_{10}$) of the number of viable bacteria (on the vertical or y axis) against the incubation time (on the horizontal or x axis). (If you are not familiar with logarithms, refer to a math book.)

The growth curve consists of the following four phases.

1. The first phase of the growth curve is the *lag phase* (A in Fig. 8-8), during which the bacteria absorb nutrients, synthesize enzymes, and prepare for cell division. The bacteria do not increase in number during the lag phase.

2. The second phase of the growth curve is the *logarithmic growth phase* (also known as the **log phase** or exponential growth phase; B in Fig. 8-8). In the log phase, the bacteria multiply so rapidly that the number of organisms doubles with each generation time (i.e., the number of bacteria increases exponentially). Growth rate is the greatest during the log phase. The log phase is always brief, unless the rapidly dividing culture is

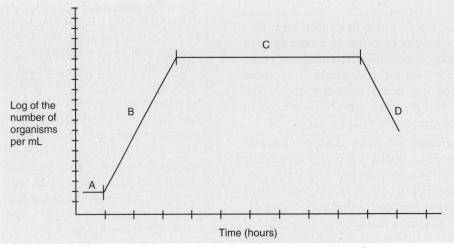

FIGURE 8-8. A population growth curve of living organisms. The logarithm of the number of bacteria per milliliter of medium is plotted against time. (*A*) Lag phase. (*B*) Logarithmic growth phase. (*C*) Stationary phase. (*D*) Death phase. (See text for details.)

maintained by constant addition of nutrients and frequent removal of waste products. When plotted on logarithmic graph paper, the log phase appears as a steeply sloped straight line.

3. As the nutrients in the liquid medium are used up and the concentration of toxic waste products from the metabolizing bacteria build up, the rate of division slows, such that the number of bacteria that are dividing equals the number that are dying. The result is the **stationary phase** (*C* in Fig. 8-8). It is during this phase that the culture is at its greatest population density.

4. As overcrowding occurs, the concentration of toxic waste products continues to increase and the nutrient supply decreases. The microorganisms then die at a rapid rate; this is the **death phase** or decline phase (*D* in Fig. 8-8). The culture may die completely, or a few microorganisms may continue to survive for months. If the bacterial species is a sporeformer, it will produce spores to survive beyond this phase. When cells are observed in old cultures of bacteria in the death phase, some of them look different from healthy organisms seen in the log phase. As a result of unfavorable conditions, morphologic changes in the cells may appear. Some cells undergo involution and assume a variety of shapes, becoming long, filamentous rods or branching or globular forms that are difficult to identify. Some develop without a cell wall and are referred to as protoplasts, spheroplasts, or L-phase variants (L-forms). When these involuted forms are inoculated into a fresh nutrient medium, they usually revert to the original shape of the healthy bacteria.

Many industrial and research procedures depend on the maintenance of an essential species of microorganism. These are continuously cultured in a controlled environment called a *chemostat* (Fig. 8-9), which regulates the supply of nutrients and the removal of waste products and excess microorganisms. Chemostats are used in industries

where yeast is grown to produce beer and wine, where fungi and bacteria are cultivated to produce antibiotics, where *E. coli* cells are grown for genetic research, and in any other process needing a constant source of microorganisms.

Culturing Obligate Intracellular Pathogens in the Laboratory

Recall from Chapter 4 that obligate intracellular pathogens are microorganisms that can only survive and multiply within living cells (called host cells). Obligate

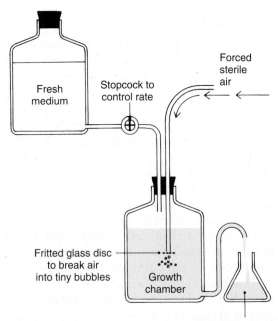

FIGURE 8-9. Chemostat used for continuous cultures. Rates of growth can be controlled either by controlling the rate at which new medium enters the growth chamber or by limiting a required growth factor in the medium.

intracellular pathogens include viruses and two groups of Gram-negative bacteria—rickettsias and chlamydias. Because obligate intracellular pathogens will not grow on artificial (synthetic) media, they present a challenge to laboratorians when large numbers of the organisms are required for diagnostic or research purposes (e.g., development of vaccines and new drugs). To grow such organisms in the laboratory, they must be inoculated into embryonated chicken eggs, laboratory animals, or cell cultures.

Culturing Fungi in the Laboratory

Fungi (including yeasts, molds, and dimorphic fungi) will grow on and in a variety of solid and liquid culture media. There is no one medium that is best for all medically important fungi. Examples of solid culture media used to grow fungi include brain heart infusion (BHI) agar, BHI agar with blood, and Sabouraud dextrose agar (SDA). Antibacterial agents are often added to the media to suppress the growth of bacteria. The low pH of SDA (pH 5.6) inhibits the growth of most bacteria; thus, SDA is selective for fungi. Laboratory personnel must exercise caution when culturing fungi, because the spores of certain fungi are highly infectious. A Class II biologic safety cabinet must be used.

Culturing Protozoa in the Laboratory

Most clinical microbiology laboratories do not culture protozoa, but techniques are available for culturing protozoa in reference and research laboratories. Examples of protozoa that can be cultured in vitro are amebae (e.g., *Acanthamoeba* spp., *Balamuthia* spp., *Entamoeba histolytica, Naegleria fowleri*), *Giardia lamblia, Leishmania* spp., *Toxoplasma gondii, Trichomonas vaginalis,* and *Trypanosoma cruzi.* Of these protozoa, it is of greatest importance to culture *Acanthamoeba, Balamuthia,* and *Naegleria fowleri* in a clinical microbiology laboratory. These amebae can cause serious (often fatal) infections of the central nervous system—infections that are difficult to diagnose by other methods. Parasitic protozoa are further discussed in Chapter 18.

Inhibiting the Growth of Microorganisms In Vitro

In certain environments, it is necessary or desirable to inhibit the growth of microbes. In hospitals, nursing homes, and other healthcare institutions, for example, it is necessary to inhibit the growth of pathogens so that they will not infect patients, staff members, or visitors. Other environments in which it is necessary or desirable to inhibit microbial growth include food and beverage processing plants, restaurants, kitchens, and bathrooms.

Definition of Terms

Before discussing the various methods used to destroy or inhibit the growth of microbes, a number of terms should be understood as they apply to microbiology.

Sterilization

Sterilization is the complete destruction of all microorganisms, including cells, spores, and viruses. When something is *sterile,* it is devoid of microbial life. Sterilization of objects can be accomplished by dry heat, autoclaving (steam under pressure), gas (ethylene oxide), various chemicals (such as formaldehyde), and certain types of radiation (e.g., ultraviolet light and gamma rays). These techniques are discussed later in this chapter.

Disinfection, Pasteurization, Disinfectants, Antiseptics, and Sanitization

Disinfection is the destruction or removal of pathogens from nonliving objects by physical or chemical methods. The heating process developed by Pasteur to kill microbes in wine—*pasteurization*—is a method of disinfecting liquids. Pasteurization is used today to eliminate pathogens from milk and most other beverages. It should be remembered that pasteurization is not a sterilization procedure, because not all microbes are destroyed.

Chemical agents are also used to eliminate pathogens. Chemicals used to disinfect inanimate objects, such as bedside equipment and operating rooms, are called ***disinfectants.*** Disinfectants are strong chemical substances that cannot be used on living tissue. ***Antiseptics*** are solutions used to disinfect skin and other living tissues. ***Sanitization*** is the reduction of microbial populations to levels considered safe by public health standards, such as those applied to restaurants.

Microbicidal Agents

The suffix *-cide* or *-cidal* refers to "killing," as in the words homicide and suicide. General terms like ***germicidal agents*** (*germicides*), ***biocidal agents*** (*biocides*), and ***microbicidal agents*** (*microbicides*) are disinfectants that kill microbes. ***Bactericidal agents*** (*bactericides*) are disinfectants that specifically kill bacteria but not necessarily bacterial endospores. Because spore coats are thick and resistant to the effects of many disinfectants, ***sporicidal agents*** are required to kill bacterial endospores. ***Fungicidal agents*** (*fungicides*) kill fungi, including fungal spores. ***Algicidal agents*** (*algicides*) are used to kill algae in swimming pools and hot tubs. ***Viricidal agents*** (or *virucidal agents*) destroy viruses. ***Pseudomonicidal agents*** kill *Pseudomonas* species, and ***tuberculocidal agents*** kill *M. tuberculosis.*

Microbistatic Agents

A ***microbistatic agent*** is a drug or chemical that inhibits growth and reproduction of microorganisms. A ***bacteriostatic agent*** is one that specifically inhibits the metabolism and reproduction of bacteria. Some of the drugs used to treat bacterial diseases are bacteriostatic, whereas others are bactericidal. Freeze-drying (lyophilization) and rapid freezing (using liquid nitrogen) are microbistatic techniques that are used to preserve microbes for future use or study.

Lyophilization is a process that combines dehydration (drying) and freezing. Lyophilized materials are frozen in a vacuum; the container is then sealed to maintain the inactive state. This freeze-drying method is widely used in industry to preserve foods, antibiotics, antisera, microorganisms, and other biologic materials. It should be remembered that lyophilization cannot be used to kill microorganisms, but, rather, is used to prevent them from reproducing and to store them for future use.

Sepsis, Asepsis, Aseptic Technique, Antisepsis, and Antiseptic Technique

Sepsis refers to the presence of pathogens in blood or tissues, whereas *asepsis* means the absence of pathogens. Various techniques, collectively referred to as *aseptic techniques,* are used to eliminate and exclude pathogens. Aseptic techniques include hand washing; the use of sterile gloves, masks, and gowns; sterilization of surgical instruments and other equipment; and the use of disinfectants, including antiseptics. *Antisepsis* is the prevention of infection. *Antiseptic technique,* developed by Joseph Lister in 1867, refers to the use of antiseptics. Antiseptic technique is a type of aseptic technique. Lister used dilute carbolic acid (phenol) to cleanse surgical wounds and equipment and a carbolic acid aerosol to prevent harmful microorganisms from entering the surgical field or contaminating the patient.

Sterile Technique

Sterile technique is practiced when it is necessary to exclude <u>all</u> microorganisms from a particular area, so that the area will be sterile. Earlier in this chapter, you learned of the importance of using sterile technique in the microbiology laboratory when inoculating culture media. In Chapter 12, you will learn how sterile technique is used in other areas of the hospital (e.g., in the operating room).

Using Physical Methods to Inhibit Microbial Growth

The methods used to destroy or inhibit microbial life are either physical or chemical, and sometimes both types are used. The physical methods commonly used in hospitals, clinics, and laboratories to destroy or control pathogens include heat, the combination of heat and pressure, desiccation, radiation, sonic disruption, and filtration.

Heat

Heat is the most practical, efficient, and inexpensive method of sterilization of those inanimate objects and materials that can withstand high temperatures. Because of these advantages, it is the means most frequently used.

Two factors — *temperature* and *time* — determine the effectiveness of heat for sterilization. There is considerable variation from organism to organism in their susceptibility to heat; pathogens usually are more susceptible than nonpathogens. Also, the higher the temperature, the shorter the time required to kill the organisms. The *thermal death point* (TDP) of any particular species of microorganism is the lowest temperature that will kill all the organisms in a standardized pure culture within a specified period. The *thermal death time* (TDT) is the length of time necessary to sterilize a pure culture at a specified temperature.

In practical applications of heat for sterilization, one must consider the material in which a mixture of microorganisms and their spores may be found. Pus, feces, vomitus, mucus, and blood contain proteins that serve as a protective coating to insulate the pathogens; when these substances are present on bedding, bandages, surgical instruments, and syringes, very high temperatures are required to destroy vegetative (growing) microorganisms and spores. In practice, the most effective procedure is to wash away the protein debris with strong soap, hot water, and a disinfectant, and then sterilize the equipment or materials with heat.

Dry Heat. Dry heat baking in a thermostatically controlled oven provides effective sterilization of metals, glassware, some powders, oils, and waxes. These items must be baked at 160° to 165°C for 2 hours or at 170° to 180°C for 1 hour. An ordinary oven of the type found in most homes may be used if the temperature remains constant. The effectiveness of dry heat sterilization depends on how deeply the heat penetrates throughout the material, and the items to be baked must be positioned so that the hot air circulates freely among them.

Incineration (burning) is an effective means of destroying contaminated disposable materials. An incinerator must never be overloaded with moist or protein-laden materials, such as feces, vomitus, or pus, because the contaminating microorganisms within these moist substances may not be destroyed if the heat does not readily penetrate and burn them. Flaming the surface of metal forceps and wire bacteriologic loops is an effective way to kill microorganisms and, for many years, was a common laboratory procedure. Flaming is accomplished by briefly holding the end of the loop or forceps in the yellow portion of a gas flame (Fig. 8-10). Open flames are dangerous, however, and, for this reason, are rarely used in modern microbiology laboratories, in which sterile, disposable, plastic inoculating loops are primarily used. Today, whenever wire inoculating loops are used, heat sterilization is usually accomplished using electrical heating devices (Fig. 8-10).

Moist Heat. Heat applied in the presence of moisture, as in boiling or steaming, is faster and more effective than dry heat, and can be accomplished at a lower temperature; thus, it is less destructive to many materials that otherwise would be damaged at higher temperatures. Moist heat causes proteins to coagulate (as occurs when eggs are hard

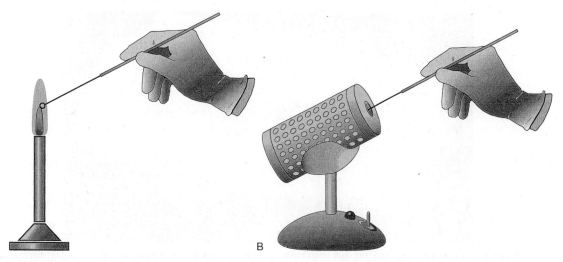

FIGURE 8-10. Dry heat sterilization. (*A*) Flaming a wire inoculating loop in a Bunsen burner flame. (*B*) Sterilizing a wire inoculating loop using an electrical heating device.

boiled). Because cellular enzymes are proteins, they are inactivated by moist heat, leading to cell death.

The vegetative forms of most pathogens are quite easily destroyed by boiling for 30 minutes. Thus, clean articles made of metal and glass, such as syringes, needles, and simple instruments, may be disinfected by boiling for 30 minutes. Because the temperature at which water boils is lower at higher altitudes, water should always be boiled for longer times at high altitudes. Boiling is not always effective, however, because heat-resistant bacterial endospores, mycobacteria, and viruses may be present. The endospores of the bacteria that cause anthrax, tetanus, gas gangrene, and botulism, as well as hepatitis viruses, are especially heat resistant and often survive boiling. Also, because thermophiles thrive at high temperatures, boiling is not an effective means of killing them.

An **autoclave** is like a large metal pressure cooker that uses steam under pressure to completely destroy all microbial life (Fig. 8-11). The increased pressure raises the temperature above the temperature of boiling water (i.e., above 100°C), and forces the steam into the materials being sterilized. Autoclaving at a pressure of 15 pounds per square inch (psi), at a temperature of 121.5°C, for 20 minutes, kills vegetative microorganisms, bacterial endospores, and viruses, as long as they are not protected by pus, feces, vomitus, blood, or other proteinaceous substances. Some types of equipment and certain materials, such as rubber, which may be damaged by high temperatures, can be autoclaved at lower temperatures for longer periods. The timing must be carefully determined based on the contents and compactness of the load. All articles must be properly packaged and arranged within the autoclave to allow steam to penetrate each package completely. Cans should remain open, bottles covered loosely with foil or cotton, and instruments wrapped in cloth. Sealed containers should not be autoclaved. Pressure-sensitive autoclave tape (Fig. 8-12) and

commercially available strips or solutions containing bacterial spores can be used as quality control measures to ensure that autoclaves are functioning properly. After autoclaving, the spores are tested to see whether they were killed.

Home canning conducted without the use of a pressure cooker does not destroy the endospores of bacteria—notably the anaerobe, *Clostridium botulinum*. Occasionally, local newspapers report cases of food poisoning resulting from the ingestion of *C. botulinum* toxins in improperly canned fruits, vegetables, and meats. Botulism food poisoning is preventable by properly washing and pressure cooking (autoclaving) food.

An effective way to disinfect clothing, bedding, and dishes is to use hot water (greater than 60°C) with deter-

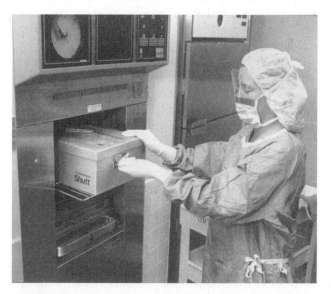

FIGURE 8-11. A large, built-in autoclave. (Photograph courtesy of Dr. Janet Duben-Engelkirk and Scott & White Hospital, Temple, TX.)

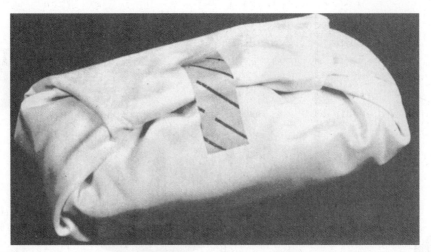

FIGURE 8-12. Pressure-sensitive autoclave tape showing dark stripes after sterilization. (Volk WA, et al. Essentials of Medical Microbiology, 4th ed. Philadelphia: JB Lippincott, 1991.)

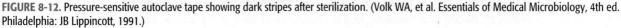

gent or soap and to agitate the solution around the items. This combination of heat, mechanical action, and chemical inhibition is deadly to most pathogens.

Cold

Most microorganisms are not killed by cold temperatures and freezing, but their metabolic activities are slowed, greatly inhibiting their growth. Refrigeration merely slows the growth of most microorganisms; it does not completely inhibit growth. Slow freezing causes ice crystals to form within cells and may rupture the cell membranes and cell walls of some bacteria; hence, slow freezing should not be used as a way to preserve or store bacteria. Rapid freezing, using liquid nitrogen, is a good way to preserve foods, biologic specimens, and bacterial cultures. It places bacteria into a state of suspended animation. Then, when the temperature is raised above the freezing point, the organisms' metabolic reactions speed up and the organisms begin to reproduce again.

Persons who are involved in the preparation and preservation of foods must be aware that thawing foods allows bacterial spores in the foods to germinate and microorganisms to resume growth. Consequently, refreezing of thawed foods is an unsafe practice, because it preserves the millions of microbes that might be present, leading to rapid deterioration of the food when it is rethawed. Also, if the endospores of *C. botulinum* or *Clostridium perfringens* were present, the viable bacteria would begin to produce the toxins that cause food poisoning.

Desiccation

For many centuries, foods have been preserved by drying. However, even when moisture and nutrients are lacking, many dried microorganisms remain viable, although they cannot reproduce. Foods, antisera, toxins, antitoxins, antibiotics, and pure cultures of microorganisms are of-ten preserved by lyophilization (freeze-drying; discussed previously).

In the hospital or clinical environment, healthcare professionals should keep in mind that dried viable pathogens may be present in dried matter, including blood, pus, fecal material, and dust that are found on floors, in bedding, on clothing, and in wound dressings. Should these dried materials be disturbed, such as by dry dusting, the microbes would be easily transmitted through the air or by contact. They would then grow rapidly if they settled in a suitable moist, warm nutrient environment such as a wound or a burn. Therefore, important precautions that must be observed include wet mopping of floors, damp dusting of furniture, rolling bed linens and towels carefully, and proper disposal of wound dressings.

Radiation

The sun is not a particularly reliable disinfecting agent because it kills only those microorganisms that are exposed to direct sunlight. The rays of the sun include the long infrared (heat) rays, the visible light rays, and the shorter ultraviolet (UV) rays. The UV rays, which do not penetrate glass and building materials, are effective only in the air and on surfaces. They do, however, penetrate cells and, thus, can cause damage to DNA. When this occurs, genes may be so severely damaged that the cell dies (especially unicellular microorganisms) or is drastically changed.

In practice, a UV lamp (often called a germicidal lamp) is useful for reducing the number of microorganisms in the air. Its main component is a low-pressure mercury vapor tube. Such lamps are found in newborn nurseries, operating rooms, elevators, entryways, cafeterias, and classrooms, where they are incorporated into louvered ceiling fixtures designed to radiate UV light across the top of the room without striking people in the room. Sterility may also be maintained by having a UV lamp placed in a hood or cabinet containing instruments, paper and cloth equipment, liquid, and other inanimate articles. Many biologic materials, such as sera, antisera, toxins, and vaccines, are sterilized with UV rays.

Those whose work involves the use of UV lamps must be particularly careful not to expose their eyes or skin to the rays, because they can cause serious burns and cellular damage. Because UV rays do not penetrate cloth, metals, and glass, these materials may be used to protect persons working in a UV environment. It has been shown that skin cancer can be caused by excessive exposure to the UV rays of the sun; thus, extensive suntanning is harmful.

X-rays and gamma and beta rays of certain wavelengths from radioactive materials may be lethal or cause mutations in microorganisms and tissue cells because they damage DNA and proteins within those cells. Studies performed in radiation research laboratories have demonstrated that these radiations can be used for the prevention of food spoilage, sterilization of heat-sensitive surgical equipment, preparation of vaccines, and treatment of some chronic diseases such as cancer, all of which are very practical applications for laboratory research. The U.S. Food and Drug Administration (FDA) approved the use of gamma rays (from cobalt-60) to process chickens and red meat in 1992 and 1997, respectively. Since then, gamma rays have been used by some food processing plants to kill pathogens (like *Salmonella* and *Campylobacter* spp.) in chickens; the chickens are labeled "irradiated" and marked with the green international symbol for radiation.

Ultrasonic Waves

In hospitals, medical clinics, and dental clinics, ultrasonic waves are a frequently used means of cleaning and sterilizing delicate equipment. Ultrasonic cleaners consist of tanks filled with liquid solvent (usually water); the short sound waves are then passed through the liquid. The sound waves mechanically dislodge organic debris on instruments and glassware. Glassware and other articles that have been cleansed in ultrasonic equipment must be washed to remove the dislodged particles and solvent and are then sterilized by another method before they are used.

Filtration

Filters of various pore sizes are used to filter or separate cells, larger viruses, bacteria, and certain other microorganisms from the liquids or gases in which they are suspended. Filters with tiny pore sizes (called micropore filters) are used in laboratories to filter bacteria and viruses out of liquids. The variety of filters is large and includes sintered glass (in which uniform particles of glass are fused), plastic films, unglazed porcelain, asbestos, diatomaceous earth, and cellulose membrane filters. Small quantities of liquid can be filtered through a filter-containing syringe, but large quantities require larger apparatuses.

A cotton plug in a test tube, flask, or pipette is a good filter for preventing the entry of microorganisms. Dry gauze

and paper masks prevent the outward passage of microbes from the mouth and nose, at the same time protecting the wearer from inhaling airborne pathogens and foreign particles that could damage the lungs. Biologic safety cabinets contain high-efficiency particulate air (HEPA) filters to protect workers from contamination. HEPA filters are also located in operating rooms and patient rooms to filter the air that enters or exits the room.

Gaseous Atmosphere

In limited situations, it is possible to inhibit growth of microorganisms by altering the atmosphere in which they are located. Because aerobes and microaerophiles require oxygen, they can be killed by placing them into an atmosphere devoid of oxygen or by removing oxygen from the environment in which they are living. Conversely, obligate anaerobes can be killed by placing them into an atmosphere containing oxygen or by adding oxygen to the environment in which they are living. For instance, wounds likely to contain anaerobes are lanced (opened) to expose them to oxygen. Another example is gas gangrene, a deep wound infection that causes rapid destruction of tissues. Gas gangrene is caused by various anaerobes in the genus *Clostridium*. In addition to debridement of the wound (removal of necrotic tissue) and the use of antibiotics, gas gangrene can be treated by placing the patient in a hyperbaric (increased pressure) oxygen chamber or in a room with high oxygen pressure. Because of the pressure, oxygen is forced into the wound, providing oxygen to the oxygen-starved tissue and killing the clostridia.

Using Chemical Agents to Inhibit Microbial Growth

Disinfectants

Chemical disinfection refers to the use of chemical agents to inhibit the growth of pathogens, either temporarily or permanently. The mechanism by which various disinfectants kill cells varies from one type of disinfectant to another. Various factors affect the efficiency or effectiveness of a disinfectant (Fig. 8-13), and these factors must be taken into consideration whenever a disinfectant is used. These factors include the following:

- Prior cleaning of the object or surface to be disinfected
- The organic load that is present, meaning the presence of organic matter (e.g., feces, blood, vomitus, pus) on the materials being treated
- The bioburden, meaning the type and level of microbial contamination
- The concentration of the disinfectant
- The contact time, meaning the amount of time that the disinfectant must remain in contact with the organisms in order to kill them (see this book's CD-ROM for "A Closer Look at Contact Time")

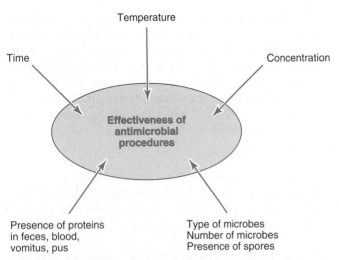

FIGURE 8-13. Factors that determine the effectiveness of any antimicrobial procedure: time, temperature, concentration, the type and number of microbes present, the presence of spores, and the presence of proteinaceous materials.

- The physical nature of the object being disinfected (e.g., smooth or rough surface, crevices, hinges)

- Temperature and pH

Directions for preparing the proper dilution of a disinfectant must be followed carefully, because too weak or too strong a concentration is usually less effective than the proper concentration. (Information about preparing dilutions can be found on this book's CD-ROM.) The items to be disinfected must first be washed to remove any proteinaceous material in which pathogens may be hidden. Although the washed article may then be clean, it is not safe to use until it has been properly disinfected. Healthcare personnel need to understand an important limitation of chemical disinfection—that many disinfectants that are effective against pathogens in the controlled conditions of the laboratory may be ineffective in the actual hospital or clinical environment. Furthermore, the stronger and more effective antimicrobial chemical agents are of limited usefulness because of their destructiveness to human tissues and certain other substances.

Almost all bacteria in the vegetative state, as well as fungi, protozoa, and most viruses, are susceptible to many disinfectants, although the mycobacteria that cause tuberculosis and leprosy, bacterial endospores, pseudomonads (*Pseudomonas* spp.), fungal spores, and hepatitis viruses are notably resistant. Therefore, chemical disinfection should never be attempted when it is possible to use proper physical sterilization techniques.

The disinfectant most effective for each situation must be chosen carefully. Chemical agents used to disinfect respiratory therapy equipment and thermometers must destroy all pathogenic bacteria, fungi, and viruses that may be found in sputum and saliva. One must be particularly aware of the oral and respiratory pathogens, including *M. tuberculosis*; species of *Pseudomonas, Staphylococcus*, and *Streptococcus*; the various fungi that cause candidiasis, blastomycosis, coccidioidomycosis, and histoplasmosis; and all respiratory viruses.

Because most disinfection methods do not destroy all bacterial endospores that are present, any instrument or dressing used in the treatment of an infected wound or a disease caused by sporeformers must be autoclaved or incinerated. Gas gangrene, tetanus, and anthrax are examples of diseases caused by sporeformers that require the healthcare worker to take such precautions. Formaldehyde and ethylene oxide, when properly used, are highly destructive to spores, mycobacteria, and viruses. Certain articles are heat sensitive and cannot be autoclaved or safely washed before disinfection; such articles are soaked for 24 hours in a strong detergent and disinfectant solution, washed, and then sterilized in an ethylene oxide autoclave. The use of disposable equipment whenever possible in these situations helps to protect patients and healthcare personnel.

The effectiveness of a chemical agent depends to some extent on the physical characteristics of the article on which it is used. A smooth, hard surface is readily disinfected, whereas a rough, porous, or grooved surface is not. Thought must be given to selection of the most suitable germicide for cleaning patient rooms and all other areas where patients are treated.

The most effective antiseptic or disinfectant should be chosen for the specific purpose, environment, and pathogen or pathogens likely to be present. The characteristics of an ideal chemical antimicrobial agent include the following:

- It should have a wide or broad antimicrobial spectrum, meaning that it should kill a wide variety of microorganisms

- It should be fast-acting, meaning that the contact time should be short

- It should not be affected by the presence of organic matter

- It must be nontoxic to human tissues and noncorrosive and nondestructive to materials on which it is used (for instance, if a tincture [e.g., alcohol–water solution] is being used, evaporation of the alcohol solvent can cause a 1% solution to increase to a 10% solution, and at this concentration, it may cause tissue damage)

- It should leave a residual antimicrobial film on the treated surface

- It must be soluble in water and easy to apply

- It should be inexpensive and easy to prepare, with simple, specific directions

- It must be stable both as a concentrate and as a working dilution, so that it can be shipped and stored for reasonable periods

- It should be odorless

How do disinfectants kill microorganisms? Some disinfectants (e.g., surface-active soaps and detergents, alcohols, and phenolic compounds) target and destroy cell membranes. Others (e.g., halogens, hydrogen peroxide, salts of heavy metals, formaldehyde, and ethylene oxide) destroy enzymes and structural proteins. Others attack cell walls or nucleic acids. Some of the disinfectants that are commonly used in hospitals are discussed in Chapter 12.

The effectiveness of phenol as a disinfectant was demonstrated by Joseph Lister in 1867, when it was used to reduce the incidence of infections after surgical procedures. The effectiveness of other disinfectants is compared with that of phenol using the *phenol coefficient test*. To perform this test, a series of dilutions of phenol and the experimental disinfectant are inoculated with the test bacteria, *Salmonella typhi* and *Staphylococcus aureus,* at 37°C. The highest dilutions (lowest concentrations) that kill the bacteria after 10 minutes are used to calculate the phenol coefficient.

Antiseptics

Most antimicrobial chemical agents are too irritating and destructive to be applied to mucous membranes and skin. Those that may be used safely on human tissues are called antiseptics. An antiseptic merely reduces the number of organisms on a surface; it does not penetrate pores and hair follicles to destroy microorganisms residing there. To remove organisms lodged in pores and folds of the skin, healthcare personnel use an antiseptic soap and scrub with a brush. To prevent resident indigenous microflora from contaminating the surgical field, surgeons wear sterile gloves on freshly scrubbed hands, and masks and hoods to cover their face and hair. Also, an antiseptic is applied at the site of the surgical incision to destroy local microorganisms.

Inhibiting the Growth of Pathogens in Our Kitchens

Many of the foods that we bring into and work with in our kitchens are contaminated with pathogens (see "Insight: Microbes in Our Food" on the CD-ROM). For example, gastrointestinal pathogens such as *E. coli* O157:H7, *Salmonella,* and *Campylobacter* are often present on poultry, ground beef, and other meat products. *Salmonella* and *Campylobacter* may also be present within and on the surface of eggs. Protozoan parasites also gain access to our kitchens by means of contaminated foods. *Toxoplasma gondii* cysts may be present in meat, especially pork or mutton, and U.S. cyclosporiasis outbreaks from 1996 to 2004 were associated with imported raspberries, basil, and snow peas.

Assuming that the meat and poultry that you serve to your family are properly and thoroughly cooked, the pathogens that are present on the surface of, or within, these foods are usually killed. They are not the problem. The real problem concerns the handling of these foods *before* cooking them. As we handle and prepare foods in the kitchen, pathogens from the foods get on our hands, countertops, plates, cutting boards, knives, and almost anything else that we touch in the kitchen.

Here is a typical scenario. You place a package of chicken breasts on a plate and then unwrap it. You then place the chicken breasts, one at a time, on a cutting board and trim away the excess fat with a knife. By the time the chicken breasts are placed into the oven, the plate, the cutting board, the knife, your hands, and anything that you have touched with your hands have become contaminated. Now you take a head of lettuce from the refrigerator, place it on the cutting board, and proceed to chop it for use in a salad. It is quite possible that any pathogens that were present on your hands, the knife, or the cutting board are now in the salad. It is not likely that you will be cooking the salad, so later when you eat it, you and your family will be ingesting live pathogens.

It is very important that you remain aware of the presence of pathogens as you prepare foods in the kitchen and take steps to eliminate contamination of yourself, your kitchen, and other foods with those pathogens. Wash your hands often, using hot water and antibacterial soap. Do not merely rinse them. In the kitchen, just as in the hospital setting, frequent and thorough handwashing is the most important way to prevent the transmission of pathogens.

Using hot water, thoroughly rinse poultry and meat blood from plates, and then place them in the dishwasher or wash them with hot, soapy water. Do not use them for anything else until after they have been washed. Always wash knives before reusing them. After working with poultry and meat, be sure to thoroughly wash countertops and cutting boards with hot, soapy water. Because bacteria can get between the slats in wooden cutting boards, consider replacing them with smooth plastic cutting boards. Use an antibacterial kitchen spray to clean countertops, refrigerator and oven handles, and anything else that you touched as you prepared the food. Remember to follow the manufacturer's directions regarding the length of time to leave the disinfectant in place before wiping it off. Because wet sponges and dishcloths are havens for pathogens, be sure to wash or replace them often. Whenever possible, people should place their sponges or dishcloths in the dishwasher each time they wash dishes and should never use dish towels to dry their hands.

Controversies Relating to the Use of Antimicrobial Agents in Animal Feed and Household Products

It has been estimated that approximately 40% of the antibiotics manufactured in the United States are used in animal feed. The reason is obvious: to prevent infectious diseases in farm animals—infections that could lead to huge economic loses for farmers and ranchers. The problem is that when antibiotics are fed to an animal, the antibiotics kill any indigenous microflora organisms that are susceptible to the antibiotics. But what survives? Any organisms that are resistant to the antibiotics. Having less competition now for space and nutrients, these drug-resistant organisms multiply and become the predominant organisms of the animal's indigenous microflora. These drug-resistant organisms are then transmitted in the animal's feces or food products (e.g., eggs, milk, and meat) obtained from the animal. Many multidrug-resistant *Salmonella* strains—strains that cause disease in animals and humans—developed in this manner. The use of antibiotic-containing animal feed is quite controversial. Microbiologists concerned about ever-increasing numbers of drug-resistant bacteria are currently attempting to eliminate or drastically reduce the practice of adding antibiotics to animal feed.

Another controversy concerns the antimicrobial agents that are being added to toys, cutting boards, hand soaps, antibacterial kitchen sprays, and many other household products. The antimicrobial agents in these products kill any organisms that are susceptible to these drugs, but what survives? Any organisms that are resistant to these agents. These drug-resistant organisms then multiply and become the predominant organisms in the home. Should a member of the household become infected with these drug-resistant and multidrug-resistant organisms, the infection will be more difficult to treat. Concerned microbiologists are currently attempting to eliminate or drastically reduce the practice of adding antimicrobial agents to household products.

Another argument against the use of antimicrobial agents in the home concerns the immune system. Many scientists believe that children must be exposed to all sorts of microorganisms during their growth and development so that their immune systems will develop correctly and be capable of properly responding to pathogens in later years. The use of household products containing antimicrobial agents might be eliminating the very organisms that are essential for proper maturation of the immune system.

◉ REVIEW OF KEY POINTS

- Microbial growth is affected by many different environmental factors, including the availability of nutrients and moisture, temperature, pH, osmotic pressure, barometric pressure, and composition of the atmosphere.
- Some microorganisms (thermophiles) prefer to live in hot temperatures, others (mesophiles) prefer moderate temperatures, and others (psychrophiles) prefer cold temperatures. Psychrotrophs are a group of psychrophiles that prefer to live at refrigerator temperature (4°C).
- Acidophiles live in acidic environments, alkaliphiles live in alkaline environments, halophiles live in salty environments, and barophiles live where there is high barometric pressure.

- The growth of microorganisms is encouraged in microbiology laboratories, research laboratories, and in various industries (e.g., antibiotic industry and certain food, beverage, and chemical industries). To culture microorganisms in the laboratory, they must be provided with appropriate nutrients, moisture, and the temperature, pH, and atmosphere that they require.
- Enriched media are necessary to grow pathogens, and especially fastidious pathogens require highly enriched media. Selective media are used to grow specific types of bacteria while inhibiting the growth of unwanted bacteria. Differential media are used to differentiate among different groups of bacteria (e.g., MacConkey agar is used to differentiate between lactose fermenters and nonlactose fermenters).
- Cell cultures, laboratory animals, or embryonated chicken eggs are required to grow obligate intracellular pathogens. They will not grow on artificial (synthetic) media.
- A population growth curve consists of four phases: lag phase, log phase, stationary phase, and death phase. Cells are healthiest and the growth rate is greatest (shortest generation time) during the logarithmic growth phase. This phase may be perpetuated in a chemostat by maintaining optimum growth conditions (i.e., by adding nutrients and removing toxic waste products and excess microorganisms).
- It is necessary or desirable to inhibit the growth of microorganisms in certain environments, such as various locations in hospitals (e.g., patients' rooms, operating rooms, intensive care units), food and beverage processing plants, restaurants, kitchens, and bathrooms.
- Sterilization is the complete destruction of all microbial life, whereas disinfection is the destruction of pathogens. Pasteurization and the use of antiseptics are examples of disinfection techniques.
- A variety of physical methods can be used to inhibit microbial growth, including dry heat, moist heat, desiccation, various types of radiation, ultrasonic waves, and filtration.
- Bacterial endospores and certain viruses are very resistant to heat and desiccation.
- A variety of chemical agents can be used to inhibit microbial growth. Bactericidal agents kill bacteria, whereas bacteriostatic agents stop bacteria from growing and dividing. Sporicidal agents kill bacterial endospores. Fungicidal agents kill fungi. Algicidal agents kill algae. Viricidal (or virucidal) agents destroy viruses. Pseudomonicidal agents kill *Pseudomonas* species, and tuberculocidal agents kill *M. tuberculosis*.
- Some disinfectants target and destroy cell walls, whereas others attack cell membranes. Others destroy enzymes, structural proteins, or nucleic acids.

- The effectiveness of a chemical disinfectant depends on many factors, including prior cleaning of the object or surface to be disinfected, the presence of organic matter (e.g., feces, blood, vomitus, pus) on the materials being treated, the type and level of microbial contamination, the concentration of the disinfectant, the contact time, the physical nature of the object being disinfected (e.g., smooth or rough surface, crevices, hinges), temperature, and pH.

- Lyophilization (freeze-drying) will not kill microbes but it does prevent microbial growth. It is a method of preserving microbes for future use. Rapid freezing, using liquid nitrogen, is another method of preserving microbes.

- Healthcare professionals must take special care not to transfer potentially pathogenic microbes from patient to patient, from themselves to patients, or from patients to themselves, by using physical and chemical methods to inhibit the growth of pathogens.

On the CD-ROM

- Insight: Microbes in Our Food
- Increase Your Knowledge
- Critical Thinking
- Additional Self-Assessment Exercises

Self-Assessment Exercises

After studying this chapter, answer the following multiple-choice questions.

1. It would be necessary to use a tuberculocidal agent to kill a particular species of:
   a. *Clostridium.*
   b. *Mycobacterium.*
   c. *Staphylococcus.*
   d. *Streptococcus.*

2. Pasteurization is an example of what kind of technique?
   a. antiseptic
   b. disinfection
   c. sterilization
   d. surgical aseptic

3. The combination of freezing and drying is known as:
   a. desiccation.
   b. lyophilization.
   c. pasteurization.
   d. tyndallization.

4. Organisms that live in and around hydrothermal vents at the bottom of the ocean are:
   a. acidophilic, psychrophilic, and halophilic.
   b. halophilic, alkaliphilic, and psychrophilic.
   c. halophilic, psychrophilic, and barophilic.
   d. halophilic, thermophilic, and barophilic.

5. When placed into a hypertonic solution, a bacterial cell will:
   a. take in more water than it releases.
   b. lyse.
   c. shrink.
   d. swell.

6. To prevent *Clostridium* infections in a hospital setting, what kind of disinfectant should be used?
   a. fungicidal
   b. pseudomonicidal
   c. sporicidal
   d. tuberculocidal

7. Sterilization can be accomplished by use of:
   a. an autoclave.
   b. antiseptics.
   c. medical aseptic techniques.
   d. pasteurization.

8. The goal of medical asepsis is to kill _____, whereas the goal of surgical asepsis is to kill _____.
   a. all microorganisms . . . . . pathogens
   b. bacteria . . . . . bacteria and viruses
   c. nonpathogens . . . . . pathogens
   d. pathogens . . . . . all microorganisms

9. Which of the following types of culture media is selective *and* differential?
   a. blood agar
   b. MacConkey agar
   c. phenylethyl alcohol agar
   d. Thayer-Martin agar

10. All the following types of culture media are enriched and selective except:
    a. blood agar.
    b. colistin-nalidixic acid agar.
    c. phenylethyl alcohol agar.
    d. Thayer-Martin agar.

USING ANTIMICROBIAL AGENTS TO CONTROL MICROBIAL GROWTH IN VIVO

LEARNING OBJECTIVES

AFTER STUDYING THIS CHAPTER, YOU SHOULD BE
ABLE TO:

- Compare and contrast chemotherapeutic agents, antimicrobial agents, and antibiotics
- State the five most common mechanisms of action of antimicrobial agents
- Differentiate between bactericidal and bacteriostatic agents
- Differentiate between narrow-spectrum and broad-spectrum antimicrobial agents
- Identify the four most common mechanisms by which bacteria become resistant to antimicrobial agents
- Define the following terms: β-lactam ring, β-lactam antibiotics, β-lactamase
- Name two β-lactamases
- State six actions that clinicians or patients can take to help in the war against drug resistance
- Explain what is meant by empiric therapy
- List six factors that a clinician would take into consideration before prescribing an antimicrobial agent for a particular patient

- State three undesirable effects of antimicrobial agents
- Explain what is meant by a superinfection and cite three diseases that can result from superinfections

INTRODUCTION

Chapter 8 contained information regarding the control of microbial growth in vitro. Another aspect of controlling the growth of microorganisms involves the use of drugs to treat (and, hopefully, to cure) infectious diseases; in other words, using drugs to control the growth of microorganisms in vivo.

Although we most often hear the term *chemotherapy* used in conjunction with cancer (i.e., cancer chemotherapy), **chemotherapy** actually refers to the use of any chemical (drug) to treat any disease or condition. The chemicals (drugs) used to treat diseases are referred to as chemotherapeutic agents. By definition, a **chemotherapeutic agent** is *any* drug used to treat *any* condition or disease.

For thousands of years, people have been discovering and using herbs and chemicals to cure infectious diseases. Native witch doctors in Central and South America long ago discovered that the herb, ipecac, aided in the treatment of dysentery, and that a quinine extract of cinchona bark was effective in treating malaria. During the 16th and 17th centuries, the alchemists of Europe searched for ways to cure smallpox, syphilis, and many other diseases that were rampant during that period of history. Many of the mercury and arsenic chemicals that were used frequently caused more damage to the patient than to the pathogen.

The chemotherapeutic agents used to treat infectious diseases are collectively referred to as antimicrobial agents. Thus, an **antimicrobial agent** is any chemical (drug) used to treat an infectious disease, either by inhibiting or killing pathogens in vivo. Drugs used to treat bacterial diseases are called **antibacterial agents,** whereas those used to treat fungal diseases are called **antifungal agents.** Drugs used to treat protozoal diseases are called **antiprotozoal agents,** and those used to treat viral diseases are called **antiviral agents.**

Some antimicrobial agents are antibiotics. By definition, an *antibiotic* is a substance produced by a microorganism that is effective in killing or inhibiting the growth of other microorganisms. Although all antibiotics are antimicrobial agents, not all antimicrobial agents are antibiotics; therefore, the terms are not synonyms and care should be taken to use the terms correctly.

HISTORICAL NOTE

The Father of Chemotherapy

The true beginning of modern chemotherapy came in the late 1800s when Paul Ehrlich, a German chemist, began his search for chemicals (referred to as "magic bullets") that would destroy bacteria, yet would not damage normal body cells. By 1909, he had tested more than 600 chemicals, without success. Finally, in that year, he discovered an arsenic compound that proved effective in treating syphilis. Because this was the 606th compound Ehrlich had tried, he called it "Compound 606." The technical name for Compound 606 is arsphenamine and the trade name was Salvarsan. Until the availability of penicillin in the early 1940s, Salvarsan and a related compound—Neosalvarsan—were used to treat syphilis. Ehrlich also found that rosaniline was useful for treating African trypanosomiasis.

○ STUDY AID

Clarifying Drug Terminology

Imagine that all *chemotherapeutic agents* are contained within one very large wooden box. Within that large box are many smaller boxes. Each of the smaller boxes contains drugs to treat one particular category of diseases. For example, one of the smaller boxes contains drugs to treat cancer; these are called cancer chemotherapeutic agents. Another of the smaller boxes contains drugs to treat hypertension (high blood pressure). Another of the smaller boxes contains drugs to treat infectious diseases; these are called *antimicrobial agents*. Now imagine that the box containing antimicrobial agents contains even smaller boxes. One of these very small boxes contains drugs to treat bacterial diseases; these are called *antibacterial agents*. Another of these very small boxes contains drugs to treat fungal diseases; these are called *antifungal agents*. Other very small boxes contain drugs to treat protozoal diseases (*antiprotozoal agents*) and drugs to treat viral infections (antiviral agents). To appropriately treat a particular disease, a clinician[a] must select a drug from the appropriate box. To treat a fungal infection, for example, the clinician must select a drug from the box containing antifungal agents.

Antibiotics are produced by certain molds and bacteria, usually those that live in soil. The antibiotics produced by soil organisms give them a selective advantage in the struggle for the available nutrients in the soil. Penicillin and cephalosporins are examples of antibiotics produced by molds, and bacitracin, erythromycin, and chloramphenicol are examples of antibiotics produced by bacteria. Although originally produced by microorganisms, many antibiotics are now synthesized or manufactured in pharmaceutical laboratories. Also, many antibiotics have been chemically modified to kill a wider variety of pathogens or reduce side effects; these modified antibiotics are called **semisynthetic antibiotics.** Semisynthetic antibiotics include semisynthetic penicillins, such as ampicillin and carbenicillin. Antibiotics are primarily antibacterial agents and are thus used to treat bacterial diseases.

---

[a]The term clinician is used throughout this chapter to refer to physicians and any other healthcare professionals who are authorized to make diagnoses and prescribe medications.

HISTORICAL NOTE

The First Antibiotics

In 1928, **Alexander Fleming,** a Scottish bacteriologist, accidentally discovered the first antibiotic when he noticed that growth of contaminant *Penicillium notatum* mold colonies on his culture plates was inhibiting the growth of *Staphylococcus* bacteria (Fig. 9-1). Fleming gave the name "penicillin" to the inhibitory substance being produced by the mold. He found that broth cultures of the mold were not toxic to laboratory animals and that they destroyed staphylococci and other bacteria. He speculated that penicillin might be useful in treating infectious diseases caused by these organisms. As was stated by Kenneth B. Raper in 1978, "Contamination of his *Staphylococcus* plate by a mold was an accident; but Fleming's recognition of a potentially important phenomenon was no accident, for Pasteur's observation that 'chance favors the prepared mind' was never more apt than with Fleming and penicillin."

During World War II, two biochemists, **Sir Howard Walter Florey** and **Ernst Boris Chain,** purified penicillin and demonstrated its effectiveness in the treatment of various bacterial infections. By 1942, the U.S. drug industry was able to produce sufficient penicillin for human use, and the search for other antibiotics began. (Earlier—in 1935—a chemist named **Gerhard Domagk** discovered that the red dye, Prontosil, was effective against streptococcal infections in mice. Further research demonstrated that Prontosil was degraded or broken down in the body into sulfanilamide, and that sulfanilamide [a sulfa drug] was the effective agent. Although sulfanilamide is an antimicrobial agent, it is not an antibiotic because it is not produced by a microorganism.) In 1944, **Selman Waksman** and his colleagues isolated streptomycin (the first antituberculosis drug) and subsequently discovered antibiotics such as chloramphenicol, tetracycline, and erythromycin in soil samples. It was Waksman who first used the term "antibiotic." For their outstanding contributions to medicine, these investigators—Ehrlich, Fleming, Florey, Chain, Waksman, and Domagk—were all Nobel Prize recipients at various times.

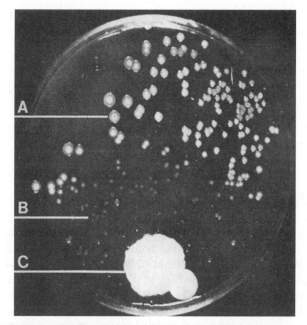

FIGURE 9-1. The discovery of penicillin by Alexander Fleming. (*A*) Colonies of *Staphylococcus aureus* (a bacterium) are growing well in this area of the plate. (*B*) Colonies are poorly developed in this area of the plate because of an antibiotic (penicillin) being produced by the colony of *Penicillium notatum* (a mold) shown at *C*. (This photograph originally appeared in the *British Journal of Experimental Pathology* in 1929.) (Koneman's Color Atlas and Textbook of Diagnostic Microbiology, 6th ed. Philadelphia: JB Lippincott, 2006.)

Ideal Qualities of an Antimicrobial Agent

The ideal antimicrobial agent should:

- Kill or inhibit the growth of pathogens
- Cause no damage to the host
- Cause no allergic reaction in the host
- Be stable when stored in solid or liquid form
- Remain in specific tissues in the body long enough to be effective
- Kill the pathogens before they mutate and become resistant to it

Unfortunately, most antimicrobial agents have some side effects, produce allergic reactions, or permit development of resistant mutant pathogens.

How Antimicrobial Agents Work

To be acceptable, an antimicrobial agent must inhibit or destroy the pathogen without damaging the host. To accomplish this, the agent must target a metabolic process or structure possessed by the pathogen but not possessed by the host (i.e., the infected person).

The five most common mechanisms of action of antimicrobial agents are as follows:

- Inhibition of cell wall synthesis
- Damage to cell membranes
- Inhibition of nucleic acid synthesis (either DNA or RNA synthesis)
- Inhibition of protein synthesis
- Inhibition of enzyme activity

Antibacterial Agents

Sulfonamide drugs inhibit production of folic acid (a vitamin) in those bacteria that require *p*-aminobenzoic acid (PABA) to synthesize folic acid. Because the sulfonamide molecule is similar in shape to the PABA molecule, bacteria attempt to metabolize sulfonamide to produce folic acid (Fig. 9-2). However, the enzymes that convert PABA to folic acid cannot produce folic acid from the sulfonamide molecule. Without folic acid, bacteria cannot produce certain essential proteins and finally die. Sulfa drugs, therefore, are called competitive inhibitors; that is, they inhibit growth of microorganisms by competing with an enzyme required to produce an essential metabolite. Sulfa drugs are *bacteriostatic,* meaning that they inhibit growth of bacteria (as opposed to a *bactericidal agent,* which kills bacteria.) Cells of humans and animals do not synthesize folic acid from PABA; they get folic acid from the food they eat. Consequently, they are unaffected by sulfa drugs.

In most Gram-positive bacteria, including streptococci and staphylococci, penicillin interferes with the synthesis and cross-linking of peptidoglycan, a component of bacterial cell walls. Thus, by inhibiting cell wall synthesis, penicillin destroys the bacteria. Why doesn't penicillin also destroy human cells? Because human cells do not have cell walls.

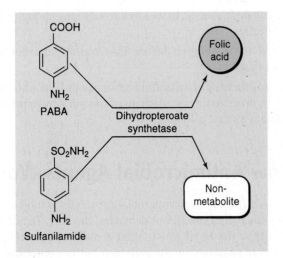

FIGURE 9-2. The effect of sulfonamide drugs. (See text for details.)

There are other antimicrobial agents that have a similar action; they inhibit a specific step that is essential to the microorganism's metabolism and, thereby, cause its destruction. Antibiotics like vancomycin, which destroys only Gram-positive bacteria, and colistin and nalidixic acid, which destroy only Gram-negative bacteria, are referred to as *narrow-spectrum antibiotics*. Those that are destructive to both Gram-positive and Gram-negative bacteria are called *broad-spectrum antibiotics*. Examples of broad-spectrum antibiotics are ampicillin, chloramphenicol, and tetracycline. Table 9-1 lists some of the antimicrobial drugs most frequently used against many common bacterial pathogens.

Antimicrobial agents work well against bacterial pathogens because the bacteria (being procaryotic) have different cellular structures and metabolic pathways that can be disrupted or destroyed by drugs that do not damage the eucaryotic host's cells. As mentioned earlier, bactericidal agents kill bacteria, whereas bacteriostatic agents stop them from growing and dividing. Bacteriostatic agents should only be used in patients whose host defense mechanisms (Chapters 15 and 16) are functioning properly (i.e., only in patients whose bodies are capable of killing the pathogen once its multiplication is stopped). Bacteriostatic agents should not be used in immunosuppressed or leukopenic patients (patients having an abnormally low number of white blood cells). Some of the mechanisms by which antibacterial agents kill or inhibit bacteria are shown in Table 9-1.

Multidrug Therapy

In some cases, a single antimicrobial agent is not sufficient to destroy all the pathogens that develop during the course of a disease; thus, two or more drugs may be used simultaneously to kill all the pathogens and to prevent resistant mutant pathogens from emerging. In tuberculosis, for example, in which multidrug-resistant strains of *Mycobacterium tuberculosis* are frequently encountered, four drugs (isoniazid, rifampin, pyrazinamide, and either ethambutol or streptomycin) are routinely prescribed, and as many as 12 drugs may be required for especially resistant strains.

Synergism Versus Antagonism

The use of two antimicrobial agents to treat an infectious disease sometimes produces a degree of pathogen killing that is far greater than that achieved by either drug alone. This is known as *synergism.* Synergism is a good thing! Many urinary, respiratory, and gastrointestinal infections respond particularly well to a combination of trimethoprim and sulfamethoxazole, a combination referred to as co-trimoxazole; brand names include Bactrim and Septra.

There are situations, however, when two drugs are prescribed (perhaps by two different clinicians who are treating the patient's infection) that actually work against

TABLE 9-1

Antibacterial Agents

MODE OF ACTION	AGENT	SOURCE	BACTERICIDAL OR BACTERIOSTATIC
Inhibition of cell wall synthesis	Bacitracin (also disrupts cell membranes)	*Bacillus subtilis* (bacterium)	Bactericidal
	Cephalosporins	*Cephalosporium* spp. (molds)	Bactericidal
	Imipenem	A semisynthetic derivative of thienamycin, produced by a *Streptomyces* sp.(bacterium)	Bactericidal
	Penicillins	*Penicillium* spp. (molds)	Bactericidal
	β-lactamase–resistant penicillins: cloxacillin, dicloxacillin, methicillin, nafcillin, oxacillin	These are semisynthetic penicillins	Bactericidal
	Extended spectrum penicillins: amoxicillin, ampicillin, carbenicillin, piperacillin, ticarcillin	These are semisynthetic penicillins	Bactericidal
	Vancomycin	*Streptomyces orientalis* (bacterium)	Bactericidal
Inhibition of protein synthesis	Chloramphenicol	*Streptomyces venezuelae* (bacterium)	Bacteriostatic
	Clindamycin	A chemical modification of lincomycin, produced by *Streptomyces lincolnensis* (bacterium)	Bacteriostatic or bactericidal, depending on drug concentration and bacterial species
	Erythromycin	*Streptomyces erythraeus* (bacterium)	Bacteriostatic (usually); bactericidal at high concentrations
	Streptomycin and other aminoglycosides	*Streptomyces* spp. (bacteria)	Bactericidal
	Tetracycline	*Streptomyces rimosus* (bacterium)	Bacteriostatic
Inhibition of nucleic acid synthesis	Rifampin	*Streptomyces mediterranei* (bacterium)	Bactericidal
	Quinolones and fluoroquinolones (e.g., ciprofloxacin, nalidixic acid, norfloxacin)	Synthetic	Bactericidal
Disruption of cell membranes	Polymyxin B and polymyxin E (colistin)	*Bacillus polymyxa* (bacterium)	Bactericidal
Inhibition of enzyme activity	Sulfonamides	Synthetic	Bacteriostatic
	Trimethoprim	Synthetic	Bacteriostatic

each other. This is known as ***antagonism.*** The extent of pathogen killing is less than that achieved by either drug alone. Antagonism is a bad thing!

Antifungal Agents

It is much more difficult to use antimicrobial drugs against fungal and protozoal pathogens, because they are eucaryotic cells; thus, the drugs tend to be more toxic to the patient. Most antifungal agents work in one of three ways:

- By binding with cell membrane sterols (e.g., nystatin and amphotericin B)
- By interfering with sterol synthesis (e.g., clotrimazole and miconazole)
- By blocking mitosis or nucleic acid synthesis (e.g., griseofulvin and 5-flucytosine)

Examples of antifungal agents are shown in Table 9-2.

TABLE 9-2

Antifungal Agents

DRUG[a]	FUNGAL DISEASE(S) THAT THE DRUG IS USED TO TREAT
Amphotericin B	Aspergillosis, blastomycosis, invasive candidiasis, coccidioidomycosis, cryptococcosis, fusariosis, histoplasmosis, mucormycosis, paracoccidioidomycosis, penicilliosis, systemic sporotrichosis
Atovaquone	*Pneumocystis* pneumonia
Echinocandins	Aspergillosis, candidiasis
Fluconazole	Blastomycosis; oropharyngeal, esophageal, and invasive candidiasis; coccidioidomycosis, cryptococcosis, fusariosis, histoplasmosis, sporotrichosis
Flucytosine	Candidiasis, chromoblastomycosis, cryptococcosis
Griseofulvin	Dermatomycosis (less toxic drugs are available, however)
Itraconazole	Aspergillosis, blastomycosis, invasive candidiasis, coccidioidomycosis, cryptococcosis, histoplasmosis, paracoccidioidomycosis, penicilliosis, pseudallescheriasis, scedosporiosis, cutaneous or systemic sporotrichosis
Ketoconazole	Blastomycosis, coccidioidomycosis, histoplasmosis, paracoccidioidomycosis
Terbinafine	Dermatomycosis
Trimethoprim-sulfamethoxazole	*Pneumocystis* pneumonia
Voriconazole	Aspergillosis, invasive candidiasis, scedosporiasis

[a]Note: this information is provided solely to acquaint readers of this book with the names of some antifungal agents, and should not be construed as advice regarding recommended therapy.

Antiprotozoal Agents

Antiprotozoal drugs are usually quite toxic to the host and work by (1) interfering with DNA and RNA synthesis (e.g., chloroquine, pentamidine, and quinacrine), or (2) interfering with protozoal metabolism (e.g., metronidazole; brand name Flagyl). Table 9-3 lists several antiprotozoal drugs and the protozoal diseases they are used to treat.

Antiviral Agents

Antiviral agents are the newest weapons in antimicrobial methodology. Until recent years, there were no drugs for the treatment of viral diseases. Antiviral agents are particularly difficult to develop and use because viruses are produced within host cells. A few drugs have been found to be effective in certain viral infections; these work by inhibiting viral replication within cells. Some antiviral agents are listed in Table 9-4.

The first antiviral agent effective against HIV (the causative agent of AIDS)—zidovudine (also known as AZT)—was introduced in 1987. A variety of additional drugs for the treatment of HIV infection were introduced during the 1990s. Certain of these antiviral agents are administered simultaneously, in combinations referred to as "cocktails." Unfortunately, such cocktails are quite expensive and some strains of HIV have become resistant to some of the drugs.

Drug Resistance

"Superbugs"

These days, it is quite common to hear about drug-resistant bacteria, or "superbugs," as they have been labeled by the press. Superbugs are microorganisms (mainly bacteria) that have become resistant to one or more antimicrobial agents. Infections caused by superbugs are much more difficult to treat. The worst of the superbugs are multidrug-resistant (i.e., pathogens that are resistant to several different antimicrobial agents). Especially troublesome superbugs include:

• Methicillin-resistant *Staphylococcus aureus* (MRSA) and methicillin-resistant *Staphylococcus epidermidis* (MRSE). These strains are resistant to all antistaphylococcal drugs except vancomycin and one or two recently developed drugs (e.g., Synercid and Zyvox). Some strains of *S. aureus,* called vancomycin-intermediate *S. aureus* (VISA), have developed resistance to the usual dosages of vancomycin, necessitating the use of higher doses to treat infections caused by these organisms.

TABLE 9-3

Antiprotozoal Agents

DRUG[a]	PROTOZOAL DISEASE(S) THAT THE DRUG IS USED TO TREAT	DRUG[a]	PROTOZOAL DISEASE(S) THAT THE DRUG IS USED TO TREAT
Amphotericin B	Primary amebic meningoencephalitis, mucocutaneous leishmaniasis	Metronidazole	Amebiasis, giardiasis, trichomoniasis
Artemisinin derivatives	Multidrug-resistant *Plasmodium falciparum* malaria	Nifurtimox	American trypanosomiasis (Chagas' disease)
Benznidazole	American trypanosomiasis (Chagas' disease)	Nitazoxanide	Giardiasis in children and cryptosporidiosis
Chloroquine phosphate or quinidine gluconate or quinine dihydrochloride	Malaria (except for chloroquine-resistant *P. falciparum* malaria and chloroquine-resistant *Plasmodium vivax* malaria)	Paromomycin	Amebiasis, cryptosporidiosis, *D. fragilis* infection, cutaneous leishmaniasis
Clindamycin plus quinine	Babesiosis	Pentamidine isethionate	African sleeping sickness (without CNS involvement), leishmaniasis
Diloxanide furoate	Amebiasis	Primaquine phosphate	Malaria
Eflornithine	African trypanosomiasis (with or without CNS involvement)	Proguanil hydrochloride	Malaria
Furazolidone	Giardiasis	Pyrimethamine plus sulfadiazine	*P. falciparum* malaria, toxoplasmosis
Halofantrine	Chloroquine-resistant *P. falciparum* malaria	Quinacrine hydrochloride	Giardiasis
Iodoquinol	Amebiasis, balantidiasis, *Dientamoeba fragilis* infection	Quinidine gluconate	*P. falciparum* malaria
Mefloquine	Chloroquine-resistant *P. falciparum* and *P. vivax* malaria	Quinine	Malaria
Melarsoprol	African trypanosomiasis (with CNS involvement)	Spiramycin	Toxoplasmosis

(continues)

TABLE 9-3

Antiprotozoal Agents *(continued)*

DRUG[a]	PROTOZOAL DISEASE(S) THAT THE DRUG IS USED TO TREAT	DRUG[a]	PROTOZOAL DISEASE(S) THAT THE DRUG IS USED TO TREAT
Stibogluconate sodium	Visceral, cutaneous, and mucocutaneous leishmaniasis	Tinidazole	Amebiasis, giardiasis, trichomoniasis
Suramin	African trypanosomiasis (with no CNS involvement)	Trimethoprim-sulfamethoxazole	Cyclosporiasis, isosporiasis
Tetracycline hydrochloride	Balantidiasis, *Dientamoeba fragilis* infection; can be used with quinine or quinidine for *P. falciparum* malaria		

[a]Note: this information is provided solely to acquaint readers of this book with the names of some antiprotozoal agents, and should not be construed as advice regarding recommended therapy.
CNS, central nervous system.

Recently, strains of *S. aureus* (called vancomycin-resistant *S. aureus* or VRSA strains) have been isolated that are resistant to even the highest practical doses of vancomycin. *S. aureus* is a very common cause of nosocomial (hospital-acquired) infections.

- Vancomycin-resistant *Enterococcus* spp. (VRE). These strains are resistant to most antienterococcal drugs,

including vancomycin. *Enterococcus* spp. are common causes of nosocomial infections, especially nosocomial urinary tract infections.

- Multidrug-resistant *Mycobacterium tuberculosis* (MRTB). Some MRTB strains are resistant to *all* antitubercular drugs and combinations of these drugs. Patients infected with these strains may have a lung or

TABLE 9-4

Antiviral Agents

VIRUS/VIRAL INFECTION(S)[a]	ANTIVIRAL AGENTS
Herpes simplex infections	Acyclovir, cidofovir, famciclovir, fomivirsen, ganciclovir, penciclovir, valganciclovir, vidarabine
Respiratory viruses	Amantadine, oseltamivir, ribavirin, rimantadine, zanamivir
Human immunodeficiency virus (HIV): nucleoside reverse-transcriptase inhibitors	Abacavir, didanosine, lamivudine, stavudine, tenofovir, zalcitabine, zidovudine
Human immunodeficiency virus (HIV): nonnucleoside reverse-transcriptase inhibitors	Delavirdine, efavirenz, nevirapine
Human immunodeficiency virus (HIV): protease inhibitors	Amprenavir, indinavir, lopinavir, nelfinavir, ritonavir, saquinavir

[a]Note: this information is provided solely to acquaint readers of this book with the names of some antiviral agents, and should not be construed as advice regarding recommended therapy.

section of lung removed—just as in the preantibiotic days—and many will die. Tuberculosis remains one of the major killers worldwide.

- Multidrug-resistant strains of *Pseudomonas* spp., *Stenotrophomonas*, *Salmonella* spp., *Shigella* spp., and *Neisseria gonorrhoeae.*
- β-Lactamase–producing strains of *Streptococcus pneumoniae* and *Haemophilus influenzae* (β-lactamases are discussed later). Some strains of these pathogens have become multiply resistant.

It is important to note that bacteria are not the only microorganisms that have developed resistance to drugs. Certain viruses (including HIV, herpes simplex viruses, and influenza viruses), fungi (both yeasts and molds), parasitic protozoa, and helminths have also become drug-resistant. Parasitic protozoa that have become drug-resistant include strains of *Plasmodium falciparum, Trichomonas vaginalis, Leishmania* spp., and *Giardia lamblia.*

How Bacteria Become Resistant to Drugs

How do bacteria become resistant to antimicrobial agents? Some bacteria are naturally resistant to a particular antimicrobial agent because they lack the specific target site for that drug (e.g., mycoplasmas have no cell walls and are, therefore, resistant to any drugs that interfere with cell wall synthesis). Other bacteria are naturally resistant because the drug is unable to cross the organism's cell wall or cell membrane and, thus, cannot reach its site of action (e.g., ribosomes). Such resistance is known as *intrinsic resistance.*

It is also possible for bacteria that were once susceptible to a particular drug to become resistant to it; this is called *acquired resistance.* Bacteria usually acquire resistance to antibiotics and other antimicrobial agents by one of four mechanisms, each of which is shown in Table 9-5 and briefly described below.

Before a drug can enter a bacterial cell, molecules of the drug must first bind (attach) to proteins on the surface of the cell; these protein molecules are called *drug-binding sites.* A chromosomal mutation can result in an alteration in the structure of the drug-binding site, so that the drug is no longer able to bind to the cell. If the drug cannot bind to the cell, it cannot enter the cell, and the organism is, therefore, resistant to the drug.

To enter a bacterial cell, a drug must be able to pass through the cell wall and cell membrane. A chromosomal mutation can result in an alteration in the structure of the cell membrane, which in turn can change the permeability of the membrane. If the drug is no longer able to pass through the cell membrane, it cannot reach its target (e.g., a ribosome or the DNA of the cell), and the organism is now resistant to the drug.

Another way in which bacteria become resistant to a certain drug is by developing the ability to produce an enzyme that destroys or inactivates the drug. Because enzymes are coded for by genes, a bacterial cell would have to acquire a new gene for the cell to be able to produce an enzyme that it never before produced. The primary way in which bacteria acquire new genes is by conjugation (Chapter 7). Often, a plasmid containing such a gene is transferred from one bacterial cell (the donor cell) to another bacterial cell (the recipient cell) during conjugation. For example, many bacteria have become resistant to penicillin because they have acquired the gene for penicillinase production during conjugation. (Penicillinase is described in a following section.) A plasmid containing multiple genes for drug resistance is

---

TABLE 9-5

Mechanisms by Which Bacteria Become Resistant to Antimicrobial Agents

MECHANISM	EFFECT
A chromosomal mutation that causes a change in the structure of a drug binding site	The drug cannot bind to the bacterial cell
A chromosomal mutation that causes a change in cell membrane permeability	The drug cannot pass through the cell membrane and thus cannot enter the cell
Acquisition (by conjugation, transduction or transformation) of a gene that enables the bacterium to produce an enzyme that destroys or inactivates the drug	The drug is destroyed or inactivated by the enzyme
Acquisition (by conjugation, transduction, or transformation) of a gene that enables the bacterium to produce a multidrug-resistance (MDR) pump	The drug is pumped out of the cell before it can damage or kill the cell

called a ***resistance factor (R-factor)***. A recipient cell that receives an R-factor becomes multidrug-resistant (i.e., it becomes a superbug). Bacteria can also acquire new genes by transduction (whereby bacteriophages carry bacterial DNA from one bacterial cell to another) and transformation (the uptake of naked DNA from the environment). (Transduction and transformation were discussed in Chapter 7.)

A fourth way in which bacteria become resistant to drugs is by developing the ability to produce multidrug-resistance (MDR) pumps (also known as MDR transporters). An MDR pump enables the cell to pump drugs out of the cell before the drugs can damage or kill the cell. The genes encoding these pumps are often located on plasmids that bacteria receive during conjugation. Bacteria receiving such plasmids become multidrug-resistant (i.e., they become resistant to several drugs).

Thus, bacteria can acquire resistance to antimicrobial agents as a result of chromosomal mutation or the acquisition of new genes by transduction, transformation, and, most commonly, by conjugation.

β-Lactamases

At the heart of every penicillin and cephalosporin molecule is a double-ringed structure, which in penicillins resembles a "house and garage" (Fig. 9-3).

The "garage" is called the ***β-lactam ring.*** Some bacteria produce enzymes that destroy the β-lactam ring; these enzymes are known as ***β-lactamases.*** When the β-lactam ring is destroyed, the antibiotic no longer works. Thus, an organism that produces a β-lactamase is resistant to antibiotics containing the β-lactam ring (collectively referred to as β-lactam antibiotics or β-lactams).

There are two types of β-lactamases: penicillinases and cephalosporinases. ***Penicillinases*** destroy the β-lactam ring in penicillins; thus, an organism that produces penicillinase is resistant to penicillins. ***Cephalosporinases*** destroy the β-lactam ring in cephalosporins; thus, an organism that produces cephalosporinase is resistant to cephalosporins. Some bacteria produce both types of β-lactamases.

To combat the effect of β-lactamases, drug companies have developed special drugs that combine a β-lactam antibiotic with a β-lactamase inhibitor (e.g., clavulanic acid, sulbactam, or tazobactam). The β-lactam inhibitor irreversibly binds to and inactivates the β-lactamase, thus enabling the companion drug to enter the bacterial cell and disrupt cell wall synthesis. Some of these special combination drugs are:

- Clavulanic acid (clavulanate) combined with amoxicillin (brand name, Augmentin)
- Clavulanic acid (clavulanate) combined with ticarcillin (Timentin)
- Sulbactam combined with ampicillin (Unasyn)
- Tazobactam combined with piperacillin (Zosyn)

What Clinicians and Patients Can Do To Help in the War Against Drug Resistance

- Education is crucial—education of healthcare professionals and, in turn, education of patients.
- Patients must stop demanding antibiotics every time they are sick or have a sick child. Patients should never pressure clinicians to prescribe antimicrobial agents. The majority of sore throats and many respiratory infections are caused by viruses, and viruses are unaffected by antibiotics. Because viruses are not killed by antibiotics, patients should not expect antibiotics when they or their children have viral infections. Instead of demanding antibiotics from clinicians, patients should be asking why one *is* being prescribed.
- It is important that clinicians not allow themselves to be pressured by patients. They should prescribe antibiotics only when warranted (i.e., only when there is a demonstrated need for them). Whenever possible, clinicians should collect a specimen for culture and have

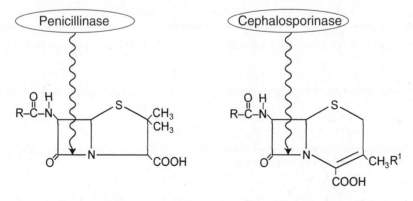

Penicillin   Cephalosporin

FIGURE 9-3. Sites of β-lactamase attack on penicillin and cephalosporin molecules. (See text for details.)

the Clinical Microbiology Laboratory perform susceptibility testing (Chapter 13) to determine which antimicrobial agents are apt to be effective.

- Clinicians should prescribe an inexpensive, narrow-spectrum drug whenever the laboratory results demonstrate that such a drug effectively kills the pathogen. According to Dr. Stuart B. Levy,[b] by some estimates, at least half of current antibiotic use in the United States is inappropriate—antibiotics are either not indicated at all or they are incorrectly prescribed as the wrong drug, the wrong dosage, or the wrong duration. Another study[c] demonstrated that colds, other upper respiratory infections, and bronchitis accounted for 21% of all antibiotic prescriptions in 1992, although these conditions typically do not benefit from antibiotics.

- Patients must take their antibiotics in the exact manner in which they are prescribed. Healthcare professionals should emphasize this to patients and do a better job explaining exactly how medications should be taken.

- It is critical that clinicians prescribe the appropriate amount of antibiotic necessary to cure the infection. Then, unless instructed otherwise, patients must take *all* their pills—even after they are feeling better. Again, this must be explained and emphasized. If treatments are cut short, there is selective killing of only the most susceptible members of a bacterial population. The more resistant variants are left behind to multiply and cause a new infection.

- Patients should always destroy any excess medications and should never keep antibiotics in their medicine cabinet. Antimicrobial agents, including antibiotics, should be taken only when prescribed and only under a clinician's supervision.

- Unless prescribed by a clinician, antibiotics should never be used in a prophylactic manner—such as to avoid "traveler's diarrhea" when traveling to a foreign country. Taking antibiotics in that manner actually *increases* the chances of developing traveler's diarrhea. The antibiotics kill some of the beneficial indigenous intestinal flora, eliminating the competition for food and space, making it easier for pathogens to gain a foothold.

- Healthcare professionals must practice good infection prevention and control procedures (Chapter 12). Frequent and proper handwashing is essential to prevent the transmission of pathogens from one patient to another. Healthcare professionals should monitor for important pathogens (such as MRSA) within healthcare settings

[b]Stuart B. Levy, M.D. The Antibiotic Paradox: How the Misuse of Antibiotics Destroys Their Curative Powers, 2nd ed. Cambridge, MA: Perseus Publishing, 2002.

[c]R. Gonzales, et al. Antibiotic prescribing for adults with colds, upper respiratory tract infections, and bronchitis by ambulatory care patients. JAMA 278:901–904, 1997.

and always isolate patients infected with multidrug-resistant pathogens.

Empiric Therapy

In some cases, a clinician must initiate therapy before laboratory results are available. This is referred to as ***empiric therapy.*** In an effort to save the life of a patient, it is sometimes necessary for the clinician to "guess" the most likely pathogen and the drug most likely to be effective. It will be an "educated guess," based on the clinician's prior experiences with the particular type of infectious disease that the patient has. Before writing a prescription for a certain antimicrobial agent, a number of factors must be taken into consideration by the clinician; some of these are listed below.

- If the laboratory has reported the identity of the pathogen, the clinician can refer to a "pocket chart" that is available in most hospitals. This pocket chart, published by the Clinical Microbiology Laboratory, contains antimicrobial susceptibility test data that have been accumulated during the past year. The pocket chart provides important information regarding drugs to which various bacterial pathogens were susceptible and resistant (Fig. 9-4).

- Is the patient allergic to any antimicrobial agents? Obviously, it would be unwise to prescribe a drug to which the patient is allergic.

- What is the age of the patient? Certain drugs are contraindicated in very young or very old patients.

- Is the patient pregnant? Certain drugs are known to be or suspected to be teratogenic (i.e., they cause birth defects).

- Is the patient an inpatient or outpatient? Certain drugs can only be administered intravenously and, therefore, cannot be prescribed for outpatients.

- If the patient is an inpatient, the clinician must prescribe a drug that is available in the hospital pharmacy (i.e., a drug that is listed in the hospital formulary).

- What is the site of the patient's infection? If the patient has cystitis (urinary bladder infection), the clinician might prescribe a drug that concentrates in the urine. Such a drug is rapidly removed from the blood by the kidneys, and high concentrations of the drug are achieved in the urinary bladder. To treat a brain abscess, the clinician would select a drug capable of crossing the blood–brain barrier.

- What other medications is the patient taking or receiving? Some antimicrobial agents will cross-react with certain other drugs, leading to a drug interaction that could be harmful to the patient.

- What other medical problems does the patient have? Certain antimicrobial agents are known to have toxic side

	E. coli	P. aeruginosa	Klebsiella	Proteus mirabilis	Enterobacter	Proteus sp.	Serratia	Citrobacter
Total isolates	615	371	253	193	107	33	40	56
Percent Sensitive								
Ampicillin	55	1	3	58	3	15	22	7
Carbenicillin	59	88	2	59	74	91	93	24
Timentin	87	81	88	99	82	97	98	93
Piperacillin	65	91	84	68	89	94	100	96
Cefazolin	95	1	83	97	11	18	0	76
Cefotetan	100	1	100	100	77	100	100	97
Ceftriaxone	100	80	100	100	90	100	100	98
Ceftazidime	100	98	95	100	86	97	100	98
Amikacin	100	100	100	100	100	100	100	100
Gentamicin	100	88	89	93	100	92	100	97
Tobramycin	100	89	94	92	100	94	100	100
Tetracycline	84	3	78	4	97	41	41	93
Trimenth-Sulfa	84	2	75	83	96	88	100	90
Nitrofurantoin	100	1	89	21	95	92	0	100
Ciprofloxacin	100	74	80	85	100	97	100	100

FIGURE 9-4. Pocket chart for aerobic Gram-negative bacteria. Illustrated here is the type of chart that clinicians carry in their pockets for use as a quick reference whenever empiric therapy is necessary. The pocket chart, which is prepared by the medical facility's Clinical Microbiology Laboratory, shows the percentage of particular organisms that were susceptible to the various drugs that were tested. The following is an example of how the pocket chart is used. A clinician is informed that *Pseudomonas aeruginosa* has been isolated from his or her patient's blood culture, but the antimicrobial susceptibility testing results on that isolate will not be available until the following day. Because therapy must be initiated immediately, the clinician refers to the pocket chart and sees that amikacin is the most appropriate drug to use (of the 371 strains of *P. aeruginosa* tested, 100% were susceptible to amikacin). [As mentioned in the text, other factors would be taken into consideration by the clinician *before* prescribing amikacin for this patient.] According to the pocket chart, which drug would be the second choice, if amikacin is not available in the hospital pharmacy? Answer: ceftazidime (98%). (Note: This chart is included for educational purposes only. It should not actually be used in a clinical setting.)

effects (e.g., nephrotoxicity, hepatotoxicity, ototoxicity). For example, a clinician would not prescribe a nephrotoxic drug to a patient who has prior kidney damage.

- Is the patient leukopenic or immunocompromised? If so, it would be necessary to use a bactericidal agent to treat the patient's bacterial infection, rather than a bacteriostatic agent. Recall that bacteriostatic agents should only be used in patients whose host defense mechanisms are functioning properly (i.e., only in patients whose bodies are capable of killing the pathogen once its multiplication is stopped). A leukopenic patient has too few white blood cells to kill the pathogen, and the immune system of an immunocompromised patient would be unable to kill the pathogen.

- The cost of the various drugs is also a major consideration. Whenever possible, clinicians should prescribe less costly, narrow-spectrum drugs, rather than expensive, broad-spectrum drugs.

Although the patient's weight will influence the dosage of a particular drug, it is usually not taken into consideration when deciding which drug to prescribe.

Undesirable Effects of Antimicrobial Agents

Listed below are some of the many reasons why antimicrobial agents should not be used indiscriminately.

- Whenever an antimicrobial agent is administered to a patient, organisms within that patient that are susceptible to the agent will die, but resistant ones will survive.

This is referred to as selecting for resistant organisms (Fig. 9-5). The resistant organisms then multiply, become dominant, and can be transmitted to other people. To prevent the overgrowth of resistant organisms, sometimes several drugs, each with a different mode of action, are administered simultaneously.

- The patient may become allergic to the agent. For example, penicillin G in low doses often sensitizes those who are prone to allergies; when these persons receive a second dose of penicillin at some later date, they may have a severe reaction known as anaphylactic shock, or they may break out in hives.

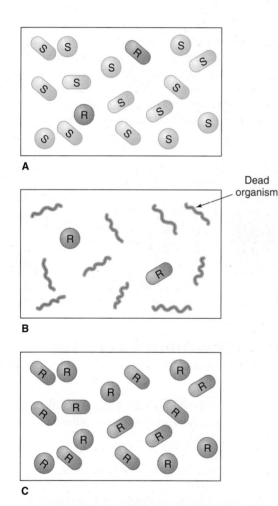

A

Dead organism

B

C

FIGURE 9-5. Selecting for drug-resistant organisms. (*A*) Indigenous microflora of a patient before initiation of antibiotic therapy. Most members of the population are susceptible (indicated by S) to the antibiotic to be administered; very few are resistant (indicated by R). (*B*) After antibiotic therapy has been initiated, the susceptible organisms are dead; only a few resistant organisms remain. (*C*) As a result of decreased competition for nutrients and space, the resistant organisms multiply and become the predominant organisms in the patient's indigenous microflora. (The same type of selection process occurs when farm animals are fed antibiotic-containing feed and when antimicrobial-containing products [e.g., toys, cutting boards] are used in our homes. Both of these topics were discussed in Chapter 8.)

- Many antimicrobial agents are toxic to humans, and some are so toxic that they are administered only for serious diseases for which no other agents are available. One such drug is chloramphenicol, which, if given in high doses for a long period, may cause a very severe type of anemia called aplastic anemia. Another is streptomycin, which can damage the auditory nerve and cause deafness. Other drugs are hepatotoxic or nephrotoxic, causing liver or kidney damage, respectively.

- With prolonged use, broad-spectrum antibiotics may destroy the normal flora of the mouth, intestine, or vagina. The person no longer has the protection of the indigenous microflora and thus becomes much more susceptible to infections caused by opportunists or secondary invaders. The resultant overgrowth by such organisms is referred to as a ***superinfection.*** A superinfection can be thought of as a "population explosion" of organisms that are usually present only in small numbers. For example, the prolonged use of oral antibiotics can result in a superinfection of *Clostridium difficile* in the colon, which can lead to such diseases as antibiotic-associated diarrhea (AAD) and pseudomembranous colitis (PMC). Yeast vaginitis often follows antibacterial therapy because many bacteria of the vaginal flora were destroyed, leading to a superinfection of the indigenous yeast, *Candida albicans.*

Concluding Remarks

In recent years, microorganisms have developed resistance at such a rapid pace that many people, including many scientists, are beginning to fear that science is losing the war against pathogens. Some strains of pathogens have arisen that are resistant to all known drugs; examples include certain strains of *M. tuberculosis* (the bacterium that causes tuberculosis), *Plasmodium* spp. (the protozoa that cause malaria), and *S. aureus* (the bacterium that causes many different types of infections, including pneumonia and postsurgical wound infections). To win the war against drug resistance, more prudent use of currently available drugs, the discovery of new drugs, and the development of new vaccines will all be necessary. Unfortunately, as someone once said, "When science builds a better mousetrap, nature builds a better mouse." To learn more about antibiotic resistance, the book by Dr. Stuart Levy (previously cited) is highly recommended.

Fortunately, antimicrobial agents are not the only in vivo weapons against pathogens. Operating within our bodies are various systems that function to kill pathogens and protect us from infectious diseases. These systems, collectively referred to as host defense systems, are discussed in Chapters 15 and 16.

○ REVIEW OF KEY POINTS

- The types of chemotherapeutic agents used to treat infectious diseases are called antimicrobial agents, some of which are antibiotics. Antimicrobial agents are often referred to simply as "drugs."

- Some antimicrobial agents are "cidal" agents, meaning that they kill pathogens, whereas others are "static" agents, meaning that they stop pathogens from growing and multiplying.

- An antibiotic is a substance produced by a microorganism (usually a soil organism) that is effective in killing or inhibiting the growth of other microorganisms. Some antibiotics (e.g., penicillins and cephalosporins) are produced by molds, whereas others (e.g., tetracycline, erythromycin, chloramphenicol) are produced by bacteria.

- The first antibiotic to be discovered (penicillin) was accidentally discovered by Alexander Fleming in 1928.

- The most common ways in which bacteria become resistant to antimicrobial agents include altering drug-binding sites, altering cell membrane permeability, developing the ability to produce an enzyme that destroys or inactivates a drug, and developing multidrug-resistance (MDR) pumps.

- β-Lactamases are bacterial enzymes that destroy the β-lactam ring in antibiotics that contain such a structure (known as β-lactam antibiotics). Examples of β-lactamases are penicillinases and cephalosporinases, which destroy the β-lactam ring in penicillins and cephalosporins, respectively. When the β-lactam ring is destroyed, the drug no longer works. Bacteria that produce penicillinases are resistant to penicillins, and those that produce cephalosporinases are resistant to cephalosporins. It is possible for an organism to produce both penicillinase and cephalosporinase.

- Empiric therapy is therapy that is initiated by a clinician before laboratory results are available (i.e., before the clinician is informed of the specific pathogen that is causing the patient's infectious disease and before any antibiotic susceptibility test results are available). Based on the patient's signs, symptoms, and history, the clinician must "guess" the most likely pathogen and the drug most likely to be effective. This is, of course, an "educated guess," based on the clinician's prior experiences with similar diseases.

- Adverse side effects of antimicrobial agents include selective pressure on microbial populations (i.e., selecting for drug-resistant organisms), patients becoming allergic to the agent, toxicity and damage to humans, and destruction of human indigenous microflora of the mouth, vagina, and intestine, leading to superinfections or increased susceptibility to infectious diseases.

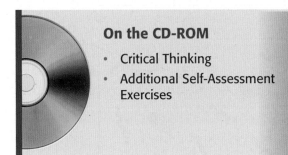

On the CD-ROM
- Critical Thinking
- Additional Self-Assessment Exercises

Self-Assessment Exercises

After studying this chapter, answer the following multiple-choice questions.

1. Which of the following is *least* likely to be taken into consideration when deciding which antibiotic to prescribe for a patient?
   a. patient's age
   b. patient's underlying medical conditions
   c. patient's weight
   d. other medications that the patient is taking

2. Which of the following is *least* likely to lead to drug resistance in bacteria?
   a. a chromosomal mutation that alters cell membrane permeability
   b. a chromosomal mutation that alters the shape of a particular drug-binding site
   c. receiving a gene that codes for an enzyme that destroys a particular antibiotic
   d. receiving a gene that codes for the production of a capsule

3. Which of the following is *not* a common mechanism by which antimicrobial agents kill or inhibit the growth of bacteria?
   a. damage to cell membranes
   b. destruction of capsules
   c. inhibition of cell wall synthesis
   d. inhibition of protein synthesis

4. Multidrug therapy is always used when a patient is diagnosed as having:
   a. an infection caused by MRSA.
   b. diphtheria.
   c. strep throat.
   d. tuberculosis.

5. Which of the following terms or names has *nothing* to do with the use of two drugs simultaneously?
   a. antagonism
   b. Salvarsan
   c. Septra
   d. synergism

6. Which of the following is *not* a common mechanism by which antifungal agents work?
   a. by binding with cell membrane sterols
   b. by blocking nucleic acid synthesis
   c. by dissolving hyphae
   d. by interfering with sterol synthesis

7. Which of the following scientists discovered penicillin?
   a. Alexander Fleming
   b. Paul Ehrlich
   c. Selman Waksman
   d. Sir Howard Walter Florey

8. Which of the following scientists is considered to be the "Father of Chemotherapy?"
   a. Alexander Fleming
   b. Paul Ehrlich
   c. Selman Waksman
   d. Sir Howard Walter Florey

9. All the following antimicrobial agents work by inhibiting cell wall synthesis except:
   a. cephalosporins.
   b. chloramphenicol.
   c. penicillin.
   d. vancomycin.

10. All the following antimicrobial agents work by inhibiting protein synthesis except:
    a. chloramphenicol.
    b. erythromycin.
    c. imipenem.
    d. tetracycline.

10

MICROBIAL ECOLOGY

LEARNING OBJECTIVES

AFTER STUDYING THIS CHAPTER, YOU SHOULD BE
ABLE TO:

- Define ecology, human ecology, and microbial ecology
- List three categories of symbiotic relationships
- Differentiate between mutualism and commensalism
  and give an example of each
- Cite an example of a parasitic relationship
- Discuss three beneficial roles of the indigenous mi-
  croflora of the human body
- Outline the nitrogen cycle; include the meanings of the
  terms nitrogen-fixation, nitrification, denitrification,
  and ammonification in the description
- Define biotechnology and cite four examples of how
  microbes are used in industry
- Name 10 foods that require microbial activity for their
  production
- Define bioremediation and cite an example

INTRODUCTION

The science of *ecology* is the systematic study of the interrelationships that exist between organisms and their
environment. If you were to take a course in human ecology, you would study the interrelationships between humans and the world around them—the nonliving world as
well as the living world. *Microbial ecology* is the study of
the numerous interrelationships between microorganisms
and the world around them; how microbes interact with
other microbes, how microbes interact with organisms
other than microbes, and how microbes interact with the
nonliving world around them. Interactions between microorganisms and animals, plants, other microbes, soil,
and our atmosphere have far-reaching effects on our lives.
We are all aware of the diseases caused by pathogens
(Chapters 17 and 18), but this is only one example of the
many ways that microbes interact with humans. Most relationships between humans and microbes are beneficial

rather than harmful. Although the "bad guys" get most of the attention in the news media, our microbial allies far outnumber our microbial enemies.

Microorganisms interact with humans in many ways and at many levels. The most intimate association that we have with microorganisms is their presence both on and within our bodies. Additionally, microbes play important roles in agriculture, various industries, disposal of industrial and toxic wastes, sewage treatment, and water purification. Microbes are essential in the fields of biotechnology, bioremediation, genetic engineering, and gene therapy (genetic engineering and gene therapy were discussed in Chapter 7).

Symbiotic Relationships Involving Microorganisms

Symbiosis

Symbiosis, or a *symbiotic relationship,* is defined as the living together or close association of two dissimilar organisms (usually two different species). The organisms that live together in such a relationship are referred to as *symbionts.* Some symbiotic relationships (called mutualistic relationships) are beneficial to both symbionts, others (commensalistic relationships) are beneficial to only one symbiont, and others (parasitic relationships) are harmful to one symbiont. Many microorganisms participate in symbiotic relationships. Various symbiotic relationships involving microbes are discussed in subsequent sections; some are illustrated in Figure 10-1.

Neutralism

The term *neutralism* is used to describe a symbiotic relationship in which neither symbiont is affected by the relationship. In other words, neutralism reflects a situation in which different microorganisms occupy the same ecologic niche, but have absolutely no effect on each other.

Commensalism

A symbiotic relationship that is beneficial to one symbiont and of no consequence (i.e., is neither beneficial nor harmful) to the other is called *commensalism.* Many of the organisms in the indigenous microflora of humans are considered to be commensals. The relationship is of obvious benefit to the microorganisms (they are provided nutrients and "housing"), but the microorganisms have no effect on the host. A *host* is defined as a living organism that harbors another living organism.

Mutualism

Mutualism is a symbiotic relationship that is beneficial to both symbionts (i.e., the relationship is mutually beneficial). Humans have a mutualistic relationship with many of the microorganisms of their indigenous microflora. An example is the intestinal bacterium *Escherichia coli,* which obtains nutrients from food materials ingested by the host and produces vitamins (such as vitamin K) that are used by the host. Vitamin K is a blood-clotting factor that is essential to humans. Also, some members of our indigenous microflora prevent colonization by pathogens and overgrowth by opportunistic pathogens (discussed further in a following section entitled "Microbial Antagonism").

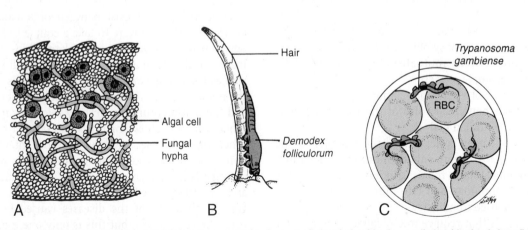

FIGURE 10-1. Various symbiotic relationships. (*A*) A lichen is an example of a mutualistic relationship (i.e., a relationship that is beneficial to both symbionts). (*B*) The tiny Demodex mites that live in human hair follicles are examples of commensals. (*C*) The flagellated protozoan that causes African sleeping sickness is a parasite (RBC, red blood cell).

As another example of a mutualistic relationship, consider the protozoa that live in the intestine of termites. Termites eat wood, but they cannot digest wood. Fortunately for them, the protozoa that live in their intestinal tract break down the large molecules in wood into smaller molecules which can be absorbed and used as nutrients by the termites. In turn, the termite provides food and a warm, moist place for the protozoa to live. Without these protozoa, the termites would die of starvation.

The lichens that you see as colored patches on rocks and tree trunks are further examples of mutualism. As discussed in Chapter 5, a lichen is composed of an alga (or a cyanobacterium) and a fungus, living so closely together that they appear to be one organism. The fungus uses some of the energy that the alga produces by photosynthesis, and the chitin in the fungal cell walls protects the alga from desiccation. Thus, both symbionts benefit from the relationship.

Parasitism

Parasitism is a symbiotic relationship that is beneficial to one symbiont (the parasite) and detrimental to the other symbiont (the host). Being detrimental to the host does not necessarily mean that the parasite causes disease. In some cases, a host can harbor a parasite, without the parasite causing harm to the host. "Smart'" parasites do not cause disease, but rather take only the nutrients they need to exist. The especially "dumb" parasites kill their hosts; then they must either find a new host or die. Nonetheless, certain parasites always cause disease, and some cause the death of the host. Parasites are discussed further in Chapter 18.

A change in conditions can cause one type of symbiotic relationship to shift to another type. For example, conditions can cause a mutualistic or commensalistic relationship between humans and their indigenous microflora to shift to a parasitic, disease-causing (pathogenic) relationship. Recall that many of the microorganisms of our indigenous microflora are opportunistic pathogens (opportunists), awaiting the opportunity to cause disease. Conditions that may enable an opportunist to cause disease include burns, lacerations, surgical procedures, or diseases that debilitate (weaken) the host or interfere with host defense mechanisms. Immunosuppressed individuals are especially susceptible to opportunistic pathogens. Opportunists can also cause disease in otherwise healthy persons if they gain access to the blood, urinary bladder, lungs, or other organs and tissues of those individuals.

Synergism (Synergistic Infections)

Sometimes, two (or more) microorganisms may "team up" to produce a disease that neither could cause by itself. This is referred to as *synergism* or a **synergistic relationship.** The diseases are referred to as ***synergistic infections,*** polymicrobial infections, or mixed infections. For example, certain oral bacteria can work together to cause a serious oral disease

○ STUDY AID

Different Uses of the Term *Synergism*

As was just explained, *synergism* can refer to the combined effects of more than one type of bacteria, as in synergistic infections. In this case, synergism is a bad thing! However, as you learned in Chapter 9, synergism can also refer to the beneficial effects of using two antibiotics simultaneously. With respect to antibiotic use, a synergistic effect is a good thing, because many more pathogens are killed by using a particular combination of two drugs than would be killed if either drug was used alone.

called acute necrotizing ulcerative gingivitis (ANUG; also known as Vincent's disease and "trench mouth"). Similarly, the disease known as bacterial vaginosis (BV) is the result of the combined efforts of several different species of bacteria.

Indigenous Microflora of Humans

A person's *indigenous microflora* or *indigenous microbiota* (sometimes referred to as "normal flora") includes all the microbes (bacteria, fungi, protozoa, and viruses) that reside on and within that person (Fig. 10-2). It has been estimated that our bodies are composed of about 10 trillion cells (including nerve cells, muscle cells, and epithelial cells), and that we have about 10 times that many microbes that live on and within our bodies (10 × 10 trillion = 100 trillion). It has also been estimated that our indigenous microflora is composed of between 500 and 1,000 different species!

A fetus has no indigenous microflora. During and after delivery, a newborn is exposed to many microorganisms from its mother, food, air, and virtually everything that touches the infant. Both harmless and helpful microbes take up residence on the baby's skin, at all body openings, and on mucous membranes that line the digestive tract (mouth to anus) and the genitourinary tract. These moist, warm environments provide excellent conditions for growth. Conditions for proper growth (moisture, pH, temperature, nutrients) vary throughout the body; thus, the types of resident flora differ from one anatomic site to another. Blood, lymph, spinal fluid, and most internal tissues and organs are normally free of microorganisms (i.e., they are sterile). Table 10-1 lists microorganisms frequently found on and within the human body.

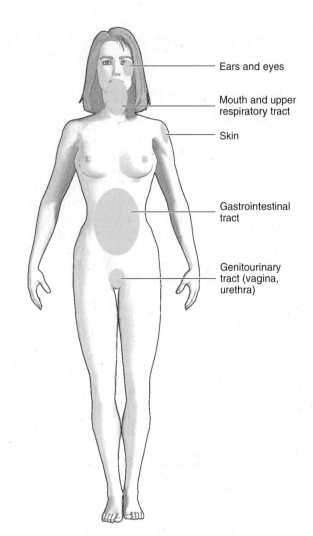

Ears and eyes

Mouth and upper respiratory tract

Skin

Gastrointestinal tract

Genitourinary tract (vagina, urethra)

FIGURE 10-2. Areas of the body where most of the indigenous microflora reside: skin, mouth, ears, eyes, upper respiratory tract, gastrointestinal tract, and genitourinary tract.

In addition to the resident microflora, transient microflora take up temporary residence on and within humans. The body is constantly exposed to microorganisms from the external environment; these transient microbes frequently are attracted to moist, warm body areas. These microbes are only temporary for many reasons: they may be washed from external areas by bathing; they may not be able to compete with the resident microflora; they may fail to survive in the acidic or alkaline environment of the site; they may be killed by substances produced by resident microflora; or they may be flushed away by bodily excretions or secretions (such as urine, feces, tears, and perspiration). Many microbes are unable to colonize (inhabit) the human body because they do not find the body to be a suitable host.

Destruction of the resident microflora disturbs the delicate balance established between the host and its microorganisms. For example, prolonged therapy with certain antibiotics often destroys many of the intestinal microflora. Diarrhea is usually the result of such an imbalance, which in turn leaves the body more susceptible to secondary invaders. When the number of usual resident microbes is greatly reduced, opportunistic invaders can more easily establish themselves within those areas. One important opportunist usually found in small numbers near body openings is the yeast, *Candida albicans,* which, in the absence of sufficient numbers of other resident microflora, may grow unchecked in the mouth, vagina, or lower intestine, causing the disease **candidiasis** (also known as moniliasis). Such an overgrowth or population explosion of an organism that is usually present in low numbers is referred to as a *superinfection.*

Microflora of the Skin

The resident microflora of the skin consists primarily of bacteria and fungi—approximately 30 different types. Although the skin is constantly exposed to air, many of the bacteria that live on the skin are anaerobes; in fact, anaerobes actually outnumber aerobes. Anaerobes live in the deeper layers of skin, hair follicles, and sweat and sebaceous glands. The most common bacteria on skin are species of *Staphylococcus* (especially *S. epidermidis* and other coagulase-negative staphylococci[a]). The number and variety of microorganisms present on the skin depends on many factors, such as the:

- Amount of moisture present
- pH
- Temperature
- Salinity
- Presence of chemical wastes such as urea and fatty acids
- Presence of other microbes, which may be producing toxic substances

Moist, warm conditions in hairy areas of the body where there are many sweat and oil glands, such as under the arms and in the groin area, stimulate the growth of many different microorganisms. Dry, calloused areas of skin have few bacteria, whereas moist folds between the toes and fingers support many bacteria and fungi. The surface of the skin near mucosal openings of the body (the mouth, eyes, nose, anus, and genitalia) is inhabited by bacteria present in various excretions and secretions.

Frequent washing with soap and water removes most of the potentially harmful transient microorganisms harbored in sweat, oil, and other secretions from moist body parts, as well as the dead epithelial cells on which they feed. Proper hygiene also serves to remove odorous organic materials present in perspiration, sebum (sebaceous gland

---

[a]Coagulase is an enzyme that causes clot formation. In the Clinical Microbiology Laboratory, the coagulase test is used to differentiate *Staphylococcus aureus* (which produces coagulase, and is referred to as being coagulase-positive) from other species of *Staphylococcus* (which do not produce coagulase, and are referred to as being coagulase-negative.)

TABLE 10-1

Anatomic Locations of Bacteria and Yeasts Found As Indigenous Microflora of Humans

	SKIN	MOUTH	NOSE AND NASOPHARYNX	OROPHARYNX	GI TRACT	GU TRACT
Anaerobic Gram-negative cocci	−	+	−	−	−	−
Anaerobic Gram-positive cocci	−	+	−	+	+	+
Bacteroides spp.	±	+	−	+	+	+
Candida spp.	+	±	−	−	−	+
Clostridium spp.	+	−	−	−	+	+
Diphtheroids	+	−	+	+	−	+
Enterobacteriaceae[a]	−	−	−	−	+	±
Enterococcus spp.	−	±	±	−	+	+
Fusobacterium spp.	−	±	±	+	+	−
Haemophilus spp.	−	−	+	+	−	−
Lactobacillus spp.	+	+	−	−	−	+
Micrococcus spp.	+	−	−	−	−	−
Neisseria meningitidis	−	−	±	±	−	−
Prevotella/ Porphyromonas spp.	−	+	−	+		
Staphylococcus spp.	+	+	+	+	+	+
Streptococcus spp.	±	+	+	+	−	−

+, commonly present; ±, less commonly present; −, absent.
[a]Sometimes referred to as enteric bacilli (includes Escherichia, Klebsiella, Proteus spp.)

secretions), and microbial metabolic by-products. Health-care professionals must be particularly careful to keep their skin and clothing as free of transient microbes as possible to help prevent personal infections and to avoid transferring pathogens to patients. These individuals should always keep in mind that most infections after burns, wounds, and surgery result from the growth of resident or transient skin microflora in these susceptible areas.

Microflora of the Ears and Eyes

The middle ear and inner ear are usually sterile, whereas the outer ear and the auditory canal contain the same types of microorganisms as are found on the skin. When a person coughs, sneezes, or blows his or her nose, these microbes may be carried along the eustachian tube and into the middle ear where they can cause infection. Infection can also develop in the middle ear when the eustachian tube does not open and close properly to maintain correct air pressure within the ear.

The external surface of the eye is lubricated, cleansed, and protected by tears, mucus, and sebum. Thus, continual production of tears and the presence of the enzyme lysozyme and other antimicrobial substances found in tears greatly reduce the numbers of indigenous microflora organisms found on the eye surfaces.

Microflora of the Respiratory Tract

The respiratory tract can be divided into the upper respiratory tract and the lower respiratory tract. The upper respiratory tract consists of the nasal passages and the throat (pharynx). The lower respiratory tract consists of the larynx (voice box), trachea, bronchi, bronchioles, and lungs.

The nasal passages and throat have an abundant and varied population of microorganisms, because these areas provide moist, warm mucous membranes that furnish excellent conditions for microbial growth. Many microorganisms found in the healthy nose and throat are harmless. Others are opportunistic pathogens, which have the potential to cause disease under certain circumstances. Some people—known as healthy **carriers**—harbor virulent (disease-causing) pathogens in their nasal passages or throats, but do not have the diseases associated with them, such as diphtheria, meningitis, pneumonia, and whooping cough. Although these carriers are unaffected by these pathogens, carriers can transmit them to susceptible persons.

The lower respiratory tract is usually free of microbes because the mucous membranes and lungs have defense mechanisms (described in Chapter 15) that efficiently remove invaders.

Microflora of the Oral Cavity (Mouth)

The anatomy of the oral cavity (mouth) affords shelter for numerous anaerobic and aerobic bacteria. Anaerobic microorganisms flourish in gum margins, crevices between the teeth, and deep folds (crypts) on the surface of the tonsils. Bacteria thrive especially well in particles of food and in the debris of dead epithelial cells around the teeth. Food remaining on and between teeth provides a rich nutrient medium for growth of the many oral bacteria. Carelessness in dental hygiene allows growth of these bacteria, with development of dental caries (tooth decay), gingivitis (gum disease), and more severe periodontal diseases.

The list of microbes that have been isolated from healthy human mouths reads like a manual of the major groups of microorganisms. It includes Gram-positive and Gram-negative bacteria (both cocci and bacilli), spirochetes, and sometimes yeasts, moldlike organisms, protozoa, and viruses. The bacteria include species of *Actinomyces, Bacteroides, Fusobacterium, Lactobacillus, Porphyromonas, Streptococcus, Neisseria,* and *Veillonella.* The most common organisms in the indigenous microflora of the mouth are various species of α-hemolytic streptococci.

Microflora of the Gastrointestinal Tract

The gastrointestinal (GI) tract (or digestive tract) consists of a long tube with many expanded areas designed for digestion of food, absorption of nutrients, and elimination of undigested materials. Excluding the oral cavity and pharynx, which have already been discussed, the GI tract includes the esophagus, stomach, small intestine, large intestine (colon), and anus. Accessory glands and organs of the GI system include the salivary glands, pancreas, liver, and gallbladder.

Gastric enzymes and the extremely acidic pH (approximately pH 1.5) of the stomach usually prevent growth of indigenous microflora, and most transient microbes (i.e., microbes consumed in foods and beverages) are killed as they pass through the stomach. There is one bacterium—a Gram-negative bacillus named *Helicobacter pylori*—that lives in some people's stomachs and is a common cause of ulcers. A few microbes, enveloped by food particles, manage to pass through the stomach during periods of low acid concentration. Also, when the amount of acid is reduced in the course of diseases such as stomach cancer, certain bacteria may be found in the stomach.

Few microflora usually exist in the upper portion of the small intestine (the duodenum) because bile inhibits their growth, but many are found in the lower parts of the small intestine (the jejunum and ileum).

The colon contains the largest number and variety of microorganisms of any colonized area of the body. It has been estimated that as many as 500 to 600 different species—primarily bacteria—live there. Because the colon is anaerobic, the bacteria living there are obligate-, aerotolerant-, and facultative anaerobes. Also, many fungi, protozoa, and viruses can live in the colon. Many of the microflora of the colon are opportunists, causing disease only when they gain access to other areas of the body (e.g., urinary bladder, bloodstream, or lesion of some type), or when the usual balance among the microorganisms is upset. *E. coli* is a good example. All humans have *E. coli* bacteria in their colon. They are opportunists, usually causing us no problems at all, but they can cause urinary tract infections (UTIs) when they gain access to the urinary bladder. In fact, *E. coli* is the most common cause of UTIs.

Many microbes are removed from the GI tract as a result of defecation. It has been estimated that about 50% of the fecal mass consists of bacteria.

Microflora of the Genitourinary Tract

The genitourinary (GU) tract (or urogenital tract) consists of the urinary tract (kidneys, ureters, urinary bladder, and urethra) and the various parts of the male and female reproductive systems.

The healthy kidney, ureters, and urinary bladder are sterile. However, the distal urethra (that part of the urethra furthest from the urinary bladder) and the external opening of the urethra harbor many microbes, including bacteria, yeasts, and viruses. As a rule, these organisms do not invade the bladder because the urethra is periodically flushed by acidic urine. Frequent urination helps to prevent UTIs. However, persistent, recurring UTIs often develop when there is an obstruction or narrowing of the urethra, which allows the invasive organisms to multiply. The most frequent causes of urethral infection (urethritis)—*Chlamydia trachomatis, Neisseria gonorrhoeae,* and mycoplasmas—are easily introduced into the urethra by sexual intercourse.

The reproductive systems of both men and women are usually sterile, with the exception of the vagina; here, the microflora varies with the stage of sexual development. During puberty and after menopause, vaginal secretions are alkaline, supporting the growth of various diphtheroids,

streptococci, staphylococci, and coliforms (*E. coli* and closely related enteric Gram-negative rods). Through the childbearing years, vaginal secretions are acidic (pH 4.0 to 5.0), encouraging the growth mainly of lactobacilli, along with a few α-hemolytic streptococci, staphylococci, diphtheroids, and yeasts. The metabolic by-products of lactobacilli, especially lactic acid, inhibit growth of the bacteria associated with bacterial vaginosis (BV). Factors that lead to a decrease in the number of lactobacilli in the vaginal microflora can lead to an overgrowth of other bacteria (e.g., *Bacteroides* spp., *Mobiluncus* spp., *Gardnerella vaginalis,* and anaerobic cocci), which in turn can lead to BV. Likewise, a decrease in the number of lactobacilli can lead to an overgrowth of yeasts, which in turn can lead to yeast vaginitis.

Beneficial and Harmful Roles of Indigenous Microflora

Humans derive many benefits from their indigenous microflora, some of which have already been mentioned. Some nutrients, particularly vitamins K and B_{12}, pantothenic acid, pyridoxine, and biotin, are obtained from secretions of certain intestinal bacteria. Evidence also indicates that indigenous microbes provide a constant source of irritants and antigens to stimulate the immune system. This causes the immune system to respond more readily by producing antibodies to foreign invaders and substances, which in turn enhances the body's protection against pathogens. The mere presence of large numbers of microorganisms at certain anatomic locations is beneficial, in that they prevent pathogens from colonizing those locations.

Microbial Antagonism

The term *microbial antagonism* means "microbes versus microbes" or "microbes against microbes." Many of the microbes of our indigenous microflora serve a beneficial role by preventing other microbes from becoming established in or colonizing a particular anatomic location. For example, the huge numbers of bacteria in our colons accomplish this by occupying space and consuming nutrients. "Newcomers" (including pathogens that we have ingested) cannot gain a foothold because of the intense competition for space and nutrients.

Other examples of microbial antagonism involve the production of antibiotics and bacteriocins. As discussed in Chapter 9, many bacteria and fungi produce antibiotics. Recall that an antibiotic is a substance produced by one microorganism that kills or inhibits the growth of another microorganism. (Actually, the term antibiotic is usually reserved for those substances produced by bacteria and fungi that have been found useful in treating infectious diseases.) Some bacteria produce proteins called bacteriocins which kill other bacteria. An example is colicin, a bacteriocin produced by *E. coli.*

Different Uses of the Term "Antagonism"

As was just explained, "antagonism," as used in the term "microbial antagonism," refers to the adverse effects that some microbes have on other microbes. However, as you learned in Chapter 9, antagonism can also refer to the adverse effects of using two antibiotics simultaneously. With respect to antibiotic use, an antagonistic effect is a bad thing, because fewer pathogens are killed by using two drugs that work against each other than would be killed if either drug was used alone.

Opportunistic Pathogens and Biotherapeutic Agents

As you know, many members of the indigenous microflora of the human body are opportunistic pathogens (opportunists), which can be thought of as organisms that are hanging around, waiting for the opportunity to cause infections. Take *E. coli* for example. Huge numbers of *E. coli* live in our intestinal tract, causing us no problems whatsoever on a day-to-day basis. They do possess the potential to be pathogenic, however, and can cause serious infections should they find their way to a site such as the urinary bladder, bloodstream, or wound. Other especially important opportunistic pathogens in the human indigenous microflora include other members of the family *Enterobacteriaceae*, *Staphylococcus aureus*, and *Enterococcus* spp.

When the delicate balance among the various species in the population of indigenous microflora is upset by antibiotics, other types of chemotherapy, or changes in pH, many complications may result. Certain microorganisms may flourish out of control, such as *C. albicans* in the vagina, leading to yeast vaginitis. Also, diarrhea and pseudomembranous colitis may occur as a result of overgrowth of *Clostridium difficile* in the colon. Cultures of *Lactobacillus* in yogurt or in medications may be prescribed to reestablish and stabilize the microbial balance. Bacteria and yeasts used in this manner are called **biotherapeutic agents** (or probiotics). Other microorganisms that have been used as biotherapeutic agents include *Bifidobacterium* spp., nonpathogenic *Enterococcus* spp., and *Saccharomyces* spp. (yeasts).

Microbial Communities

We often read about one particular microorganism as being the cause of a certain disease or as playing a specific role in nature. In reality, it is rare to find an ecologic niche in which only one type of microorganism is present or only one microorganism is causing a particular effect. In nature, microorganisms are often organized into what are known as **biofilms**—complex and tenacious communities of assorted organisms. Bacterial biofilms are virtually everywhere; examples include dental plaque, the slippery coating on a rock in a stream, and the slime that accumulates on the inner walls of various types of pipes and tubing. A bacterial biofilm consists of a variety of different species of bacteria plus a gooey polysaccharide (extracellular matrix) that the bacteria secrete. The bacteria grow in tiny clusters—called **microcolonies**—that are separated by a network of water channels. The fluid that flows through these channels bathes the microcolonies with dissolved nutrients and carries away waste products.

Biofilms have medical significance. They form on urinary catheters and permanent medical implants and have been implicated in diseases such as endocarditis, cystic fibrosis, middle ear infections, kidney stones, periodontal disease, and prostate infections. Microbes commonly associated with biofilms on indwelling medical devices include the yeast *C. albicans* and bacteria such as *S. aureus*, coagulase-negative staphylococci, *Enterococcus* spp., *Klebsiella pneumoniae*, and *Pseudomonas aeruginosa*.

Biofilms are very resistant to antibiotics and disinfectants. Antibiotics that, in the laboratory, have been shown to be effective against pure cultures of organisms within biofilms may be ineffective against those same organisms within an actual biofilm. Let's take penicillin as an example. Penicillin is an antibiotic that prevents bacteria from producing cell walls. In the laboratory, penicillin may kill actively growing cells of a particular organism, but it does not kill any cells of that organism within the biofilm that are not growing (i.e., that are not actively building cell walls). Also, any penicillinases (discussed in Chapter 9) being produced by organisms within the biofilm will inactivate the penicillin molecule, and will thus protect other organisms within the biofilm from the effects of penicillin. Therefore, some bacteria that are present within the biofilm protect other species of bacteria within the biofilm. Another example of how bacteria within a biofilm cooperate with each other involves nutrients. In some biofilms, bacteria of different species cooperate to break down nutrients that any single species cannot break down by itself. In some cases, one species within a biofilm feeds on the metabolic wastes of another.

Research has shown that bacteria within biofilms produce many different types of proteins that those same organisms do not produce when they are grown in pure culture. Some of these proteins are involved in the formation of the extracellular matrix and microcolonies. It is thought that bacteria in biofilms can communicate with each other. Experiments with *P. aeruginosa* have demonstrated that when a sufficient number of cells accumulate, the concentrations of certain signaling molecules becomes high enough to trigger changes in the activity of dozens of genes. Whereas in the past, scientists studied ways to control individual species of bacteria, they are now concentrating their efforts on ways to attack and control biofilms.

Agricultural Microbiology

There are many uses for microorganisms in agriculture. They are used extensively in the field of genetic engineering to create new or genetically altered plants. Such genetically engineered plants might grow larger, be better tasting, or be more resistant to insects, plant diseases, or extremes in temperature. Some microorganisms are used as pesticides. Many microorganisms are decomposers, which return minerals and other nutrients to soil. In addition, microorganisms play major roles in elemental cycles, such as the carbon, oxygen, nitrogen, phosphorous, and sulfur cycles.

Role of Microbes in Elemental Cycles

Bacteria are exceptionally adaptable and versatile. They are found on the land, in all waters, in every animal and plant, and even inside other microorganisms (in which case they are referred to as **endosymbionts**). Some bacteria and fungi serve a valuable function by recycling back into the soil the nutrients from dead, decaying animals and plants, as was briefly discussed in Chapter 1. Free-living fungi and bacteria that decompose dead organic matter into inorganic materials are called saprophytes. The inorganic nutrients that are returned to the soil are used by chemotrophic bacteria and plants for synthesis of biologic molecules necessary for their growth. The plants are eaten by animals, which eventually die and are recycled again with the aid of saprophytes. The cycling of elements by microorganisms is sometimes referred to as biogeochemical cycling.

Good examples of the cycling of nutrients in nature are the nitrogen, carbon, oxygen, sulfur, and phosphorus cycles, in which microorganisms play very important roles. In the nitrogen cycle (Fig. 10-3), free atmospheric nitrogen gas (N_2) is converted by **nitrogen-fixing bacteria** and cyanobacteria into ammonia (NH_3) and the ammonium ion (NH_4^+). Then, chemolithotrophic soil bacteria, called **nitrifying bacteria,** convert ammonium ions into nitrite ions (NO_2^-) and nitrate ions (NO_3^-). Plants then use the nitrates to build plant proteins; these proteins are eaten by animals, which then use them to build animal proteins. Excreted nitrogen-containing animal waste products (such as urea in urine) are converted by certain bacteria to ammonia by a process known as **ammonification.** Also, dead plant and animal nitrogen-containing debris and fecal material are transformed by saprophytic fungi and bacteria into ammonia, which in turn is converted into nitrites and nitrates for recycling by plants. To replenish the free nitrogen in the air, a group of bacteria called **denitrifying bacteria** convert nitrates to atmospheric nitrogen gas (N_2). The cycle goes on and on.

Some nitrogen-fixing bacteria (e.g., *Rhizobium* and *Bradyrhizobium* spp.) live in and near the root nodules of plants called legumes, such as alfalfa, clover, peas, soybeans, and peanuts (Fig. 10-4). These plants are often used in crop-rotation techniques by farmers to return nitrogen compounds to the soil for use as nutrients by cash crops. Nitrifying soil bacteria include *Nitrosomonas, Nitrosospira, Nitrosococcus, Nitrosolobus,* and *Nitrobacter* spp. Denitrifying bacteria include certain species of *Pseudomonas* and *Bacillus.*

Other Soil Microorganisms

In addition to the bacteria that play essential roles in elemental cycles, there are a multitude of other microorganisms in soil—bacteria (including cyanobacteria), fungi (primarily molds), algae, protozoa, viruses, and viroids. Many of the soil microorganisms are decomposers.

A variety of human pathogens live in soil, including various *Clostridium* spp. (e.g., *Clostridium tetani,* the causative agent of tetanus; *Clostridium botulinum,* the causative agent of botulism; and the various *Clostridium* spp. that cause gas gangrene). The spores of *Bacillus anthracis* (the causative

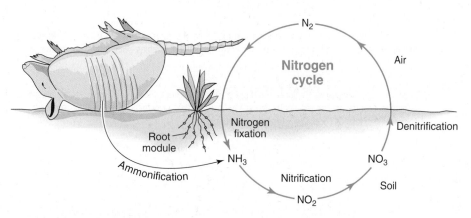

FIGURE 10-3. The nitrogen cycle. (See text for details.)

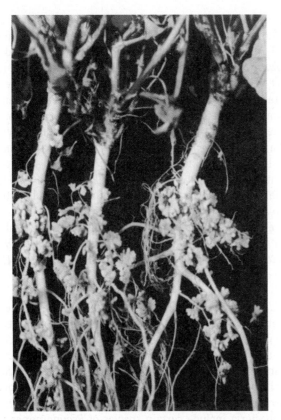

FIGURE 10-4. Nodules on the roots of a legume. These root nodules contain nitrogen-fixing bacteria, such as *Rhizobium* species. (Lechavelier HA, Pramer D. The Microbes. Philadelphia: JB Lippincott, 1970.)

agent of anthrax) may also be present in soil, where they can remain viable for many years. Various yeasts (e.g., *Cryptococcus neoformans*) and fungal spores present in soil may cause human diseases after inhalation of the dust that results from overturning dirt.

The types and amounts of microorganisms living in soil depend on many factors, including the amount of decaying organic material, available nutrients, moisture content, amount of oxygen available, pH, temperature, and the presence of waste products of other microbes.

Infectious Diseases of Farm Animals

Farmers, ranchers, and agricultural microbiologists are concerned about the many infectious diseases of farm animals—diseases that may be caused by a wide variety of pathogens (e.g., viruses, bacteria, protozoa, fungi, and helminths). Not only is there the danger that some of these diseases could be transmitted to humans (discussed in Chapter 11), but these diseases are also of obvious economic concern to farmers and ranchers. Fortunately, vaccines are available to prevent many of these diseases. Although a discussion of these diseases is beyond the scope of this introductory microbiology book, it is important for microbiology students to be aware of their existence. (Likewise, microbiology students should realize that there are many infectious diseases of wild animals, zoo animals, and pets; topics that, because of space limitations, also cannot be addressed in this book.) Table 10-2 lists a few of the many infectious diseases of farm animals and the causative agents of those diseases.

TABLE 10-2

Infectious Diseases of Farm Animals

CATEGORY	DISEASES
Prion diseases	Bovine spongiform encephalopathy ("mad cow disease"), scrapie
Viral diseases	Blue tongue (sore muzzle), bovine viral diarrhea (BVD), equine encephalomyelitis (sleeping sickness), equine infectious anemia, foot-and-mouth disease, infectious bovine rhinotracheitis, influenza, rabies, swine pox, vesicular stomatitis, warts
Bacterial diseases	Actinomycosis ("lumpy jaw"), anthrax, blackleg, botulism, brucellosis ("Bang's disease"), campylobacteriosis, distemper (strangles), erysipelas, foot rot, fowl cholera, leptospirosis, listeriosis, mastitis, pasteurellosis, pneumonia, redwater (bacillary hemoglobinuria), salmonellosis, tetanus ("lock jaw"), tuberculosis, vibriosis
Fungal diseases	Ringworm
Protozoal diseases	Anaplasmosis, bovine trichomoniasis, cattle tick fever (babesiosis), coccidiosis, cryptosporidiosis

Microbial Diseases of Plants

Microbes cause thousands of different types of plant diseases, often resulting in huge economic losses. Most plant diseases are caused by fungi, viruses, viroids, and bacteria. Not only are living plants attacked and destroyed, but microbes (primarily fungi) also cause the rotting of stored grains and other crops. Plant diseases have interesting names such as blights, cankers, galls, leaf spots, mildews, mosaics, rots, rusts, scabs, smuts, and wilts. Three especially infamous plant diseases are Dutch elm disease (which, since its importation into the United States in 1930, has destroyed about 70% of the elm trees in North America), late blight of potatoes (which resulted in the Great Potato Famine in Ireland, 1845–1849), and wheat rust (which destroys tons of wheat annually). Table 10-3 contains the names of a few of the many plant diseases caused by microorganisms.

Biotechnology

The U.S. Congress defines *biotechnology* as "any technique that uses living organisms (or parts of organisms) to make or modify products, to improve plants or animals, or to develop microorganisms for specific uses." (Biotechnology for the 21st century: Realizing the promise. Washington, D.C.: U.S. Government Printing Office, 1993.) Microbes are used in a variety of industries, including the production of certain foods and beverages, food additives, amino acids, enzymes, chemicals, vitamins (such as vitamins B_{12} and C), vaccines, and antibiotics, as well as in the mining of ores such as copper and uranium.

Microorganisms are used in the production of foods such as acidophilus milk, bread, butter, cocoa, coffee, cottage cheese, cultured buttermilk, fish sauces, green olives,

TABLE 10-3

Examples of Plant Diseases Caused by Microorganisms

DISEASE	PATHOGEN	DISEASE	PATHOGEN
Bean mosaic disease	Virus	Late blight of potatoes	Fungus (a water mold)
Black spot of roses	Fungus	Mushroom root rot	Fungus
Blue mold of tobacco	Fungus (a water mold)	Potato spindle tuber	Viroid
Brown patch of lawns	Fungus	Powdery mildews	Fungi
Chestnut blight	Fungus	Tobacco mosaic disease	Virus
Citrus exocortis	Viroid	Various leaf spots	Bacteria and fungi
Cotton root rot	Fungus	Various rots	Fungi
Crown gall	Bacteria	Various rusts	Fungi
Downy mildew of grapes	Fungus (a water mold)	Various smuts	Fungi
Dutch elm disease	Fungus	Wheat mosaic disease	Virus
Ergot	Fungus	Wheat rust	Fungus

kimchi (from cabbage), meat products (e.g., country-cured hams, sausage, salami), olives, pickles, poi (fermented taro root), sauerkraut, sour cream, soy sauce, tofu, various ripened cheeses (e.g., Brie, Camembert, Cheddar, Colby, Edam, Gouda, Gruyere, Limburger, Muenster, Parmesan, Romano, Roquefort, Swiss), vinegar, and yogurt. Microbes (yeasts) are also used in the production of alcoholic beverages, such as ale, beer, bourbon, brandy, cognac, rum, rye whiskey, sake (rice wine), Scotch whiskey, vodka, and wine.

Two amino acids produced by microbes are used in the artificial sweetener called aspartame (NutraSweet). Microbes are also used in the commercial production of amino acids (e.g., alanine, aspartate, cysteine, glutamate, glycine, histidine, lysine, methionine, phenylalanine, tryptophan) that are used in the food industry. Certain bacteria and molds are used in the production of vitamins (e.g., riboflavin and vitamin B_{12}).

Microbial enzymes used in industry include amylases, cellulase, collagenase, lactase, lipase, pectinase, and proteases. Microbes can be used in the large-scale production of chemicals such as acetic acid, acetone, butanol, citric acid, ethanol, formic acid, glycerol, isopropanol, and lactic acid, as well as biofuels such as hydrogen and methane. They can also be used in the mining of arsenic, cadmium, cobalt, copper, nickel, uranium, and other metals in a process known as leaching or bioleaching.

Many antibiotics are produced in pharmaceutical company laboratories by fungi and bacteria. Penicillins and cephalosporins are examples of antibiotics produced by fungi. Examples of antibiotics produced by bacteria are bacitracin, chloramphenicol, erythromycin, polymyxin B, streptomycin, tetracycline, and vancomycin. Genetically engineered bacteria and yeasts are used in the production of human insulin, human growth hormone, interferon, hepatitis B vaccine, and other important substances (discussed in Chapter 7).

Bioremediation

The term *bioremediation* refers to the use of microorganisms to clean up various types of wastes, including industrial wastes and other pollutants (e.g., herbicides and pesticides). Some of the microbes used in this manner have been genetically engineered to digest specific wastes. For example, genetically engineered, petroleum-digesting bacteria were used to clean up the 11 million–gallon oil spill in Prince William Sound, Alaska, in 1989. At a government defense plant in Savannah River, Georgia, scientists have used naturally occurring bacteria known as methanotrophs to remove highly toxic solvents such as trichloroethylene and tetrachloroethylene (collectively referred to as TCEs) from the soil. The methanotrophs, which normally consume methane in the environment, were more or less "tricked" into decomposing the TCEs. In addition, microbes are used extensively in composting, sewage treatment, and water purification (see Chapter 11).

◉ REVIEW OF KEY POINTS

- Microbial ecology is the study of the interrelationships among microorganisms and the living and nonliving world around them.

- Most relationships between humans and microbes are beneficial rather than harmful.

- Microbes play important roles in agriculture, industrial processes, sewage treatment, and water purification, as well as in the fields of genetic engineering, gene therapy, and bioremediation.

- A mutualistic relationship is of benefit to both parties (both symbionts), whereas a commensalistic relationship is of benefit to one symbiont and of no consequence to the other (i.e., neither beneficial nor harmful). A parasitic relationship is beneficial to the parasite and detrimental to the host. Although many parasites cause disease, others do not.

- Synergism is a mutualistic relationship in which two organisms work together to produce a result that neither could accomplish alone. Synergistic infections include trench mouth and bacterial vaginosis.

- Relatively few types of microbes become human indigenous microflora because the human body is not a suitable host for most environmental microorganisms.

- Destruction of the resident microflora disturbs the delicate balance established between a host and its microorganisms.

- A usually harmless opportunist may cause complications when an abnormal situation occurs, such as entry of the organism into a wound, the bloodstream, or an organ (e.g., the urinary bladder), or after destruction of much of the indigenous microflora by antibiotic therapy.

- Frequent washing with soap and water removes most of the potentially harmful transient microbes found in sweat and other human body secretions.

- Many benefits are derived by humans from the symbiotic relationships established with their indigenous microflora.

- Inorganic nutrients, returned to the soil by saprophytes, are used by chemotrophic bacteria and plants for synthesis of biologic molecules necessary for growth. The plants are eaten by animals, which eventually die and are recycled again with the aid of saprophytes.

- Biotechnology includes the industrial use of microbes in the production of certain foods and beverages, food additives, chemicals, amino acids, enzymes, vitamins B_{12} and C, and antibiotics, as well as in the refining of ores to obtain copper, uranium, and gold.

- Bioremediation includes the use of microbes to dispose of industrial and toxic wastes and other environmental pollutants, such as pesticides, herbicides, and petroleum spills. Many of the microbes used in bioremediation are found in nature, but others are genetically engineered to digest specific wastes.

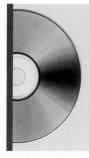

On the CD-ROM

- Critical Thinking
- Additional Self-Assessment Exercises

Self-Assessment Exercises

After studying this chapter, answer the following multiple-choice questions.

1. A symbiont could be a(n):
   a. commensal.
   b. opportunist.
   c. parasite.
   d. all of the above

2. The greatest number and variety of indigenous microflora of the human body live in or on the:
   a. colon.
   b. genitourinary tract.
   c. mouth.
   d. skin.

3. *Escherichia coli* living in the human colon can be considered to be a(n):
   a. endosymbiont.
   b. opportunist.
   c. symbiont in a mutualistic relationship.
   d. all of the above

4. Which of the following sites of the human body does not have indigenous microflora?
   a. bloodstream
   b. colon
   c. distal urethra
   d. vagina

5. Which of the following would be present in highest numbers in the indigenous microflora of the human mouth?
   a. α-hemolytic streptococci
   b. β-hemolytic streptococci
   c. *Candida albicans*
   d. *Staphylococcus aureus*

6. Which of the following would be present in highest numbers in the indigenous microflora of the skin?
   a. *Candida albicans*
   b. coagulase-negative staphylococci
   c. *Enterococcus* spp.
   d. *Escherichia coli*

7. The indigenous microflora of the external ear canal is most like the indigenous microflora of the:
   a. colon
   b. mouth
   c. skin
   d. distal urethra

8. Which of the following are *least* likely to play a role in the nitrogen cycle?
   a. indigenous microflora
   b. nitrifying and denitrifying bacteria
   c. nitrogen-fixing bacteria
   d. bacteria living in the root nodules of legumes

9. Microorganisms are used in which of the following industries?
   a. antibiotic
   b. chemical
   c. food, beer, and wine
   d. all of the above

10. The term that best describes a symbiotic relationship in which two different microorganisms occupy the same ecologic niche, but have absolutely no effect on each other is:
    a. commensalism.
    b. mutualism.
    c. neutralism.
    d. parasitism.

EPIDEMIOLOGY AND PUBLIC HEALTH

LEARNING OBJECTIVES

AFTER STUDYING THIS CHAPTER, YOU SHOULD BE ABLE TO:

- Define epidemiology
- Differentiate among infectious, communicable, and contagious diseases; cite an example of each
- Differentiate between the incidence of a disease and the prevalence of a disease
- Differentiate among sporadic, endemic, nonendemic, epidemic, and pandemic diseases
- Name three diseases that are currently considered to be pandemics
- List the six components of the chain of infection in the proper order
- Identify three examples of living reservoirs and three examples of nonliving reservoirs
- List five modes of infectious disease transmission
- List four examples of potential biological warfare (bw) or bioterrorism agents
- Outline the steps involved in water treatment
- Explain what is meant by a coliform count and state its importance

Epidemiology

Introduction

Both *pathology* and *epidemiology* can be loosely defined as the study of disease, but they involve different aspects of disease. Whereas a pathologist studies the structural and functional manifestations of disease and is involved in diagnosing diseases in individuals, an *epidemiologist* studies the factors that determine the frequency, distribution, and determinants of diseases in human populations. With respect to infectious diseases, these factors include the characteristics of various pathogens; susceptibility of different human populations resulting from overcrowding, lack of immunization, nutritional status, inadequate sanitation procedures, and other factors; locations (reservoirs) where pathogens are lurking; and the various ways in which infectious diseases are transmitted. It could be said that epidemiologists are concerned with the who, what, where, when, and why of infectious diseases: Who becomes infected? What pathogens are causing the infections? Where do the pathogens come from? When do certain diseases occur? Why do some diseases occur in certain places but not in others? How are pathogens transmitted? Do some diseases occur only at certain times of the year? If so, why? Epidemiologists also develop ways to prevent, control, or eradicate diseases in populations. Epidemiologists are concerned with *all* types of diseases—not just infectious diseases. However, only infectious diseases are discussed in this chapter. (See "Insight: Epidemiologists" on the CD-ROM for information about this profession.)

Epidemiologic Terminology

Sometimes it seems like epidemiologists speak a language all their own. They frequently use terms such as communicable, contagious, and zoonotic diseases; the incidence, morbidity rate, prevalence, and mortality rate of a particular disease; and adjectives such as sporadic, endemic, epidemic, and pandemic to describe the status of a particular infectious disease in a given population. The following sections briefly examine these terms.

Communicable and Contagious Diseases

As previously stated, an infectious disease is a disease that is caused by a pathogen. If the infectious disease is transmissible from one human to another (i.e., person-to-person), it is called a **communicable disease.** Although it might seem like splitting hairs, a **contagious disease** is defined as a communicable disease that is *easily transmitted* from one person to another. Example: Assume that you are in the front row of a movie theater. One person seated in the back row has gonorrhea and another has influenza, both of which are communicable diseases. The person with influenza is coughing and sneezing throughout the movie, creating an aerosol of influenza viruses. Thus, even though you are seated far away from the person with influenza, you might very well develop influenza as a result of inhalation of the aerosols produced by that person. Influenza is a contagious disease. On the other hand, it is highly unlikely that you would contract gonorrhea as a result of your movie-going experience. Gonorrhea is not a contagious disease.

Zoonotic Diseases

Infectious diseases that humans acquire from animal sources are called zoonotic diseases or zoonoses (sing., zoonosis). These diseases are discussed later in this chapter.

Incidence and Morbidity Rate

The **incidence** of a particular disease is defined as the number of new cases of that disease in a defined population during a specific time period, for example, the number of new

cases of hantavirus pulmonary syndrome in the United States during 2005. The incidence of a disease is similar to the **morbidity rate** for that disease, which is usually expressed as the number of new cases of a particular disease that occurred during a specified time period per a specifically defined population (usually per 1,000, 10,000, or 100,000 population), for example, the number of new cases of a particular disease in 2005 per 100,000 U.S. population.

Prevalence

There are two types of **prevalence:** period prevalence and point prevalence. The *period prevalence* of a particular disease is the number of cases of the disease existing in a given population during a specific time period (e.g., the total number of cases of gonorrhea that existed in the U.S. population during 2005). The *point prevalence* of a particular disease is the number of cases of the disease existing in a given population at a particular moment in time (e.g., the number of cases of malaria in the U.S. population at this moment).

HISTORICAL NOTE

The Broad Street Pump

In the mid-19th century, a British physician by the name of John Snow designed and conducted an epidemiologic investigation of a cholera outbreak in London. He carefully compared households affected by cholera with households that were unaffected, and concluded that the primary difference between them was their source of drinking water. At one point in his investigation, he ordered the removal of the handle of the Broad Street water pump, thus helping to end an epidemic that had killed more than 500 people. People were unable to pump (and, therefore, unable to drink) the contaminated water. Snow published a paper, *On the Communication of Cholera by Impure Thames Water,* in 1884, and a book, *On the Mode of Communication of Cholera,* in 1885. He concluded that cholera was spread via fecally contaminated water. The water at the Broad Street pump was being contaminated with sewage from the adjacent houses (Fig. 11-1). Snow is considered by many to be the "Father of Epidemiology."

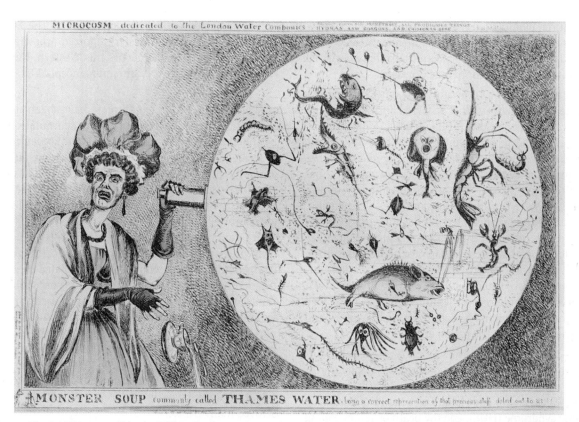

FIGURE 11-1. *Thames Water,* an etching by William Heath, c. 1828. A satire on the contamination of the water supply. A London commission reported in 1828 that the Thames River water at Chelsea was "charged with the contents of the great common-sewers, the drainings of the dunghills and laystalls, [and] the refuse of hospitals, slaughterhouses, and manufactures." (Zigrosser C. Medicine and the Artist [Ars Medica]. New York: Dover Publications, Inc., 1970. By permission of the Philadelphia Museum of Art.)

Mortality Rate

Mortality refers to death. The ***mortality rate*** (also known as the *death rate*) is the ratio of the number of people who died of a particular disease during a specified time period per a specified population (usually per 1,000, 10,000, or 100,000 population), for example, the number of people who died of a particular disease in 2005 per 100,000 U.S. population.

Sporadic Diseases

A ***sporadic disease*** is one that occurs only occasionally (sporadically) within the population of a particular geographic area. In the United States, sporadic diseases include botulism, cholera, gas gangrene, plague, tetanus, and typhoid fever. Quite often, certain diseases occur only sporadically because they are kept under control as a result of immunization programs and sanitary conditions. It is possible for outbreaks of these controlled diseases to occur, however, whenever vaccination programs and other public health programs are neglected.

Endemic Diseases

Endemic diseases are diseases that are always present within the population of a particular geographic area. The number of cases of the disease may fluctuate over time, but the disease never dies out completely. Endemic infectious diseases of the United States include bacterial diseases such as tuberculosis, staphylococcal and streptococcal infections, sexually transmitted diseases like gonorrhea and syphilis, and viral diseases such as the common cold, influenza, chickenpox, and mumps. In some parts of the United States, plague (caused by a bacterium called *Yersinia pestis*) is endemic among rats, prairie dogs, and other rodents, but is not endemic among humans. Plague in humans is only occasionally observed in the United States, and is, therefore, a sporadic disease. The actual incidence of an endemic disease at any particular time depends on a balance among several factors, including the environment, genetic susceptibility of the population, behavioral factors, number of people who are immune, virulence of the pathogen, and reservoir or source of infection.

Epidemic Diseases

Endemic diseases may on occasion become ***epidemic diseases.*** An epidemic (or outbreak) is defined as a greater than usual number of cases of a disease in a particular region, usually occurring within a relatively short period of time. An epidemic does not necessarily involve a large number of people, although it might. If a dozen people develop staphylococcal food poisoning shortly after their return from a church picnic, then that constitutes an epidemic—a small one, to be sure, but an epidemic nonetheless.

Listed here are a few of the epidemics that have occurred in the United States within the past 35 years:

- **1976.** Epidemic of a respiratory disease (Legionnaire's disease or legionellosis) that occurred during an American Legion convention in Philadelphia, Pennsylvania, which resulted in approximately 220 hospitalizations and 34 deaths. The pathogen (*Legionella pneumophila,* a Gram-negative bacillus) was present in the water being circulated through the air-conditioning system of the hotel where the affected Legionnaires were staying. Aerosols of the organism were inhaled by occupants of some of the rooms in the hotel. Subsequent epidemics of legionellosis have occurred in other hotels, hospitals, cruise ships, and supermarkets. The supermarket outbreaks were associated with the misting of vegetables. Virtually all epidemics of legionellosis have involved contaminated water or colonized water pipes and aerosols containing the pathogen.

- **1992–1993.** Epidemic involving *Escherichia coli* O157: H7-contaminated hamburger meat in the Pacific northwest, which resulted in approximately 500 diarrheal cases, 45 cases of kidney failure as a result of hemolytic uremic syndrome (HUS), and the death of several young children. *E. coli* O157:H7 is a particularly virulent serotype of *E. coli;* it is also known as enterohemorrhagic *E. coli*. In this epidemic, the source of the *E. coli* was cattle feces. The ground beef used to make the hamburgers had been contaminated with cattle feces during the slaughtering process. The hamburgers had not been cooked long enough, or at a high enough temperature, to kill the bacteria.

- **1993.** Epidemic of hantavirus pulmonary syndrome (HPS) on Indian reservations in the four-corners region (where the borders of Colorado, New Mexico, Arizona, and Utah all meet), which resulted in approximately 50 to 60 cases, including 28 deaths. The particular hantavirus strain (now called Sin Nombre virus) was present in the urine and feces of deer mice, some of which had gained entrance to the homes of villagers. Aerosols of the virus were produced when residents swept up house dust containing the rodent droppings. The pathogen was then inhaled by individuals in those homes.

- **1993.** Epidemic of cryptosporidiosis (a diarrheal disease) in Milwaukee, Wisconsin, which resulted from drinking water that was contaminated with the oocysts of *Cryptosporidium parvum* (a protozoan parasite). This epidemic is described more fully later in this chapter.

- **2002.** Epidemic of West Nile virus (WNV) infections throughout the United States. More than 4,100 human cases occurred during that year, resulting in 284 deaths. In addition, more than 16,000 birds died as a result of WNV infections, and more than 14,500 horses were infected with WNV during 2002. The 2002 WNV epidemic was the largest recognized arboviral meningoencephalitis epidemic in the Western Hemisphere and the largest WNV meningoencephalitis epidemic ever recorded.

These and other epidemics have been identified through constant surveillance and accumulation of data by the Centers for Disease Control and Prevention (CDC; described later in this chapter). Epidemics usually follow a specific pattern, in which the number of cases of a disease increases to a maximum and then decreases rapidly, because the number of susceptible and exposed individuals is limited.

Epidemics may occur in communities that have not been previously exposed to a particular pathogen. People from populated areas who travel into isolated communities frequently introduce a new pathogen to susceptible inhabitants of that community; then the disease spreads like wildfire. Over the years, there have been many such examples. The syphilis epidemic in Europe in the early 1500s might have been caused by a highly virulent spirochete carried back from the West Indies by Columbus' men in 1492. Also, measles, smallpox, and tuberculosis introduced to Native Americans by early explorers and settlers almost destroyed many tribes.

In communities in which normal sanitation practices are relaxed, allowing fecal contamination of water supplies and food, epidemics of typhoid fever, cholera, giardiasis, and dysentery often occur. Visitors to these communities should be aware that they are especially susceptible to these diseases, because they never developed a natural immunity by being exposed to them during childhood.

Influenza ("flu") epidemics occur in many areas during certain times of the year and involve most of the population because the immunity developed in prior years is usually temporary. Thus, the disease recurs each year among those who are not revaccinated or naturally resistant to the infection. Epidemics of influenza cause approximately 20,000 deaths per year in the United States.

Ebola virus has caused several epidemics of hemorrhagic fever in Africa (Sudan and the Republic of the Congo in 1976; Sudan in 1979; Kikwit and the Republic of the Congo in 1995; Gabon in 1994 and 1996; Uganda in 2000; several outbreaks in Gabon and the Republic of the Congo between 2001 and 2003). The 2000 outbreak in Uganda (425 cases, 224 deaths) was the largest Ebola epidemic ever recorded. Between 50 and 90% of infected patients have died in these epidemics. The source of the virus is not yet known.

In a hospital setting, a relatively small number of infected patients can constitute an epidemic. If a higher than usual number of patients on a particular ward should suddenly become infected by a particular pathogen, this would constitute an epidemic, and the situation must be brought to the attention of the Hospital Infection Control Committee (discussed in Chapter 12).

Pandemic Diseases

A ***pandemic disease*** is a disease that is occurring in epidemic proportions in many countries simultaneously—sometimes worldwide. The 1918 Spanish flu pandemic was the most devastating pandemic of the 20th century, and is the catastrophe against which all modern pandemics are measured. That pandemic killed more than 20 million people worldwide, including 500,000 in the United States. Almost every nation on Earth was affected. Influenza pandemics are often named for the point of origin or first recognition, such as the Taiwan flu, Hong Kong flu, London flu, Port Chalmers flu, and the Russian flu.

According to the World Health Organization (WHO), infectious diseases are responsible for approximately half the deaths that occur in developing countries; approximately half of those are caused by three infectious diseases—HIV/AIDS, tuberculosis, and malaria—each of which is currently occurring in pandemic proportions. Together, these three diseases cause more than 300 million illnesses and more than 5 million deaths per year.

HIV/AIDS. Although the first documented evidence of human immunodeficiency virus (HIV) infection in humans can be traced to an African serum sample collected in 1959, it is possible that humans were infected with HIV before that date. The acquired immunodeficiency syndrome (AIDS) epidemic began in the United States around 1979, but the epidemic was not detected until 1981. It was not until 1983 that the virus that causes AIDS was discovered. HIV is thought to have been transferred to humans from other primates (chimpanzees in the case of HIV-1, and sooty mangabeys in the case of HIV-2). Additional information about AIDS can be found in Chapter 17. The following statistics, which should prove sobering to anyone who thought that AIDS was "on the run," were obtained from the WHO and CDC web sites (www.who.org; www.cdc.gov):

- The total number of people living with HIV, worldwide, rose in 2004 to reach its highest level ever—an estimated 39.4 million people. Table 11-1 shows the distribution of HIV-infected individuals at the end of 2004.

TABLE 11-1

Estimated Number of People Living With HIV Infection/AIDS at the End of 2004

GEOGRAPHIC AREA	ESTIMATED NUMBER
Sub-Saharan Africa	25.4 million
South and Southeast Asia	7.1 million
Latin America	1.7 million
Eastern Europe and Central Asia	1.4 million
East Asia	1.1 million
North America	1 million
Western Europe	610,000
North Africa and Middle East	540,000
Caribbean	440,000
Oceania	35,000

Source: World Health Organization (WHO), Geneva (www.who.org).

HISTORICAL NOTE

AIDS in the United States

It has been stated that the AIDS epidemic in the United States officially began with publication of the June 5, 1981, issue of *Morbidity and Mortality Weekly Report*. That issue contained a report of five cases of *Pneumocystis carinii* pneumonia (PCP) in male patients at the UCLA Medical Center. The PCP infections were later shown to be the result of a disease syndrome, which in September 1982 was first called acquired immunodeficiency syndrome (AIDS). It was not until 1983 that the virus that causes AIDS—now called human immunodeficiency virus (HIV)—was discovered. By the end of December 2003, a total of 524,060 Americans (more than had died in World Wars I and II combined) had died of AIDS. (Note: *Pneumocystis carinii* was recently renamed. It is now called *Pneumocystis jiroveci*.).

- An estimated 4.9 million people worldwide acquired HIV infection in 2004.

- The global AIDS epidemic killed 3.1 million people worldwide in 2004.

- Sub-Saharan Africa is the worst affected region, with 25.4 million people living with HIV at the end of 2004. This represents 64% of all people living with HIV worldwide.

- Southern Africa accounts for one third of all AIDS deaths globally.

- As of December 2003, a total of 929,985 U.S. cases had been reported to the CDC, including 920,566 adult and adolescent cases and 9,419 cases in children younger than age 13.

- As of December 2003, the total number of U.S. deaths of persons with AIDS was 524,060, including 518,568 adults and adolescents and 5,492 children younger than age 13.

- During 2003, 43,171 new U.S. AIDS cases (43,112 adult cases and 59 cases in children younger than 13) and 18,017 U.S. AIDS deaths were reported to the CDC.

- According to the CDC, an estimated 1,039,000 to 1,185,000 persons in the U.S. were living with HIV/AIDS at the end of 2003, with 24 to 27% undiagnosed and unaware of their HIV infection.

Tuberculosis. Another current pandemic is tuberculosis. To complicate matters, many strains of *Mycobacterium tuberculosis* (the bacterium that causes tuberculosis) have developed resistance to the drugs that are used to treat tuberculosis. Tuberculosis caused by these strains is known as multidrug-resistant tuberculosis (MDRTB). Some strains of *M. tuberculosis* have developed resistance to every drug and every combination of drugs that has ever been used to treat tuberculosis. Additional information about tuberculosis can be found in Chapter 17. The following statistics were obtained from the WHO and CDC web sites:

- Among infectious diseases, tuberculosis (TB) remains the second leading killer of adults in the world, with more than 2 million TB-related deaths each year.

- Overall, one third of the world's population is currently infected with *M. tuberculosis*.

- Someone in the world becomes newly infected with *M. tuberculosis* every second.

- Excluding individuals infected with HIV, between 5 and 10% of people who are infected with *M. tuberculosis* become sick or infectious at some time during their life.

- Left untreated, each person with active TB will infect on average between 10 and 15 people every year.

- TB is the leading cause of death among people infected with HIV. Worldwide, tuberculosis causes about 13% of AIDS deaths.

- During 2003, TB caused an estimated 1.75 million deaths worldwide. In that year, 14,874 new U.S. cases of TB were reported to the CDC.

Malaria. Malaria is the world's most important tropical parasitic disease, killing more people than any other communicable disease, except tuberculosis. Additional information about malaria can be found in Chapter 18. The following statistics were obtained from the WHO and CDC web sites:

- 41% of the world's population live in malaria-endemic areas.

- Worldwide prevalence of malaria is estimated to be between 300 and 500 million clinical cases each year.

- An estimated 700,000 to 2.7 million people die of malaria annually; 75% of them are African children.

- In 2002, malaria was the fourth leading cause of death in children in developing countries (after perinatal conditions, lower respiratory infections, and diarrheal diseases).

- During 2004, 1,458 new U.S. cases of malaria were reported to the CDC. Most U.S. cases are imported (i.e., acquired by people who have lived or traveled in malaria-endemic countries).

- Mosquitoborne malaria does occur in the United States. Between 1957 and 2003, 63 such outbreaks have occurred. In virtually all cases, the mosquitoes became infected by biting persons who had acquired malaria outside the United States.

Interactions Among Pathogens, Hosts, and the Environment

Whether an infectious disease occurs depends on many factors, some of which are listed below:

1. Factors pertaining to the pathogen:
   - Virulence of the pathogen (virulence will be discussed in Chapter 14; for now, think of virulence as a measure or degree of pathogenicity; some pathogens are more virulent than others).
   - Way for the pathogen to enter the body (i.e., is there a portal of entry?).
   - Number of organisms that enter the body (i.e., will there be a sufficient number to cause infection?).

2. Factors pertaining to the host (i.e., the person who may become infected):
   - Health status (e.g., is the person hospitalized? does he or she have any underlying illnesses? has the person undergone invasive medical or surgical procedures or catheterization? does he or she have any prosthetic devices?).
   - Nutritional status.
   - Other factors pertaining to the susceptibility of the host (e.g., age, lifestyle [behavior], socioeconomic level, travel, hygiene, substance abuse, immune status).

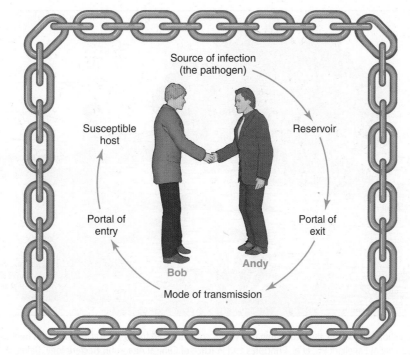

FIGURE 11-2. The six components in the infectious disease process; also known as the chain of infection.

3. Factors pertaining to the environment:
   - Physical factors such as geographic location, climate, heat, cold, humidity, and season of the year.
   - Availability of appropriate reservoirs (discussed later in this chapter), intermediate hosts (discussed in Chapter 18), and vectors (discussed later in this chapter).
   - Sanitary and housing conditions; adequate waste disposal.
   - Availability of potable (drinkable) water.

Chain of Infection

There are six components in the infectious disease process (also known as the chain of infection). They are illustrated in Figure 11-2 and are briefly described here:

1. There must first be a pathogen. As an example, let us assume that the pathogen is a cold virus.
2. There must be a source of the pathogen (i.e., a reservoir). In Figure 11-2, the infected person on the right ("Andy") is the reservoir. Andy has a cold.
3. There must be a portal of exit (i.e., a way for the pathogen to escape from the reservoir). When Andy blows his nose, cold viruses get onto his hands.
4. There must be a mode of transmission (i.e., a way for the pathogen to travel from Andy to another person). In Figure 11-2, the cold virus is being transferred by direct contact between Andy and his friend ("Bob")—by shaking hands.

5. There must be a portal of entry (i.e., a way for the pathogen to gain entry into Bob). When Bob rubs his nose, the cold virus is transferred from his hand to the mucous membranes of his nose.
6. There must be a susceptible host. For example, Bob would not be a susceptible host (and would, therefore, not develop a cold) if he had previously been infected by that particular cold virus and had developed immunity to it.

Reservoirs of Infection

The sources of microorganisms that cause infectious diseases are many and varied. They are known as ***reservoirs of infection*** or simply *reservoirs*. A reservoir is any site where the pathogen can multiply or merely survive until it is transferred to a host. Reservoirs may be living hosts or inanimate objects or materials (Fig. 11-3).

Living Reservoirs

Living reservoirs include humans, household pets, farm animals, wild animals, certain insects, and certain arachnids (ticks and mites). The human and animal reservoirs may or may not actually be experiencing illness caused by the pathogens they are harboring.

Human Carriers

The most important reservoirs of human infectious diseases are other humans—people with infectious diseases as well as carriers. A carrier is a person who is colonized with

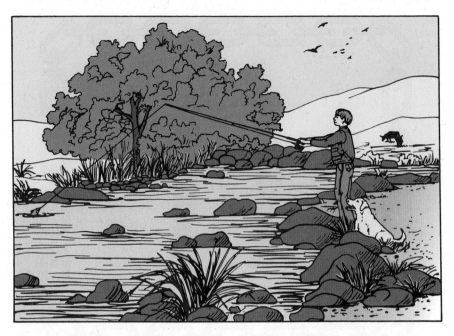

FIGURE 11-3. Reservoirs of infection include soil, dust, contaminated water, contaminated foods, insects, and infected humans, domestic animals, and wild animals. (Reproduced courtesy of Engelkirk PG, et al. Principles and Practice of Clinical Anaerobic Bacteriology. Belmont, CA: Star Publishing Co., 1992.)

a particular pathogen, but the pathogen is not currently causing disease in that person. However, the pathogen can be transmitted from the carrier to others, who may then become ill. There are several types of carriers. *Passive carriers* carry the pathogen without ever having had the disease. An *incubatory carrier* is a person who is capable of transmitting a pathogen during the incubation period of a particular infectious disease. *Convalescent carriers* harbor and can transmit a particular pathogen while recovering from an infectious disease (i.e., during the convalescence period). *Active carriers* have completely recovered from the disease, but continue to harbor the pathogen indefinitely (see the following Historical Note for an example). Respiratory secretions or feces are usually the vehicles by which the pathogen is transferred, either directly from the carrier to a susceptible individual or indirectly through food or water. Human carriers are very important in the spread of staphylococcal and streptococcal infections as well as in the spread of hepatitis, diphtheria, dysentery, meningitis, and sexually transmitted diseases (STDs).

Animals

As previously stated, infectious diseases that humans acquire from animal sources are called zoonotic diseases or zoonoses. Many pets and other animals are important reservoirs of zoonoses. Zoonoses are acquired by direct contact with the animal, by inhalation or ingestion of the pathogen, or by injection of the pathogen by an arthropod. Measures for the control of zoonotic diseases include the use of personal protective equipment when handling animals, animal vaccinations, proper use of pesticides, isolation or destruction of infected animals, and proper disposal of animal carcasses and waste products.

Dogs, cats, bats, skunks, and other animals are known reservoirs of rabies. The rabies virus is usually transmitted to a human through the saliva that is injected when one of these rabid animals bites the human. Cat and dog bites often transfer bacteria from the mouths of animals into tissues, where severe infections may result. Toxoplasmosis, a protozoan disease caused by *Toxoplasma gondii,* can be contracted by ingesting oocysts from cat feces that are present in litter boxes or sand boxes, as well by ingesting cysts that are present in infected raw or undercooked meats. Toxoplasmosis may cause severe brain damage to, or death of, the fetus when contracted by a woman during her first trimester (first 3 months) of pregnancy. The diarrheal disease, salmonellosis, is frequently acquired by ingesting *Salmonella* bacteria from the feces of turtles, other reptiles, and poultry. A variant form of Creutzfeldt-Jakob (CJ) disease in humans may be acquired by ingestion of prion-infected beef from cows with bovine spongiform encephalopathy (BSE or "mad cow disease"). Persons skinning rabbits can become infected with the bacterium *Francisella tularensis* and develop tularemia. Contact with dead animals or animal hides could result in the inhalation of the spores of *Bacillus anthracis,* leading to inhalation anthrax, or the spores could enter a cut, leading to cutaneous anthrax. Ingestion of the spores could lead to gastrointestinal anthrax. Psittacosis or "parrot fever" is a respiratory infection that may be acquired from infected birds (usually parakeets and parrots).

The most prevalent zoonotic infection in the United States is Lyme disease (discussed below), one of many arthropodborne zoonoses. (Arthropodborne diseases are diseases that are transmitted by arthropods.) Other zoonoses that occur in the United States include anthrax, brucellosis, campylobacteriosis, cryptosporidiosis, echinococcosis, ehrlichiosis, hantavirus pulmonary syndrome (HPS), leptospirosis, pasteurellosis, plague, psittacosis, Q fever, rabies, ringworm, Rocky Mountain spotted fever, salmonellosis, toxoplasmosis, tularemia, and various viral encephalitides (e.g., Western equine encephalitis, Eastern equine encephalitis, St. Louis encephalitis, California encephalitis, West Nile virus encephalitis). Some of the more than 200 known zoonoses are listed in Table 11-2. For a discussion of nosocomial (hospital-acquired) zoonoses, see the Insight section on this topic under Chapter 12 of this book's CD-ROM.

Arthropods

Many different types of arthropods serve as reservoirs of infection, including insects (e.g., mosquitoes, biting flies, lice, and fleas), and arachnids (e.g., mites and ticks). When involved in the transmission of infectious diseases, these arthropods are referred to as **vectors.** The arthropod vector first takes a blood meal from an infected person or animal and then transfers the pathogens to a healthy individual. Take Lyme disease, for example, which is the most common arthropodborne disease in the United States. First, a tick takes a blood meal from an infected deer or mouse. The tick is now infected with *Borrelia burgdorferi,* the spirochete that causes Lyme disease. Some time later, the tick takes a blood meal from a human and, in the process, injects the bacteria into the human. Ticks are especially notorious vectors. In the United States, there are at least 10 infectious diseases that are transmitted by ticks (see the following Study Aid). Other arthropodborne infectious diseases are shown in Table 11-3. Chapter 18 contains additional information about arthropods.

Nonliving Reservoirs

Nonliving or inanimate reservoirs of infection include air, soil, dust, food, milk, water, and fomites (defined below). Air can become contaminated by dust or respiratory secretions of humans expelled into the air by breathing, talking, sneezing, and coughing. The most highly contagious diseases include colds and influenza, in which the respiratory viruses can be transmitted through the air on droplets of respiratory tract secretions. Air currents and air vents can transport respiratory pathogens throughout healthcare facilities and other buildings. Dust particles can carry spores of certain bacteria and dried bits of human and animal excretions containing pathogens. Bacteria cannot multiply in

---

HISTORICAL NOTE

"Typhoid Mary"—An Infamous Carrier

Mary Mallon was a domestic employee—a cook—who worked in the New York City area in the early 1900s. Mary had recovered from typhoid fever earlier in life. Although no longer ill, she was a carrier. *Salmonella typhi,* the causative agent of typhoid fever, was still living in her gallbladder and passing in her feces. Apparently, Mary's hygienic practices were inadequate, and she would transport the *Salmonella* bacteria via her hands from the restroom to the kitchen, where she then unwittingly introduced them into foods that she prepared. After several typhoid fever outbreaks were traced to her, Mary was offered the choice of having her gallbladder removed surgically or being jailed. She opted for the latter and spent several years in jail. Mary was released from jail after promising never to cook professionally again. However, the lure of the kitchen was too great. She changed her name and resumed her profession in a variety of hotels, restaurants, and hospitals. As in the past, "everywhere that Mary went, typhoid fever was sure to follow." She was again arrested and spent her remaining years quarantined in a New York City hospital. Mary Mallon died in 1938 at the age of 70.

○ STUDY AID

Tickborne Diseases of the United States

Viral diseases:
    Colorado tick fever
    Powassan virus encephalitis
Bacterial diseases:
    Human granulocytic ehrlichiosis
    Human monocytic ehrlichiosis
    Lyme disease
    Q fever
    Rocky Mountain spotted fever
    Tickborne relapsing fever
    Tularemia
Protozoal disease:
    Babesiosis
(In addition to serving as vectors in these infectious diseases, ticks can cause tick paralysis.)

TABLE 11-2

Examples of Zoonotic Diseases

CATEGORY	DISEASE	PATHOGEN	ANIMAL RESERVOIR(S)	MODE OF TRANSMISSION
Viral diseases	Avian influenza ("bird flu")	An influenza virus	Birds	Direct or indirect contact with infected birds
	Equine encephalitis	Various arboviruses	Birds, small mammals	Mosquito bite
	Hantavirus pulmonary syndrome	Hantaviruses	Rodents	Inhalation of contaminated dust or aerosols
	Lassa fever	Lassa virus	Wild rodents	Inhalation of contaminated dust or aerosols
	Marburg disease	Marburg virus	Monkeys	Contact with blood or tissues from infected monkeys
	Rabies	Rabies virus	Rabid dogs, cats, skunks, foxes, wolves, raccoons, coyotes, bats	Animal bite or inhalation
	Yellow fever	Yellow fever virus	Monkeys	*Aedes aegypti* mosquito bite
	West Nile virus encephalitis	West Nile virus	Birds	Mosquito bite
Bacterial diseases	Anthrax	*Bacillus anthracis*	Cattle, sheep, goats	Inhalation, ingestion, entry through cuts, contact with mucous membranes
	Bovine tuberculosis	*Mycobacterium bovis*	Cattle	Ingestion
	Brucellosis	*Brucella* spp.	Cattle, swine, goats	Inhalation, ingestion of contaminated milk, entry through cuts, contact with mucous membranes
	Campylobacter infection	*Campylobacter* spp.	Wild mammals, cattle, sheep, pets	Ingestion of contaminated food and water
	Cat-scratch disease	*Bartonella henselae*	Domestic cats	Cat scratch, bite, or lick
	Ehrlichiosis	*Ehrlichia* spp.	Deer, mice	Tick bite
	Endemic typhus	*Rickettsia typhi*	Rodents	Flea bite
	Leptospirosis	*Leptospira* spp.	Cattle, rodents, dogs	Contact with contaminated animal urine
	Lyme disease	*Borrelia burgdorferi*	Deer, rodents	Tick bite
	Pasteurellosis	*Pasteurella multocida*	Oral cavities of animals	Bites, scratches
	Plague	*Yersinia pestis*	Rodents	Flea bite
	Psittacosis (ornithosis, parrot fever)	*Chlamydophila psittaci*	Parrots, parakeets, other pet birds, pigeons, poultry	Inhalation of contaminated dust and aerosols
	Relapsing fever	*Borrelia* spp.	Rodents	Tick bite
	Rickettsial pox	*Rickettsia akari*	Rodents	Mite bite
	Rocky Mountain spotted fever	*Rickettsia rickettsii*	Rodents, dogs	Tick bite
	Salmonellosis	*Salmonella* spp.	Poultry, livestock, reptiles	Ingestion of contaminated food, handling reptiles
	Scrub typhus	*Orientia tsutsugamushi*	Rodents	Mite bite
	Tularemia	*Francisella tularensis*	Wild mammals	Entry through cuts, inhalation, tick or deer fly bite
	Q fever	*Coxiella burnetii*	Cattle, sheep, goats	Tick bite, air, mild contact with infected animals

(continues)

TABLE 11-2

Examples of Zoonotic Diseases *(continued)*

CATEGORY	DISEASE	PATHOGEN	ANIMAL RESERVOIR(S)	MODE OF TRANSMISSION
Fungal diseases	Tinea (ringworm) infections	Various dermatophytes	Various animals including dogs	Contact with infected animals
Protozoal diseases	African trypanosomiasis	Subspecies of *Trypanosoma brucei*	Cattle, wild game animals	Tsetse fly bite
	American trypanosomiasis (Chagas' disease)	*Trypanosoma cruzi*	Numerous wild and, domestic animals including dogs, cats, wild rodents	Trypomastigotes in the feces of reduviid bug are rubbed into bite wound or the eye
	Babesiosis	*Babesia microti*	Deer, mice, voles	Tick bite
	Leishmaniasis	*Leishmania* spp.	Rodents, dogs	Sandfly bite
	Toxoplasmosis	*Toxoplasma gondii*	Cats, pigs, sheep, rarely cattle	Ingestion of oocysts in cat feces or cysts in raw or undercooked meat
Helminth diseases	Echinococcosis (hydatid disease)	*Echinococcus granulosis*	Dogs	Ingestion of eggs
	Dog tapeworm infection	*Dipylidium caninum*	Dogs, cats	Ingestion of flea containing the larval stage
	Rat tapeworm infection	*Hymenolepis diminuta*	Rodents	Ingestion of beetle containing the larval stage

the air, but can easily be transported by airborne particles to a warm, moist, nutrient-rich site, where they can multiply. Also, some fungal respiratory diseases (e.g., histoplasmosis) are frequently transferred by dust containing yeasts or spores. Soil contains the spores of the *Clostridium* species that cause tetanus, botulism, and gas gangrene. Any of these diseases can follow the introduction of spores into an open wound.

Food and milk may be contaminated by careless handling, which allows pathogens to enter from soil, dust particles, dirty hands, hair, and respiratory secretions. If these pathogens are not destroyed by proper processing and cooking, food poisoning can develop. In the United States, foodborne diseases cause approximately 76 million illnesses, 300,000 hospitalizations, and 5,000 deaths per year. Diseases frequently transmitted through foods and water are amebiasis (caused by the ameba, *Entamoeba histolytica*), botulism (caused by the bacterium, *Clostridium botulinum*), cholera (caused by the bacterium, *Vibrio cholerae*), *Clostridium perfringens* food poisoning, infectious hepatitis (caused by hepatitis A virus), staphylococcal food poisoning, typhoid fever (caused by the bacterium, *Salmonella typhi*), and trichinosis (a helminth disease, caused by ingesting *Trichinella spiralis* larvae in pork). Other common foodborne and waterborne pathogens are shown in Table 11-4.

Human and animal fecal matter from outhouses, cesspools, and feed lots is often carried into water supplies. Improper disposal of sewage and inadequate treatment of drinking water contribute to the spread of fecal and soil pathogens. *Fomites* are inanimate objects capable of transmitting pathogens. Fomites found within healthcare settings include patients' gowns, bedding, towels, eating and drinking utensils, and hospital equipment, such as bedpans, stethoscopes, latex gloves, electronic thermometers, and electrocardiographic electrodes, which become contaminated by pathogens from the respiratory tract, intestinal tract, or the skin of patients. Even telephones, doorknobs, and computer keyboards can serve as fomites. Great care must be taken by healthcare personnel to prevent transmission of pathogens from living and nonliving reservoirs to hospitalized patients.

Modes of Transmission

Healthcare professionals must be thoroughly familiar with the sources (reservoirs) of potential pathogens and pathways for their transfer. A hospital staphylococcal epidemic may begin when aseptic conditions are relaxed and a *Staphylococcus aureus* carrier transmits the pathogen to

TABLE 11-3

Arthropods That Serve As Vectors of Human Infectious Diseases

VECTORS	DISEASE(S)
Black flies (*Simulium* spp.)	Onchocerciasis ("river blindness") (H)
Cyclops spp.	Fish tapeworm infection (H), guinea worm infection (H)
Fleas	Dog tapeworm infection (H), endemic typhus (B), murine typhus (B), plague (B)
Lice	Epidemic relapsing fever (B), epidemic typhus (B), trench fever (B)
Mites	Rickettsial pox (B), scrub typhus (B)
Mosquitoes	Dengue fever (V), filariasis ("elephantiasis") (H), malaria (P), viral encephalitis (V), yellow fever (V)
Reduviid bugs	American trypanosomiasis (Chagas' disease) (P)
Sand flies (*Phlebotomus* spp.)	Leishmaniasis (P)
Ticks	Babesiosis (P), Colorado tick fever (V), ehrlichiosis (B), Lyme disease (B), relapsing fever (B), Rocky Mountain spotted fever (B), tularemia (B)
Tsetse flies (*Glossina* spp.)	African trypanosomiasis (P)

B, bacterial disease; *P*, protozoal disease; *H*, helminth disease; *V*, viral disease.

susceptible patients (e.g., babies, surgical patients, or debilitated persons). Such an infection could quickly spread throughout the entire hospital population.

The five principal modes by which transmission of pathogens occurs are contact (either direct or indirect contact), airborne, droplet, vehicular, and vectors (Fig. 11-4 and Table 11-5). Vehicular transmission involves contaminated inanimate objects ("vehicles"), such as food, water, dust, and fomites. Vectors are various types of biting insects and arachnids.

Communicable diseases—infectious diseases that are transmitted from person to person—are usually transmitted in the following ways:

- Direct skin-to-skin contact. For example, the common cold virus is frequently transmitted from the hand of someone who just blew his or her nose to another person by hand shaking. Within hospitals, this mode of

transfer is particularly prevalent, which is why it is so important for healthcare professionals to wash their hands before and after every patient contact. Frequent handwashing will prevent the transfer of pathogens from one patient to another.

- Direct mucous membrane–to–mucous membrane contact by kissing or sexual intercourse. Most STDs are transmitted in this manner. STDs include syphilis, gonorrhea, and infections caused by chlamydia, herpes, and HIV. Chlamydial genital infections are especially common in the United States; in fact, they are the most common nationally notifiable infectious diseases in the United States. (Nationally notifiable infectious diseases are discussed later in this chapter.)

- Indirectly by airborne droplets of respiratory secretions, usually produced as a result of sneezing or

TABLE 11-4

Pathogens Commonly Transmitted Via Food and Water[a]

PATHOGEN	VEHICLE	COMMENTS
Campylobacter jejuni (bacterium)	Chickens	
Cryptosporidium parvum (protozoan)	Drinking water	Highly resistant to disinfectants used to purify drinking water
Cyclospora cayetanensis (protozoan)	Drinking water, raspberries	
E. coli O157:H7 (bacterium)	Meats, produce contaminated by manure in growing fields (e.g., sprouts), drinking water	
Giardia lamblia (also called *Giardia intestinalis*) (protozoan)	Drinking water	Moderately resistant to disinfectants used to purify drinking water
Listeria monocytogenes (bacterium)	Soft cheeses and deli meats	
Salmonella enteritidis (bacterium)	Eggs	
Salmonella typhimurium DT-104 (bacterium)	Unpasteurized milk	Resistant to many antibiotics
Shigella spp. (bacteria)	Drinking water	

[a]Additional pathogens transmitted in food and water are mentioned in the text.

coughing. Most contagious airborne diseases are caused by respiratory pathogens carried to susceptible people in droplets of respiratory secretions. Some respiratory pathogens may settle on dust particles and be carried long distances through the air and into a building's ventilation or air-conditioning system. Improperly cleaned inhalation therapy equipment can easily transfer these pathogens from one patient to another. Diseases that may be transmitted in this manner include colds, influenza, measles, mumps, chickenpox, smallpox, and pneumonia.

- Indirectly by contamination of food and water by fecal material. Many infectious diseases are transmitted by restaurant food handlers who fail to wash their hands after using the restroom.

- Indirectly by arthropod vectors. Arthropods such as mosquitoes, flies, fleas, lice, ticks, and mites can transfer a variety of pathogens from person to person.

- Indirectly by fomites that become contaminated by respiratory secretions, blood, urine, feces, vomitus, or exudates from hospitalized patients. Fomites such as stethoscopes and latex gloves are sometimes the vehicles

by which pathogens are transferred from one patient to another. Examples of fomites are shown in Figure 11-5.

- Indirectly by transfusion of contaminated blood or blood products from an ill person or by **parenteral injection** (injection directly into the bloodstream) using nonsterile syringes and needles. One reason why disposable sterile tubes, syringes, and various other types of single-use hospital equipment have become very popular is that they are effective in preventing bloodborne infections (e.g., hepatitis, syphilis, malaria, AIDS, systemic staphylococcal infections) that result from reuse of equipment. Individuals using illegal intravenous drugs commonly transmit these diseases to each other by sharing needles and syringes, which easily become contaminated with the blood of an infected person.

Public Health Agencies

Public health agencies at all levels constantly strive to prevent epidemics and to identify and eliminate any that do occur. One way in which healthcare personnel participate

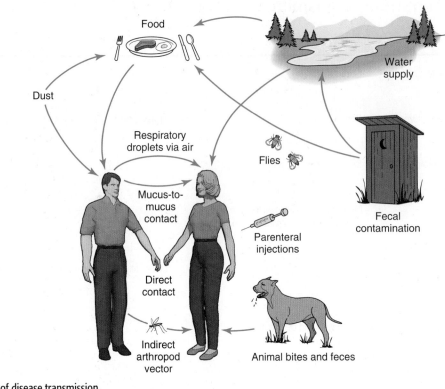

FIGURE 11-4. Modes of disease transmission.

in this massive program is by reporting cases of communicable diseases to the proper agencies. They also help by educating the public, explaining how diseases are transmitted, explaining proper sanitation procedures, identifying and attempting to eliminate reservoirs of infection, carrying out measures to isolate diseased persons, participating in immunization programs, and helping to treat sick persons. Through measures such as these, smallpox and poliomyelitis have been totally or nearly eliminated in most parts of the world.

World Health Organization (WHO)

The World Health Organization (WHO), a specialized agency of the United Nations, was founded in 1948. Its missions are to promote technical cooperation for health among nations, carry out programs to control and eradicate diseases, and improve the quality of human life. When an epidemic strikes, such as the 2000 Ebola outbreak in Uganda, teams of epidemiologists are sent to the site to investigate the situation and assist in bringing the outbreak under control. Because of this assistance, many countries have been successful in their fight to control smallpox, diphtheria, malaria, trachoma, and numerous other diseases. At one time, smallpox killed about 40% of those infected and caused scarring and blindness in many others. In 1980, the WHO announced that smallpox had been completely eradicated from the face of the earth; hence, routine

smallpox vaccination is no longer required.[a] More recently, the WHO has been attempting to eradicate polio and dracunculiasis (Guinea worm infection); to eliminate leprosy, neonatal tetanus, and Chagas' disease; and to control onchocerciasis ("river blindness"). WHO definitions of control, elimination, and eradication of disease are presented in Table 11-6. The WHO is currently attempting to eradicate polio. Thus far, polio has been eradicated from the Western Hemisphere (including the United States). Certification of total eradication requires that no wild poliovirus be found through optimal surveillance for at least 3 years.

Centers for Disease Control and Prevention (CDC)

In the United States, a federal agency called the U.S. Department of Health and Human Services administers the Public Health Service and the Centers for Disease Control and Prevention (CDC), which assist state and local health departments in the application of all aspects of epidemiology. Many microbiologists and epidemiologists work at the CDC headquarters in Atlanta, Georgia. Microbiologists at

---

[a]*Because smallpox virus is a potential bioterrorism agent, public health authorities have authorized the manufacture and stockpiling of smallpox vaccine, to be administered in the event of an emergency.*

TABLE 11-5

Common Routes of Transmission of Infectious Diseases

ROUTE OF EXIT	ROUTE OF TRANSMISSION OR ENTRY	DISEASES
Skin	Skin discharge → air → respiratory tract	Chickenpox, colds, influenza, measles, staph and strep infections
	Skin to skin	Impetigo, eczema, boils, warts, syphilis
Respiratory	Aerosol droplet inhalation	Colds, influenza, pneumonia, mumps, measles, chickenpox, tuberculosis
	Nose or mouth → hand or object → nose	
Gastrointestinal	Feces → hand → mouth	Gastroenteritis, hepatitis, salmonellosis, shigellosis, typhoid fever, cholera, giardiasis, amebiasis
	Stool → soil, food, or water → mouth	
Salivary	Direct salivary transfer	Herpes cold sore, infectious mononucleosis, strep throat
Genital secretions	Urethral or cervical secretions	Gonorrhea, herpes, *Chlamydia* infection
	Semen	Cytomegalovirus infection, AIDS, syphilis, warts
Blood	Transfusion or needlestick injury	Hepatitis B, cytomegalovirus infection, malaria, AIDS
	Insect bite	Malaria relapsing fever
Zoonotic	Animal bite	Rabies
	Contact with animal carcasses	Tularemia, anthrax
	Arthropod	Rocky Mountain spotted fever, Lyme disease, typhus, viral encephalitis, yellow fever, malaria, plague

the CDC are able to work with the most dangerous pathogens known to science because of the elaborate containment facilities that are located there. CDC epidemiologists travel to areas of the United States and elsewhere in the world, wherever and whenever an epidemic is occurring, to investigate and attempt to control the epidemic.

When the CDC was first established as the Communicable Disease Center in Atlanta, Georgia, in 1946, its focus was communicable diseases. The two most important infectious diseases in the United States at that time were malaria and typhus. Since then, the CDC's scope has been expanded greatly, and it now consists of 12 centers, institutes, and offices, one of which is the National Center for Infectious Diseases (NCID). Approximately 9,000 employees are employed by the CDC, in 170 occupations. The

CDC's overall mission is "to promote health and quality of life by preventing and controlling diseases, injury, and disability. . . . The CDC strives to protect people's health and safety, provide reliable health information, and improve health through strong partnerships." (www.cdc.gov) The NCID mission is "to prevent illness, disability, and death caused by infectious diseases in the United States and around the world." (www.cdc.gov/ncidod)

Certain infectious diseases, referred to as nationally notifiable diseases, must be reported to the CDC by all 50 states. (As of January 2003, there were 60 nationally notifiable diseases; most of them are discussed in Chapters 17 and 18.) Ten of the most common nationally notifiable infectious diseases in the United States are listed in Table 11-7.

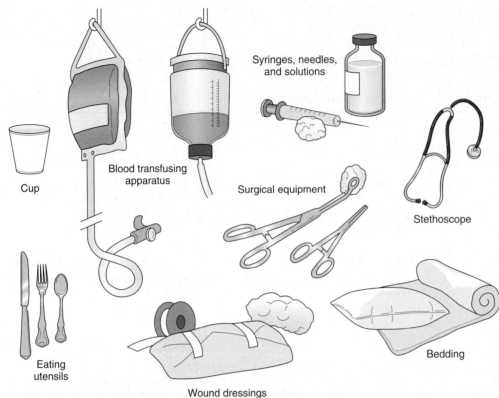

Cup

Blood transfusing apparatus

Syringes, needles, and solutions

Surgical equipment

Stethoscope

Eating utensils

Wound dressings

Bedding

FIGURE 11-5. Various medical instruments and apparatus that may serve as inanimate vectors of infection (fomites).

The CDC prepares a weekly publication entitled *Morbidity and Mortality Weekly Report* (*MMWR*), which contains timely information about infectious disease outbreaks in the United States and other parts of the world, as well as cumulative statistics regarding the number of cases of nationally notifiable infectious diseases that have occurred in the United States during the current year. Students of the health sciences are encouraged to read *MMWR*, which is accessible at the CDC web site (www.cdc.gov).

Through the efforts of these public health agencies, working with local physicians, nurses, other healthcare professionals, educators, and community leaders, many diseases are no longer endemic in the United States. Some of the diseases that no longer pose a serious threat to U.S. communities include cholera, diphtheria, malaria, polio, smallpox, and typhoid fever.

The prevention and control of epidemics is a never-ending community goal. To be effective, it must include measures to:

- Increase host resistance through the development and administration of vaccines that induce active immunity and maintain it in susceptible persons.

TABLE 11-6

WHO Definitions of Epidemiologic Terms Relating to Infectious Diseases

TERM	DEFINITION
Control of an infectious disease	Ongoing operations or programs aimed at reducing the incidence or prevalence of that disease
Elimination of an infectious disease	The reduction of case transmission to a predetermined very low level (e.g., to a level below one case per million population)
Eradication of an infectious disease	Achieving a status where no further cases of that disease occur anywhere and where continued control measures are unnecessary

TABLE 11-7

Ten of the Most Common Nationally Notifiable Infectious Diseases in the United States

RANKING	DISEASE	NO. OF U.S. CASES REPORTED (2004)
1	Genital chlamydial infections	929,462
2	Gonorrhea	330,132
3	AIDS	44,108
4	Salmonellosis	41,660
5	Syphilis (all stages)	33,401
6	Chickenpox	26,659
7	Whooping cough	25,827
8	Giardiasis	20,636
9	Lyme disease	19,804
10	Tuberculosis	14,517

Source: Centers for Disease Control (CDC), Atlanta, GA (www.cdc.gov).

- Ensure that persons who have been exposed to a pathogen are protected against the disease (e.g., through injections of gamma globulin or antisera).
- Segregate, isolate, and treat those who have contracted a contagious infection to prevent the spread of pathogens to others.
- Identify and control potential reservoirs and vectors of infectious diseases; this control may be accomplished by prohibiting healthy carriers from working in restaurants, hospitals, nursing homes, and other institutions where they may transfer pathogens to susceptible people, and by instituting effective sanitation measures to control diseases transmitted through water supplies, sewage, and food (including milk).

Bioterrorism and Biological Warfare Agents

Sad to say, pathogenic microorganisms sometimes wind up in the hands of mentally deranged people who want to use them to cause harm to others. In times of war, the use of microorganisms in this manner is called biological warfare, and the microbes are referred to as ***biological warfare (bw) agents.*** However, the danger does not just exist during times of war. There is always a possibility that members of terrorist or radical hate groups might use pathogens to create fear, chaos, illness, and death. These pathogens are referred to as **bioterrorism agents.**

Four of the pathogens most often discussed as potential bw and bioterrorism agents are *Bacillus anthracis, Clostridium botulinum,* smallpox virus (*Variola major*), and *Yersinia pestis,* the causative agents of anthrax, botulism, smallpox, and plague, respectively. If disseminated in some type of aerosol, either *B. anthracis* spores or *Y. pestis* bacilli could result in numerous, severe, and potentially fatal pulmonary infections. In addition, entry of *B. anthracis* into wounds could cause cutaneous anthrax, and ingestion of the organisms could result in intestinal anthrax. Anthrax infections involve significant hemorrhage and serous effusions (fluid which has escaped from blood or lymphatic vessels) in various organs and body cavities and are frequently fatal.

Clostridium botulinum spores could be added to water supplies or food. Botulinal toxin is odorless and tasteless, and only a tiny quantity of the toxin needs be ingested to cause potentially fatal cases of botulism. Since 1980, when

HISTORICAL NOTE

Biological Warfare Agents

The use of pathogens as biological warfare agents dates back thousands of years. Ancient Romans threw carrion (decaying dead bodies) into wells to contaminate the drinking water of their enemies. In the Middle Ages, the bodies of plague victims were catapulted over city walls in an attempt to infect the inhabitants of the cities. Early North American explorers provided Native Americans with blankets and handkerchiefs that were contaminated with smallpox and measles viruses.

the WHO announced that smallpox had been eradicated, civilians no longer receive smallpox vaccinations. Thus, throughout the world, huge numbers of people are highly susceptible to the virus. Although there are no reservoirs for smallpox virus in nature, preserved samples of the virus exist in a few medical research laboratories throughout the world. There is always the danger that smallpox virus, or any of the other pathogens mentioned here, could fall into the wrong hands. Other pathogens viewed as potential bw agents are the causative agents of brucellosis, Q fever, tularemia, viral encephalitis, and viral hemorrhagic fevers. Table 11-8 contains a listing of potential bioterrorism agents that, according to the CDC, pose the greatest threats to civilians—pathogens with which public health agencies must be prepared to cope.

In 1996, 45 laboratory employees in a large Texas medical center developed severe, acute diarrheal illness caused by *Shigella dysenteriae* type 2, a rare cause of diarrhea in the United States. An investigation revealed that a portion of the laboratory's stock culture of this organism had been deliberately used to contaminate muffins and doughnuts, which had been anonymously left in the laboratory break room and subsequently eaten by laboratory employees. It is not known whether the culprit was ever apprehended.

An instance of biological terrorism (*bioterrorism*) occurred in a small Oregon town in 1984. Members of a religious cult purposely contaminated salad bars at two restaurants with *Salmonella typhimurium* in an attempt to sicken local citizens and thus prevent them from voting in an upcoming election. They also contaminated the

---

TABLE 11-8

Critical Biological Agent Categories for Public Health Preparedness[a]

CATEGORY	BIOLOGICAL AGENT(S)	DISEASE
Category A—Agents having the greatest potential for adverse public health impact; most require broad-based public health preparedness efforts	*Variola major*	Smallpox
	Bacillus anthracis	Anthrax
	Yersinia pestis	Plague
	Clostridium botulinum	Botulism (botulinal toxins)
	Francisella tularensis	Tularemia
	Filoviruses and arenaviruses (e.g., Ebola virus, Lassa virus)	Viral hemorrhagic fevers
Category B—Agents having a moderate to high potential for large-scale dissemination or a heightened general public health awareness that could cause mass public fear and civil disruption	*Coxiella burnetii*	Q fever
	Brucella spp.	Brucellosis
	Burkholderia mallei	Glanders
	Burkholderia pseudomallei	Melioidosis
	Alphaviruses (Venezuela equine, eastern equine, and western equine encephalitis viruses)	Encephalitis
	Rickettsia prowazekii	Typhus fever
	Toxins (e.g., ricin [from the castor oil plant], staphylococcal enterotoxin B)	Toxic syndromes
	Chlamydophila psittaci	Psittacosis
	Food safety treats (e.g., *Salmonella* spp., *Escherichia coli* O157:H7)	
	Water safety treats (e.g., *Vibrio cholerae*, *Cryptosporidium parvum*)	
Category C—Agents currently not believed to present a high bioterrorism risk to public health, but could emerge as future threats	Emerging threat agents (e.g., Nipah virus, hantavirus)	

[a]From Rotz LD, et al. Public health assessment of potential biologicalal terrorism agents. Emerg Infect Dis 2002;8:225–230 (prepared and published by the National Center for Infectious Diseases, Centers for Disease Control and Prevention, based on unclassified information).

drinking water of two county commissioners. More than 750 people became ill, including the two commissioners, but no deaths occurred. The Japanese cult that released nerve gas in the Tokyo subway system in 1995, killing 12 people and injuring about 3,800, has also attempted to develop botulinal toxin, anthrax, cholera, and Q fever for bioterrorism use. During the late 1990s, there were a number of anthrax threats in the United States, but, fortunately, most turned out to be hoaxes.

Then, in fall 2001, letters containing *Bacillus anthracis* spores were mailed to several politicians and members of the news media. According to the CDC, a total of 18 cases of anthrax resulted: 11 cases of inhalation anthrax (with five fatalities) and 7 cases of cutaneous anthrax (with no fatalities). Undoubtedly, many additional cases were prevented as a result of prompt prophylactic (preventative) antibiotic therapy.

To minimize the danger of potentially deadly microorganisms falling into the wrong hands, the U.S. Antiterrorism and Effective Death Penalty Act of 1996 makes the CDC responsible for controlling shipment of those pathogens and toxins deemed most likely to be used as bw agents. Authorities must constantly be on the alert for possible theft of these pathogens from biological supply houses and legitimate laboratories. In addition, vaccines, antitoxins, and other antidotes must be available wherever the threat of the use of these biological agents is high (e.g., in various potential war zones).

The American Society for Microbiology has recommended that all clinical microbiology laboratories be staffed with individuals who are familiar with the likely agents of bioterrorism and have been trained to detect, identify, and safely handle these agents. What individuals can do to prepare for bioterrorist attacks is discussed in "Insight: Preparing for a Bioterrorist Attack" on the CD-ROM.

Water Supplies and Sewage Disposal

Water is the most essential resource necessary for the survival of humanity. The main sources of community water supplies are surface water from rivers, natural lakes, and reservoirs, as well as groundwater from wells. However, two general types of water pollution (i.e., chemical pollution and biological pollution) are present in our society, making it increasingly difficult to provide safe water supplies.

Chemical pollution of water occurs when industrial installations dump waste products into local waters without proper pretreatment, when pesticides are used indiscriminately, and when chemicals are expelled in the air and carried to earth by rain ("acid rain"). The main source of biological pollution is waste products of humans—fecal material and garbage—that swarm with pathogens. The

causative agents of cholera, typhoid fever, bacterial and amebic dysentery, giardiasis, cryptosporidiosis, infectious hepatitis, and poliomyelitis can all be spread through contaminated water.

Waterborne epidemics today are the result of failure to make use of available existing knowledge and technology. In those countries that have established safe sanitary procedures for water purification and sewage disposal, outbreaks of typhoid fever, cholera, and dysentery occur only rarely.

In spring 1993, a waterborne epidemic of cryptosporidiosis (a diarrheal disease) affected more than 400,000 people in Milwaukee, Wisconsin. This was the largest waterborne epidemic that has ever occurred in the United States. The oocysts of *Cryptosporidium parvum* (a protozoan) were present in cattle feces, which, when the winter snow melted, were washed off Wisconsin's numerous dairy farms into Lake Michigan. Milwaukee uses the water of Lake Michigan as its drinking water supply. Although the lake water had been treated, the tiny oocysts passed through the filters that were being used at that time. Thus, the *Cryptosporidium* oocysts were present in the city's drinking water, and people became infected when they drank the water. The epidemic caused the death of more than 100 immunosuppressed individuals.

Sources of Water Contamination

Rainwater falling over large areas collects in lakes and rivers and, thus, is subject to contamination by soil microbes and raw fecal material. For example, an animal feed lot located near a community water supply source harbors innumerable pathogens, which are washed into lakes and rivers. A city that draws its water from a local river, processes it, and uses it, but then dumps inadequately treated sewage into the river at the other side of town, may be responsible for a serious health problem in another city downstream on the same river. The city downstream must then find some way to rid its water supply of the pathogens. In many communities, untreated raw sewage and industrial wastes are dumped directly into local waters. Also, a storm or a flood may result in contamination of the local drinking water with sewage (Fig. 11-6).

Groundwater from wells also can become contaminated. To prevent such contamination, the well must be dug deep enough to ensure that the surface water is filtered through soil before it reaches the level of the well. Outhouses, septic tanks, and cesspools must be situated in such a way that surface water passing through these areas does not carry fecal microbes directly into the well water. With the growing popularity of trailer homes, a new problem has arisen because of trailer sewage disposal tanks that are located too near a water supply. In some very old cities, where cracked underground water pipes lie alongside leaking sewage pipes, sewage can enter the water pipes, thus contaminating the water just before it enters people's homes.

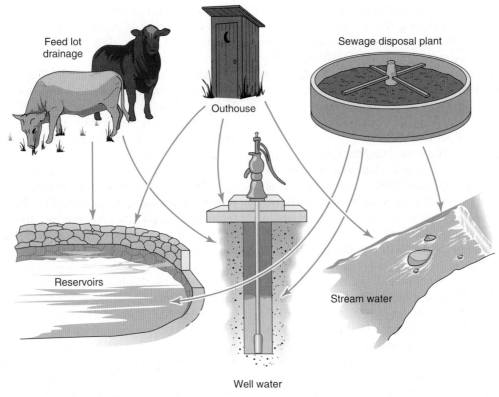

FIGURE 11-6. Sources of water contamination.

Water Treatment

Water must be properly treated to make it safe for human consumption. It is interesting to trace the many steps involved in such treatment (Fig. 11-7). The water first is filtered to remove large pieces of debris such as twigs and leaves. Next, the water remains in a holding tank, where additional debris settles to the bottom of the tank; this phase of the process is known as sedimentation or settling. Alum (aluminum potassium sulfate) is then added to coagulate smaller pieces of debris, which then settle to the bottom; this phase is known as coagulation or flocculation. The water is then filtered through sand or diatomaceous earth filters to remove the remaining bacteria, protozoan cysts and oocysts, and other small particles. In some water treatment facilities, charcoal filters or membrane filtration systems are also used. Membrane filtration will remove tiny *Giardia lamblia* cysts and *Cryptosporidium parvum* oocysts. Finally, chlorine gas or sodium hypochlorite is added to a final concentration of 0.2 to 1.0 part per million (ppm); this kills most remaining bacteria. In some water treatment facilities, ozone (O_3) treatment or ultraviolet (UV) light may be used in place of chlorination.

Small communities in rural areas may be financially unable to construct water treatment plants that incorporate all of the above-mentioned steps. Some may rely on chlorination alone. Unfortunately, the levels of chlorine routinely used for water treatment do not kill some pathogens, such as *Giardia* cysts and *Cryptosporidium* oocysts. Other communities use all the water treatment steps, but fail to use filters having a small enough pore size to trap tiny pathogens such as *Cryptosporidium* oocysts (which are about 4 to 6 μm in diameter).

In the laboratory, water can be tested for fecal contamination by checking for the presence of coliform bacteria (**coliforms**). *Coliforms* are *E. coli* and other lactose-fermenting members of the Family Enterobacteriaceae, such as *Enterobacter* and *Klebsiella* spp. These bacteria normally live in the intestinal tracts of animals and humans; thus, their presence in drinking water is an indication that the water was fecally contaminated. Water is considered potable (safe to drink) if it contains 1 coliform or less per 100 mL of water.

If one is unsure about the purity of drinking water, boiling it for 20 minutes destroys most pathogens that are present. It can then be cooled and consumed. Boiling will kill *Giardia* cysts and *Cryptosporidium* oocysts, but there are some bacterial spores and viruses that can withstand long periods of boiling. The most common causes of waterborne outbreaks in the United States are *Giardia lamblia, Cryptosporidium parvum, E. coli* O157:H7, *Shigella,* and a virus called Norwalk-like virus.

Sewage Treatment

Raw sewage consists mainly of water, fecal material (including intestinal pathogens), and garbage and bacteria from the drains of houses and other buildings. When

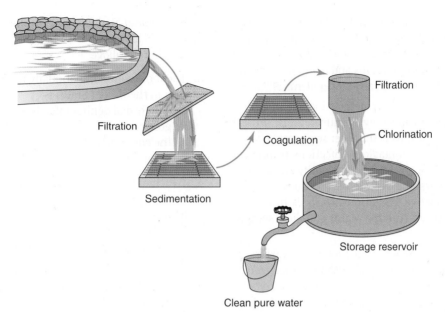

Filtration

Coagulation

Filtration

Chlorination

Sedimentation

Storage reservoir

Clean pure water

FIGURE 11-7. Steps in water treatment. (See text for details.)

sewage is adequately treated in a disposal plant, the water it contains can be returned to lakes and rivers to be recycled.

Primary Sewage Treatment. In the sewage disposal plant, large debris is first filtered out (called screening), skimmers remove floating grease and oil, and floating debris is shredded or ground. Then, solid material settles out in a primary sedimentation tank. Flocculating substances can be added to cause other solids to settle out. The material that accumulates at the bottom of the tank is called primary sludge.

Secondary Sewage Treatment. The liquid (called primary effluent) then undergoes secondary treatment, which includes aeration or trickling filtration. The purpose of aeration is to encourage the growth of aerobic microbes, which oxidize the dissolved organic matter to CO_2 and H_2O. Trickling filters accomplish the same thing (i.e., conversion of dissolved organic matter to CO_2 and H_2O by microbes), but in a different manner. After either aeration or trickling filtration, the activated sludge is transferred to a settling tank, where any remaining solid material settles out. The remaining liquid (called secondary effluent) is filtered and disinfected (usually by chlorination), so that the effluent water can be returned to rivers or oceans.

Tertiary Sewage Treatment. In some desert cities, where water is in short supply, the effluent water from the sewage disposal plant is further treated (referred to as tertiary sewage treatment), so that it can be returned directly to the drinking water system; this is a very expensive process. Tertiary sewage treatment involves the addition of chemicals, filtration (using fine sand or charcoal), chlorination, and sometimes distillation. In other cities, effluent water is used to irrigate lawns; however, it is expensive to install a separate water system for this purpose. In some communities, the sludge is heated to kill bacteria, then dried and used as fertilizer.

REVIEW OF KEY POINTS

- Epidemiology is the study of the frequency and distribution of diseases and contributing factors (e.g., virulence of pathogens; susceptibility of a population because of overcrowding, lack of immunization, or inadequate sanitation; reservoirs of infection; and various modes of transmission). Epidemic, endemic, pandemic, and sporadic diseases are epidemiologic terms used to describe the prevalence of a disease in an area at a particular time.

- The sources of pathogens are known as reservoirs of infection (or simply, reservoirs); they may be living reservoirs (e.g., humans, animals, or arthropods) or nonliving reservoirs (e.g., air, soil, dust, food, water, or inanimate objects found in the home, office, or hospital).

- The principal modes of transmission of pathogens are by way of contact (either direct or indirect contact), airborne, droplet, vehicular, and vectors. The primary ways in which communicable diseases are transmitted are direct skin-to-skin or mucous membrane–to–mucous membrane contact, and indirectly by airborne droplets of respiratory secretions, contamination of food and water by fecal material, arthropod vectors, fomites, and transfusion of contaminated blood or blood products from an ill person, or by parenteral injection (injection directly into the bloodstream) using nonsterile syringes and needles.

- To eradicate certain diseases and prevent epidemics, epidemiologists must consider the virulence of the pathogens, susceptibility of the population, sanitation practices, reservoirs of infection, and ways in which pathogens are transmitted.

- The World Health Organization, the Centers for Disease Control and Prevention, and public health and community groups, at all levels, must work together to coordinate preventive health programs and maintain constant surveillance of sources and causes of epidemics.

- Prevention and control of epidemics include measures to increase host resistance by immunizations; protect people from exposure to pathogens; segregate, isolate, and treat those with contagious infections to prevent the spread of pathogens to others; identify and control potential reservoirs and vectors of infectious diseases; and institute effective sanitation measures to control diseases transmitted through water supplies, sewage, and food.

- The four most likely potential biological warfare or bioterrorism agents are *Bacillus anthracis, Clostridium botulinum,* smallpox virus (*Variola major*), and *Yersinia pestis,* the causative agents of anthrax, botulism, smallpox, and plague, respectively.

- The major steps in water treatment are sedimentation (settling), coagulation (flocculation), filtration, and chlorination.

On the CD-ROM

- Insight
  - Epidemiologists
  - Preparing for a Bioterrorist Attack
- Increase Your Knowledge
- Microbiology—Hollywood Style
- Critical Thinking
- Additional Self-Assessment

Self-Assessment Exercises

After studying this chapter, answer the following multiple-choice questions.

1. Which of the following terms best describes chlamydial genital infection in the United States?
   a. arthropodborne disease
   b. epidemic disease
   c. pandemic disease
   d. sporadic disease

2. Which of the following are considered reservoirs of infection?
   a. carriers
   b. contaminated food and drinking water
   c. rabid animals
   d. all of the above

3. The most common nationally notifiable infectious disease in the United States is:
   a. chlamydial genital infections.
   b. gonorrhea.
   c. the common cold.
   d. tuberculosis.

4. Which of the following arthropods is the vector of Lyme disease?
   a. flea
   b. mite
   c. mosquito
   d. tick

5. The most common zoonotic disease in the United States is:
   a. Lyme disease.
   b. plague.
   c. rabies.
   d. Rocky Mountain spotted fever.

6. Which one of the following organisms is *not* one of the four most likely potential biological warfare or bioterrorism agents?
   a. *Bacillus anthracis*
   b. Ebola virus
   c. *Variola major*
   d. *Yersinia pestis*

7. All of the following are major steps in the treatment of a community's drinking water except:
   a. boiling.
   b. filtration.
   c. flocculation.
   d. sedimentation.

8. The largest waterborne epidemic ever to occur in the United States occurred in which of the following cities?
   a. Chicago
   b. Los Angeles
   c. Milwaukee
   d. New York City

9. Typhoid fever is caused by a species of:
   a. *Campylobacter.*
   b. *Escherichia.*
   c. *Salmonella.*
   d. *Shigella.*

10. Which of the following associations is incorrect?
   a. ehrlichiosis. . .tick
   b. malaria. . .mosquito
   c. plague. . .flea
   d. Rocky Mountain spotted fever. . .mite

12

HEALTHCARE EPIDEMIOLOGY: NOSOCOMIAL INFECTIONS AND INFECTION CONTROL

LEARNING OBJECTIVES

AFTER STUDYING THIS CHAPTER, YOU SHOULD BE
ABLE TO:

- Differentiate among nosocomial, community-acquired, and iatrogenic infections
- List the seven pathogens that most commonly cause nosocomial infections
- State the four most common types of nosocomial infections
- List six types of patients who are especially vulnerable to nosocomial infections
- State the three major contributing factors in nosocomial infections
- Differentiate between medical and surgical asepsis
- State the most important and effective way to reduce the number of nosocomial infections
- Differentiate between standard precautions and trans-mission-based precautions and state the three types of transmission-based precautions
- Differentiate between source and protective (reverse) isolation
- Cite three important considerations in the handling of each of the following: food, eating utensils, fomites, and sharps
- List six responsibilities of the Infection Control Committee
- State three ways in which the Clinical Microbiology Laboratory participates in infection control

INTRODUCTION

The Society for Healthcare Epidemiology of America (SHEA) defines healthcare epidemiology as "any activity designed to study and/or improve patient care outcomes in any type of healthcare institution or setting. Healthcare epidemiology. . .includes a variety of disciplines and activities directed at enhancing the quality of health care and preventing and controlling adverse outcomes. Among these activities are epidemiologic and laboratory investigation,

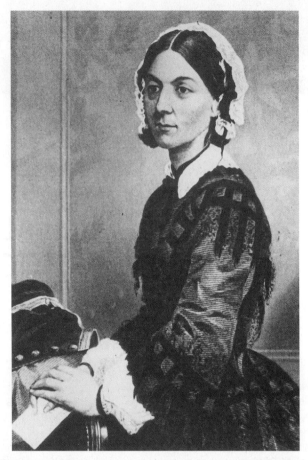

FIGURE 12-1. Florence Nightingale. (From Taylor C, et al. Fundamentals of Nursing: The Art and Science of Nursing Care, 4th ed. Philadelphia: Lippincott Williams & Wilkins, 2001. Courtesy of the Center for the Study of the History of Nursing, University of Pennsylvania.)

HISTORICAL NOTE

Florence Nightingale (1820–1910)

Although born in and named for Florence, Italy, Florence Nightingale (Fig. 12-1) was raised in England. Because her wealthy father was a strong believer in education for women, she received an excellent education in mathematics, history, economics, astronomy, science, philosophy, and several languages. As a young child, she cared for sick and injured pets, and, when a bit older, she cared for ill servants. In 1849, she started formal studies of the European hospital system.

In 1853, Nightingale became superintendent of the Hospital for Invalid Gentlewomen in London. In 1854, she volunteered for service in the Crimean War (a 2-year war over the domination of southeast Europe, in which England, France, Turkey, and Sardinia defeated Russia). She assumed direction of all nursing operations at the war front, and as a result of her insistence on sanitary measures, the mortality rates among the sick (owing to cholera, dysentery, and typhoid fever) and wounded were drastically reduced. After the war, she returned to England and received a commission to study the sanitary conditions of the British army. In 1858, she published *Notes on the Matters Affecting the Health, Efficiency, and Hospital Administration of the British Army,* the first detailed study of the housing and health of soldiers. In 1860, she founded the Nightingale School Home for Nurses at St. Thomas's Hospital in London—this marked the beginning of professional education in nursing. She had a talent for collecting, arranging, and presenting facts and figures, and used the statistical morbidity and mortality data that she collected to improve hospital conditions. She helped to reform the health and living conditions of the British army, the sanitary conditions and administration of hospitals, and the nursing profession. Florence Nightingale is regarded as the founder of modern nursing.

surveillance, risk reduction programs focused on device and procedure management, policy development and implementation, education and information dissemination, and cost-benefit assessment of prevention and control programs" (from the SHEA web site; www.shea-online.org).

The importance of microbiology to those who work in health-related occupations can never be overemphasized. Whether working in a hospital, nursing home, or medical or dental clinic, or caring for sick persons in their homes, all healthcare professionals must follow standardized procedures to prevent the spread of communicable diseases. Thoughtless or careless actions when providing patient care can cause serious infections that otherwise could have been prevented.

Nosocomial Infections

Definitions

Infectious diseases (infections) can be divided into two categories: (1) those that are acquired within hospitals or other healthcare facilities (called hospital-acquired infections or nosocomial infections) and (2) those that are acquired outside of healthcare facilities (called community-acquired infections). A hospitalized patient may have either type of infection. According to the Centers for Disease Control and Prevention (CDC), community-acquired infections are those that are present or incubating at the time of hospital admission. All other hospital-associated infections are considered nosocomial, including those that erupt within 14 days of hospital discharge. Iatrogenic infections (iatrogenic literally meaning "physician-induced") or diseases are the result of medical or surgical treatment and are, thus, caused by surgeons, other physicians, or other healthcare personnel. Examples of iatrogenic infections are post-surgical wound infections and urinary tract infections that result from urinary catheterization of patients.

Frequency of Nosocomial Infections

It is sad to think that a patient who enters a hospital for one problem could develop an infection while in the hospital and perhaps die of that infection. Yet, this is an all too common occurrence. Of the approximately 40 million hospitalizations per year in the United States, an estimated 2 million hospitalized patients (about 5% of the total) acquire nosocomial infections. In 1995, approximately 88,000 deaths were related to nosocomial infections—about one death every 6 minutes—and nosocomial infections added an estimated $4.5 billion to the cost of health care in the United States that year. Of course, as bad as this is, the current nosocomial rates are considerably lower than they were in the past (Fig. 12-2).

Pathogens Most Often Involved in Nosocomial Infections

The hospital setting harbors many pathogens and potential pathogens. They live on and in healthcare professionals, other hospital employees, visitors to the hospital, and patients themselves. Some live in dust, whereas others live in wet or moist areas like sink drains, showerheads, whirlpool baths, mop buckets, flower pots, and even food from the kitchen. To make matters worse, the bacterial pathogens that lurk around in hospital settings are usually drug-resistant strains and, quite often, are multidrug resistant.

The following seven bacteria or groups of bacteria are the most common causes of nosocomial infections in the United States:

- Gram-positive cocci (during 1990–1996, the following three Gram-positive cocci caused 34% of the nosocomial infections in the United States):
  Staphylococcus aureus
  Coagulase-negative staphylococci
  Enterococcus spp.
- Gram-negative bacilli (during 1990–1996, the following four Gram-negative bacilli caused 32% of the nosocomial infections in the United States):
  Escherichia coli
  Pseudomonas aeruginosa
  Enterobacter spp.
  Klebsiella spp.

Although some of the pathogens that cause nosocomial infections come from the external environment, most come from the patients themselves—their own indigenous microflora that enter a surgical incision or otherwise gain entrance to areas of the body other than those where they normally reside. Urinary catheters, for example, provide a "superhighway" for indigenous microflora organisms to gain access to the urinary bladder.

Approximately 70% of nosocomial infections involve drug-resistant bacteria, which are common in hospitals and nursing homes as a result of the many antimicrobial agents that are used there. The drugs place selective pressure on the microbes, meaning that only those that are resistant to the drugs will survive. These resistant organisms then multiply and predominate (refer to Fig. 9-5).

Pseudomonas infections are especially hard to treat, as are infections caused by multidrug-resistant

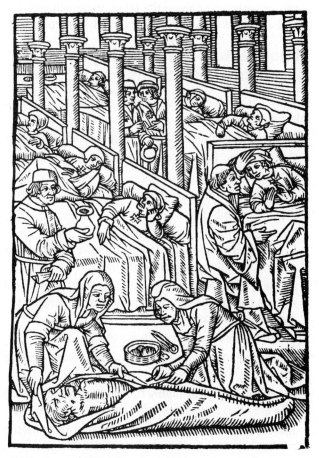

FIGURE 12-2. Hospital interior. Woodcut from Saint-Gelais, Le Vergier d'Honneur, Paris, Jehan Petit, c. 1500. Seen here are a sick man being attended to by a physician, a man receiving spiritual consolation, a corpse being prepared for burial, and, in the background, a well man, about to leave the hospital, receiving a word of advice from a physician. (Zigrosser C. Medicine and the Artist [Ars Medica]. New York: Dover Publications, Inc., 1970. By permission of the Philadelphia Museum of Art.).

Mycobacterium tuberculosis (MDRTB), vancomycin-resistant *Enterococcus* spp. (VRE), and methicillin-resistant strains of *Staphylococcus aureus* (MRSA) and *Staphylococcus epidermidis* (MRSE). However, bacteria are not the only pathogens that have become drug resistant. Viruses (such as HIV), fungi (such as various *Candida* spp.), and protozoa (such as malarial parasites) have also developed drug resistance.

In 2001, the CDC launched a campaign to prevent antimicrobial resistance in healthcare settings. Table 12-1 contains the 12 steps that the CDC has recommended to prevent antimicrobial resistance among hospitalized adults.

Most Common Types of Nosocomial Infections

The four most common types of nosocomial infections, listed in descending order of frequency, are:

1. Urinary tract infections (UTIs)
2. Surgical wound infections (also referred to as postsurgical wound infections)
3. Lower respiratory tract infections (primarily pneumonia)
4. Bloodstream infections (septicemia)

Other common nosocomial infections are the gastrointestinal diseases caused by *Clostridium difficile* (referred to as *Clostridium difficile*-associated diseases). *C. difficile* is a common member of the indigenous microflora of the colon, where it exists in relatively small numbers. Although *C. difficile* produces two types of toxins (an enterotoxin and a cytotoxin), the concentrations of these toxins are too low to cause disease when only small numbers of *C. difficile* are present. However, superinfections of *C. difficile* can occur when a patient receives oral antibiotics that kill off susceptible members of the gastrointestinal flora. (Superinfections are described in Chapter 9.) *C. difficile,* which is resistant to many orally administered antibiotics, then increases in number, leading to increased concentrations of the toxins. The enterotoxin causes a disease known as antibiotic-associated diarrhea (AAD). The cytotoxin causes a disease known as pseudomembranous colitis (PMC), in which sections of the lining of the colon slough off, resulting in bloody stools. Both AAD and PMC are common in hospitalized patients.

Nosocomial zoonoses are a recently recognized problem in hospitals (see "Insight: Nosocomial Zoonoses" on the CD-ROM).

Patients Most Likely To Develop Nosocomial Infections

Patients most likely to develop nosocomial infections are immunosuppressed patients—patients whose immune systems have been weakened by age, underlying diseases, or medical or surgical treatments. Contributing factors include an aging population, increasingly aggressive medical and therapeutic interventions, and an increase in the number of implanted prosthetic devices, organ transplantations, xenotransplantations (the transplantation of animals organs or tissues into humans), and vascular and urinary catheterizations. The highest infection rates are in intensive care unit (ICU) patients. Nosocomial infection rates are three times higher in adult and pediatric ICUs than elsewhere in the hospital. Listed here are the most vulnerable patients in a hospital setting:

- Elderly patients.
- Women in labor and delivery.
- Premature infants and newborns.
- Surgical and burn patients.
- Diabetic and cancer patients.
- Patients receiving treatment with steroids, anticancer drugs, antilymphocyte serum, and radiation.
- Immunosuppressed patients (i.e., patients whose immune systems are not functioning properly).
- Patients who are paralyzed or are undergoing renal dialysis or catheterization; quite often, these patients' normal defense mechanisms are not functioning properly.

Major Factors Contributing to Nosocomial Infections

The three major factors that combine to cause nosocomial infections (Fig. 12-3) are:

- An ever-increasing number of drug-resistant pathogens.
- The failure of healthcare personnel to follow infection control guidelines.
- An increased number of immunocompromised patients.

Additional contributing factors are:

- The indiscriminate use of antimicrobial agents, which has resulted in an increase in the number of drug-resistant and multidrug-resistant pathogens.
- A false sense of security about antimicrobial agents, leading to a neglect of aseptic techniques and other infection control procedures.
- Lengthy, more complicated types of surgery.
- Overcrowding of hospitals and other healthcare facilities, as well as shortages of staff.
- Increased use of less-highly trained healthcare workers, who are often unaware of infection control procedures.
- Increased use of anti-inflammatory and immunosuppressant agents, such as radiation, steroids, anticancer chemotherapy, and antilymphocyte serum.
- Overuse and improper use of indwelling medical devices.

Medical devices that support or monitor basic body functions contribute greatly to the success of modern medical treatment. However, by bypassing normal defensive

TABLE 12-1

Twelve Steps to Prevent Antimicrobial Resistance Among Hospitalized Adults

Prevent Infection

Step 1. Vaccinate	Give influenza vaccine and *Streptococcus pneumoniae* vaccine to at-risk patients before discharge. Healthcare workers should receive the influenza vaccine annually.
Step 2. Get the catheters out	Use catheters only when essential. Use the correct catheter. Use proper insertion and catheter-care protocols. Remove catheters when they are no longer essential.

Diagnose and Treat Infection Effectively

Step 3. Target the pathogen	Culture the patient. Target empiric therapy to likely pathogens and your facility's antibiogram information. Target definitive therapy to known pathogens and antimicrobial susceptibility test results.
Step 4. Access the experts	Consult infectious disease experts for patients with serious infections.

Use Antimicrobials Wisely

Step 5. Practice antimicrobial control	Engage in local antimicrobial control efforts.
Step 6. Use local data	Know your facility's antibiogram. Know your patient population.
Step 7. Treat infection, not contamination	Use proper antisepsis for blood and other cultures. Culture the blood, not the skin or catheter hub. Use proper methods to obtain and process all cultures.
Step 8. Treat infection, not colonization	Treat pneumonia, not the tracheal aspirate. Treat bacteremia, not the catheter tip or hub. Treat urinary tract infection, not the indwelling catheter.
Step 9. Know when to say "no" to vancomycin	Treat infection, not contaminants or colonization. Fever in a patient with an intravenous catheter is not a routine indication for vancomycin.
Step 10. Stop antimicrobial treatment	When infection is cured. When cultures are negative and infection is unlikely. When infection is not diagnosed.

Prevent Transmission

Step 11. Isolate the pathogen	Use standard infection control precautions. Contain infectious body fluids. (Follow airborne, droplet, and contact precautions.) When in doubt, consult infection control experts.
Step 12. Break the chain of contagion	Stay home when you (the healthcare worker) are sick. Keep your hands clean. Set an example.

Source: Centers for Disease Control (CDC), Atlanta, GA (www.cdc.gov/drugresistance/healthcare/ha/12steps_HA.htm). This web site also discusses steps to prevent antimicrobial resistance among dialysis patients, surgical patients, hospitalized children, and long-term care patients.

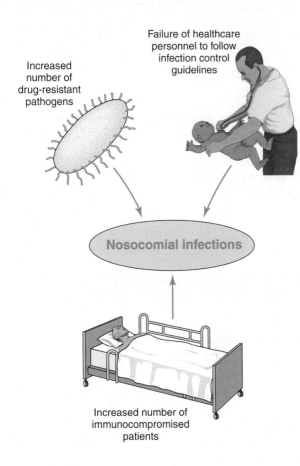

Increased
number of
drug-resistant
pathogens

Failure of healthcare
personnel to follow
infection control
guidelines

Nosocomial infections

Increased number of
immunocompromised
patients

FIGURE 12-3. The three major contributing factors in nosocomial infections.

barriers, these devices provide microorganisms access to normally sterile body fluids and tissues. The risk of bacterial or fungal infection is related to the degree of debilitation of the patient and the design and management of the device. It is advisable to discontinue the use of urinary catheters, vascular catheters, respirators, and hemodialysis on individual patients as soon as medically feasible.

What Can Be Done To Reduce the Number of Nosocomial Infections?

It is critical for all healthcare workers to be aware of the problem of nosocomial infections and to take appropriate measures to minimize the number of such infections that occur within healthcare facilities. The primary way to reduce the number of nosocomial infections is strict compliance with infection control guidelines (these guidelines are described in a subsequent section).

Handwashing is the single most important measure to reduce the risks of transmitting pathogens from one patient to another or from one anatomic site to another on the same patient. Handwashing, as it specifically pertains

to healthcare personnel, is discussed in a subsequent section ("Standard Precautions"). Presented here are commonsense, everyday, handwashing guidelines that pertain to everyone:

- Wash your hands before you:
  - Prepare or eat food.
  - Treat a cut or wound or tend to someone who is sick.
  - Insert or remove contact lenses.
- Wash your hands after you:
  - Use the restroom.
  - Handle uncooked foods, particularly raw meat, poultry, or fish.
  - Change a diaper.
  - Cough, sneeze, or blow your nose.
  - Touch a pet, particularly reptiles and exotic animals.
  - Handle garbage.
  - Tend to someone who is sick or injured.
- Wash your hands in the following manner:
  - Use warm or hot, running water.
  - Use soap (preferably an antibacterial soap).
  - Wash all surfaces thoroughly, including wrists, palms, back of hands, fingers, and under fingernails (preferably with a nail brush).
  - Rub hands together for at least 10 to 15 seconds.
  - When drying, begin with your forearms and work toward your hands and fingertips, and pat your skin rather than rubbing to avoid chapping and cracking.

(These handwashing guidelines were originally published by the Bayer Corporation and the American Society for Microbiology.)

Other means of reducing the incidence of nosocomial infections include disinfection and sterilization techniques, air filtration, use of ultraviolet lights, isolating especially infectious patients, and wearing gloves, masks, and gowns whenever appropriate.

Infection Control

"Infection control" pertains to the numerous measures that are taken to prevent infections from occurring in healthcare settings. These preventive measures include actions taken to eliminate or contain reservoirs of infection, interrupt the transmission of pathogens, and protect persons (patients, employees, and visitors) from becoming infected—in short, they are ways to break various links in the chain of infection (refer to Fig. 11-2).

Ever since the discoveries and observations of Ignaz Semmelweis and Joseph Lister (see the following Historical Notes) in the 19th century, it has been known that wound contamination is not inevitable and that pathogens can be

Contributions of Joseph Lister

Joseph Lister (1827–1912), a British surgeon, made significant contributions in the areas of antisepsis ("against infection") and asepsis ("without infection"). During the 1860s, he instituted the practice of using phenol (carbolic acid) as an antiseptic to reduce microbial contamination of open surgical wounds. Lister routinely applied a dilute phenol solution to all wounds and insisted that anything coming in contact with the wounds (e.g., surgeons' hands, surgical instruments, and wound dressings) be immersed in phenol. In 1870, he instituted the practice of performing surgical procedures within a phenol mist. Although this practice probably killed microbes that were present in the air, it proved unpopular with the surgeons and nurses who inhaled the irritating phenol mist. Later contributions by Lister included such aseptic techniques as steam sterilization of surgical instruments; the use of sterile masks, gloves, and gowns by members of the surgical team; and the use of sterile drapes and gauze sponges in the operating room. Lister's antiseptic and aseptic techniques greatly reduced the incidence of surgical wound infections and surgical mortality. Because phenol is quite caustic and toxic, it was later replaced by other antiseptics.

prevented from reaching vulnerable areas, a concept referred to as asepsis. Asepsis, which literally means "without infection," includes any actions (referred to as aseptic techniques) taken to prevent infection or break the chain of infection. There are two types of asepsis: medical asepsis and surgical asepsis. The techniques used to achieve asepsis depend on the site, circumstances, and environment.

Medical Asepsis

Once basic cleanliness is achieved, it is not difficult to maintain asepsis. Medical asepsis, or clean technique, involves procedures and practices that reduce the number and transmission of pathogens. Medical asepsis includes all the precautionary measures necessary to prevent direct transfer of pathogens from person to person and indirect transfer of pathogens through the air or on instruments, bedding, equipment, and other inanimate objects (fomites). Medical aseptic techniques include frequent and thorough

handwashing; personal grooming; proper cleaning of supplies and equipment; disinfection; proper disposal of needles, contaminated materials, and infectious waste; and sterilization. Disinfectants that are commonly used in hospitals are shown in Table 12-2.

Surgical Asepsis

Surgical asepsis, or sterile technique, includes practices used to render and keep objects and areas sterile (i.e., free of microorganisms). Note the differences between medical and surgical asepsis: (1) medical asepsis is a clean technique, whereas surgical asepsis is a sterile technique, and (2) the goal of medical asepsis is to exclude pathogens, whereas the goal of surgical asepsis is to exclude all microorganisms.

Surgical aseptic techniques are practiced in operating rooms, labor and delivery areas, certain areas of the hospital laboratory, and at patients' bedsides. For example, invasive procedures, such as drawing blood, injecting medications, urinary catheter insertion, cardiac catheterization, and lumbar punctures, must be performed using strict surgical aseptic precautions. Other surgical aseptic techniques include scrubbing hands and fingernails before entering the operating room; using sterile gloves, masks, gowns, and shoe covers; using sterile solutions and dressings; using sterile drapes and creating a sterile field; and using heat-sterilized surgical instruments.

The surgical site of the patient's skin must be shaved and thoroughly cleansed and scrubbed with soap and antiseptic. If the surgery is to be extensive, the surrounding area is covered with a sterile plastic film or sterile cloth drapes so that a sterile surgical field is established. The surgeon and all surgical assistants must scrub their hands for 10 minutes with a disinfectant soap and cover their clothes, mouth, and hair, because these might shed microorganisms onto the operative site. These coverings include sterile gloves, gowns, caps, masks, and shoe covers (Figs. 12-4 and 12-5). All instruments, sutures, and dressings must be sterile. As soon as they become contaminated, they must be thoroughly cleaned and sterilized for reuse, or disposed of properly. All needles, syringes, and other sharp items of equipment ("sharps") must be disposed of by placing them into appropriate puncture-proof "sharps" containers.

Floors, walls, and all equipment in the operating room must be thoroughly cleaned and disinfected before and after each use. Proper ventilation must be maintained to ensure that fresh, filtered air is circulated throughout the room at all times.

Standard Precautions

In a healthcare setting, one is not always aware of which patients are infected with HIV, hepatitis B virus (HBV), or other communicable pathogens. Thus, to prevent transmission of pathogens, standard precautions (as defined by the CDC in

TABLE 12-2

Disinfectants Commonly Used in Hospitals

DISINFECTANT	MODE OF ACTION AND SPECTRUM	USES
Alcohols (e.g., 60 to 90% solutions of ethyl, isopropyl, and benzyl alcohols)	Cause denaturation of proteins; bactericidal, tuberculocidal, fungicidal, virucidal, but not sporicidal	For disinfection of thermometers, rubber stoppers, external surfaces of stethoscopes, endoscopes, and certain other equipment
Chorine and chlorine compounds (Clorox, Halazone, hypochlorites, Warexin)	Thought to cause inhibition of key enzymatic reactions, protein denaturation, and inactivation of nucleic acids; bactericidal, tuberculocidal, fungicidal, virucidal, sporicidal	For disinfection of countertops, floors, blood spills, needles, syringes; water treatment
Formaldehyde (formalin is 37% formaldehyde by weight)	Alters the structure of proteins and purine bases; bactericidal, tuberculocidal, fungicidal, virucidal, sporicidal	Limited uses because of irritating fumes, pungent odor, and potential carcinogenicity; used for preserving anatomic specimens
Glutaraldehyde	Interferes with DNA, RNA, and protein synthesis; bactericidal, fungicidal, virucidal, sporicidal; relatively slow tuberculocidal activity	For disinfection of medical equipment such as endoscopes, tubing, dialyzers, and anesthesia and respiratory therapy equipment; has a pungent odor and is irritating to eyes, throat, and nose; may cause respiratory irritation, asthma, rhinitis, and contact dermatitis
Hydrogen peroxide	Produces destructive free radicals that attack membrane lipids, DNA, and other essential cell components; bactericidal, tuberculocidal, fungicidal, virucidal, sporicidal	For disinfection of inanimate surfaces; limited clinical use; contact with eyes may cause serious eye damage
Iodine (iodine solutions or tinctures) and iodophors (e.g., povidone-iodine, Wescodyne, Betadine, Isodine, Ioprep, Surgidine)	Thought to disrupt protein and nucleic acid structure and synthesis; bactericidal, tuberculocidal, virucidal; may require prolonged contact times to be fungicidal and sporicidal	Primarily for use as antiseptics; also for disinfection of rubber stoppers, thermometers, endoscopes
Orthophthaldehyde	Mode of action unknown; bactericidal, tuberculocidal, fungicidal, virucidal, sporicidal	Stains skin, clothing, environmental surfaces; limited clinical use
Peracetic acid (peroxyacetic acid)	Thought to disrupt cell wall permeability and alter the structure of proteins; bactericidal, tuberculocidal, fungicidal, virucidal, sporicidal	Used in an automated machine to chemically sterilize immersible medical, surgical, and dental instruments, including endoscopes and arthroscopes; concentrate can cause serious eye and skin damage
Combination of peracetic acid and hydrogen peroxide	Mode of action as described above for hydrogen peroxide and peracetic acid; bactericidal, tuberculocidal, fungicidal, virucidal, but not sporicidal	For disinfection of hemodialyzers

(continued)

TABLE 12-2

Disinfectants Commonly Used in Hospitals *(continued)*

DISINFECTANT	MODE OF ACTION AND SPECTRUM	USES
Phenol (carbolic acid) and phenolics (e.g., xylenols, *o*-phenylphenol, hexylresorcinol, hexachlorophene, cresol, Lysol)	Disrupts cell walls and inactivates essential enzyme systems; bactericidal, tuberculocidal, fungicidal, virucidal, but not sporicidal	For decontamination of the hospital environment, including laboratory surfaces, and for noncritical medical and surgical items; residual disinfectant on porous surfaces may cause tissue irritation
Quaternary ammonium compounds (a variety of organically substituted ammonium compounds, such as dodecyl dimethyl ammonium chloride)	Inactivate energy-producing enzymes, denaturation of disruption of cell membranes; bactericidal, fungicidal, and virucidal to lipophilic viruses; generally not tuberculocidal, sporicidal, or virucidal to hydrophilic viruses	For disinfection of noncritical surfaces such as floors, furniture, and walls; should not be used as antiseptics

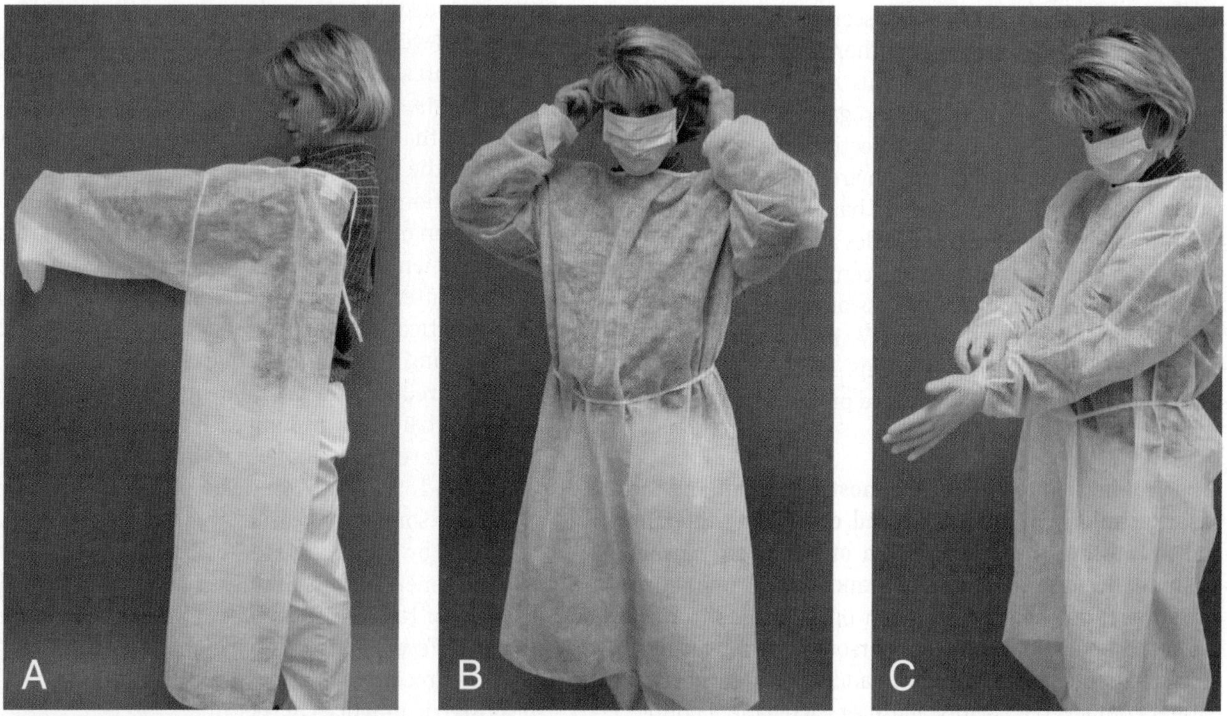

FIGURE 12-4. Healthcare professional donning sterile gown (*A*), mask (*B*), and gloves (*C*). (McCall RE, Tankersley CM. Phlebotomy Essentials, 3rd ed. Philadelphia: Lippincott Williams & Wilkins, 2003.)

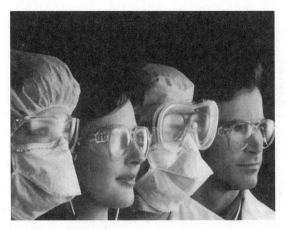

FIGURE 12-5. Various pieces of personal protective equipment, including masks, goggles, hair protection, and disposable gowns.

1996[a]) are used for the care of all hospitalized patients, regardless of their diagnosis or presumed infection status. Standard precautions incorporate the major features of universal precautions (which were instituted in 1985 to reduce the risk of transmission of bloodborne pathogens) and body substance isolation (instituted in 1987 to reduce the risk of transmission of pathogens from moist body substances). Standard precautions are designed to reduce the risk of transmission of bloodborne and other pathogens in hospitals and apply to blood; all body fluids, secretions, and excretions except sweat, regardless of whether they contain visible blood; nonintact skin; and mucous membranes. Standard precautions provide guidelines regarding handwashing; wearing of gloves, masks, eye protection, and gowns; cleaning of patient-care equipment; environmental control (including cleaning and disinfection); handling of soiled linens; handling and disposal of used needles and other "sharps"; resuscitation devices; and patient placement. Standard precautions will protect healthcare professionals and their patients from becoming infected with HIV, HBV, and most other pathogens. The sign shown in Fig. 12-6 summarizes the most important aspects of Standard precautions.

Handwashing

It cannot be said too often: the most important and most basic technique in preventing and controlling infections and preventing the transmission of pathogens is handwashing. Because contaminated hands are a prime cause of cross-infection (i.e., transmission of pathogens from one patient to another), healthcare personnel caring for hospitalized patients must wash their hands thoroughly between patient contacts (i.e., before and after each patient contact). In addition, hands should be washed between tasks and procedures on the same patient to prevent cross-contamination of different body sites. Hands must be washed after

[a] Information in this chapter on standard and transmission-based precautions is from *Guideline for Isolation Precautions in Hospitals.* Centers for Disease Control and Prevention, Atlanta, GA, 1996.

HISTORICAL NOTE

The Father of Handwashing

Ignaz Philipp Semmelweis (1818–1865) has been referred to as the "Father of Handwashing," the "Father of Hand Disinfection," and the "Father of Hospital Epidemiology." Semmelweis, a Hungarian physician, was employed in the maternity department of a large Viennese hospital during the 1840s. Many of the women whose babies were delivered in one of the hospital's clinics became ill and died of a disease known as puerperal fever (also known as childbed fever), the cause of which was unknown at the time. (It is now known that puerperal fever is caused by *Streptococcus pyogenes.*) Semmelweis observed that physicians and medical students often went directly from an autopsy room to the obstetrics clinic to assist in the delivery of a baby. Although they washed their hands with soap and water on entering the clinic, Semmelweis noted that their hands still had a disagreeable odor. He concluded that the puerperal fever that the women later developed was caused by "cadaverous particles" present on the hands of the physicians and students. In May 1847, Semmelweis instituted a policy that stated that "all students or doctors who enter the wards for the purpose of making an examination must wash their hands thoroughly in a solution of chlorinated lime which will be placed in convenient basins near the entrance of the wards." Thereafter, the maternal mortality rate dropped dramatically. This was the first evidence that cleansing contaminated hands with an antiseptic agent reduces nosocomial infections more effectively than handwashing with plain soap and water. It is interesting to note that Oliver Wendell Holmes (1809–1894), an American physician, had concluded some years earlier that puerperal fever was spread by healthcare workers' hands. However, the recommendations Holmes made in his historical essay of 1843, entitled *The Contagiousness of Puerperal Fever,* met with opposition (as did Semmelweis's recommendations) and had little impact on obstetric practices of the time.

touching blood, body fluids, secretions, excretions, and contaminated items, even when gloves are worn. Hands must be washed immediately after gloves are removed.

A plain (nonantimicrobial) soap may be used for routine handwashing, but an antimicrobial or antiseptic

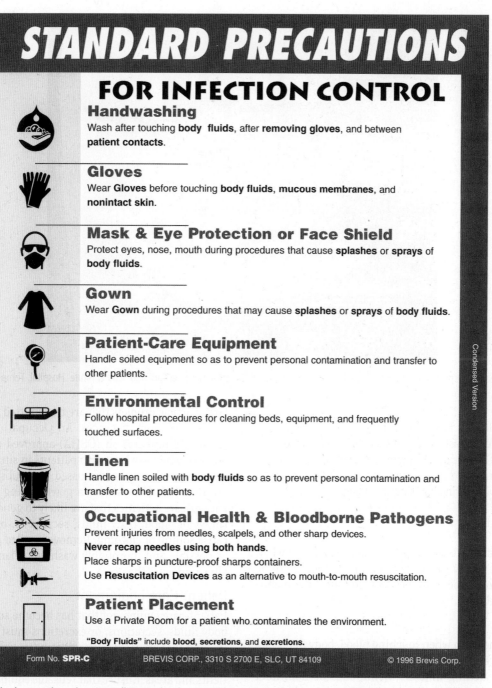

FIGURE 12-6. Standard precautions sign. (McCall RE, Tankersley CM. Phlebotomy Essentials, 3rd ed. Philadelphia: Lippincott Williams & Wilkins, 2003. Courtesy of the Brevis Corp., Salt Lake City, UT.)

agent should be used in certain circumstances (e.g., before entering an operating room or to control outbreaks within the hospital). After lathering, hands should be rubbed briskly for at least 10 to 15 seconds, using friction (Fig. 12-7). Interlace fingers and rub the palms and backs of the hands at least five times, using a circular motion. Be sure to clean beneath fingernails. After rinsing, hands should be dried thoroughly, using either paper towels or an air dryer. A clean, unused paper towel should be used to turn off the hand faucet. According to the CDC, alcohol-based handrubs can be used in settings where hand-

Helpful Hints Regarding Handwashing

To make sure that you have washed your hands sufficiently, rub your soapy hands and interlaced fingers together for as long as it takes you to sing the birthday song ("Happy Birthday to You") twice through, or all verses of "Twinkle, Twinkle, Little Star" once. Alternatively, you could use a quick-drying alcohol foam, gel,

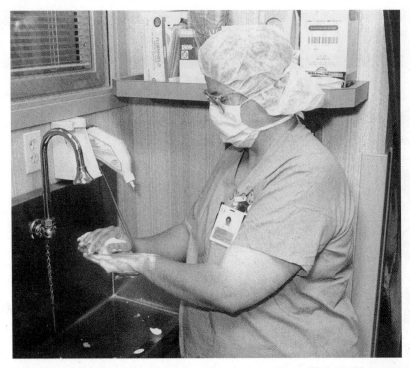

FIGURE 12-7. Healthcare professional washing her hands. (Courtesy of Dr. Janet Duben-Engelkirk and Scott & White Hospital, Temple, TX.)

or lotion. Studies have shown that these convenient products are at least as effective as old-fashioned soap and water. They are quick, they dry in about 15 seconds, and by using them, you eliminate the possibility of someone overhearing you singing off key!

washing facilities are inadequate or unavailable, or when hands are not visibly soiled. The volume of handrub to be used varies from product to product, so follow the manufacturer's directions.

Gloves

Gloves must be worn when touching blood, body fluids, secretions, excretions, and contaminated items, as well as just before touching mucous membranes or nonintact skin. Gloves must be changed between tasks and procedures on the same patient whenever there is risk of transferring microorganisms from one body site to another. Always remove gloves promptly after use and before going to another patient. Thoroughly wash your hands immediately after removing gloves; there is always the possibility that the gloves contained small tears in them or that your hands became contaminated while removing the gloves.

Masks, Eye Protection, Face Shields, and Gowns

Always wear a mask and eye protection or a face shield during procedures and patient-care activities that are likely to generate splashes or sprays of blood, body fluids, secretions, or excretions. A surgical mask will protect the wearer from

large particle droplets that are transmitted by close contact and travel short distances. An Occupational Safety and Health Administration (OSHA)-approved respirator must be worn when working with patients in situations in which airborne precautions (discussed in a subsequent section) are required. Always wear a gown during procedures and patient-care activities that are likely to generate splashes or sprays of blood, body fluids, secretions, or excretions, or cause soiling of clothing. Remove a soiled gown as quickly as possible and thoroughly wash your hands immediately after removing the gown.

Patient-Care Equipment

Patient-care equipment that has become soiled with blood, body fluids, secretions, or excretions must be handled in a manner that prevents contaminating yourself or your clothing and prevents transfer of microorganisms to other patients and areas. Ensure that reusable equipment is not used for the care of another patient until it has been appropriately cleaned, disinfected, or sterilized. Properly dispose of single-use items. Visibly contaminated articles should be bagged.

Environmental Control

The hospital must have, and employees must comply with, adequate procedures for the routine care, cleaning, and disinfection of environmental surfaces, beds, bed rails, bedside equipment, and other frequently touched surfaces.

Linens

Linens that have become soiled with blood, body fluids, secretions, or excretions must be handled, transported, and processed in a manner that prevents contaminating yourself or your clothing and prevents transfer of microorganisms to other patients and areas.

Occupational Health and Bloodborne Pathogens

Needlestick injuries and injuries resulting from broken glass and other "sharps" are the primary manner in which healthcare professionals become infected with pathogens such as HIV and HBV. Thus, standard precautions include guidelines regarding the safe handling of such items. Preferably, used needles should not be resheathed. If resheathing is deemed appropriate, never resheath needles using both hands. Use either a one-handed scoop technique (Fig. 12-8) or a mechanical device that eliminates the danger of sticking yourself with the needle. Do not remove used needles from disposable syringes by hand and do not attempt to bend or break used needles. Place used disposable syringes, needles, scalpel blades, broken glass, and other sharps in appropriate puncture-resistant containers. Such containers should be located in areas where such sharps are likely to be used.

Patient Placement

Whenever possible, use private rooms for patients who might contaminate the hospital environment or who do not (or cannot be expected to) assist in maintaining appropriate hygiene or environmental control.

Transmission-Based Precautions

The five main routes of transmission of pathogens are contact (either direct or indirect contact), airborne, droplet, vehicular, and vectors. Within a hospital, pathogens are transmitted by three major routes: airborne, droplet, and contact. Transmission-based precautions are designed for patients known or suspected to be infected with highly transmissible or epidemiologically important pathogens for which additional precautions beyond standard precautions are required to interrupt transmission within hospitals. There are three types of transmission-based precautions, which may be used either singly or in combination: airborne precautions, droplet precautions, and contact precautions. **Please note that these transmission-based precautions are to be used in addition to the standard precautions already being used.**

Airborne Precautions

Airborne transmission involves either airborne droplet nuclei or dust particles containing a pathogen. Airborne droplet nuclei are small-particle residues (5 μm or less in diameter) of evaporated droplets containing microorganisms; because of their small size, they remain suspended in air for long periods. Airborne precautions (Fig. 12-9) apply to patients known or suspected to be infected with epidemiologically important pathogens that can be transmitted by the airborne route (e.g., *Mycobacterium tuberculosis,* rubeola virus, varicella virus). In addition to standard precautions, the patient is placed in a private room having negative air pressure and from which air is either discharged outdoors or (if recirculated) passed through high-efficiency particulate air (HEPA) filters. If a private room is not available, the patient may be placed in a room with a patient having active infection with the same pathogen, but with no other infection. Persons entering the patient's room must wear respiratory protection unless they are known to be immune to the pathogen. Figure 12-10 shows the type N95 respirator that must be worn when entering the room of a patient with known or suspected tuberculosis. A surgical mask is placed on the patient whenever it is necessary to transport the patient from the room. Pathogens transmitted by airborne transmission are listed in Table 12-3.

Droplet Precautions

Technically, droplet transmission is a form of contact transmission. However, in droplet transmission, the mechanism of transfer is quite different than either direct or indirect contact transmission. Droplets are produced primarily as a result of coughing, sneezing, and talking, as well as during hospital procedures such as suctioning and bronchoscopy. Transmission occurs when droplets (larger than 5 μm in diameter) containing microorganisms are propelled a short distance through the air and become deposited on another person's conjunctiva, nasal mucosa, or

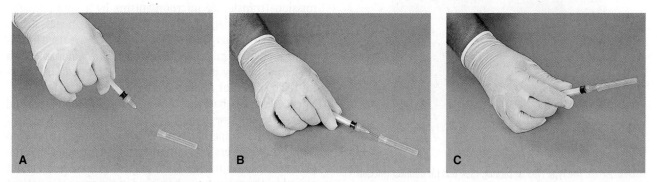

FIGURE 12-8. One-handed scoop technique for resheathing needles. (*A*) Lining up the needle with the cap. Note that the needle is lying on a flat surface. (*B*) Lifting cap onto needle. (*C*) Covering needle with cap. (Taylor CT, et al. Fundamentals of Nursing: The Art and Science of Nursing Care, 4th ed. Philadelphia: Lippincott Williams & Wilkins, 2001.)

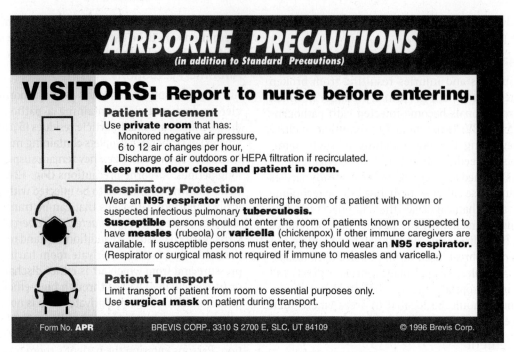

FIGURE 12-9. Airborne precautions sign. (McCall RE, Tankersley CM. Phlebotomy Essentials, 3rd ed. Philadelphia: Lippincott Williams & Wilkins Publishers, 2003. Courtesy of the Brevis Corp., Salt Lake City, UT.)

mouth. Because of their size, droplets do not remain suspended in the air. Droplet precautions (Fig. 12-11) must be used for patients known or suspected to be infected with microorganisms transmitted by droplets that can be generated in the ways previously mentioned; examples include meningococcal meningitis, multidrug-resistant pneumococcal meningitis or pneumonia, whooping cough, strep throat, streptococcal pneumonia, and influenza. In addi-

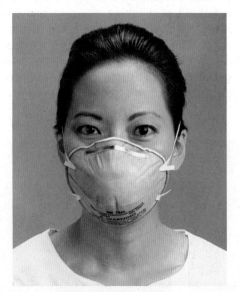

FIGURE 12-10. The type N95 respirator. (See text for details.) (McCall RE, Tankersley CM. Phlebotomy Essentials, 3rd ed. Philadelphia: Lippincott Williams & Wilkins, 2003. Courtesy of 3M Occupational Health and Environmental Safety Division, St. Paul, MN.)

tion to standard precautions, the patient is placed in a private room. If a private room is not available, the patient may be placed in a room with a patient having active infection with the same pathogen but with no other infection. Special air handling and ventilation are not required to prevent droplet transmission. Persons working within 3 feet of the patient must wear a mask. A surgical mask is placed on the patient whenever it is necessary to transport the patient from the room. Pathogens transmitted by droplet transmission are listed in Table 12-3.

Contact Precautions

Contact transmission is the most important and frequent mode of transmission of nosocomial infections. Contact transmission is divided into two subgroups: direct-contact transmission (transfer of microorganisms by body surface–to–body surface contact) and indirect-contact transmission (transfer of microorganisms by a contaminated intermediate object, such as instruments, needles, and dressings). Contact precautions (Fig. 12-12) are used for patients known or suspected to be infected or colonized with epidemiologically important pathogens that can be transmitted by direct or indirect contact; examples include multidrug-resistant bacteria, *Clostridium difficile*-associated diseases, respiratory syncytial virus (RSV) infection in children, scabies, impetigo, chickenpox or shingles, and viral hemorrhagic fevers. In addition to standard precautions, the patient is placed in a private room. If a private room is not available, the patient may be placed in a room with a patient having active infection with the same pathogen but with no other infection. In addition to wearing gloves as outlined

TABLE 12-3

Infectious Diseases Requiring Transmission-Based Precautions

TYPES OF TRANSMISSION-BASED PRECAUTIONS	INFECTIOUS DISEASES
Airborne precautions	Chickenpox; disseminated shingles or shingles in immunocompromised patients; measles (rubeola); pulmonary or laryngeal tuberculosis
Droplet precautions	Adenovirus infection in infants and young children; adenovirus pneumonia; epiglottitis caused by *Haemophilus influenzae;* German measles; Group A streptococcal infections in infants and children; *H. influenzae* or *Neisseria meningitidis* meningitis or pneumonia; influenza; meningococcemia; mumps; *Mycoplasma* pneumonia; parvovirus B19 infections; pertussis (whooping cough); pharyngeal diphtheria; pharyngitis, pneumonia, or scarlet fever in infants and young children; pneumonic plague
Contact precautions	Acute viral (hemorrhagic) conjunctivitis; adenovirus infection in infants and young children; adenovirus pneumonia; cellulitis with uncontrolled drainage; chickenpox, *Clostridium difficile* infections; congenital rubella; cutaneous diphtheria; disseminated shingles or shingles in immunocompromised patients; enterohemorrhagic O157:H7 *E. coli;* hepatitis A; *Shigella* or rotavirus infections in diapered or incontinent patients; enteroviral infections in infants and young children; gastrointestinal, respiratory, skin, wound, or burn infections or colonization with multidrug-resistant organisms; hemorrhagic fevers (e.g., Lassa and Ebola viruses); impetigo; lice (pediculosis); major draining abscesses, major infected decubitus ulcer; Marburg virus disease; major staphylococcal or Group A streptococcal skin, wound, or burn infections; neonatal or mucocutaneous herpes simplex infections; parainfluenza virus respiratory infection in infants and young children; respiratory syncytial virus infection in infants, young children, and immunocompromised adults; scabies; staphylococcal furunculosis in infants and young children

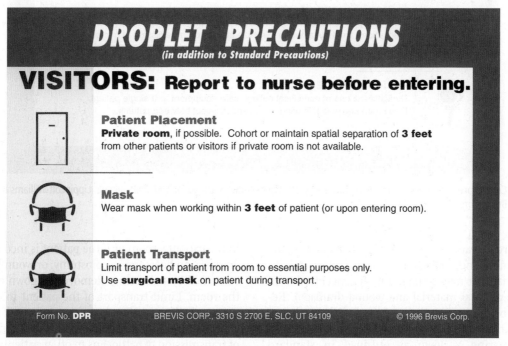

FIGURE 12-11. Droplet precautions sign. (McCall RE, Tankersley CM. Phlebotomy Essentials, 3rd ed. Philadelphia: Lippincott Williams & Wilkins, 2003. Courtesy of the Brevis Corp., Salt Lake City, UT.)

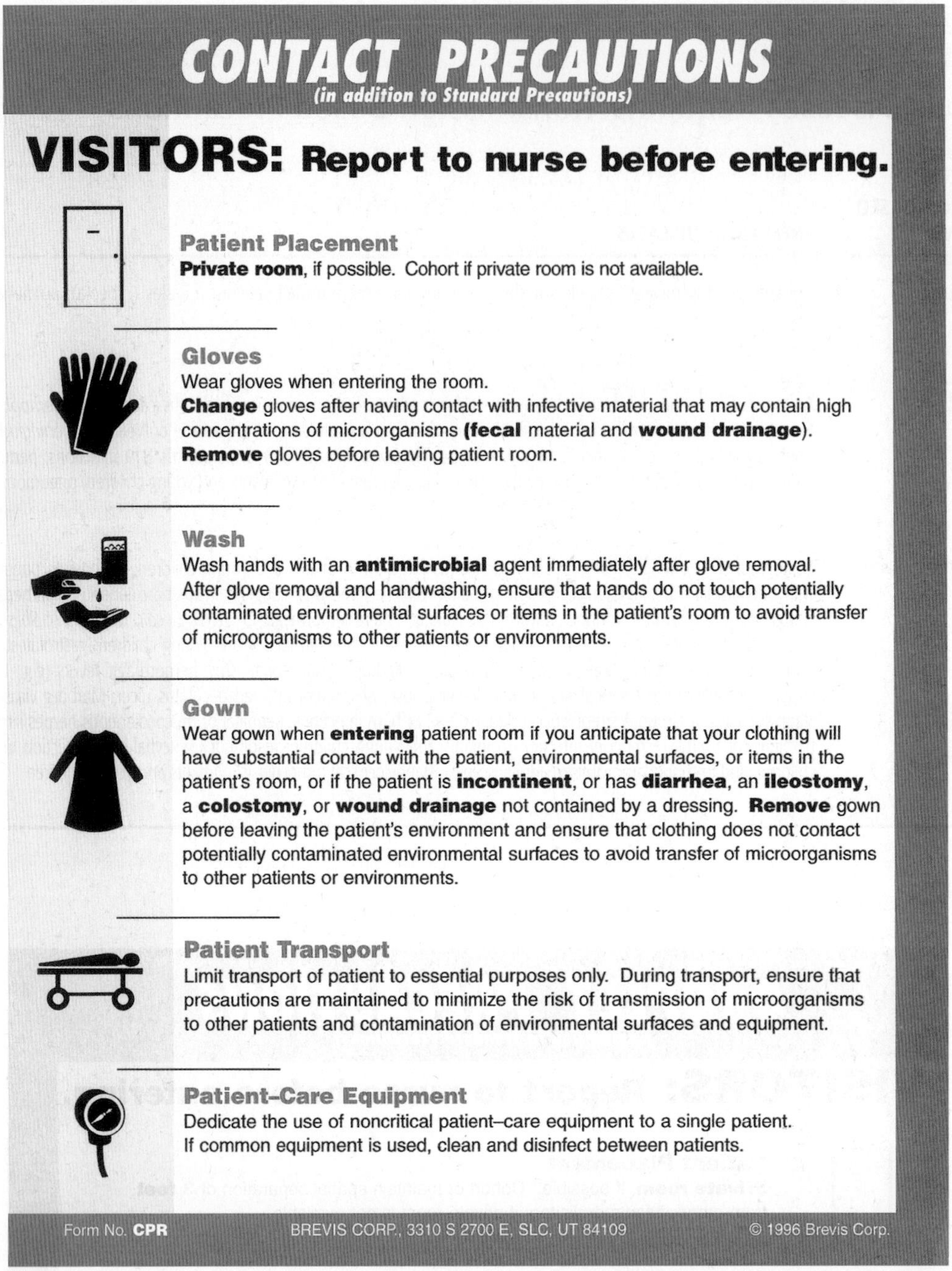

CONTACT PRECAUTIONS
(in addition to Standard Precautions)

VISITORS: Report to nurse before entering.

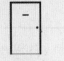

Patient Placement
Private room, if possible. Cohort if private room is not available.

Gloves
Wear gloves when entering the room.
Change gloves after having contact with infective material that may contain high concentrations of microorganisms **(fecal** material and **wound drainage)**.
Remove gloves before leaving patient room.

Wash
Wash hands with an **antimicrobial** agent immediately after glove removal. After glove removal and handwashing, ensure that hands do not touch potentially contaminated environmental surfaces or items in the patient's room to avoid transfer of microorganisms to other patients or environments.

Gown
Wear gown when **entering** patient room if you anticipate that your clothing will have substantial contact with the patient, environmental surfaces, or items in the patient's room, or if the patient is **incontinent**, or has **diarrhea**, an **ileostomy**, a **colostomy**, or **wound drainage** not contained by a dressing. **Remove** gown before leaving the patient's environment and ensure that clothing does not contact potentially contaminated environmental surfaces to avoid transfer of microorganisms to other patients or environments.

Patient Transport
Limit transport of patient to essential purposes only. During transport, ensure that precautions are maintained to minimize the risk of transmission of microorganisms to other patients and contamination of environmental surfaces and equipment.

Patient–Care Equipment
Dedicate the use of noncritical patient–care equipment to a single patient. If common equipment is used, clean and disinfect between patients.

Form No. **CPR**   BREVIS CORP, 3310 S 2700 E, SLC, UT 84109   © 1996 Brevis Corp.

FIGURE 12-12. Contact precautions sign. (McCall RE, Tankersley CM. Phlebotomy Essentials, 3rd ed. Philadelphia: Lippincott Williams & Wilkins, 2003. Courtesy of the Brevis Corp., Salt Lake City, UT

under standard precautions, wear gloves when entering the patient's room. Change gloves after having contact with infective material that may contain a high concentration of pathogens (e.g., fecal material and wound drainage). Remove gloves before leaving the room and wash hands immediately with an antimicrobial or antiseptic agent. In addition to wearing a gown as outlined in standard precautions, wear a gown when entering the patient's room if you anticipate that your clothing will have substantial contact with the patient, environmental surfaces, or items in the patient's room or if the patient is incontinent or has diarrhea, an ileostomy, a colostomy, or wound drainage not contained by a dressing. Remove the gown before leaving the room. Limit transport of the patient to essential purposes only. If the patient is transported out of the room, ensure that precautions are maintained to minimize the risk of transmission of pathogens to other patients and contamination of environmental surfaces or equipment. When possible, dedicate the use of noncritical patient-care equipment to a single patient to avoid sharing between patients. If this is not possible, then such equipment must be adequately cleaned and disinfected before use for another patient. Pathogens transmitted by contact transmission are listed in Table 12-3.

Source Isolation

When patients with tuberculosis or other contagious diseases are placed into isolation to protect other people from becoming infected, it is known as source isolation (Fig. 12-13). These isolation rooms are usually under negative pressure to prevent room air from entering the hallway when the door is opened, and air that is evacuated from such rooms passes through HEPA filters to remove pathogens.

Protective Isolation

Certain patients are especially vulnerable to infection; among them are patients with severe burns, those who have leukemia, patients who have received a transplant, immunosuppressed persons, those receiving radiation treatments, and leukopenic patients (those having abnormally low white blood cell counts). Premature infants are also highly susceptible to infection. All such patients are protected through an isolation procedure known as protective isolation (also referred to as reverse isolation or neutropenic isolation), where patients are placed in a total protected environment (TPE). The TPE includes a private room in which vented air entering the room is passed through HEPA filters. The room is under positive pressure to prevent hallway air from entering when the door is opened (Fig. 12-14). The room must be thoroughly cleaned and disinfected before the patient is admitted. All items coming in contact with the patient must be disinfected or sterilized. Persons entering the room must wear sterile gowns, masks, gloves, caps, and shoe covers to prevent introducing microorganisms into the room from their

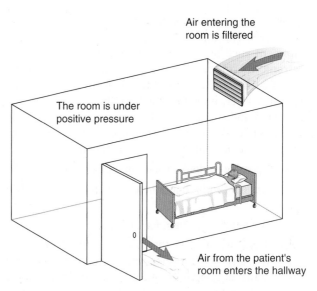

Air entering the room is filtered

The room is under positive pressure

Air from the patient's room enters the hallway

FIGURE 12-14. Protective isolation. (See text for details.)

clothes or respiratory tracts. Proper handwashing procedures must be followed before entering the room.

Handling Food and Eating Utensils

Contaminated food provides an excellent environment for the growth of pathogens. Most often, human carelessness, especially neglecting the practice of handwashing, is responsible for this contamination. Foodborne pathogens and the diseases they cause are discussed in Chapter 11. Regulations for safe handling of food and eating utensils are not difficult to follow. They include:

- Using high-quality, fresh food.
- Properly refrigerating and storing food.
- Properly washing, preparing, and cooking food.
- Properly disposing of uneaten food.
- Thoroughly washing hands and fingernails before handling food and after visiting a restroom.
- Properly disposing of nasal and oral secretions in tissues and then thoroughly washing hands and fingernails.
- Covering hair and wearing clean clothes and aprons.
- Providing periodic health examinations for kitchen workers.
- Prohibiting anyone with a respiratory or gastrointestinal disease from handling food or eating utensils.
- Keeping all cutting boards and other surfaces scrupulously clean.
- Rinsing and then washing cooking and eating utensils in a dishwasher in which the water temperature is greater than 80°C.

Handling Fomites

As previously described, fomites are any nonliving or inanimate objects other than food that may harbor and transmit

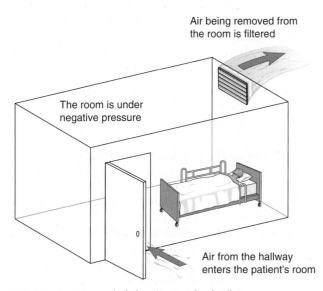

Air being removed from the room is filtered

The room is under negative pressure

Air from the hallway enters the patient's room

FIGURE 12-13. Source isolation. (See text for details.)

microbes. Examples of fomites are patients' gowns, bedding, towels, and eating and drinking utensils; and hospital equipment such as bedpans, stethoscopes, latex gloves, electronic thermometers, and electrocardiographic electrodes that become contaminated by pathogens from the respiratory tract, intestinal tract, or the skin of patients. Telephones and computer keyboards in patient-care areas can also serve as fomites. Transmission of pathogens by fomites can be prevented by observing the following rules:

- Use disposable equipment and supplies wherever possible.
- Disinfect or sterilize equipment as soon as possible after use.
- Use individual equipment for each patient.
- Use electronic or glass thermometers fitted with one-time use, disposable covers or use disposable, single-use thermometers; electronic and glass thermometers must be cleaned or sterilized on a regular basis, following manufacturer's instructions.
- Empty bedpans and urinals, wash them in hot water, and store them in a clean cabinet between uses.
- Place bed linen and soiled clothing in bags to be sent to the laundry.

Medical Waste Disposal

General Regulations

According to OSHA standards, medical wastes must be disposed of properly. These standards include the following:

- Any receptacle used for decomposable solid or liquid waste or refuse must be constructed so that it does not leak and must be maintained in a sanitary condition. This receptacle must be equipped with a solid, tight-fitting cover, unless it can be maintained in a sanitary condition without a cover.
- All sweepings, solid or liquid wastes, refuse, and garbage shall be removed to avoid creating a menace to health and shall be removed as often as necessary to maintain the place of employment in a sanitary condition.
- The medical facility's infection control program must address the handling and disposal of potentially contaminated items.

Disposal of Sharps

Sharps should be handled and disposed of in the following manner:

- Preferably, needles shall not be resheathed, purposely bent or broken by hand, removed from disposable syringes, or otherwise manipulated by hand.
- Should it be necessary to resheath needles, never do so using both hands. Always use either a one-handed scoop technique or a mechanical device that eliminates the danger of sticking yourself with the needle.
- After use, needles, disposable syringes, scalpel blades,

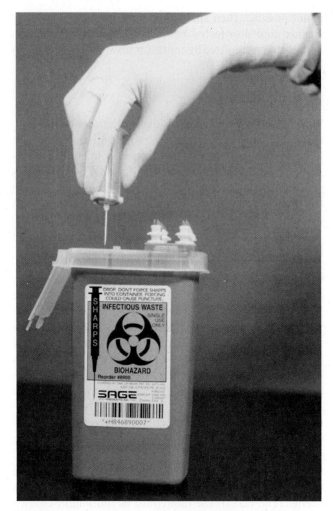

FIGURE 12-15. A type of sharps container. (McCall RE, Tankersley CM. Phlebotomy Essentials, 2nd ed. Philadelphia: Lippincott Williams & Wilkins, 1998. Courtesy of Sage Products, Inc., Crystal Lake, IL.)

and other sharp items must be placed in puncture-resistant containers for disposal of sharps (Fig. 12-15).

- Sharps containers must be easily accessible to all personnel needing them and must be located in all areas where needles are commonly used, as in areas where blood is drawn, including patient rooms, emergency rooms, intensive care units, and surgical suites.
- Sharps containers must be constructed in such a manner that the contents will not spill if knocked over and will not cause injuries.

Infection Control Committees and Infection Control Professionals

All healthcare facilities should have some type of formal infection control program in place. Its functions will vary slightly from one type of healthcare facility to another. In a hospital setting, the infection control program is usually under the jurisdiction of the hospital's Infection Control Committee (ICC) or Epidemiology Service. The ICC is composed of representatives from most of the hospital's departments, including medical and surgical services, pathology, nursing, hospital administration, risk management, pharmacy, housekeeping, food services, and central supply. The chairperson is usually an Infection Control Professional (ICP; see "Insight: Infection Control Professionals" on the CD-ROM), such as a physician (e.g., an epidemiologist or infectious disease specialist), an infection control nurse, a microbiologist, or some other person knowledgeable about infection control.

The ICC periodically reviews the hospital's infection control program and the incidence of nosocomial infections. It is a policy-making and review body that may take drastic action (e.g., instituting quarantine measures) when epidemiologic circumstances warrant. Other ICC responsibilities include patient surveillance, environmental surveillance, investigation of outbreaks and epidemics, and education of the hospital staff regarding infection control.

Although every department of the hospital endeavors to maintain aseptic conditions, the total environment is constantly bombarded with microbes from outside the hospital. These must be controlled for the protection of the patients. Hospital personnel (usually ICPs) entrusted with this aspect of health care diligently and constantly work to maintain the proper environment. In the event of an epidemic, the ICP notifies city, county, and state health authorities so they can assist in ending the epidemic.

Role of the Microbiology Laboratory in Hospital Epidemiology and Infection Control

Clinical Microbiology Laboratory (CML) personnel participate in infection control in three major ways:

- By monitoring the types and numbers of pathogens isolated from hospitalized patients. In most hospitals, such monitoring is accomplished using computers and appropriate software programs.
- By notifying the appropriate ICP should an unusual pathogen or an unusually high number of isolates of a common pathogen be detected. The ICP will then initiate an investigation of the outbreak.
- By processing environmental samples, including samples from hospital employees, that have been collected from within the affected ward(s). It is hoped that this will pinpoint the exact source of the pathogen that is causing the outbreak. Examples of environmental samples include air samples, nasal swabs from healthcare personnel, and swabs of sink drains, whirlpool tubs, respiratory therapy equipment, bed rails, and ventilation grates and ducts.

Assume that there is an epidemic of *Klebsiella pneumoniae* infections on the pediatric ward and that *K. pneumoniae* has been isolated from a certain environmental sample collected on that ward. How do CML personnel determine that the *K. pneumoniae* that has been isolated from the environmental sample is the same strain of *K. pneumoniae*

that has been isolated from the patients? Traditionally, the two most commonly used methods have been by biotype and antibiogram. If the two strains produce the exact same biochemical test results, they are said to have the same biotype. If they produce the exact same susceptibility and resistance patterns when antimicrobial susceptibility testing is performed, they are said to have the same antibiogram. Having the same biotype and antibiogram is evidence (but not absolute proof) that they are the same strain. Because of the limitations of phenotypic methods (such as biotypes and antibiograms), however, most hospitals are currently using what is known as molecular epidemiology, in which genotypic (as opposed to phenotypic) typing methods are used. Most often, these methods involve genotyping of plasmid or chromosomal DNA. Genotypic methods provide more accurate data than phenotypic methods. If the two isolates of *K. pneumoniae* in the above example have exactly the same genotype (i.e., possess exactly the same genes), they are the same strain; therefore, the source of the epidemic has been found. Action will then be taken to eliminate the source.

Concluding Remarks

A nosocomial infection can add several weeks to a patient's hospital stay and may lead to serious complications and even death. From an economic viewpoint, insurance companies rarely reimburse hospitals and other healthcare facilities for the costs associated with nosocomial infections. Insurance companies take the position that nosocomial infections are the fault of the healthcare facility and, therefore, that the facility should bear any additional patient costs related to such infections. Sadly, cross-infections transmitted by hospital personnel, including physicians, are all too common; this is particularly true when hospitals and clinics are overcrowded and the staff is overworked. However, nosocomial infections can be avoided through proper education and disciplined compliance with infection control practices.

All healthcare workers must fully comprehend the problem of nosocomial infections, must be completely knowledgeable about infection control practices, and must personally do everything in their power to prevent nosocomial infections from occurring.

ⓞ REVIEW OF KEY POINTS

- Infections that are acquired in the hospital (or any other healthcare setting) are called nosocomial infections, whereas those that are acquired elsewhere are called community-acquired infections. Iatrogenic infections or diseases are the result of medical or surgical treatment by surgeons, other physicians, and other healthcare personnel.

- Nosocomial infections occur all too frequently. Some of the factors causing nosocomial infections are an ever-increasing number of drug-resistant pathogens, lack of awareness of routine infection control measures, neglect of aseptic techniques and safety precautions, lengthy complicated surgeries, overcrowding of hospitals, shortage of hospital staff, an increased number of immunosuppressed patients, and the overuse and improper use of indwelling medical devices.

- The seven most common causes of nosocomial infections in the United States are *Staphylococcus aureus,* coagulase-negative staphylococci, *Enterococcus* spp., *Escherichia coli, Pseudomonas aeruginosa, Enterobacter* spp., and *Klebsiella* spp.

- The four most common types of nosocomial infections are urinary tract infections (UTIs), surgical wound infections (also referred to as postsurgical wound infections), lower respiratory tract infections (primarily pneumonia), and bloodstream infections (septicemia).

- The patients most susceptible to nosocomial infections are women in delivery, newborn infants, and immunosuppressed, surgical, cancer, diabetic, paralyzed, and burn patients. Reverse isolation techniques are designed to protect the most vulnerable patients, such as those with severe burns, leukemia, or transplants, those who are undergoing radiation treatments, and other immunosuppressed persons.

- Medical asepsis is a clean technique, the goal of which is to exclude pathogens. Surgical asepsis is a sterile technique, the goal of which is to exclude all microorganisms.

- Medical aseptic techniques include proper handwashing and personal hygiene of hospital personnel; wearing of gloves, masks, and gowns when appropriate; proper cooking and storing of food; sanitary methods for handling food and eating utensils; proper disposal of waste products and contaminated materials; proper use of isolation rooms; proper washing and sterilizing of hospital equipment; proper use of disposable equipment; and proper use of disinfectants and antiseptics.

- Surgical aseptic techniques include scrubbing hands and fingernails before entering the operating room; using sterile gloves, masks, gowns, and shoe covers; using sterile solutions and dressings; using sterile drapes and creating a sterile field; using heat-sterilized surgical instruments; and using surgical aseptic precautions during invasive procedures, such as drawing blood, injecting medications, inserting urinary catheters, and performing cardiac catheterization and lumbar punctures.

- All healthcare personnel must follow the same procedures to prevent the spread of communicable diseases. They must prevent cross-infections from themselves to susceptible patients; from hospitalized, contagious patients to susceptible patients; and from hospitalized, contagious patients to themselves. Healthcare personnel must use precautions that will protect them from bloodborne pathogens such as hepatitis B virus and HIV.

- Standard precautions must be used for the care of all patients. They are designed to reduce the risk of transmission of bloodborne and other pathogens. They apply to mucous membranes, nonintact skin, blood, and all body secretions and excretions except sweat, regardless of whether they contain visible blood.

- Transmission-based precautions (airborne precautions, droplet precautions, and contact precautions) are used in addition to standard precautions to protect healthcare personnel and hospital patients from airborne, droplet, and contact modes of pathogen transmission.

- Patients with highly infectious diseases are placed in source isolation to protect other persons (patients, hospital employees, and visitors) from becoming infected. Protective (reverse) isolation is used to protect highly susceptible patients (e.g., premature babies, patients with severe burns or leukemia, patients who have received a transplant, immunosuppressed persons, patients receiving radiation treatments, and leukopenic patients) from becoming infected.

- Every hospital should have an Infection Control Committee (ICC) that is responsible for ensuring that the hospital is in compliance with all applicable infection control regulations. Other duties of the ICC are to periodically review the hospital's infection control program and the incidence of nosocomial infections, patient surveillance, environmental surveillance, investigation of outbreaks and epidemics, education of the hospital staff regarding infection control, and notification of appropriate city, county, and state health authorities in the event of an outbreak in the hospital.

- Clinical Microbiology Laboratory (CML) personnel participate in infection control by monitoring the types and numbers of pathogens isolated from hospitalized patients, notifying the appropriate ICP should an unusual pathogen or an unusually high number of isolates of a common pathogen be detected, and processing environmental samples that have been collected from within the affected ward(s) during an outbreak in the hospital.

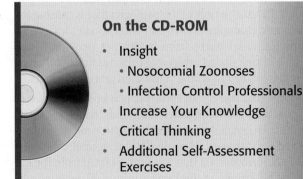

On the CD-ROM

- Insight
  - Nosocomial Zoonoses
  - Infection Control Professionals
- Increase Your Knowledge
- Critical Thinking
- Additional Self-Assessment Exercises

Self-Assessment Exercises

After studying this chapter, answer the following multiple-choice questions.

1. A nosocomial infection is one that:
   a. develops during hospitalization or erupts within 14 days of hospital discharge.
   b. affects only the nose.
   c. is acquired in the community.
   d. the patient has at the time of hospital admission.

2. An example of a fomite would be:
   a. a drinking glass used by a patient.
   b. bandages from an infected wound.
   c. soiled bed linens.
   d. all of the above.

3. Which of the following Gram-positive bacteria is most likely to be the cause of a nosocomial infection?
   a. *Clostridium difficile*
   b. *Staphylococcus aureus*
   c. *Streptococcus pneumoniae*
   d. *Streptococcus pyogenes*

4. Which of the following Gram-negative bacteria is least likely to be the cause of a nosocomial infection?
   a. a *Klebsiella* species
   b. a *Salmonella* species
   c. *Escherichia coli*
   d. *Pseudomonas aeruginosa*

5. Protective (reverse) isolation would be appropriate for a patient:
   a. infected with MRSA.
   b. with leukopenia.
   c. with pneumonic plague.
   d. with tuberculosis.

6. Which of the following is not part of standard precautions?
   a. handwashing between patient contacts
   b. placing a patient in a private room having negative air pressure
   c. properly disposing of needles, scalpels, and other sharps
   d. wearing gloves, masks, eye protection, and gowns when appropriate

7. A patient suspected of having tuberculosis has been admitted to the hospital. Which one of the following is not appropriate?
   a. droplet precautions
   b. source isolation
   c. standard precautions
   d. use of a type N95 respirator by healthcare professional who are caring for the patient

8. Which of the following statements about medical asepsis is false?
   a. Disinfection is a medical aseptic technique.
   b. Handwashing is a medical aseptic technique.
   c. Medical asepsis is considered a clean technique.
   d. The goal of medical asepsis is to exclude all microorganisms from an area.

9. Which of the following statements about source isolation is false?
   a. Air entering the room is passed through HEPA filters.
   b. The room is under negative air pressure.
   c. Source isolation is appropriate for patients with meningococcal meningitis, whooping cough, or influenza.
   d. Transmission-based precautions will be necessary.

10. Contact precautions are required for patients with:
    a. *Clostridium difficile*-associated diseases.
    b. infections caused by multidrug-resistant bacteria.
    c. viral hemorrhagic fevers.
    d. all of the above.

13

DIAGNOSING INFECTIOUS DISEASES

LEARNING OBJECTIVES

AFTER STUDYING THIS CHAPTER, YOU SHOULD BE
ABLE TO:

* Discuss the role of healthcare professionals in the collection of clinical specimens
* List the types of clinical specimens that are submitted to
 the Clinical Microbiology Laboratory for the diagnosis
 of infectious diseases
* Discuss general precautions that must be observed during the collection and handling of clinical specimens
* Describe the proper procedures for obtaining blood,
 urine, cerebrospinal fluid, sputum, throat, wound, GC,
 and fecal specimens for submission to the Clinical
 Microbiology Laboratory
* State the information that must be included on specimen labels and laboratory request slips

* Outline the organization of the Pathology Department
 and the Clinical Microbiology Laboratory
* Compare and contrast the anatomical and clinical
 pathology divisions of the Pathology Department
* Identify the various types of personnel that work in
 anatomical and clinical pathology

INTRODUCTION

The proper diagnosis of an infectious disease requires
(1) taking a complete patient history, (2) conducting a thorough physical examination of the patient, (3) carefully
evaluating the patient's signs and symptoms, and (4) im-
plementing the proper selection, collection, transport, and
processing of appropriate clinical specimens. The latter

topics—those involving clinical specimens—are discussed in this chapter. The other topics are beyond the scope of this book.

Clinical Specimens

The various types of specimens (e.g., blood, urine, feces, cerebrospinal fluid) that are collected from patients and used to diagnose or follow the progress of infectious diseases are referred to as **clinical specimens.** The most common types of clinical specimens that are sent to the hospital's microbiology laboratory (hereafter referred to as the Clinical Microbiology Laboratory or CML) are listed in Table 13-1. It is extremely important that these specimens are of the highest possible quality and that they are collected in a manner that does not jeopardize either the patient or the person collecting the specimen.

TABLE 13-1

Types of Clinical Specimens Submitted to the Clinical Microbiology Laboratory

TYPE OF SPECIMEN	TYPE(S) OF INFECTIOUS DISEASE THAT THE SPECIMEN IS USED TO DIAGNOSE	TYPE OF SPECIMEN	TYPE(S) OF INFECTIOUS DISEASE THAT THE SPECIMEN IS USED TO DIAGNOSE
Blood	B, F, P, V	"Scotch tape prep"	P
Bone marrow	B	Skin scrapings	F
Bronchial and bronchoalveolar washes	V	Skin snip	P
Cerebrospinal fluid (CSF)	B, F, P, V	Sputum	B, F, P
Cervical and vaginal swabs	B	Synovial (joint) fluid	B
Conjunctival swab or scraping	B, V	Throat swabs	B, V
Feces and rectal swabs	B, P, V	Tissue (biopsy and autopsy) specimens	B, F, P, V
Hair clippings	F	Urethral discharge material	B
Nail (fingernail and toenail) clippings	F	Urine	B, P, V
Nasal swabs	B	Urogenital secretions (e.g., vaginal discharge material, prostatic secretions)	B, P
Pus from a wound or abscess	B	Vesicle fluid or scraping	V

B, bacterial infections; F, fungal infections; P, parasitic infections; V, viral infections.

Role of Healthcare Professionals in the Submission of Clinical Specimens

A close working relationship among the members of the healthcare team is essential for the proper diagnosis of infectious diseases. When an attending physician suspects that a patient has a particular infectious disease, appropriate clinical specimens must be obtained and certain diagnostic tests may be requested. The doctor, nurse, medical technologist, or other qualified healthcare professional must select the appropriate specimen, collect it properly, and then properly transport it to the laboratory where it is processed. Laboratory findings must then be conveyed to the attending physician as quickly as possible to facilitate the prompt diagnosis and treatment of the infectious disease.

Healthcare professionals who collect and transport clinical specimens should exercise extreme caution during the collection and transport of clinical specimens to avoid sticking themselves with needles, cutting themselves with other types of sharps, or coming in contact with any type of specimen. Healthcare personnel who collect clinical specimens must strictly adhere to the safety policies known as standard precautions (Chapter 12). According to the Clinical and Laboratory Standards Institute (CLSI), "All specimens should be collected or transferred into a leakproof primary container with a secure closure. Care should be taken by the person collecting the specimen not to contaminate the outside of the primary container....Within the institution, the primary container should be placed into a second container, which will contain the specimen if the primary container breaks or leaks in transit to the laboratory." (CLSI Document M29-A3, 2005.) Within the laboratory, all specimens are handled carefully, following standard precautions, and ultimately disposed of as infectious waste.

Importance of High-Quality Clinical Specimens

Specimens submitted to the CML must be of the highest possible quality. High-quality clinical specimens are required to achieve accurate, *clinically relevant laboratory results* (i.e., results that provide information about the patient's infectious disease). It has often been stated that the quality of the laboratory work performed in the CML can be only as good as the quality of specimens that are received. It is impossible for the CML to obtain and report high-quality test results if the laboratory receives poor-quality specimens or the wrong types of specimens.

The three components of specimen quality are (1) proper specimen selection (i.e., the correct type of specimen must be submitted), (2) proper specimen collection, and (3) proper transport of the specimen to the laboratory. The laboratory must provide written guidelines regarding specimen selection, collection, and transport in the form of

---

○ STUDY AID

Three Components of Specimen Quality

1. Proper selection of the specimen (i.e., to determine the proper specimen)
2. Proper collection of the specimen
3. Proper transport of the specimen to the laboratory

---

a book (although the name of the book varies from one institution to the next, it is referred to in this book as the **"Laboratory Policies and Procedures Manual"** or Lab P&P Manual, for short). Copies of the Lab P&P Manual must be available to every ward, floor, clinic, and department. Often, it is accessible through the hospital's computer system. However, **the person who collects the specimen is ultimately responsible for its quality.**

It would not be feasible in a book of this size to provide a complete discussion of the proper methods for selecting, collecting, and transporting clinical specimens. Only a few important concepts are discussed here. See "Insight: Specimen Quality and Clinical Relevance" on the CD-ROM for additional details.

When clinical specimens are improperly collected and handled, (1) the etiologic (causative) agent may not be found or may be destroyed, (2) overgrowth by indigenous microflora may mask the pathogen, and (3) contaminants may interfere with the identification of pathogens and the diagnosis of the infectious disease.

Proper Selection, Collection, and Transport of Clinical Specimens

When collecting clinical specimens for microbiology, these general precautions should be taken:

- The specimen must be properly selected. That is, it must be the appropriate type of specimen for diagnosis of the suspected infectious disease.

- The specimen must be properly and carefully collected. Whenever possible, specimens must be collected in a manner that will eliminate or minimize contamination of the specimen with indigenous microflora.

- The material should be collected from a site where the suspected pathogen is most likely to be found and where the least contamination is likely to occur.

- Whenever possible, specimens should be obtained before antimicrobial therapy has begun. If this is not possible, the laboratory should be informed as to which antimicrobial agent(s) the patient is receiving.

- The acute stage of the disease (when the patient is experiencing the symptoms of the disease) is the most appropriate time to collect most specimens. Some viruses, however, are more easily isolated during the prodromal or onset stage of disease.

- Specimen collection should be performed with care and tact to avoid harming the patient, causing discomfort, or causing undue embarrassment. If the patient is to collect the specimen, such as sputum or urine, the patient must be given clear and detailed collection instructions.

- A sufficient quantity of the specimen must be obtained to provide enough material for all required diagnostic tests. The amount of specimen to collect should be specified in the Lab P&P Manual.

- All specimens should be placed or collected into a sterile container to prevent contamination of the specimen by indigenous microflora and airborne microbes. Appropriate types of collection devices and specimen containers should be specified in the Lab P&P Manual.

- Specimens should be protected from heat and cold and promptly delivered to the laboratory so that the results of the analyses will validly represent the number and types of organisms present at the time of collection. If delivery to the laboratory is delayed, some delicate pathogens might die; therefore, certain types of specimens must be rushed to the laboratory immediately after collection. Certain specimens must be placed on ice during delivery to the laboratory, whereas other specimens should never be refrigerated or placed on ice because of the fragile and sensitive nature of the pathogens. Obligate anaerobes die when exposed to air. Any indigenous microflora in the specimen may overgrow, inhibit, or kill pathogens. Specimen transport instructions should be contained in the Lab P&P Manual.

- Hazardous specimens must be handled with even greater care to avoid contamination of the courier, patients, and healthcare professionals. Such specimens must be placed in a sealed plastic bag for immediate and careful transport to the laboratory.

- Whenever possible, sterile, disposable specimen containers should be used. If reusable containers are used, they should be cleaned, sterilized, and properly stored to avoid contamination of the specimen by microbes and potentially harmful chemicals.

- The specimen container must be properly labeled and accompanied by an appropriate request slip containing adequate instructions. As a minimum, labels should contain the patient's name, hospital identification number, and room number; the requesting physician's name; the culture site; and the date and time of collection. As a minimum, request slips must contain the patient's name, age, sex, and hospital identification number; the name of the requesting physician; specific information about the type of specimen and the site from which it was collected; the date and time of collection; the initials of the person who collected the specimen; and information about any antimicrobial agents that the patient is receiving. The laboratory should always be given sufficient clinical information to aid in performing appropriate analyses. For example, the request slip that accompanies a wound specimen should not merely state "wound"; rather, it should state the specific type of wound (e.g., burn wound, dog bite wound, postsurgical wound infection).

- Specimens should be collected and delivered to the laboratory as early in the day as possible to give the technologists sufficient time to process the material, especially when the hospital or clinic does not have 24-hour laboratory service.

Types of Clinical Specimens Usually Required To Diagnose Infectious Diseases

Specific techniques for the collection and transport of clinical specimens vary from institution to institution and are contained in the institution's Lab P&P Manual. Only a few of the most important considerations are mentioned here.

Blood

Blood is usually sterile. The presence of bacteria in the bloodstream (**bacteremia**) may indicate a disease, although temporary or transient bacteremias may occur after oral surgery, tooth extraction, or even aggressive tooth brushing. Bacteremia may occur during certain stages of many infectious diseases. These diseases include bacterial meningitis, typhoid fever and other salmonella infections, pneumococcal pneumonia, urinary infections, endocarditis, brucellosis, tularemia, plague, anthrax, syphilis, and wound infections caused by β-hemolytic streptococci, staphylococci, and other invasive bacteria. **Septicemia** is a serious disease characterized by chills, fever, prostration, and the presence of bacteria or their toxins in the bloodstream. The most severe types of septicemia are those caused by Gram-negative bacilli, owing to the endotoxin that is released from their cell walls. Endotoxin can induce fever and septic shock, which can be fatal. To diagnose either bacteremia or septicemia, it is recommended that at least three blood cultures be collected during a 24-hour period.

To prevent contamination of the blood specimen with indigenous skin flora, extreme care must be taken to use sterile technique when collecting blood for culture. The

-Emias

The suffix *-emia* refers to the bloodstream, often the presence of something in the bloodstream. **Toxemia** refers to the presence of toxins in the bloodstream; bacteremia, the presence of bacteria; **fungemia,** the presence of fungi; **viremia,** the presence of viruses; **parasitemia,** the presence of parasites. Septicemia, however, is an actual disease, quite often a serious, life-threatening disease. Septicemia is defined as chills, fever, prostration (extreme fatigue), and the presence of bacteria or their toxins in the bloodstream. **Meningococcemia** is a specific type of septicemia, in which the bloodstream contains *Neisseria meningitidis* (also known as **meningococci**). **Leukemia** is also a disease—actually, there are several different types of leukemias. In all types, there is a proliferation of abnormal white blood cells (**leukocytes**) in the blood. Some types of leukemia are known to be caused by viruses.

person drawing the blood must wear sterile gloves, and gloves must be changed between patients. After locating a suitable vein, disinfect the skin with 70% isopropyl alcohol and then with an iodophor. (It should be noted that the protocol for skin disinfection varies from one medical facility to another. For example, some facilities use isopropyl alcohol alone; some use tincture of iodine alone; some use povidone-iodine alone; some use a combination of ethyl alcohol and povidone-iodine.)

When disinfecting the site, use a concentric swabbing motion, starting at the point at which you intend to insert the needle and working outward from that point. Allow the iodophor to dry. Apply a tourniquet and then withdraw the appropriate amount of blood. Do not touch the site after it has been disinfected. Traditionally, the blood has been injected into two blood culture bottles (one aerobic bottle and one anaerobic bottle), but there are many different types of blood culture systems currently available. Always disinfect the rubber tops of blood culture bottles before insertion of the needle. Inject the volume of blood specified for the type of blood culture being used. After venipuncture, remove the iodophor from the skin with alcohol. The blood culture bottle(s) should be transported promptly to the laboratory for incubation at 37°C. Blood culture bottles should not be refrigerated.

Urine

Urine is ordinarily sterile while it is in the urinary bladder. However, during urination, it becomes contaminated by indigenous microflora of the distal urethra (the portion of the urethra farthest from the bladder). Contamination can be reduced by collecting a **clean-catch, midstream urine (CCMS urine)**. "Clean-catch" refers to the fact that the area around the external opening of the urethra is cleansed by washing with soap and rinsing with water before urinating. This removes the indigenous microflora that live in the area. "Midstream" refers to the fact that the initial portion of the urine stream is directed into a toilet or bedpan, and then the urine stream is directed into a sterile container. Thus, the microorganisms that live in the distal urethra are flushed out of the urethra by the initial portion of the urine stream, into the toilet or bedpan, rather than into the specimen container. In some circumstances, the physician may prefer to collect a catheterized specimen or use the suprapubic needle aspiration technique to obtain a sterile sample of urine. In the latter technique, a needle is inserted through the abdominal wall into the urinary bladder, and a syringe is used to withdraw urine from the bladder. To prevent continued bacterial growth, all urine specimens must be processed within 30 minutes of collection, or refrigerated at 4°C until they can be analyzed. Refrigerated urine specimens should be cultured within 24 hours. Failure to refrigerate a urine specimen will cause an inflated colony count (described below), which could lead to an incorrect diagnosis of a urinary tract infection (UTI).

There are actually three parts to a urine culture: (1) a colony count, (2) isolation and identification of the pathogen, and (3) antimicrobial susceptibility testing. The colony count is a way of estimating the number of viable bacteria that are present in the urine specimen. A calibrated loop is used to perform the colony count. A **calibrated loop** is a bacteriologic loop that has been manufactured so that it contains a precise volume of urine. There are two types of calibrated loops: those calibrated to contain 0.01 mL of fluid, and those calibrated to contain 0.001 mL of fluid. The calibrated loop is dipped into the CCMS urine specimen. Then the volume of urine within the calibrated loop is inoculated over the entire surface of a blood agar plate, which is then incubated overnight at

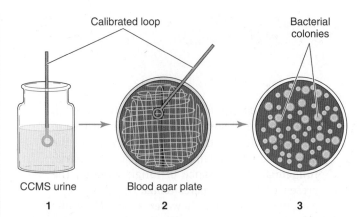

FIGURE 13-1. Obtaining a urine colony count. (*1*) A calibrated loop is dipped into a clean-catch, midstream (CCMS) urine specimen. (*2*) The volume of urine contained within the calibrated loop is spread over the entire surface of a blood agar plate, which is then incubated overnight at 37°C. (*3*) The colonies are counted after the plate is removed from the incubator. (See text for additional details.)

Clinical Procedure:

Collecting a Clean-Catch, MidStream Urine Specimen

Instructions for Female Patients

1. Sit comfortably on the toilet and swing one knee to the side as far as you can.

2. Spread your genital area with one hand and hold it spread open while you wash and rinse the area and collect the specimen.

3. Wash your genital area, using the cleaning materials supplied. Wipe yourself as carefully as you can from front to back, between the folds of skin.

4. After washing, rinse with a water-moistened pad with the same front-to-back motion. Use each pad only once, and then throw it away.

5. Hold the specimen collection cup with your fingers on the outside; do not touch the rim. Pass a small amount of urine into the toilet before passing urine into the cup. Fill the cup approximately half full.

6. Place the lid on the cup carefully and tightly, and give it to the nurse or laboratory assistant.

Instructions for Male Patients

1. Retract the foreskin (if uncircumcised).

2. Wash the glans (the head of the penis), using the cleaning materials supplied.

3. After washing, rinse with a water-moistened pad. Use each pad only once, and then throw it away.

4. Hold the specimen collection cup with your fingers on the outside; do not touch the rim. Pass a small amount of urine into the toilet before passing urine into the cup. Fill the cup approximately half full.

5. Place the lid on the cup carefully and tightly, and give it to the nurse or laboratory assistant.

37°C (Fig. 13-1). After incubation, the colonies are counted and this number is then multiplied by the dilution factor (either 100 or 1,000) to obtain the number of colony-forming units (CFU) per milliliter of urine. (The dilution factor is 100 if a 0.01-mL calibrated loop was used, or 1,000 if a 0.001-mL calibrated loop was used.) A CFU count that is 100,000 (1×10^5) CFU/mL or higher is indicative of a UTI, although high colony counts may also be caused by contamination of the urine specimen with indigenous microflora during specimen collection or failure to refrigerate the specimen between collection and

transport to the laboratory. The mere presence of bacteria in the urine (***bacteriuria***) is not significant, as urine always becomes contaminated with bacteria during urination (voiding). However, the presence of two or more bacteria per $\times 1,000$ microscopic field of a Gram-stained urine smear is indicative of a UTI with 100,000 or more CFU per milliliter.

Cerebrospinal Fluid

Meningitis, encephalitis, and meningoencephalitis are rapidly fatal diseases that can be caused by a variety of microbes, including bacteria, fungi, protozoa, and viruses. ***Meningitis*** is inflammation or infection of the membranes (meninges) that surround the brain and spinal column. ***Encephalitis*** is inflammation or infection of the brain. ***Meningoencephalitis*** is inflammation or infection of both the brain and the meninges. To diagnose these diseases, ***cerebrospinal fluid*** (also referred to as spinal fluid or CSF) must be collected into a sterile tube by a lumbar puncture (spinal tap) under surgically aseptic conditions (Fig.13-2). This technically difficult procedure is performed by a physician. CSF specimens must be rushed to the laboratory and must not be refrigerated.

Because of the extremely serious nature of central nervous system (CNS) infections, the CSF will be treated as a STAT (emergency) specimen in the CML, and a workup of the specimen will be initiated immediately. Information obtained as a result of examining a Gram stain of the spinal fluid sediment will be reported by telephone to the physician immediately; this is what is known as a ***preliminary report.*** Preliminary reports are laboratory reports that are communicated (usually by telephone) to the requesting physician before the availability of the final report. Preliminary reports containing CSF Gram stain observations frequently enable physicians to make diagnoses and initiate therapy, and often save patients' lives.

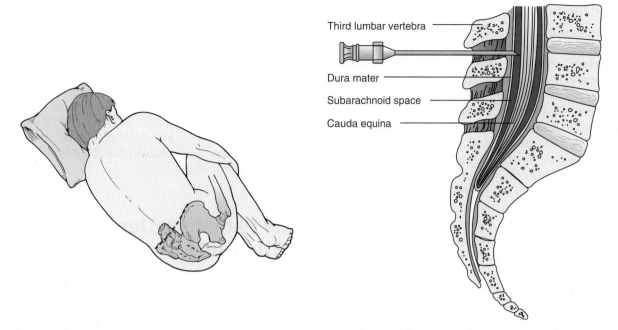

Third lumbar vertebra

Dura mater

Subarachnoid space

Cauda equina

FIGURE 13-2. Technique of lumbar puncture. (Taylor C, et al. Fundamentals of Nursing, 2nd ed. Philadelphia: JB Lippincott, 1993.)

Sputum

Sputum is pus that accumulates deep within the lungs of a patient with pneumonia, tuberculosis, or other lower respiratory infection. Unfortunately, many of the sputum specimens that are submitted to the CML are actually saliva. A laboratory workup of a patient's saliva will not provide clinically relevant information about the patient's lower respiratory infection and will be a waste of time, effort, and money. This situation can be avoided if someone (most often, a nurse) takes a moment to explain to the patient what is required. (Example: "The next time you cough up some of that thick, greenish material from your lungs, Mr. Smith, please spit it into this container.") If proper mouth hygiene is maintained, the sputum will not be severely contaminated with oral flora. If tuberculosis is suspected, extreme care in collecting and handling the specimen should be exercised because one could easily be infected with the pathogens. Usually, sputum specimens may be refrigerated for several hours without loss of the pathogens.

The physician may wish to obtain a better quality specimen by bronchial aspiration through a bronchoscope or by a process known as transtracheal aspiration. Needle biopsy of the lungs may be necessary for diagnosis of *Pneumocystis jiroveci* pneumonia (as in patients with AIDS) and for certain other pathogens. Although once classified as a protozoan, *P. jiroveci* is currently considered to be a fungus.

Throat Swabs

Routine throat swabs are collected to determine whether a patient has strep throat. If any other pathogen (e.g.,

Neisseria gonorrhoeae or *Corynebacterium diphtheriae*) is suspected by the physician to be causing the patient's pharyngitis, a specific culture for that pathogen must be noted on the request slip, so that the appropriate culture media will be inoculated. There is an art to the proper collection of a throat swab, as described in the following box.

Clinical Procedure:

Proper Technique for Obtaining a Throat Swab Specimen

1. Using a tongue depressor to hold the patient's tongue down, observe the back of the throat and tonsillar area for localized areas of inflammation (redness) and exudate.

2. Remove a Dacron or calcium alginate swab from its packet.

3. Under direct observation, carefully but firmly rub the swab over any areas of inflammation or exudate or over the tonsils and posterior pharynx. Do not touch the cheeks, teeth, or gums with the swab as you withdraw it from the mouth.

4. Insert the swab back into its packet and crush the transport medium vial in the transport container.

5. Transport the swab to the laboratory as soon as possible. If transport will be delayed beyond 1 hour, refrigerate the swab.

Wound Specimens

Whenever possible, a wound specimen should be an aspirate (i.e., pus that has been collected using a small needle and syringe assembly), rather than a swab specimen. Specimens collected by swab are frequently contaminated with indigenous microflora and often dry out before they can be processed in the CML. The person collecting the specimen should always indicate the type of wound infection (e.g., dog bite, postsurgical, or burn wound infection) on the request slip and the anatomical site from which the specimen was obtained. This provides valuable information that will enable CML personnel to inoculate appropriate types of media and be on the lookout for specific organisms. For example, *Pasteurella multocida* is frequently isolated from dog bite wound infections, but this Gram-negative bacillus is rarely encountered in other types of specimens. Merely stating "wound" on the request slip is insufficient.

GC Cultures

The initials GC represent an abbreviation for **gonococci,** a term referring to *Neisseria gonorrhoeae.* As mentioned earlier, *N. gonorrhoeae* is a fastidious bacterium that is microaerophilic and capnophilic. Only Dacron, calcium alginate, or nontoxic cotton swabs should be used to collect GC specimens. Ordinary cotton swabs contain fatty acids, which can be toxic to *N. gonorrhoeae.* When attempting to diagnose gonorrhea, swabs (vaginal, cervical, urethral, throat, and rectal) should be inoculated immediately onto Thayer-Martin or Martin-Lewis medium and incubated in a carbon dioxide (CO_2) environment. Alternatively, they should be inoculated into a tube or bottle (e.g., Transgrow) that contains an appropriate culture medium and an atmosphere containing 5 to 10% CO_2. To prevent loss of the CO_2, the bottle should be held in an upright position while inoculating. These cultures should be incubated at 37°C overnight and then shipped to a microbiology laboratory for positive identification of *N. gonorrhoeae.* If it is necessary to transport a swab specimen, the swab should be placed into a transport medium for shipment. Never refrigerate GC swabs because the low temperature might kill the *N. gonorrhoeae.*

Fecal Specimens

Ideally, fecal specimens (stool specimens) should be collected at the laboratory and processed immediately to prevent a decrease in temperature, which allows the pH to drop, causing the death of many *Shigella* and *Salmonella* species. Alternatively, the specimen may be placed in a container with a preservative that maintains a pH of 7.0.

Because the colon is anaerobic, fecal bacteria are obligate-, aerotolerant-, and facultative anaerobes. However, fecal specimens are cultured anaerobically only when *Clostridium difficile*-associated disease is suspected or to diagnose clostridial food poisoning. In intestinal infections, the pathogens frequently overwhelm the normal microflora, so that they are the predominant organisms seen in smears and cultures. A combination of direct microscopic examination, culture, biochemical tests, and immunologic tests may be performed to identify Gram-negative and Gram-positive bacteria (e.g., enteropathogenic *Escherichia coli, Salmonella* spp., *Shigella* spp., *Clostridium perfringens, C. difficile, Vibrio cholerae, Campylobacter* spp., and *Staphylococcus* spp.), fungi (*Candida*), intestinal protozoa (*Giardia, Entamoeba*), and intestinal helminths.

The Pathology Department ("The Lab")

The clinical specimens just described are submitted to the Clinical Microbiology Laboratory. Within a hospital setting, the Clinical Microbiology Laboratory is an integral part of the Pathology Department (which is frequently referred to simply as "the lab"). Because virtually all healthcare personnel will interact in some way(s) with the Pathology Department, they should understand how it is organized and the types of laboratory tests that are performed there.

The Pathology Department is under the direction of a **pathologist** (a physician who has had extensive, specialized training in **pathology,** the study of the structural and functional manifestations of disease). As shown in Figure 13-3, the Pathology Department consists of two major divisions: Anatomical Pathology and Clinical Pathology.

Anatomical Pathology

Most pathologists work in Anatomical Pathology, where they perform autopsies in the morgue and examine diseased organs, stained tissue sections, and cytology specimens. Other healthcare professionals employed in Anatomical Pathology include cytogenetic technologists, cytotechnologists, histologic technicians, histotechnologists, and pathologist's assistants.

In addition to the morgue, Anatomical Pathology houses the Histopathology Laboratory, the Cytology Laboratory, and the Cytogenetics Laboratory. In some Pathology Departments, the Electron Microscopy Laboratory is also located in Anatomical Pathology.

Clinical Pathology

In addition to the Clinical Microbiology Laboratory (discussed later in this chapter), Clinical Pathology consists of several other laboratories: the Clinical Chemistry Laboratory (or Clinical Chemistry/Urinalysis Laboratory); the Hematology Laboratory (or Hematology/Coagulation

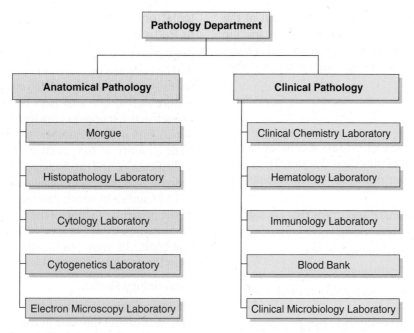

FIGURE 13-3. Organization of a typical pathology department.

Laboratory); the Blood Bank (or Immunohematology Laboratory); and the Immunology Laboratory (described in Chapter 16). In the Clinical Microbiology Laboratory of smaller hospitals, immunodiagnostic procedures are performed in the Immunology Section (sometimes called the Serology Section).

Personnel working in Clinical Pathology include pathologists; specialized scientists such as chemists and microbiologists, who have graduate degrees in their specialty areas; **clinical laboratory scientists** (also known as *medical technologists* or MTs), who have 4-year baccalaureate degrees; and **clinical laboratory technicians** (also known as *medical laboratory technicians* or MLTs), who have 2-year associate degrees (see "Insight: Medical Laboratory Professions" on the CD-ROM).

The Clinical Microbiology Laboratory

Organization

Depending on the size of the hospital, the Clinical Microbiology Laboratory (hereafter referred to as the CML) may be under the direction of a pathologist, a microbiologist (having either a master's degree or doctorate in clinical microbiology), or, in smaller hospitals, a medical technologist who has had many years of experience working in microbiology. Most of the actual bench work that is performed in the CML is performed by MTs and MLTs.

As shown in Figure 13-4, the CML is divided into various sections, which, to a large degree, correspond to the various

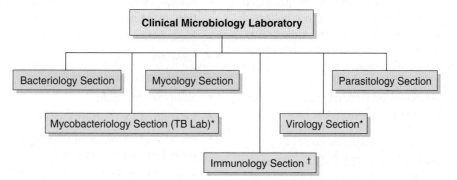

FIGURE 13-4. Organization of a typical clinical microbiology laboratory. (*) Virology and Mycobacteriology Sections are usually found only in larger hospitals and medical centers; smaller hospitals usually do not have these sections; instead, virology and mycobacteriology specimens are sent to a reference laboratory. (†) Usually only smaller hospitals have an Immunology Section, in which immunodiagnostic procedures are performed; larger hospitals and medical centers usually have an Immunology Laboratory, which performs a much wider variety of immunologic procedures, and would function independently of the Clinical Microbiology Laboratory.

categories of microorganisms. With the exception of the Immunology Section, the responsibilities of the specific sections of the CML are described in this chapter. Procedures performed in the Immunology Section are described in Chapter 16.

Responsibilities

The primary mission of the CML is to assist clinicians in the diagnosis and treatment of infectious diseases. To accomplish this mission, the four major, day-to-day responsibilities of the CML are to:

- Process the various clinical specimens that are submitted to the CML (described below).
- Isolate pathogens from those specimens.
- Identify (speciate) the pathogens.
- Perform antimicrobial susceptibility testing when appropriate to do so.

The exact steps in the processing of clinical specimens vary from one specimen type to another and also depend on the specific section of the CML to which the specimen is submitted. In general, processing includes the following steps:

- Examining the specimen macroscopically and recording pertinent observations (e.g., cloudiness or the presence of blood, mucus, or an unusual odor).
- Examining the specimen microscopically and recording pertinent observations (e.g., the presence of white blood cells or microorganisms).
- Inoculating appropriate culture media in an attempt to isolate the pathogen(s) from the specimen and get them growing in pure culture in the laboratory.

The CML is sometimes called on to assume an additional responsibility, namely the processing of environmental samples (i.e., samples collected from within the hospital environment). Such samples are processed by the CML whenever there is an outbreak or epidemic within the hospital, in an attempt to locate the source of the pathogen involved. Environmental samples include those collected from appropriate hospital sites (e.g., floors, sink drains, showerheads, whirlpool baths, respiratory therapy equipment) and employees (e.g., nasal swabs, material from open wounds).

Frequently, CML personnel are the first people to recognize that an outbreak is occurring within the hospital. For example, CML personnel might note an unusually high number of isolates of a particular pathogen from specimens submitted from a particular ward. The CML would notify the Hospital Infection Control Committee (see Chapter 12) of the unusually high number of isolates, and the committee would then be responsible for collecting appropriate environmental samples and submitting them to the CML for processing.

Isolation and Identification (Speciation) of Pathogens

In an effort to isolate bacteria (including mycobacteria) and fungi (yeasts and molds) from clinical specimens, the specimens are inoculated into liquid culture media or onto solid culture media. The goal is to get any pathogens that are present in the specimen growing in pure culture (by themselves), and in large number, so that there will be a sufficient quantity of the organism to inoculate appropriate identification and antimicrobial susceptibility testing systems. Specific types of media were discussed in Chapter 8. The manner in which pathogens are identified depends on the particular section of the CML that the specimen was submitted to. (Note: As previously mentioned, throughout this book, the term "to identify an organism" means to learn the organism's name, i.e., to speciate it.)

Bacteriology Section

The overall responsibility of the Bacteriology Section of the CML is to assist clinicians in the diagnosis of bacterial diseases. In the Bacteriology Section, various types of clinical specimens are processed, bacterial pathogens are isolated from the specimens, tests are performed to identify the bacterial pathogens, and antimicrobial susceptibility testing is performed whenever it is appropriate to do so. Once they are isolated from clinical specimens, bacterial pathogens are identified by gathering clues (phenotypic characteristics). Thus, CML professionals are very much like detectives and crime scene investigators (Fig. 13-5), gathering clues about a pathogen until they are finally able to identify it.

The various phenotypic characteristics (clues) useful in identifying bacteria include the following:

- Gram reaction (i.e., Gram-positive or Gram-negative)
- cell shape (e.g., cocci, bacilli, curved, spiral-shaped, filamentous, branching)
- morphologic arrangement of cells (e.g., pairs, tetrads, chains, clusters)
- growth or no growth on various types of plated media
- colony morphology (e.g., color, general shape, elevation, margin)
- presence or absence of a capsule
- motility
- number and location of flagella
- ability to sporulate
- location of spores (terminal or subterminal)
- presence or absence of various enzymes (e.g., catalase, coagulase, oxidase, urease)
- ability to catabolize various carbohydrates and amino acids (miniaturized biochemical test systems—"minisystems"—are often used for this purpose; see Figs. 13-6 and 13-7)
- ability to reduce nitrate

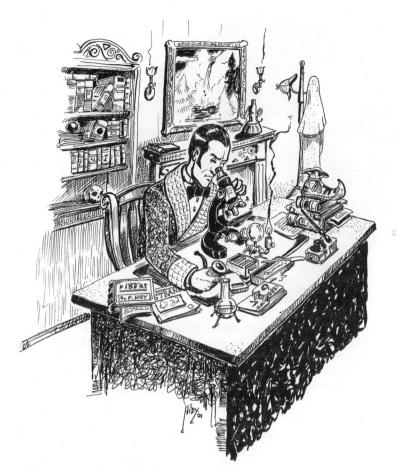

FIGURE 13-5. Clinical Microbiology Laboratory professionals are very much like detectives and crime scene investigators, gathering clues about a pathogen until they have enough information to identify (speciate) it.

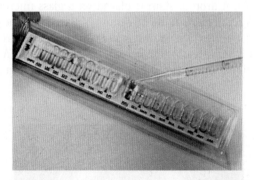

FIGURE 13-6. Shown here is a minisystem (API-20E) used to identify members of the family *Enterobacteriaceae*. Each of the 20 chambers contains a different substrate. If the organism is capable of breaking down a particular substrate, a change in pH will occur; this will cause the pH indicator to change color. Thus, a color change indicates a positive test result. No color change indicates a negative test result. (Koneman EW, et al. Color Atlas and Textbook of Diagnostic Microbiology, 5th ed. Philadelphia: Lippincott Williams & Wilkins, 1997.)

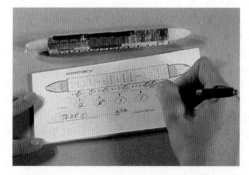

FIGURE 13-7. Shown here is a minisystem (Enterotube II) used to identify members of the family *Enterobacteriaceae*. As with the API-20E strip, color changes represent positive test results. By totaling the numerical values of the positive tests, a five-digit code number is generated. The identity of the organism is then determined by looking the number up in a code book. (Koneman EW, et al. Color Atlas and Textbook of Diagnostic Microbiology, 5th ed. Philadelphia: Lippincott Williams & Wilkins, 1997.)

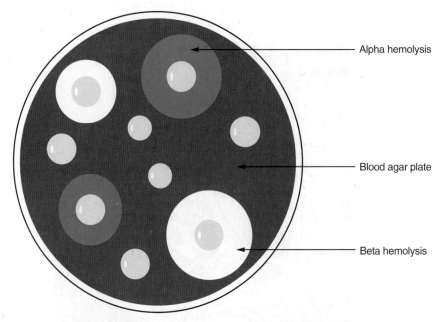

- Alpha hemolysis
- Blood agar plate
- Beta hemolysis

FIGURE 13-8. Diagram illustrating the three types of hemolysis that can be observed on a blood agar plate: alpha hemolysis (a green zone around the bacterial colony), beta hemolysis (a clear zone around the bacterial colony), and gamma hemolysis (neither a green nor a clear zone around the bacterial colony). α-Hemolytic bacteria produce an enzyme that causes a partial breakdown of hemoglobin in the red blood cells in the medium, which results in a green color. β-Hemolytic bacteria produce an enzyme that completely destroys (lyses) the red blood cells, thus producing a clear zone. γ-Hemolytic bacteria (also referred to as nonhemolytic bacteria) produce neither of these enzymes and, therefore, cause no change in the red blood cells.

- ability to produce indole from tryptophan
- atmospheric requirements
- type of hemolysis produced (Fig. 13-8)

Mycology Section

The overall responsibility of the Mycology Section of the CML is to assist clinicians in the diagnosis of fungal infections (mycoses). In the Mycology Section, various types of clinical specimens are processed, fungal pathogens are isolated, and tests are performed to identify the fungal pathogens. In general, the specimens processed in the Mycology Section are the same types of specimens that are processed in the Bacteriology Section. However, three types are specimens are much more commonly submitted to the Mycology Section than to the Bacteriology Section: hair clippings, nail clippings, and skin scrapings.

A potassium hydroxide preparation (KOH prep) is performed on hair clippings, nail clippings, and skin scrapings. (See CD-ROM Appendix 5 for details of the KOH preparation.) The KOH acts as a clearing agent, by dissolving keratin in the specimens. This enables the technologist to see into the specimens when they are examined microscopically, and to determine whether there are any fungal elements (e.g., yeasts or hyphae) in the specimen. Specimens will also be inoculated onto Sabouraud dextrose agar, a selective medium for fungi. Bacteria do not grow on this medium because of the low pH (pH 5.6), but most molds grow quite well.

When isolated from clinical specimens, yeasts are identified by using a variety of biochemical tests, primarily by

their ability to catabolize various carbohydrates. Molds are identified using a combination of rate of growth and macroscopic and microscopic observations, *not* by performing biochemical tests. Macroscopic observations are things that you can learn about the mycelium by looking at it with the naked eye—like color, texture, and topography (see Figs. 13-9 and 13-10).

To examine a mold microscopically, a tease mount is prepared. A drop of stain is placed on a glass microscope slide. A small piece of the mycelium is placed into the drop. Teasing needles (also known as dissecting needles) are used to gently pull (tease) the piece of mycelium apart. A glass coverslip is added, and the tease mount preparation is ex-

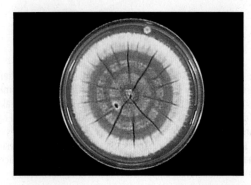

FIGURE 13-9. A colony (mycelium) of the mold *Aspergillus fumigatus,* a common cause of pulmonary infections in immunosuppressed patients. (Koneman EW, et al. Color Atlas and Textbook of Diagnostic Microbiology, 5th ed. Philadelphia: Lippincott Williams & Wilkins, 1997.)

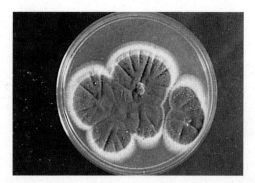

FIGURE 13-10. Colonies (mycelia) of a *Penicillium* species. Although penicillin is derived from *Penicillium,* this mold can also cause infections in immunosuppressed patients. (Koneman's Color Atlas and Textbook of Diagnostic Microbiology, 6th ed. Philadelphia: Lippincott Williams & Wilkins, 2006.)

amined under the microscope. The stain that is used in the tease mount is lactophenol cotton blue (LPCB), containing lactic acid, phenol, and cotton blue. The lactic acid preserves morphology. The phenol kills the organisms, so they will not be infectious. The cotton blue stains the mycelial structures blue.

When the tease mount preparation is examined microscopically, the first thing to determine is whether the mold has septate or aseptate hyphae (described in Chapter 5). Next, the technologist will look for spores and the structures on or within which the spores are produced. The appearance of these structures further enables the technologist to identify the mold (refer back to Fig. 5-5).

Susceptibility testing of fungi is not currently performed in most CMLs, although, because of the ever-growing problem of drug resistance in fungi, it is likely that such testing will become routine in the near future.

Parasitology Section

The overall responsibility of the Parasitology Section of the CML is to assist clinicians in the diagnosis of parasitic diseases—specifically, infections caused by endoparasites (parasites that live within the body), such as parasitic protozoa and helminths (parasitic worms). In general, parasitic infections are diagnosed by observing and recognizing various parasite life cycle stages (e.g., trophozoites and cysts of protozoa; microfilariae, eggs, and larvae of helminths) in clinical specimens. Parasites are identified primarily by the characteristic appearance (e.g., size, shape, internal details) of the various life cycle stages that are seen in clinical specimens. Sometimes, whole worms or segments of worms are observed in fecal specimens. Parasites are described in detail in Chapter 18.

Virology Section

The overall responsibility of the Virology Section of the CML is to assist clinicians in the diagnosis of viral diseases. Many viral diseases are diagnosed using immunodiagnostic

procedures (described in Chapter 16). Other techniques used to identify viral pathogens are:

- observation of intracytoplasmic or intranuclear viral inclusion bodies in specimens by cytologic or histologic examination
- observation of viruses in specimens using electron microscopy
- molecular techniques such as nucleic acid probes and polymerase chain reaction assays (described on the CD-ROM)
- virus isolation by use of cell cultures; viruses are identified primarily by the type(s) of cell lines that they are able to infect and the physical changes (called cytopathic effect or CPE) that they cause in the infected cells

Mycobacteriology Section

The primary responsibility of the Mycobacteriology Section (or "TB Lab," as it is often called) of the CML is to assist clinicians in the diagnosis of tuberculosis. In the Mycobacteriology Section, various types of specimens (primarily sputum specimens) are processed, acid-fast staining is performed, mycobacteria are isolated and identified, and susceptibility testing is performed. *Mycobacterium* spp. are identified using a combination of growth characteristics (e.g., growth rate, colony pigmentation, photoreactivity, and morphology) and a variety of biochemical tests. *Mycobacterium tuberculosis*, the primary cause of human tuberculosis, is a very slow-growing organism. Fortunately, the acid-fast stain (described in Chapter 4) enables rapid presumptive diagnosis of tuberculosis.

Additional information pertaining to the CML, including molecular diagnostic procedures, antimicrobial susceptibility testing, quality assurance and quality control in the CML, and safety in the CML, can be found in CD-ROM Appendix 4: "Responsibilities of the Clinical Microbiology Laboratory."

⊙ REVIEW OF KEY POINTS

- To avoid becoming infected, extreme care must be taken by those involved in collecting, handling, and processing clinical specimens, particularly, blood, urine, cerebrospinal fluid, sputum, mucous membranes, and fecal specimens. Always follow the safety precautions known as standard precautions.

- The quality of work performed by the Clinical Microbiology Laboratory (CML) can only be as good as the quality of the clinical specimens that are submitted to the CML.

- The three components of specimen quality are proper selection, proper collection, and proper transport of the specimen.

- The person who collects the specimen is ultimately responsible for its quality.

- The laboratory is responsible for publishing a book (often referred to as the Lab P&P Manual) that contains instructions for the proper selection, collection, and transport of clinical specimens.

- When collecting blood specimens for culture, the venipuncture site must be thoroughly cleansed and disinfected to prevent contamination of the specimen with indigenous skin flora.

- Aspirates (i.e., pus that has been collected using a needle and syringe assembly) are the preferred type of wound specimen. Specimens collected by swab are frequently contaminated with indigenous microflora and often dry out before they can be processed in the CML. The type of wound should always be indicated on the request slip.

- All clinical specimens must be labeled properly, and laboratory request slips must contain all necessary information.

- The proper specimen to diagnose urinary tract infections (UTIs) is a clean-catch, midstream urine (CCMS urine). Urine specimens must be refrigerated until they can be transported to the laboratory.

- Because meningitis is such a serious and often rapidly fatal disease, cerebrospinal fluid (CSF) specimens are processed immediately on their receipt in the CML. Important information that is learned about the specimen is immediately reported to the requesting physician; this is known as a preliminary report. Such reports often save patients' lives.

- Routine throat swabs are collected to determine whether a patient has strep throat. If any other pathogen (e.g., *Neisseria gonorrhoeae* or *Corynebacterium diphtheriae*) is suspected to be causing the patient's pharyngitis, a specific culture for that pathogen must be noted on the request slip.

- *Neisseria gonorrhoeae* is a fastidious bacterium that is both microaerophilic and capnophilic. Therefore, when attempting to diagnose gonorrhea, swabs (vaginal, cervical, urethral, throat, and rectal swabs) should be inoculated immediately onto a highly enriched and highly selective medium (such as Thayer-Martin or Martin-Lewis medium) and incubated in a carbon dioxide (CO_2) atmosphere.

- The primary mission of the Clinical Microbiology Laboratory (CML) is to assist physicians in the diagnosis of infectious diseases.

- The major responsibilities of those employed in the CML are (1) processing clinical specimens, (2) isolating pathogens from specimens, (3) identifying pathogens, and (4) performing antimicrobial susceptibility testing.

- Environmental samples, collected from various sites within the hospital, are processed by the CML whenever an outbreak is suspected within the hospital.

On the CD-ROM

- Insight
  - Specimen Quality and Clinical Relevance
  - The Medical Laboratory Professions
- Increase Your Knowledge
- Critical Thinking
- Additional Self-Assessment Exercises

Self-Assessment Exercises

After studying this chapter, answer the following multiple-choice questions.

1. Assuming that a clean-catch, midstream urine was processed in the CML, which of the following colony counts is (are) indicative of a urinary tract infection?
   a. 10,000 CFU/mL
   b. 100,000 CFU/mL
   c. >100,000 CFU/mL
   d. both b and c

2. Which of the following statements is *not* true about the disk-diffusion method of antimicrobial susceptibility testing? (Note: information about susceptibility testing can be found on the CD-ROM that accompanies this book.)
   a. A pure culture of the organism is required.
   b. It is also known as the "Kirby-Bauer test."
   c. The plate should be incubated in a CO_2 incubator for 12 hours.
   d. The test should be performed in the exact manner described by the CLSI.

3. Which of the following statements about cerebrospinal fluid (CSF) specimens is false?
   a. They are collected only by physicians.
   b. They are treated as STAT (emergency) specimens in the laboratory.
   c. They should always be refrigerated.
   d. They should be rushed to the laboratory after collection.

4. All clinical specimens submitted to the CML must be:
   a. properly and carefully collected.
   b. properly labeled.
   c. properly transported to the laboratory.
   d. all of the above.

5. Which of the following methods of antimicrobial susceptibility testing is the most accurate? (Note: information about susceptibility testing can be found on the CD-ROM that accompanies this book.)
   a. agar dilution method
   b. disk-diffusion method
   c. macro broth dilution method
   d. micro broth dilution method

6. Which of the following methods of antimicrobial susceptibility testing is the most popular method in the United States? (Note: information about susceptibility testing can be found on the CD-ROM that accompanies this book.)
   a. agar dilution method
   b. disk-diffusion method
   c. macro broth dilution method
   d. micro broth dilution method

7. Who is primarily responsible for the quality of specimens submitted to the CML?
   a. microbiologist who is in charge of the CML
   b. pathologist who is in charge of "the lab"
   c. person who collects the specimen
   d. person who transports the specimen to the CML

8. Which of the following is *not* one of the four major, day-to-day responsibilities of the CML?
   a. identify (speciate) pathogens
   b. isolate pathogens from clinical specimens
   c. perform antimicrobial susceptibility testing when appropriate
   d. process environmental samples

9. Which of the following sections is *least* likely to be found in the CML of a small hospital?
   a. Bacteriology Section
   b. Mycology Section
   c. Parasitology Section
   d. Virology Section

10. In the Mycology Section of the CML, molds are identified by _____.
    a. biochemical test results
    b. macroscopic observations
    c. microscopic observations
    d. a combination of b and c

14

PATHOGENESIS OF INFECTIOUS DISEASES

LEARNING OBJECTIVES

AFTER STUDYING THIS CHAPTER, YOU SHOULD BE ABLE TO:

- Cite four reasons why an individual might not develop an infectious disease after exposure to a pathogen
- Discuss the four periods or phases in the course of an infectious disease
- Differentiate between localized and systemic infections
- Explain the differences among acute, subacute, and chronic diseases
- Explain what is meant by "symptoms of a disease" and cite several examples
- Explain what is meant by "signs of a disease" and cite several examples
- Cite several examples of latent infections
- Differentiate between primary and secondary infections

- List six steps in the pathogenesis of an infectious disease
- Define virulence and virulence factors
- List three bacterial structures that serve as virulence factors
- List six bacterial exoenzymes that serve as virulence factors
- Differentiate between endotoxins and exotoxins
- List six bacterial exotoxins and the diseases they cause
- Describe three mechanisms by which pathogens escape the immune response

INTRODUCTION

By definition, a microorganism is an organism that is too small to be seen with the unaided eye. How is it possible for such tiny organisms to cause disease in plants and animals, which are gigantic in comparison to microbes? This chapter will attempt to answer that question, with emphasis on disease in humans.

The prefix *path-* refers to disease. Examples of words containing this prefix are *pathogen* (a microbe capable of causing disease), *pathology* (the study of the structural and functional manifestations of disease), *pathologist* (a physician who has specialized in pathology), ***pathogenicity*** (the ability to cause disease), and ***pathogenesis*** (the steps or mechanisms involved in the development of a disease).

Infection Versus Infectious Disease

As discussed previously in this book, an infectious disease is a disease caused by a microbe, and the microbes that cause infectious diseases are collectively referred to as pathogens. The word *infection* tends to be confusing because it is used in different ways by different people. Most commonly, infection is used as a synonym for infectious disease. For example, saying "the patient has an ear infection" is the same thing as saying "the patient has an infectious disease of the ear." Because this is how the word *infection* is used by physicians, nurses, the mass media, and most other people, this is how *infection* is used in this book.

Many microbiologists, however, reserve use of the word *infection* to mean colonization by a pathogen (i.e., when a pathogen lands on or enters a person's body and establishes residence there, then the person is infected with that pathogen). That pathogen may or may not go on to cause disease in the person. In other words, a person can be infected with a certain pathogen, but not have the infectious disease caused by that pathogen (recall the discussion of carriers in Chapter 11).

Why Infection Does Not Always Occur

Many people who are exposed to pathogens do not get sick. Listed below are some of the many reasons that could explain this:

- The microbe may land at an anatomic site where it is unable to multiply. For example, when a respiratory pathogen lands on the skin, it may be unable to grow there because the skin lacks the necessary warmth, moisture, and nutrients required for growth of that particular microorganism. Additionally, the low pH and presence of fatty acids make the skin a hostile environment for certain organisms.

- Many pathogens must attach to specific receptor sites (described later) before they are able to multiply and

cause damage. If they land at a site where such receptors are absent, they are unable to cause disease.

- Antibacterial factors that destroy or inhibit the growth of bacteria (e.g., the lysozyme that is present in tears, saliva, and perspiration) may be present at the site where a pathogen lands.

- The indigenous microflora of that site (e.g., the mouth, vagina, or intestine) may inhibit growth of the foreign microbe by occupying space and using up available nutrients. This is a type of *microbial antagonism,* in which one microbe or group of microbes wards off another.

- The indigenous microflora at the site may produce antibacterial factors (proteins called ***bacteriocins***) that destroy the newly arrived pathogen. This is also a type of microbial antagonism.

- The individual's nutritional and overall health status often influences the outcome of the pathogen–host encounter. A person who is in good health, with no underlying medical problems, would be less likely to become infected than a person who is malnourished or in poor health.

- The person may be immune to that particular pathogen, perhaps as a result of prior infection with that pathogen or having been vaccinated against that pathogen. Immunity and vaccination are discussed in Chapter 16.

- Phagocytic white blood cells (phagocytes) present in the blood and other tissues may engulf and destroy the pathogen before it has an opportunity to multiply, invade, and cause disease.

Four Periods or Phases in the Course of an Infectious Disease

Once a pathogen has gained entrance to the body, the course of an infectious disease has four periods or phases (Fig. 14-1).

1. **The incubation period** is the time that elapses between arrival of the pathogen and the onset of symptoms. The length of the incubation period is influenced by many factors, including the overall health and nutritional status of the host, the immune status of the host (i.e., whether the host is immunocompetent or immunosuppressed), the virulence of the pathogen, and the number of pathogens that enter the body.

2. **The prodromal period** is the time during which the patient feels "out of sorts," but is not yet experiencing actual symptoms of the disease. Patients may feel like they are "coming down with something," but are not yet sure what it is.

3. **The period of illness** is the time during which the patient experiences the typical symptoms associated with that particular disease (e.g., sore throat, headache,

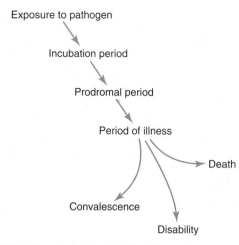

FIGURE 14-1. The course of an infectious disease.

sinus congestion). Communicable diseases are most easily transmitted during this third period.

4. **The convalescent period** is the time during which the patient recovers. For certain infectious diseases, especially viral respiratory diseases, the convalescent period can be quite long. Although the patient may recover from the illness itself, permanent damage may be caused by destruction of tissues in the affected area. For example, brain damage may follow encephalitis or meningitis, paralysis may follow poliomyelitis, and deafness may follow ear infections.

Localized Versus Systemic Infections

Once an infectious process is initiated, the disease may remain localized to one site or it may spread. Pimples, boils, and abscesses are examples of *localized infections.* If the pathogens are not contained at the original site of infection, they may be carried to other parts of the body by way of lymph, blood, or, in some cases, phagocytes. When the infection has spread throughout the body, it is referred to as either a *systemic infection* or a *generalized infection.* For example, the bacterium that causes tuberculosis—*Mycobacterium tuberculosis*—may spread to many internal organs, a condition known as miliary tuberculosis.

Acute, Subacute, and Chronic Diseases

A disease may be described as being acute, subacute, or chronic. An *acute disease* has a rapid onset, usually followed by a relatively rapid recovery; measles, mumps, and influenza are examples. A *chronic disease* has an insidious (slow) onset and lasts a long time; examples are

tuberculosis, leprosy (Hansen disease), and syphilis. Sometimes a disease having a sudden onset can develop into a long-lasting disease. Some diseases, such as bacterial endocarditis, come on more suddenly than a chronic disease, but less suddenly than an acute disease; they are referred to as *subacute diseases.*

Symptoms of a Disease Versus Signs of a Disease

A *symptom of a disease* is defined as some evidence of a disease that is experienced or perceived by the patient; something that is subjective. Examples of symptoms include any type of ache or pain, a ringing in the ears (tinnitus), blurred vision, nausea, dizziness, itching, and chills. Diseases, including infectious diseases, may be either symptomatic or asymptomatic. A *symptomatic disease* (or clinical disease) is a disease in which the patient is experiencing symptoms. An *asymptomatic disease* (or subclinical disease) is a disease that the patient is unaware of because he or she is not experiencing any symptoms.

In its early stages, gonorrhea is usually symptomatic in male patients (who develop a urethral discharge and experience pain while urinating), but asymptomatic in female patients. Only after several months, during which the organism may have caused extensive damage to her reproductive organs, is pain experienced by the infected woman. In trichomoniasis (caused by the protozoan, *Trichomonas vaginalis*), the situation is reversed. Infected women are usually symptomatic (experiencing vaginitis), whereas infected men are usually asymptomatic. These two sexually transmitted diseases (STDs) are especially difficult to control because people are often unaware that they are infected and unknowingly transmit the pathogens to others during sexual activities.

A *sign of a disease* is defined as some type of objective evidence of a disease. For example, while palpating a patient, a physician might discover a lump or an enlarged liver (hepatomegaly) or spleen (splenomegaly). Other signs of disease include abnormal heart or breath sounds, blood pressure, pulse rate, and laboratory results as well as abnormalities that appear on radiographs, ultrasound studies, or computed tomography (CT) scans.

Latent Infections

An infectious disease may go from being symptomatic to asymptomatic, and then some time later, go back to being symptomatic. Such diseases are referred to as *latent infections*. Herpes virus infections, such as cold sores (fever blisters), genital herpes infections, and shingles, are examples of latent infections. Cold sores occur intermittently, but

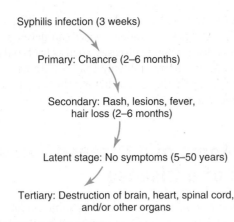

Syphilis infection (3 weeks)

Primary: Chancre (2–6 months)

Secondary: Rash, lesions, fever,
hair loss (2–6 months)

Latent stage: No symptoms (5–50 years)

Tertiary: Destruction of brain, heart, spinal cord,
and/or other organs

FIGURE 14-2. Stages of syphilis.

the patient continues to harbor the herpes virus between cold sore episodes. The virus remains dormant within cells of the nervous system until some type of stress acts as a trigger. The stressful trigger may be a fever, sunburn, extreme cold, or emotional stress. A person who had chickenpox as a child may harbor the virus throughout his or her lifetime and then, later in life, as the immune system weakens, that person may develop shingles. Shingles, a painful infection of the nerves, is considered a latent manifestation of chickenpox.

If not successfully treated, syphilis progresses through primary, secondary, latent, and tertiary stages (Fig. 14-2). During the primary stage, the patient has an open lesion called a chancre, which contains the spirochete *Treponema pallidum*. A few weeks after the spirochete enters the bloodstream, the chancre disappears, and the symptoms of the secondary stage arise, including rash, fever, and mucous membrane lesions. These symptoms also disappear after a few weeks, and the disease enters a latent stage, which may last from 1 to 50 years. During this time, the patient has few or no symptoms. In tertiary syphilis, the spirochetes cause destruction of the organs in which they have been hiding—the brain, heart, and bone tissue.

Primary Versus Secondary Infections

One infectious disease may commonly follow another, in which case the first disease is referred to as a ***primary infection*** and the second disease is referred to as a ***secondary infection.*** For example, serious cases of bacterial pneumonia frequently follow relatively mild viral respiratory infections. During the primary infection, the virus causes damage to the ciliated epithelial cells that line the respiratory tract. The function of these cells is to move foreign materials up and out of the respiratory tract and into the throat where they can be swallowed. While coughing, the patient may inhale some saliva, containing an opportunistic pathogen,

such as *Streptococcus pneumoniae* or *Haemophilus influenzae.* Because the ciliated epithelial cells were damaged by the virus, they are unable to clear the bacteria from the lungs. The bacteria then multiply and cause pneumonia. In this example, the viral infection is the primary infection and bacterial pneumonia is the secondary infection.

Steps in the Pathogenesis of Infectious Diseases

In general, the pathogenesis of infectious diseases often follows this sequence:

1. **Entry** of the pathogen into the body. Portals of entry include penetration of skin or mucous membranes by the pathogen, inoculation of the pathogen into bodily tissues by an arthropod, inhalation (into the respiratory tract), ingestion (into the gastrointestinal tract), introduction of the pathogen into the genitourinary tract, or introduction of the pathogen directly into the blood (e.g., through blood transfusion or the use of shared needles by intravenous drug abusers).

2. **Attachment** of the pathogen to some tissue(s) within the body.

3. **Multiplication** of the pathogen. The pathogen may multiply in one location of the body, resulting in a localized infection (e.g., an abscess), or it may multiply throughout the body (a systemic infection).

4. **Invasion or spread** of the pathogen.

5. **Evasion of host defenses.**

6. **Damage to host tissue(s).** The damage may be so extensive as to cause the death of the patient.

It is important to understand that not all infectious diseases involve <u>all</u> these steps. For example, once ingested, some exotoxin-producing intestinal pathogens are capable of causing disease without adhering to the intestinal wall or invading tissue.

Virulence

The words *virulent* and ***virulence*** tend to be confusing because they are used in several different ways. Sometimes virulent is used as a synonym for pathogenic. For example, there may be virulent (pathogenic) strains and *avirulent* (nonpathogenic) strains of a particular species. The **virulent strains** are capable of causing disease, whereas the **avirulent strains** are not. For example, toxigenic strains of *Corynebacterium diphtheriae* (i.e., strains that produce diphtheria toxin) are virulent, whereas nontoxigenic strains are not. Encapsulated strains of *S. pneumoniae* can cause disease, but nonencapsulated strains of *S. pneumoniae* cannot. As will be discussed in a subsequent section, piliated strains of certain pathogens are able to cause disease, whereas non-piliated strains are not; thus, the piliated strains are virulent, but the nonpiliated strains are avirulent.

Sometimes virulence is used to express a measure or degree of pathogenicity. Although all pathogens cause disease, some are more virulent than others (i.e., they are better able to cause disease). For example, it only takes about 10 *Shigella* cells to cause shigellosis (a diarrheal disease), but it takes between 100 and 1,000 *Salmonella* cells to cause salmonellosis (another diarrheal disease). Thus, *Shigella* is considered to be more virulent than *Salmonella*. In some cases, certain strains of a particular species are more virulent than others. For example, the "flesh-eating" strains of *Streptococcus pyogenes* are more virulent than other strains of *S. pyogenes* because they produce certain necrotizing enzymes that are not produced by the other strains. Similarly, only certain strains of *S. pyogenes* produce **erythrogenic toxin** (the cause of scarlet fever); these strains are considered more virulent than the strains of *S. pyogenes* that do not produce erythrogenic toxin. Strains of *Staphylococcus aureus* that produce toxic shock syndrome toxin-1 (TSST-1) are considered more virulent than strains of *S. aureus* that do not produce this toxin.

Sometimes virulence is used in reference to the severity of the infectious diseases that are caused by the pathogens.

Used in this manner, one pathogen is more virulent than another if it causes a more serious disease.

Virulence Factors (Attributes That Enable Pathogens to Attach, Escape Destruction, and Cause Disease)

The physical attributes or properties of pathogens that enable them to escape various host defense mechanisms and cause disease are called ***virulence factors.*** Virulence factors are phenotypic characteristics that, like all phenotypic characteristics, are dictated by the organism's genotype. Toxins are obvious virulence factors, but other virulence factors are not so obvious. Some virulence factors are shown in Figure 14-3.

Attachment

Perhaps you have noticed that certain pathogens infect dogs but not humans, whereas others infect humans but not dogs. Perhaps you have wondered why certain pathogens cause respiratory infections whereas others cause gastrointestinal

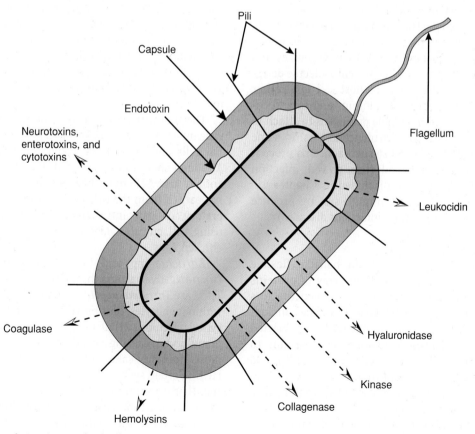

FIGURE 14-3. Virulence factors (see text for details).

infections. Part of the explanation has to do with the type or types of cells to which the pathogen is able to attach. To cause disease, some pathogens must be able to anchor themselves to cells after they have gained access to the body.

Receptors and Adhesins

The general terms **receptor** and *integrin* are used to describe the molecule on the surface of a host cell that a particular pathogen is able to recognize and attach to. Often, these receptors are glycoprotein molecules. A particular pathogen can only attach to cells bearing the appropriate receptor. Thus, certain viruses cause respiratory infections because they are able to recognize and attach to certain receptors that are present on cells that line the respiratory tract. Because those particular receptors are not present on cells lining the gastrointestinal tract, the virus is unable to cause gastrointestinal infections. Similarly, certain viruses cause infections in dogs, but not in humans, because dog cells possess a receptor that human cells lack.

S. pyogenes cells have an adhesin (called protein F) on their surfaces that enables this pathogen to adhere to a protein—fibronectin—that is found on many host cell surfaces. HIV (the virus that causes AIDS) is able to attach to cells bearing a surface receptor called CD4. Such cells are known as CD4$^+$ cells. A category of lymphocytes called T-helper cells (the primary target cells for HIV) are examples of CD4$^+$ cells.

The general terms **adhesin** and *ligand* are used to describe the molecule on the surface of a pathogen that is able to recognize and bind to a particular receptor. For example, the adhesin on the envelope of HIV that recognizes and binds to the CD4 receptor is a glycoprotein molecule designated gp120. (Entry of HIV into a host cell is a rather complex event, requiring several adhesins and several coreceptors.) Because adhesins enable pathogens to attach to host cells, they are considered virulence factors. In some cases, antibodies directed against such adhesins prevent the pathogen from attaching and, thus, prevent infection by that pathogen. (As will be discussed in Chapter 16, antibodies are proteins that our immune systems produce to protect us from pathogens and infectious diseases.)

Bacterial Fimbriae (Pili)

Bacterial fimbriae (pili) are long, thin, hairlike, flexible projections composed primarily of an array of proteins called pilin. Fimbriae are considered to be virulence factors because they enable bacteria to attach to surfaces, including various tissues within the human body. Fimbriated (piliated) strains of *Neisseria gonorrhoeae* are able to anchor themselves to the inner walls of the urethra and cause urethritis. Should nonfimbriated (nonpiliated) strains of *N. gonorrhoeae* gain access to the urethra, they are flushed out by urination and are thus unable to cause urethritis. Therefore, with respect to urethritis, fimbriated

strains of *N. gonorrhoeae* are virulent and nonfimbriated strains are avirulent.

Similarly, fimbriated strains of *Escherichia coli* that gain access to the urinary bladder are able to anchor themselves to the inner walls of the bladder and cause cystitis; thus, with respect to cystitis, fimbriated strains of *E. coli* are virulent. Should nonfimbriated strains of *E. coli* gain access to the urinary bladder, they are flushed out by urination and are unable to cause cystitis; thus, nonfimbriated strains are avirulent.

The fimbriae of group A, β-hemolytic streptococci (*S. pyogenes*) contain molecules of M-protein. M-protein serves as a virulence factor in two ways: (1) it enables the bacteria to adhere to pharyngeal cells, and (2) it protects the cells from being phagocytized by white blood cells (i.e., the M-protein serves an antiphagocytic function).

Other bacterial pathogens possessing fimbriae are *Vibrio cholerae, Salmonella* spp., *Shigella* spp., *Pseudomonas aeruginosa,* and *Neisseria meningitidis.* Because bacterial fimbriae enable bacteria to colonize surfaces, they are sometimes referred to as colonization factors.

Obligate Intracellular Pathogens

Certain pathogens, such as *Rickettsia* and *Chlamydia* spp. (all of which are Gram-negative bacteria), *must* live within host cells to survive and multiply; they are referred to as **obligate intracellular pathogens** (or obligate intracellular parasites). Rickettsias invade and live within endothelial cells and vascular smooth muscle cells. Rickettsias are capable of synthesizing proteins, nucleic acids, and adenosine triphosphate (ATP), but are thought to require an intracellular environment because they possess an unusual membrane transport system; they are said to have leaky membranes.

The different species and serotypes of chlamydias invade different types of cells, including conjunctival epithelial cells and cells of the respiratory and genital tracts. Although chlamydias produce ATP molecules, they preferentially use ATP molecules produced by host cells; this has earned them the title of "energy parasites." In the laboratory, obligate intracellular pathogens are propagated using cell cultures, laboratory animals, or embryonated chicken eggs.

Ehrlichia spp. and *Anaplasma phagocytophilum* are Gram-negative bacteria that closely resemble *Rickettsia* spp. They are **intraleukocytic pathogens.** *Ehrlichia* spp. live within monocytes, causing a disease known as human monocytic ehrlichiosis (HME). *A. phagocytophilum* lives within granulocytes, causing a condition known as human anaplasmosis (formerly called human granulocytic ehrlichiosis or HGE). Certain sporozoan protozoa, such as the *Plasmodium* spp. that cause human malaria and the *Babesia* spp. that cause human babesiosis, are **intraerythrocytic pathogens** (i.e., they live within erythrocytes).

Brucella abortus, Francisella tularensis, Legionella pneumophila, Listeria monocytogenes, Salmonella spp., and Yersinia pestis) are able to survive by means of mechanisms that are not yet understood.

Capsules

Bacterial capsules are considered to be virulence factors because they serve an antiphagocytic function (i.e., they

Pathogens That Routinely Multiply Within Macrophages

CATEGORY OF PATHOGENS	EXAMPLES	DISEASE(S)
Viruses	Herpes viruses	Genital herpes, herpes labialis (cold sores or fever blisters)
	HIV	AIDS
	Rubeola virus	Measles
	Poxviruses	Smallpox, monkeypox
Rickettsias	*Rickettsia rickettsii*	Rocky Mountain spotted fever
	Rickettsia prowazeki	Epidemic (louseborne) typhus
Other bacteria	*Brucella* spp.	Brucellosis
	Legionella pneumophila	Legionellosis
	Listeria monocytogenes	Listeriosis
	Mycobacterium leprae	Hansen disease (leprosy)
	Mycobacterium tuberculosis	Tuberculosis
Protozoa	*Leishmania* spp.	Leishmaniasis
	Toxoplasma gondii	Toxoplasmosis
	Trypanosoma cruzi	Chagas' disease (American trypanosomiasis)
Fungi	*Cryptococcus neoformans*	Cryptococcosis

The Word *Facultative*

Wherever the word *facultative* appears in this book, it implies a choice. For example, the term *facultative anaerobe* was introduced in Chapter 4. Such an organism can live either in the presence or absence of oxygen; it has a choice! In this chapter, the term *facultative intracellular pathogen* is introduced. Such an organism can live either extracellularly or intracellularly (within host cells); it has a choice! The term *facultative parasite* will be introduced in Chapter 18. Such an organism can live either a free-living or parasitic existence; it has a choice!

Facultative Intracellular Pathogens

Some pathogens, referred to as **facultative intracellular pathogens** (or facultative intracellular parasites), are capable of both an intracellular and extracellular existence. Many facultative intracellular pathogens that can be grown in the laboratory on artificial culture media are also able to survive within phagocytes. How facultative intracellular pathogens are able to survive within phagocytes is discussed in the next section. Phagocytosis is discussed in greater detail in Chapter 15.

Intracellular Survival Mechanisms

As will be discussed in Chapter 15, phagocytes play an important role in our defenses against pathogens. The two most important categories of phagocytes in the human body (referred to as professional phagocytes) are macrophages and neutrophils. Once phagocytized, most pathogens are destroyed within the phagocytes by hydrolytic enzymes (e.g., lysozyme, proteases, lipases, DNAse, RNase, myeloperoxidase), hydrogen peroxide, superoxide anions, and other mechanisms. However, certain pathogens are able to survive and multiply within phagocytes after being ingested (Table 14-1).

Some pathogens (such as the bacterium, *M. tuberculosis*) have a cell wall composition that resists digestion. Mycobacterial cell walls contain waxes, and it is thought that these waxes protect the organisms from digestion. Other pathogens (like the protozoan, *Toxoplasma gondii*) prevent the fusion of lysosomes (vesicles that contain digestive enzymes) with the phagocytic vacuole (phagosome). Other pathogens (such as the bacterium, *Rickettsia rickettsii*) produce phospholipases that destroy the phagosome membrane, thus preventing lysosome-phagosome fusion. Other pathogens (such as the bacteria,

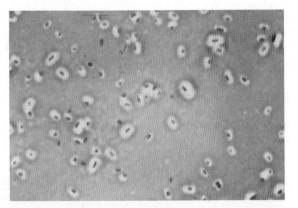

FIGURE 14-4. Photomicrograph of *Streptococcus pneumoniae.* After the bacteria were treated with a specific antibody to enhance visibility of their capsules (known as a Quellung reaction, which is discussed in Chapter 16), a dye was added to the preparation. The bacteria and the background have stained pink, but the capsules appear as colorless "halos" around the bacterial cells. (Koneman's Color Atlas and Textbook of Diagnostic Microbiology, 6th ed. Philadelphia: Lippincott Williams & Wilkins, 2006.)

protect encapsulated bacteria from being phagocytized by phagocytic white blood cells). Phagocytes are unable to attach to encapsulated bacteria because they lack surface receptors for the polysaccharide material of which the capsule is made. If they cannot adhere to the bacteria, they cannot ingest them. Because encapsulated bacteria that gain access to the bloodstream or tissues are protected from phagocytosis, they are able to multiply, invade, and cause disease. Nonencapsulated bacteria, on the other hand, are phagocytized and killed. Encapsulated bacteria include *S. pneumoniae* (Fig. 14-4), *Klebsiella pneumoniae,* *H. influenzae,* and *N. meningitidis.* The capsule of the yeast, *Cryptococcus neoformans,* is also considered to be a virulence factor.

Flagella

Bacterial flagella are considered virulence factors because flagella enable flagellated (motile) bacteria to invade aqueous areas of the body that nonflagellated (nonmotile) bacteria are unable to reach. Perhaps flagella also enable bacteria to avoid phagocytosis—it is more difficult for phagocytes to catch a moving target.

Exoenzymes

Although pili, capsules, and flagella are considered virulence factors, they really do not explain how bacteria and other pathogens actually <u>cause</u> disease. **The major mechanisms by which pathogens cause disease are the exoenzymes or toxins that they produce.** Some pathogens (e.g., certain strains of *S. pyogenes*) produce exoenzymes <u>and</u> toxins.

Some pathogens release enzymes (called exoenzymes) that enable them to evade host defense mechanisms, invade,

or cause damage to body tissues. These exoenzymes include necrotizing enzymes, coagulase, kinases, hyaluronidase, collagenase, hemolysins, and lecithinase.

Necrotizing Enzymes

Many pathogens produce exoenzymes that destroy tissues; these are collectively referred to as necrotizing enzymes. Notorious examples are the flesh-eating strains of *S. pyogenes,* which produce proteases and other enzymes that cause very rapid destruction of soft tissue, leading to a disease called necrotizing fasciitis. The *Clostridium* species that cause gas gangrene (myonecrosis) produce a variety of necrotizing enzymes, including proteases and lipases.

Coagulase

An important identifying feature of *S. aureus* in the laboratory is its ability to produce a protein called **coagulase.** Although coagulase ends in *-ase* like the names of many enzymes, it is technically not an enzyme. Coagulase binds to prothrombin, forming a complex called staphylothrombin. The protease activity of thrombin is activated in this complex, causing the conversion of fibrinogen to fibrin. In the body, coagulase may enable *S. aureus* to clot plasma and thereby to form a sticky coat of fibrin around themselves for protection from phagocytes, antibodies, and other host defense mechanisms.

Kinases

Kinases (also known as fibrinolysins) have the opposite effect of coagulase. Sometimes the host will cause a fibrin clot to form around pathogens in an attempt to wall them off and prevent them from invading deeper into body tissues. Kinases are enzymes that lyse (dissolve) clots; therefore, pathogens that produce kinases are able to escape from clots. **Streptokinase** is the name of a kinase produced by streptococci, and **staphylokinase** is the name of a kinase produced by staphylococci. Streptokinase has been used to treat patients with coronary thrombosis. Because *S. aureus* produces both coagulase and staphylokinase, not only can *S. aureus* cause the formation of clots, but it can also dissolve them.

Hyaluronidase

The "spreading factor," as **hyaluronidase** is sometimes called, enables pathogens to spread through connective tissue by breaking down **hyaluronic acid,** the polysaccharide "cement" that holds tissue cells together. Hyaluronidase is secreted by several pathogenic species of *Staphylococcus, Streptococcus,* and *Clostridium.*

Collagenase

The enzyme **collagenase,** produced by certain pathogens, breaks down collagen (the supportive protein found in tendons, cartilage, and bones). This enables the pathogens to invade tissues. *Clostridium perfringens,* a major cause of gas gangrene, spreads deeply within the body by secreting both collagenase and hyaluronidase.

Hemolysins

Hemolysins are enzymes that cause damage to the host's red blood cells (erythrocytes). Not only does the lysis (bursting or destruction) of red blood cells harm the host, but it also provides the pathogens with a source of iron. In the laboratory, the effect an organism has on the red blood cells in blood agar enables differentiation between alpha-hemolytic (α-hemolytic) and beta-hemolytic (β-hemolytic) bacteria. The hemolysins produced by α-hemolytic bacteria cause a partial breakdown of hemoglobin in the red blood cells, resulting in a green zone around the colonies of α-hemolytic bacteria. The hemolysins produced by β-hemolytic bacteria cause complete lysis of the red blood cells, resulting in a clear zone around the colonies of β-hemolytic bacteria (see Fig. 13.8). Hemolysins are produced by many pathogenic bacteria, but the type of hemolysis produced by an organism is of most importance when attempting to speciate a *Streptococcus* in the laboratory.

Lecithinase

C. perfringens, the major cause of gas gangrene, is able to rapidly destroy extensive areas of tissue, especially muscle tissue. One of the enzymes produced by *C. perfringens* is called **lecithinase,** which breaks down phospholipids collectively referred to as **lecithin.** This enzyme is destructive to cell membranes of red blood cells and other tissues.

Toxins

The ability of pathogens to damage host tissues and cause disease may depend on the production and release of various types of poisonous substances, referred to as toxins. The two major categories of toxins are endotoxins and exotoxins. **Endotoxins,** which are integral parts of the cell walls of Gram-negative bacteria, can cause a number of adverse physiologic effects. **Exotoxins,** on the other hand, are toxins that are produced within cells and then released from the cells.

Endotoxin

Septicemia (often referred to as sepsis) is a very serious disease consisting of chills, fever, prostration (extreme exhaustion), and the presence of bacteria or their toxins in the bloodstream. Septicemia caused by Gram-negative bacteria, sometimes referred to as Gram-negative sepsis, is an especially serious type of septicemia. The cell walls of Gram-negative bacteria contain lipopolysaccharide (LPS), the lipid portion of which is called lipid-A or endotoxin. Endotoxin can cause serious, adverse, physiologic effects such as fever and shock. Substances that cause fever are known as **pyrogens.**

Shock is a life-threatening condition resulting from very low blood pressure and an inadequate blood supply to body tissues and organs, especially the kidneys and brain. The type of shock that results from Gram-negative sepsis is known as **septic shock.** Symptoms include reduced mental alertness, confusion, rapid breathing, chills, fever, and warm, flushed skin. As shock worsens, several organs begin to fail, including the kidneys, lungs, and heart. Blood clots may form within blood vessels. More than 500,000 cases of sepsis occur annually in the United States; approximately half of these are caused by Gram-negative bacteria. There is a 30 to 35% mortality rate associated with Gram-negative sepsis.

Exotoxins

Exotoxins are poisonous proteins that are secreted by a variety of pathogens; they are often named for the target organs that they affect. The most potent exotoxins are **neurotoxins,** which affect the central nervous system. The neurotoxins produced by *Clostridium tetani* and *Clostridium botulinum*—tetanospasmin and botulinal toxin—cause tetanus and botulism, respectively. Tetanospasmin affects control of nerve transmission, leading to a spastic, rigid type of paralysis in which the patient's muscles are contracted. Botulinal toxin also blocks nerve impulses but by a different mechanism, leading to a generalized, flaccid type of paralysis in which the patient's muscles are relaxed. Both diseases are often fatal. See this book's CD-ROM for "A Closer Look at Botulinal Toxin."

Other types of exotoxins, called **enterotoxins,** are toxins that affect the gastrointestinal tract, often causing diarrhea and sometimes vomiting. Examples of bacterial pathogens that produce enterotoxins are *Bacillus cereus,* certain serotypes of *E. coli, Clostridium difficile, C. perfringens, Salmonella* spp., *Shigella* spp., *V. cholerae,* and some strains of *S. aureus.* In addition to releasing an enterotoxin (called toxin A), *C. difficile* also produces a cytotoxin (called toxin B) that damages the lining of the colon, leading to a condition known as pseudomembranous colitis.

Symptoms of toxic shock syndrome are caused by exotoxins secreted by certain strains of *S. aureus* and, less commonly, *S. pyogenes.* Staphylococcal toxic shock syndrome toxin (TSST-1) primarily affects the integrity of capillary walls. **Exfoliative toxin** (or epidermolytic toxin) of *S. aureus* causes the epidermal layers of skin to slough away, leading to a disease known as scalded skin syndrome. *S. aureus* also produces a variety of toxins that destroy cell membranes.

Erythrogenic toxin, produced by some strains of *S. pyogenes,* causes scarlet fever. **Leukocidins** are toxins that destroy white blood cells (leukocytes). Thus, leukocidins (which are produced by some staphylococci, streptococci, and clostridia) cause destruction of the very cells that the body sends to the site of infection to ingest and destroy pathogens.

Diphtheria toxin, produced by toxigenic strains of *C. diphtheriae,* inhibits protein synthesis. It kills mucosal epithelial cells and phagocytes and adversely affects the heart and nervous system. The toxin is actually coded for by a bacteriophage gene. Thus, only *C. diphtheriae* cells that are "infected" with that particular bacteriophage are able to produce diphtheria toxin. Other exotoxins that inhibit protein synthesis are *P. aeruginosa* exotoxin A, Shiga toxin (produced by *Shigella* spp.), and the Shiga-like toxins produced by certain serotypes of *E. coli*.

Mechanisms by Which Pathogens Escape Immune Responses

Immunology, the study of the immune system, is discussed in detail in Chapter 16. A primary role of the immune system is to recognize and destroy pathogens that invade our bodies. However, there are many ways in which pathogens avoid being destroyed by immune responses. Several mechanisms will be mentioned here; others are beyond the scope of this book.

Antigenic Variation

As discussed in Chapter 16, antigens are foreign molecules that evoke an immune response—often stimulating the immune system to produce antibodies. Some pathogens are able to periodically change their surface antigens, a phenomenon known as antigenic variation. About the time that the host has produced antibodies in response to the pathogen's surface antigens, those antigens are shed and new ones appear in their place. Examples of pathogens capable of antigenic variation are influenza viruses, HIV, *Borrelia recurrentis* (the causative agent of relapsing fever), *N. gonorrhoeae*, and the trypanosomes that cause African trypanosomiasis. Trypanosomes can keep up their antigenic variation for 20 years, never presenting the same appearance twice.

Camouflage and Molecular Mimicry

Adult schistosomes (trematodes that cause schistosomiasis) are able to conceal their foreign nature by coating themselves with host proteins—a sort of camouflage. In molecular mimicry, the pathogen's surface antigens closely resemble host antigens and are therefore not recognized as being foreign. Although there is little evidence to prove that molecular mimicry leads to a subdued immune response against the pathogens, it is known that the hyaluronic acid capsule of streptococci is almost identical to the hyaluronic acid component of human connective tissue. It is also interesting that in mycoplasmal pneumonia, antibodies produced by the host against antigens of *Mycoplasma pneumoniae* can cause damage to the host's heart, lung, brain, and red blood cells.

Destruction of Antibodies

Several bacterial pathogens, including *H. influenzae*, *N. gonorrhoeae*, and streptococci, produce an enzyme (IgA protease) that destroys IgA antibodies. Thus, these pathogens are capable of destroying some of the antibodies that the host's immune system has produced in an attempt to destroy them.

Table 14-2 contains a recap of bacterial virulence factors.

TABLE 14-2

Recap of Bacterial Virulence Factors

VIRULENCE FACTOR	COMMENTS
Bacterial structures:	
Flagella	Enable bacteria to gain access to anatomic areas that nonmotile bacteria cannot reach; may enable bacteria to "escape" from phagocytes
Capsules	Serve an antiphagocytic function
Pili	Enable bacteria to attach to surfaces
Enzymes:	
Coagulase	Enables bacteria to produce clots within which to "hide"
Kinases	Enable bacteria to dissolve clots
Hyaluronidase	Dissolves hyaluronic acid, enabling bacteria to penetrate deeper into tissues
Lecithinase	Destroys cell membranes
Necrotizing enzymes	Cause massive destruction of tissues
Toxins:	
Endotoxin	Released from the cell walls of Gram-negative bacteria; causes fever and septic shock
Exotoxins	Produced within the cell, but then released from the cell
Neurotoxins	Cause damage to the central nervous system; tetanospasmin and botulinal toxin are examples
Enterotoxins	Cause gastrointestinal disease
Clostridium difficile toxin B	The cytotoxin that causes pseudomembranous colitis
Staphylococcus aureus TSST-1	The toxin that causes most cases of toxic shock syndrome
Exfoliative toxin	Produced by some strains of *S. aureus;* causes scalded skin syndrome
Erythrogenic toxin	Produced by some strains of *Streptococcus pyogenes;* causes scarlet fever
Diphtheria toxin	Produced by toxigenic strains of *Corynebacterium diphtheriae;* causes diphtheria
Leukocidins	Cause the destruction of leukocytes

◉ REVIEW OF KEY POINTS

- Although most people, including most healthcare professionals, use the terms *infection* and *infectious disease* synonymously, microbiologists define infection as colonization by a pathogen. Once colonized by a pathogen, the person is said to be infected with that pathogen, regardless of whether the pathogen is causing disease.

- When individuals are exposed to pathogens, these microbes may or may not cause disease, depending on a number of factors (including the person's nutritional health and immune status, as well as the virulence of the pathogen).

- *Pathogenicity* is the ability of a microbe to cause disease, whereas *pathogenesis* refers to the actual steps that are involved in the development of a disease. Sometimes (but not always) pathogenesis follows this sequence: entry of the pathogen into the body → attachment → multiplication → invasion or spread → evasion of host defenses → damage to host tissue(s).

- When the body loses its battle with a pathogen, clinical disease results, accompanied by characteristic signs and symptoms. *Signs* of a disease are various types of objective evidence of a disease (e.g., increased or decreased blood pressure, elevated body temperature, abnormal pulse rate, abnormalities that are discovered by palpation, and abnormal test results). *Symptoms* of a disease are various types of subjective evidence of disease that are experienced or perceived by patients (e.g., aches or pains, chills, anorexia, nausea, and itching).

- Some pathogens manifest themselves periodically, remaining dormant between episodes. The diseases caused by such pathogens are referred to as latent infections, examples being syphilis and various types of herpes infections (e.g., cold sores, genital herpes, shingles).

- An infection may be acute, subacute, or chronic; localized or systemic; and symptomatic or asymptomatic. As the disease progresses, it may change from one stage to another.

- The four phases of an infectious disease are the incubation period, prodromal period, period of illness, and convalescent period. In some cases, the period of illness is followed by disability or death. A primary infection may set the stage for a secondary infection caused by another pathogen.

- Virulence is a measure or degree of pathogenicity. Different species or even different strains of the same species vary in their ability to cause disease; thus, some are more virulent than others. Some strains of a particular species may be virulent, whereas other strains of the same species are avirulent.

- *Virulence factors* are the phenotypic characteristics of a microorganism that enable it to cause disease. Some virulence factors are structural features (e.g., capsules, flagella, pili) that enable pathogens to avoid phagocytosis and reach and attach to various tissues within the host.

- The two major virulence factors by which bacteria cause disease are exoenzymes and toxins. Exoenzymes that are virulence factors include coagulase, kinases, hyaluronidase, collagenase, hemolysins, lecithinase, and necrotizing enzymes. These exoenzymes enable pathogens to evade host defenses, invade, and cause damage to body tissues.

- Toxins include endotoxins (found in the cell walls of Gram-negative bacteria) and exotoxins (toxins that are released from the cells that produce them). Examples of exotoxins are neurotoxins (which cause paralysis), enterotoxins (which cause gastrointestinal disease), TSST-1 (which causes toxic shock syndrome), exfoliative or epidermolytic toxin (which causes scalded skin syndrome), erythrogenic toxin (which causes scarlet fever), leukocidins (which destroy leukocytes), and diphtheria toxin (which causes diphtheria).

- The two most important categories of phagocytes in the human body are macrophages and neutrophils. Although their primary function is to ingest and destroy pathogens, some pathogens are able to survive within phagocytes. Some prevent fusion of the phagosome with a lysosome. Others have a cell wall structure that resists the digestion process.

- Some pathogens are able to escape immune responses. The mechanisms by which they are able to accomplish this include antigenic variation, camouflage, molecular mimicry, and destruction of antibodies.

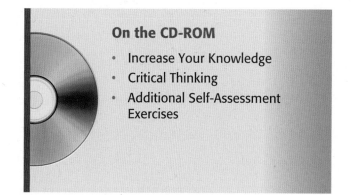

On the CD-ROM
- Increase Your Knowledge
- Critical Thinking
- Additional Self-Assessment Exercises

Self-Assessment Exercises

After studying this chapter, answer the following multiple-choice questions.

1. Which of the following virulence factors enable(s) bacteria to attach to tissues?
   a. capsules
   b. endotoxin
   c. flagella
   d. pili

2. Neurotoxins are produced by:
   a. *Clostridium botulinum* and *Clostridium tetani.*
   b. *Clostridium difficile* and *Clostridium perfringens.*
   c. *Pseudomonas aeruginosa* and *Mycobacterium tuberculosis.*
   d. *Staphylococcus aureus* and *Streptococcus pyogenes.*

3. Which of the following pathogens produce enterotoxins?
   a. *Bacillus cereus* and certain serotypes of *Escherichia coli*
   b. *Clostridium difficile* and *Clostridium perfringens*
   c. *Salmonella* spp. and *Shigella* spp.
   d. all of the above

4. A bloodstream infection with _____ could result in the release of endotoxin into the bloodstream.
   a. *Clostridium difficile* or *Clostridium perfringens*
   b. *Neisseria gonorrhoeae* or *Escherichia coli*
   c. *Staphylococcus aureus* or *Mycobacterium tuberculosis*
   d. *Staphylococcus aureus* or *Streptococcus pyogenes*

5. Communicable diseases are most easily transmitted during the:
   a. incubation period.
   b. period of convalescence.
   c. period of illness.
   d. prodromal period.

6. Enterotoxins affect cells in the:
   a. central nervous system.
   b. gastrointestinal tract.
   c. genitourinary tract.
   d. respiratory tract.

7. Which of the following bacteria is *least* likely to be the cause of septic shock?
   a. *Escherichia coli*
   b. *Haemophilus influenzae*
   c. *Mycoplasma pneumoniae*
   d. *Neisseria meningitidis*

8. Which of the following produces both a cytotoxin *and* an enterotoxin?
   a. *Clostridium botulinum*
   b. *Clostridium difficile*
   c. *Clostridium tetani*
   d. *Corynebacterium diphtheriae*

9. Which of the following virulence factors enable(s) bacteria to avoid phagocytosis by white blood cells?
   a. capsule
   b. cell membrane
   c. cell wall
   d. pili

10. Which of the following can cause toxic shock syndrome?
    a. *Clostridium difficile* and *Clostridium perfringens*
    b. *Mycoplasma pneumoniae* and *Mycobacterium tuberculosis*
    c. *Neisseria gonorrhoeae* and *Escherichia coli*
    d. *Staphylococcus aureus* and *Streptococcus pyogenes*

15

NONSPECIFIC HOST DEFENSE MECHANISMS

LEARNING OBJECTIVES

AFTER STUDYING THIS CHAPTER, YOU SHOULD BE ABLE TO:

- Define the following terms: host defense mechanisms, antibody, antigen, lysozyme, microbial antagonism, colicin, bacteriocins, superinfection, pyrogen, interferon, complement cascade, complement, opsonization, inflammation, vasodilation, phagocytosis, and chemotaxis
- Briefly describe the three lines of defense used by the body to combat pathogens and give one example of each
- Explain what is meant by "nonspecific host defense mechanisms" and how they differ from "specific host defense mechanisms"
- Identify three ways by which the digestive system is protected from pathogens
- Describe how interferons function as host defense mechanisms
- Name three cellular and chemical responses to microbial invasion

- Describe the major benefits of complement activation
- List the four cardinal (main) signs and symptoms associated with inflammation
- Discuss the four primary purposes of the inflammatory response
- Outline the four steps in phagocytosis
- Identify the three major categories of leukocytes and the three categories of granulocytes
- Cite four ways in which pathogens escape destruction by phagocytes
- Categorize the disorders and conditions that affect the body's nonspecific host mechanisms

INTRODUCTION

In Chapter 14, you discovered the ways in which pathogens cause infectious diseases. In this chapter and the next, you will learn how our bodies fight pathogens in an attempt to prevent the infectious diseases that they cause.

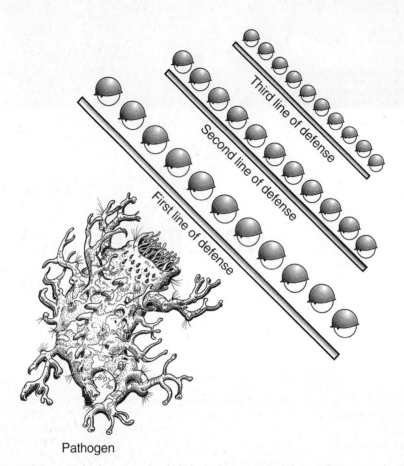

Pathogen

FIGURE 15-1. Lines of defense. Host defense mechanisms—ways in which the body protects itself from pathogens—can be thought of as an entrenched army consisting of three lines of defense. (See text for details.) (With permission from the Colorado Association for Continuing Medical Laboratory Education, Denver, CO.)

Humans and animals have survived on earth for hundreds of thousands of years because they have many built-in or naturally occurring mechanisms of defense against pathogens and the infectious diseases that they cause. The ability of any animal to resist these invaders and recover from disease is attributable to many complex interacting functions within the body.

Host defense mechanisms—ways in which the body protects itself from pathogens—can be thought of as an army consisting of three lines of defense (Fig. 15-1). If the enemy (the pathogen) breaks through the first line of defense, it will encounter and, it is hoped, be stopped by the second line of defense. If the enemy manages to break through and escape the first two lines of defense, there is a third line of defense ready to attack it.

The first two lines of defense are nonspecific; these are ways in which the body attempts to destroy *all* types of substances that are foreign to it, including pathogens. The third line of defense, the immune response, is very specific. In the third line of defense (or **specific host defense mechanisms**), special proteins called *antibodies* are usually produced in the body in response to the presence of foreign substances. These foreign substances are called *antigens* because they stimulate the production of specific antibodies; they are

*"anti*body *gen*erating" substances. The antibodies that are produced are very specific, in that they usually can only recognize and attach to the antigen that stimulated their production. Immune responses are discussed in greater detail in Chapter 16. The various categories of host defense mechanisms are summarized in Figure 15-2.[a]

Nonspecific Host Defense Mechanisms

Nonspecific host defense mechanisms are general and serve to protect the body against many harmful substances. One of the nonspecific host defenses is the innate, or inborn, resistance observed among some species of animals and some persons who have a natural resistance to certain diseases. Innate or inherited characteristics make these people and animals more resistant to some diseases than to others. The exact factors that produce this innate resistance

[a]Some immunologists consider both the second and third lines of defense as parts of the immune system. They refer to the second line of defense as *innate immune responses* and the third line of defense as *acquired immune responses.*

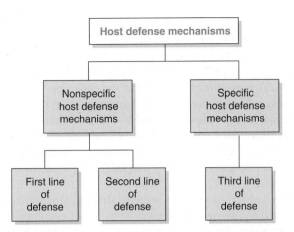

FIGURE 15-2. Categories of host defense mechanisms. (With permission from the Colorado Association for Continuing Medical Laboratory Education, Denver, CO.)

are not well understood, but are probably related to chemical, physiologic, and temperature differences between the species as well as the general state of physical and emotional health of the person and environmental factors that affect certain races, but not others.

Although we are usually unaware of it, our bodies are constantly in the process of defending us against microbial invaders. We encounter pathogens and potential pathogens many times per day, every day of our lives. Usually, our bodies successfully ward off or destroy the invading microbes. Nonspecific host defense mechanisms discussed in this chapter include mechanical and physical barriers to invasion, chemical factors, microbial antagonism by our indigenous microflora, fever, the inflammatory response (inflammation), and phagocytic white blood cells (phagocytes).

First Line of Defense

Skin and Mucous Membranes As Physical Barriers

The intact, unbroken skin that covers our bodies represents a nonspecific host defense mechanism, in that it serves as a physical or mechanical barrier to pathogens. Very few pathogens are able to penetrate intact skin. Although certain helminth infections (e.g., hookworm infection and schistosomiasis) are acquired by penetration of the skin by parasites, it is unlikely that many, if any, bacteria are capable of penetrating intact skin. In most cases, it is only when the skin is cut, abraded (scratched), or burned that pathogens gain entrance or when they are injected through the skin (e.g., by arthropods or the sharing of needles by intravenous drug abusers). Even the tiniest of cuts (a paper cut, for example) can serve as a portal of entry for pathogens.

Although they are composed of only a single layer of cells, mucous membranes also serve as a physical or mechanical barrier to pathogens. Most pathogens can only

pass through when these membranes are cut or scratched. As is true for skin, even the tiniest of cuts can serve as portals of entry for pathogens. The sticky mucus that is produced by goblet cells within the mucous membranes serves to entrap invaders; thus, it is considered part of the first line of defense.

Cellular and Chemical Factors

Not only does skin provide a physical barrier, but there are several additional factors that account for the skin's ability to resist pathogens. The dryness of most areas of skin inhibits colonization by many pathogens. Also, the acidity (approximately pH 5.0) and temperature ($<37°C$) of the skin inhibit the growth of pathogens. The oily sebum that is produced by sebaceous glands in the skin contains fatty acids, which are toxic to some pathogens. Perspiration serves as a nonspecific host defense mechanism by flushing organisms from pores and the surface of the skin. Perspiration also contains the enzyme, *lysozyme,* which degrades peptidoglycan in bacterial cell walls (especially Gram-positive bacteria). Even the sloughing off of dead skin cells removes potential pathogens from the skin.

In addition to being sticky, the mucus produced at mucous membranes contains a variety of substances (e.g., lysozyme, lactoferrin, and lactoperoxidase) that can kill bacteria or inhibit their growth. As previously mentioned, lysozyme destroys bacterial cell walls by degrading peptidoglycan. Lactoferrin is a protein that binds iron, a mineral that is required by all pathogens. Because they are unable to compete with lactoferrin for free iron, the pathogens are deprived of this essential nutrient. Lactoperoxidase is an enzyme that produces superoxide radicals, highly reactive forms of oxygen, which are toxic to bacteria.

Because mucosal cells are among the most rapidly dividing cells in the body, they are constantly being produced and released from mucous membranes. Bacteria that are adhering to the cells are often expelled along with the cells to which they are attached.

The respiratory system would be particularly accessible to invaders that could ride in on dust or other particles inhaled with each breath were it not for the hair, mucous membranes, and irregular chambers of the nose that serve to trap much of the inhaled debris. Also, the cilia (mucociliary covering) present on epithelial cells of the posterior nasal membranes, nasal sinuses, bronchi, and trachea sweep the trapped dust and microbes upward toward the throat, where they are swallowed or expelled by sneezing and coughing. Damage to these ciliated epithelial cells (e.g., damage caused by smoking, other pollutants, and bacterial or viral respiratory infections) can increase a person's susceptibility to bacterial respiratory infections. Phagocytes in the mucous membranes may also be involved in this mucociliary clearance mechanism.

Lysozyme and other enzymes that lyse or destroy bacteria are present in nasal secretions, saliva, and tears. Even the swallowing of saliva can be thought of as a nonspecific host defense mechanism, because thousands of bacteria are removed from the oral cavity every time we swallow. Humans swallow approximately 1 L of saliva per day.

To a certain extent, the following factors protect the digestive system from bacterial colonization and are therefore considered to be nonspecific host defense mechanisms:

- Digestive enzymes.
- Acidity of the stomach (approximately pH 1.5).
- Alkalinity of the intestines.

Bile, which is secreted from the liver into the small intestine, lowers the surface tension and causes chemical changes in bacterial cell walls and membranes that make bacteria easier to digest. As a result of the combination of stomach acid, bile salts, and the rapid flow of its contents, the small intestine is relatively free of bacteria. Many invading microorganisms are trapped in the sticky, mucous lining of the digestive tract, where they may be destroyed by bactericidal enzymes and phagocytes. Peristalsis and the expulsion of feces serve to remove bacteria from the intestine. Bacteria make up about 50% of feces.

The urinary tract is usually sterile in healthy persons, with the exception of indigenous microorganisms that colonize the distal urethra (that part of the urethra furthest from the urinary bladder). Microorganisms are continually flushed from the urethra by frequent urination and expulsion of mucus secretions. Many urinary bladder infections result from infrequent urination, including the failure to urinate after intercourse. Conditions that obstruct urine flow (e.g., benign prostatic hyperplasia [BPH]) also increase the chances of developing cystitis. The low pH of vaginal fluid usually inhibits colonization of the vagina by pathogens. However, women who are taking certain oral contraceptives are particularly susceptible to some infections because the contraceptives increase the pH of the vagina.

Microbial Antagonism

When resident microbes of the indigenous microflora prevent colonization by new arrivals to a particular anatomical site, it is known as *microbial antagonism* and is another example of a nonspecific host defense mechanism. The inhibitory capability of the indigenous microflora has been attributed to the following factors:

- Competition for colonization sites.
- Competition for nutrients.
- Production of substances that kill other bacteria.

It is thought that the indigenous microflora of the skin, oral cavity, upper respiratory tract, and colon play a major role as a nonspecific host defense mechanism by preventing pathogens and potential pathogens from colonizing these sites. The effectiveness of microbial antagonism is frequently decreased after prolonged administration of broad-spectrum

antibiotics. The antibiotics reduce or eliminate certain members of the indigenous microflora (e.g., the vaginal and gastrointestinal flora), leading to overgrowth by bacteria or fungi that are resistant to the antibiotic(s) being administered. This overgrowth or "population explosion" of organisms is called a *superinfection*. A superinfection of *Candida albicans* in the vagina may lead to the condition known as yeast vaginitis. A superinfection of *Clostridium difficile* in the colon may lead to *C. difficile*-associated diseases known as antibiotic-associated diarrhea (AAD) and pseudomembranous colitis (PMC).

Some bacteria produce proteins that kill other bacteria; collectively, these antibacterial substances are known as *bacteriocins*. An example is *colicin,* which is produced by certain strains of *Escherichia coli*. Similar antibacterial substances are produced by some strains of *Pseudomonas* and *Bacillus* species as well as by certain other bacteria. Bacteriocins have a narrower range of activity than do antibiotics, but they are more potent than antibiotics.

Second Line of Defense

Pathogens able to penetrate the first line of defense are usually destroyed by nonspecific cellular and chemical responses, collectively referred to as the second line of defense. A complex sequence of events develops involving production of fever, production of interferons, activation of the complement system, inflammation, chemotaxis, and phagocytosis. Each of these responses is discussed in this chapter.

Transferrin

Transferrin, a glycoprotein synthesized in the liver, has a high affinity for iron. Its normal function is to store and deliver iron to host cells. Like lactoferrin (mentioned earlier), transferrin serves as a nonspecific host defense mechanism by sequestering iron and depriving pathogens of this essential nutrient. Studies have shown that transferrin levels in the blood increase dramatically in response to systemic bacterial infections.

Fever

Normal body temperature fluctuates between 36.2°C and 37.5°C (97.2°F and 99.5°F), with an average of about 37°C (98.6°F). A body temperature greater than 37.8°C (100°F) is generally considered to be a fever. Substances that stimulate the production of fever are called *pyrogens* or *pyrogenic substances.* Pyrogens may originate either outside or inside the body. Those from outside the body include pathogens and various pyrogenic substances that they produce or release (e.g., endotoxin). Interleukin 1 (IL-1) is an example of a pyrogen that is produced within the body (i.e., it is an endogenous pyrogen). The resulting increased body temperature (fever) is considered to be a nonspecific host defense mechanism. It augments the host's defenses in the following ways:

- by stimulating white blood cells (leukocytes) to deploy and destroy invaders

- by reducing available free plasma iron, which limits the growth of pathogens that require iron for replication and synthesis of toxins

- by inducing the production of IL-1, which causes the proliferation, maturation, and activation of lymphocytes in the immunologic response

Elevated body temperatures also slow down the rate of growth of certain pathogens and can even kill some especially fastidious pathogens.

The following scenario illustrates one way in which fever develops during an infectious disease:

1. A patient has septicemia caused by Gram-negative bacteria (referred to as "Gram-negative sepsis").

2. The bacteria release endotoxin into the patient's bloodstream. (Endotoxin is part of the cell wall structure of Gram-negative bacteria; it is the lipid component of lipopolysaccharide.)

3. Phagocytes ingest (phagocytize) the endotoxin.

4. The ingested endotoxin stimulates the phagocytes to produce IL-1, an endogenous pyrogen. IL-1 is produced primarily by macrophages.

5. IL-1 stimulates the hypothalamus (a part of the brain referred to as the body's thermostat) to produce prostaglandins.

6. Once metabolized, the prostaglandins cause the hypothalamic thermostat to be set at a higher level.

7. The increased thermostatic reading sends out signals to the nerves surrounding peripheral blood vessels. This causes the vessels to contract, thus conserving heat.

8. The increased body heat, resulting from vasoconstriction, continues until the temperature of the blood supplying the hypothalamus matches the elevated thermostat reading. The thermostat can be reset to the normal body temperature when the concentration of endogenous pyrogen decreases.

There are, of course, detrimental aspects of fever—especially prolonged high fevers. These include increased heart rate, increased metabolic rate, increased caloric demand, and mild to severe dehydration.

Interferons

Interferons are small, antiviral proteins produced by virus-infected cells. They are called interferons because they "interfere" with viral replication. The three known types of interferon, referred to as alpha (α), beta (β), and gamma (γ) interferons, are induced by different stimuli, including viruses, tumors, bacteria, and other foreign cells. The different types of interferons are produced by different type of cells. α-Interferon is produced by B lymphocytes (B cells), monocytes, and macrophages; β-interferon, by fibroblasts and other virus-infected cells; and γ-interferon, by activated T lymphocytes (T cells) and natural killer cells (NK cells).

The interferons produced by a virus-infected cell are unable to save that cell from destruction, but once they are released from that cell, they attach to the membranes of surrounding cells and prevent viral replication from occurring in those cells. Thus, the spread of the infection is inhibited, allowing other body defenses to fight the disease more effectively. In this way, many viral diseases (e.g., colds, influenza, and measles) are limited in duration. Similarly, the acute phase of herpes simplex cold sores is of limited duration. The herpesvirus then enters a latent phase and hides in nerve ganglion cells where it is protected until the person's defenses are down; the cycle of disease and latency is repeated over and over.

Interferons are not virus-specific, meaning that they are effective against a variety of viruses, not just the particular type of virus that stimulated their production. Interferons are species-specific, however, meaning that they are effective only in the species of animal that produced them. Thus, rabbit interferons are only effective in rabbits and could not be used to treat viral infections in humans. Human interferons are industrially produced by genetically engineered bacteria (bacteria into which human interferon genes have been inserted) and are used experimentally to treat certain viral infections (e.g., warts, herpes simplex, hepatitis B and C) and cancers (e.g., leukemias, lymphomas, Kaposi's sarcoma in AIDS patients). In addition to interfering with viral multiplication, interferons also activate certain lymphocytes (NK cells) to kill virus-infected cells. NK cells are discussed in Chapter 16.

In addition to the beneficial aspects of the interferons that are produced in response to certain viral infections, they actually cause the nonspecific flulike symptoms (malaise, myalgia, chills, fever) that are associated with many viral infections.

The Complement System

Complement is not a single entity, but rather a group of approximately 30 different proteins (including nine proteins designated as C1 through C9) that are found in normal blood plasma. These proteins make up what is called "the complement system"—so named because it is complementary to the action of the immune system. The proteins of the complement system, sometimes collectively referred to as complement components, interact with each other in a stepwise manner, known as the *complement cascade.* A discussion of the somewhat complex steps in the complement cascade is beyond the scope of this book. What is of primary importance is that activation of the complement system is considered a nonspecific host defense mechanism; it assists in the destruction of many different pathogens. The major consequences of complement activation are listed here:

- initiation and amplification of inflammation
- attraction of phagocytes to sites where they are needed (chemotaxis; discussed later)
- activation of leukocytes
- lysis of bacteria and other foreign cells
- increased phagocytosis by phagocytic cells (opsonization)

See this book's CD-ROM for "A Closer Look at the Complement System."

Opsonization is a process by which phagocytosis is facilitated by the deposition of *opsonins* (e.g., antibodies or certain complement fragments) onto the surface of particles or cells. In some cases, phagocytes are unable to ingest certain particles or cells (e.g., encapsulated bacteria) until opsonization occurs. One of the products formed during the complement cascade, called C3b, is an opsonin. It is deposited on the surface of microorganisms. Neutrophils and macrophages possess surface molecules (receptors) that can recognize and bind to C3b.

Complement fragments C3a, C4a, and C5a cause mast cells to degranulate and release histamine, leading to increased vascular permeability and smooth muscle contraction. (Mast cells are discussed in Chapter 16.) C5a also acts as a chemoattractant (chemotactic agent) for neutrophils and macrophages. Chemoattractants are discussed in a subsequent section.

There are a variety of hereditary complement deficiencies that interfere with activities of the complement system. Some of these inherited deficiencies are associated with defects in activation of the classical pathway. A deficiency of C3 leads to a defect in activation of both the classical and alternative pathways. Defects of properdin factors impair activation of the alternative pathway. Any of these defects leads to increased susceptibility to pyogenic (pus-producing) staphylococcal and streptococcal infections.

Acute-Phase Proteins

Plasma levels of molecules collectively referred to as acute-phase proteins increase rapidly in response to infection, inflammation, and tissue injury. They serve as host defense mechanisms by enhancing resistance to infection and promoting the repair of damaged tissue. Acute-phase proteins include C-reactive protein (which is used as a laboratory marker for, or indication of, inflammation), serum amyloid A protein, protease inhibitors, and coagulation proteins.

Cytokines

Cytokines are chemical mediators that are released from many different types of cells in the human body. They enable cells to communicate with each other. They act as chemical messengers both within the immune system (discussed in Chapter 16) and between the immune system and other systems of the body. A cell is able to "sense" the presence of a cytokine if it possesses appropriate surface receptors that can recognize the cytokine. The cytokine mediates (causes) some type of response in a cell that is able to sense its presence. Some cytokines are chemoattractants (to be discussed later), recruiting phagocytes to locations where they are needed. Others, like interferons (previously discussed), have a direct role in host defense.

Inflammation

The body normally responds to any local injury, irritation, microbial invasion, or bacterial toxin by a complex series of events collectively referred to as *inflammation* or the *inflammatory response* (Fig. 15-3). The three major events in acute inflammation are:

- an increase in the diameter of capillaries (*vasodilation*), which increases blood flow to the site
- increased permeability of the capillaries, allowing the escape of plasma and plasma proteins
- egress (exit) of leukocytes from the capillaries and their accumulation at the site of injury

The primary purposes of the inflammatory response (Fig. 15-4) are to:

- localize an infection
- prevent the spread of microbial invaders
- neutralize any toxins being produced at the site
- aid in the repair of damaged tissue

During the inflammatory process, many nonspecific host defense mechanisms come into play. These interrelated physiologic reactions result in the four cardinal (main) signs and symptoms of inflammation: redness, heat, swelling (*edema*), and pain. There is often pus formation, and occasionally there is a loss of function of the damaged area (e.g., an inflamed elbow might prevent bending of the arm).

A complex series of physiologic events occurs immediately after the initial damage to the tissue. One of the initial events is vasodilation at the site of injury, mediated by vasoactive agents (e.g., histamine and prostaglandins) released from damaged cells. Vasodilation allows more blood to flow to the site, bringing redness and heat. Additional heat results from increased metabolic activities in the tissue cells at the site. Vasodilation causes the endothelial cells that line the capillaries to stretch and separate, resulting in increased permeability. Plasma escapes from the capillaries into the surrounding area, causing the site to become *edematous* (swollen). Sometimes the swelling is severe enough to interfere with the bending of a particular joint (e.g., knuckle, elbow, knee, ankle), leading to a loss of function.

A variety of chemotactic agents (discussed later) are produced at the site of inflammation, leading to an influx of

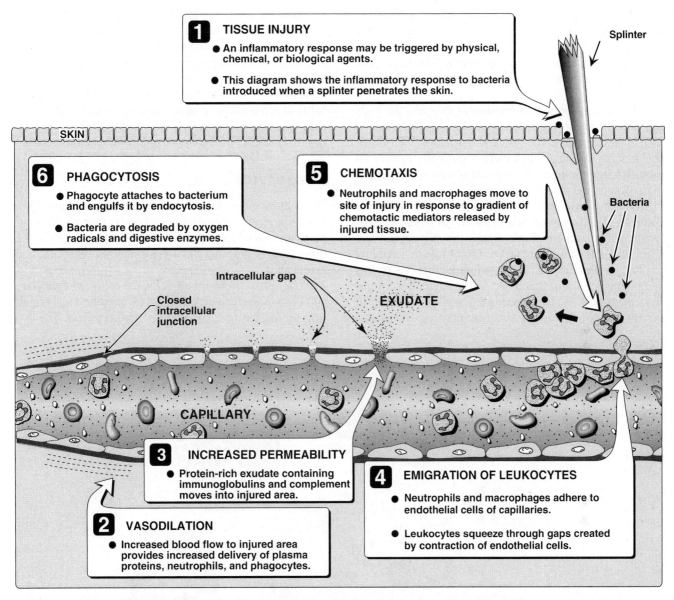

FIGURE 15-3. Sequence of events in inflammation. (Harvey RA, Champe PA (eds.). Lippincott Illustrated Reviews: Microbiology. Philadelphia: Lippincott Williams & Wilkins, 2001.)

phagocytes. The pain or tenderness that accompanies inflammation may result from actual damage of the nerve fibers because of the injury, irritation by microbial toxins or other cellular secretions (such as prostaglandins), or increased pressure on nerve endings because of the edema.

The accumulation of fluid, cells, and cellular debris at the inflammation site is referred to as an ***inflammatory exudate.*** If the exudate is thick and greenish-yellow, containing many live and dead leukocytes, it is known as a ***purulent exudate*** or *pus.* However, in many inflammatory responses, such as arthritis or pancreatitis, there is no exudate and no invading microorganisms. When ***pyogenic microorganisms*** (pus-producing microorganisms), such as staphylococci and streptococci, are present, additional pus is

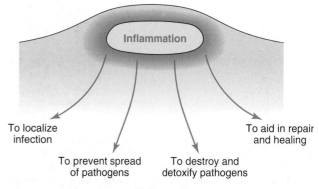

FIGURE 15-4. The purposes of inflammation.

produced as a result of the killing effect of the bacterial toxins on phagocytes and tissue cells. Although most pus is greenish-yellow, the exudate is often bluish-green in infections caused by *Pseudomonas aeruginosa*. This is caused by the bluish-green pigment (called pyocyanin) produced by this organism.

When the inflammatory response is over and the body has won the battle, the phagocytes clean up the area and help to restore order. The cells and tissues can then repair the damage and begin to function normally again in a homeostatic (equilibrated) state, although some permanent damage and scarring may result.

The lymphatic system—including lymph (the fluid component of the lymphatic system), lymphatic vessels, lymph nodes, and lymphatic organs (tonsils, spleen, and thymus gland)—also plays an important role in defending the body against invaders. The primary functions of this system include draining and circulating intercellular fluids from the tissues and transporting digested fats from the digestive system to the blood. Also, macrophages, B cells, and

T cells in the lymph nodes serve to filter the lymph by removing foreign matter and microbes, and by producing antibodies and other factors to aid in the destruction and detoxification of any invading microorganisms.

The body continually wages war against damage, injury, malfunction, and microbial invasion. The outcome of each battle depends on the person's age, hormonal balance, genetic resistance, and overall state of physical and mental health, as well as the virulence of the pathogens involved.

Phagocytosis

The cellular elements of blood are shown in Figure 15-5. The three major categories of leukocytes that are found in blood are monocytes, lymphocytes, and granulocytes. The three types of granulocytes are eosinophils, basophils, and neutrophils.

Phagocytic white blood cells are called ***phagocytes,*** and the process by which phagocytes surround and engulf (ingest) foreign material is called ***phagocytosis.*** The two

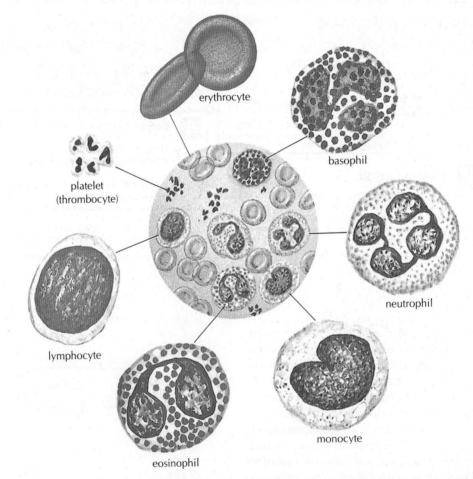

FIGURE 15-5. Cellular elements of the blood, as seen in a Wright's-stained peripheral blood smear. Wright's stain contains two dyes: eosin (a reddish-orange acidic dye, which stains basic substances) and methylene blue (a dark blue dye, which stains acidic substances). Eosinophil granules stain reddish-orange because their contents are basic and, therefore, attract the acidic dye. Basophil granules stain dark blue because their contents are acidic and, therefore, attract the basic dye. The contents of neutrophil granules are neutral (neither basic nor acidic) and, therefore attract neither the acidic dye nor the basic dye. (McCall RE, Tankersley CM. Phlebotomy Essentials, 2nd ed. Philadelphia: Lippincott-Raven Publishers, 1998.)

Cellular Elements of Blood

Erythrocytes (red blood cells)
Thrombocytes (platelets)
Leukocytes (white blood cells)
    Granulocytes
        Basophils
        Eosinophils
        Neutrophils
    Monocytes/Macrophages
    Lymphocytes
        B cells
        T cells
            Helper T cells (T_H cells)
            Cytotoxic T cells (T_C cells)
        Natural killer cells (NK cells)

TABLE 15-1

Four Steps in Phagocytosis

STEP	BRIEF DESCRIPTION
1. Chemotaxis	Phagocytes are attracted by chemotactic agents to the site where they are needed
2. Attachment	A phagocyte attaches to an object
3. Ingestion	Pseudopodia surround the object, and it is taken into the cell
4. Digestion	The object is broken down and dissolved by digestive enzymes and other mechanisms

most important groups of phagocytes in the human body are macrophages and neutrophils; they are sometimes called "professional phagocytes," because phagocytosis is their major function. Macrophages serve as a "clean-up crew" to rid the body of unwanted and often harmful substances, such as dead cells, unused cellular secretions, debris, and microorganisms.

Granulocytes are named for the prominent cytoplasmic granules that they possess. Phagocytic granulocytes include *neutrophils* and *eosinophils.* Neutrophils (also known as polymorphonuclear cells, polys, and PMNs) are much more efficient at phagocytosis than eosinophils. An abnormally high number of eosinophils in the peripheral bloodstream is known as *eosinophilia.* Examples of conditions that cause eosinophilia are allergies and helminth infections. A third type of granulocyte, *basophils,* are also involved in allergic and inflammatory reactions, although they are not phagocytes. Basophil granules contain histamine and other chemical mediators. Basophils are discussed in Chapter 16.

Macrophages develop from a type of leukocyte called *monocytes* during the inflammatory response to infections. Those that leave the bloodstream and migrate to infected areas are called *wandering macrophages. Fixed macrophages* (also known as *histocytes* or *histiocytes*) remain in tissues and organs and serve to trap foreign debris. Macrophages are extremely efficient phagocytes. They are found in tissues of the *reticuloendothelial system (RES).* This nonspecific defensive system includes cells in the liver (Kupffer cells), spleen, lymph nodes, and bone marrow as well as the lungs (alveolar or dust cells), blood vessels, intestines, and brain (microglia). The principal function of the entire RES is the engulfment and removal of foreign

and useless particles, living or dead, such as excess cellular secretions, dead and dying leukocytes, erythrocytes, and tissue cells as well as foreign debris and microorganisms that gain entrance to the body.

The four steps in phagocytosis are discussed below and are summarized in Table 15-1.

Chemotaxis

Phagocytosis begins when phagocytes move to the site where they are needed. This directed migration is called *chemotaxis* and is the result of chemical attractants called *chemotactic agents* (also called chemotactic factors, chemotactic substances, and chemoattractants). Chemotactic agents that are produced by various cells of the human body are called *chemokines.*[a] Chemotactic agents are produced during the complement cascade and inflammation. The phagocytes move along a concentration gradient, meaning that they move from areas of low concentrations of chemotactic agents to the area of highest concentration. The area of highest concentration is the site where the chemotactic agents are being produced or released—often the site of inflammation. Thus, the phagocytes are attracted to the site where they are needed. Different types of chemotactic agents attract different types of leukocytes; some attract monocytes, others neutrophils, and still others eosinophils.

[a]Various types of cells within the human body, including cells of the immune system, communicate with each other. They do so by means of chemical messages—proteins known as cytokines. If the cytokines are chemotactic agents, attracting leukocytes to areas where they are needed, they are referred to as chemokines.

Attachment

The next step in phagocytosis is attachment of the phagocyte to the object (e.g., a yeast or bacterial cell) to be ingested. Phagocytes can only ingest objects to which they can attach. As previously mentioned, opsonization is sometimes necessary to enable phagocytes to attach to certain particles (e.g., encapsulated bacteria). The particle becomes coated with opsonins (either complement fragments or antibodies). Because the phagocyte possesses surface molecules (receptors) for complement fragments and antibodies, the phagocyte can now attach to the particle (Fig. 15-6).

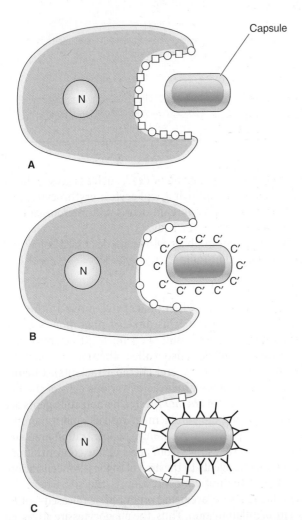

Capsule

A

B

C

FIGURE 15-6. Opsonization. (*A*) The phagocyte shown here is unable to attach to the encapsulated bacterium because there are no molecules (receptors) on the surface of the phagocyte that can recognize or attach to the polysaccharide capsule. (*B*) Complement fragments (represented by the symbol C′) have been deposited onto the surface of the capsule. (In this example, the opsonins are complement fragments.) Now the phagocyte can attach to the bacterium because there are receptors (represented by ○ on the phagocyte's surface that can recognize and bind to complement fragments. (*C*) Antibodies (the Y-shaped molecules) have attached to the capsule. (In this example, the opsonins are antibodies.) Now the phagocyte can attach to the bacterium because there are receptors (represented by □ on the phagocyte's surface that can recognize and bind to the Fc region of antibody molecules. (See text for additional details.) N = nucleus.

Ingestion

The phagocyte then surrounds the object with pseudopodia, which fuse together, and the object is ingested (phagocytized or phagocytosed) (Fig. 15-7). Phagocytosis is one type of endocytosis, the process of ingesting material from outside a cell. Within the cytoplasm of the phagocyte, the object is contained within a membrane-bound vesicle called a ***phagosome.***

Digestion

The phagosome next fuses with a nearby lysosome to form a digestive vacuole (***phagolysosome***), within which killing and digestion occur (Fig. 15-8). Recall from Chapter 3 that lysosomes are membrane-bound vesicles containing digestive enzymes. Digestive enzymes found within lysosomes include lysozyme, β-lysin, lipases, proteases, peptidases, DNAses, and RNases, which degrade carbohydrates, lipids, proteins, and nucleic acids.

Other mechanisms also participate in the destruction of phagocytized microorganisms. In neutrophils, for example, a membrane-bound enzyme called NADPH oxidase reduces oxygen to very destructive products such as superoxide anions, hydroxyl radicals, hydrogen peroxide, and singlet oxygen. These highly reactive reduction products assist in the destruction of the ingested microbes. Another killing mechanism involves the enzyme myeloperoxidase. After lysosome fusion, myeloperoxidase is released, which in the presence of hydrogen peroxide and chloride ion, produces a potent microbicidal agent called hypochlorous acid.

Figures 15-9 and 15-10 depict various stages in the phagocytosis of *Giardia lamblia* trophozoites by rat leukocytes. *G. lamblia* (also known as *Giardia intestinalis*) is a flagellated protozoan parasite that causes a diarrheal disease known as giardiasis. These electron micrographs were taken during a laboratory research project involving opsonization of *Giardia* trophozoites.

Mechanisms by Which Pathogens Escape Destruction by Phagocytes

During the initial phases of infection, capsules serve an antiphagocytic function, protecting encapsulated bacteria from being phagocytized. Some bacteria produce an exoenzyme (or toxin) called *leukocidin*, which kills phagocytes. As mentioned in Chapter 14, not all bacteria engulfed by phagocytes are destroyed within phagolysosomes. For example, waxes in the cell wall of *Mycobacterium tuberculosis* protect the organism from digestion. The bacteria are even able to multiply within the phagocytes and are transported within them to other parts of the body. Other pathogens that are able to survive within phagocytes include bacteria such as *Rickettsia rickettsii, Legionella pneumophila, Brucella abortus, Coxiella burnetii, Listeria monocytogenes,* and *Salmonella,* as well as protozoan parasites such as *Toxoplasma gondii, Trypanosoma cruzi,* and *Leishmania* spp. The mechanism by which each pathogen evades digestion by lysosomal enzymes differs from one pathogen to another; in some cases, the

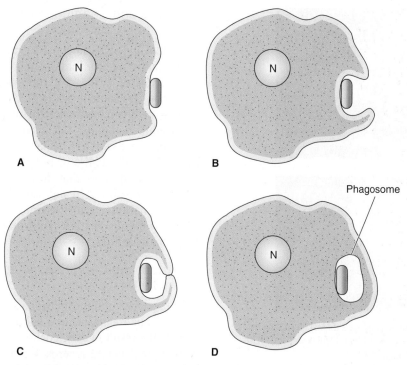

FIGURE 15-7. The ingestion phase of phagocytosis. (*A*) A phagocyte has attached to a bacterial cell. (*B*) Pseudopodia extend around the bacterial cell. (*C*) The pseudopodia meet and fuse together. (*D*) The bacterial cell, surrounded by a membrane, is now inside the phagocyte. The membrane-bound structure, containing the ingested bacterial cell, is called a phagosome. N = nucleus.

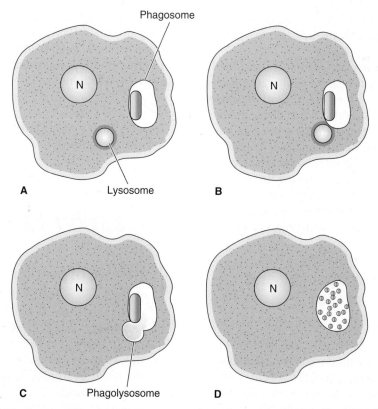

FIGURE 15-8. The digestion phase of phagocytosis. (*A*) A lysosome, containing digestive enzymes, approaches a phagosome. (*B*) The lysosome membrane fuses with the phagosome membrane. (*C*) The lysosome and phagosome become a single membrane-bound vesicle, known as a phagolysosome. The phagolysosome contains the ingested bacterial cell plus digestive enzymes. (*D*) The bacterial cell is digested within the phagolysosome. N = nucleus.

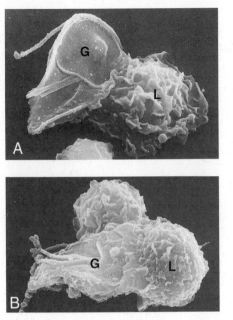

FIGURE 15-9. Scanning electron micrographs (SEMs) illustrating the phagocytosis of *Giardia* trophozoites (G) by rat leukocytes (L). (SEMs courtesy of S. Erlandsen and P. Engelkirk.)

mechanism is not yet understood. These pathogens may remain dormant within phagocytes for months or years before they escape to cause disease. Thus, these types of virulent pathogens usually win the battle with phagocytes. Unless antibodies or complement fragments are present to aid in the destruction of these pathogens, the infection may progress unchecked.

Ehrlichia and *Anaplasma* spp., closely related to rickettsias, are obligate, intracellular, Gram-negative bacteria that live within leukocytes (i.e., they are *intraleukocytic pathogens*). These organisms cause two endemic, tickborne diseases in the United States. *Ehrlichia* spp. cause human monocytic ehrlichiosis (HME), a condition in which the bacteria infect monocytic phagocytes. *Anaplasma* spp. cause human anaplasmosis (or human granulocytic ehrlichiosis [HE], as it is sometimes called), a condition in which the bacteria infect granulocytes. The bacteria are somehow able to prevent the fusion of lysosomes with phagosomes.

Disorders and Conditions That Adversely Affect Phagocytic and Inflammatory Processes

Leukopenia

Some patients have an abnormally low number of circulating leukocytes—a condition known as *leukopenia.* (Although the terms *leukopenia* and *neutropenia* are often used synonymously, they are not synonyms. Technically, neutropenia is an abnormally low number of circulating neutrophils; neutropenia = neutrophilic leukopenia.) Leukopenia may result from bone marrow injury as a result of ionizing radiation or drugs, nutritional deficiencies, or congenital stem cell defects.

Disorders and Conditions Affecting Leukocyte Motility and Chemotaxis

The inability of leukocytes to migrate in response to chemotactic agents may be related to a defect in the production of actin, a structural protein associated with motility. Some drugs (e.g., corticosteroids) can also inhibit the chemotactic activity of leukocytes. Decreased neutrophil chemotaxis also occurs in the inherited childhood disease known as Chediak-Higashi syndrome (CHS). In addition, the PMNs of individuals with CHS contain abnormal lysosomes that do not readily fuse with phagosomes, resulting in decreased bactericidal activity. CHS is characterized by symptoms such as albinism, central nervous system abnormalities, and recurrent bacterial infections.

Disorders and Conditions Affecting Intracellular Killing by Phagocytes

The phagocytes of some individuals are capable of ingesting bacteria, but are incapable of killing certain species. This is usually the result of deficiencies in myeloperoxidase or an inability to generate superoxide anion, hydrogen peroxide, or hypochlorite. Chronic granulomatous disease (CGD) is an often-fatal genetic disorder that is characterized by repeated bacterial infections. The PMNs of individuals with CGD can ingest bacteria but cannot kill certain species. In one form of CGD, the person's PMNs are unable to produce hydrogen peroxide. In another hereditary disorder, the individual's PMNs completely lack myeloperoxidase. Their PMNs do possess other microbicidal mechanisms, however, so these individuals usually do not experience recurrent infections.

Additional Factors

Table 15-2 lists some additional factors that can impair host defense mechanisms.

○ STUDY AID

Beware of Similar Sounding Words

When a patient has an abnormally low number of circulating leukocytes, the condition is known as **leukopenia**. When a patient has an abnormally high number of circulating leukocytes, the condition is known as **leukocytosis** (which is usually the result of an infection). **Leukemia** is a type of cancer in which there is a proliferation of abnormal leukocytes in the blood. Actually, there are several different types of leukemia, classified by the dominant type of leukocyte.

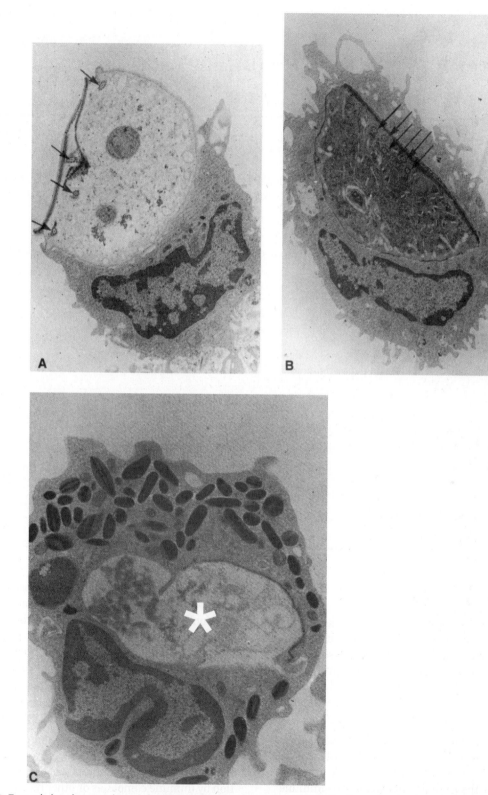

FIGURE 15-10. Transmission electron micrographs (TEMs) illustrating the phagocytosis of *Giardia* trophozoites by rat leukocytes. (*A*) Attachment. (*B*) Ingestion. (*C*) Digestion. Note the cross-sections of flagella (arrows) in A and B, and the phagolysosome (*) and darkly stained granules in the eosinophil shown in C. (TEMs courtesy of S. Koester and P. Engelkirk.)

TABLE 15-2

Additional Factors That Can Impair Host Defense Mechanisms

FACTOR	COMMENTS
Nutritional status	Malnutrition is accompanied by decreased resistance to infections
Increased iron levels	High concentrations of iron make it easier for bacteria to satisfy their iron requirements; high concentrations of iron reduce the chemotactic and phagocytic activities of phagocytes; increased iron levels may result from a variety of conditions or habits
Stress	People living under stressful conditions are more susceptible to infections than people living under less stressful conditions
Age	Newborn infants lack a fully developed immune system; the efficiency of the immune system and other host defenses declines after age 50
Cancer and cancer chemotherapy	Cancer chemotherapeutic agents kill healthy cells and malignant ones
AIDS	Destruction of the AIDS patient's helper T cells (T_H cells) decreases the patient's ability to produce antibodies to certain pathogens (discussed in Chapter 16)
Drugs	Steroids and alcohol, for example
Various genetic defects	B-cell and T-cell deficiencies, for example

REVIEW OF KEY POINTS

- Certain human host defense mechanisms are classified as nonspecific, whereas others are classified as specific. Nonspecific host defense mechanisms serve to protect the body from a variety of foreign substances or pathogens. Specific host defense mechanisms are directed against a particular foreign substance or pathogen that has entered the body.

- Another way to categorize host defense mechanisms is to divide them into first, second, and third lines of defense. The first and second lines of defense are nonspecific, whereas the third line of defense (the immune system) is specific.

- The first line of defense includes innate or inborn resistance; physical barriers such as intact skin and intact mucous membranes; chemical, physiologic, and temperature barriers; microbial antagonism by indigenous microflora; and overall nutritional status and state of health.

- The second line of defense includes nonspecific cellular and chemical responses such as inflammation, fever, interferon production, activation of the complement system, iron balance, cellular secretions, activation of blood proteins, chemotaxis, phagocytosis, neutralization of toxins, and the cleanup and repair of damaged tissues.

- Interferons are small, antiviral proteins that prevent viral multiplication in virus-infected cells and serve to limit viral infections.

- The complement system involves approximately 30 different blood proteins that interact in a stepwise manner known as the complement cascade. Complement activation by immune complexes or other mechanisms aids in the initiation and amplification of inflammation, attraction and activation of leukocytes, lysis of bacteria and other foreign cells, and enhanced phagocytosis (opsonization).

- Fever is a nonspecific host defense mechanism that augments host defenses by stimulating leukocytes to deploy and destroy invaders, reducing available free plasma iron, and inducing the production of IL-1, which causes the proliferation, maturation, and activation of lymphocytes in the immunologic response. Elevated body temperatures also slow down the rate of growth of certain pathogens and kill especially fastidious pathogens. Substances that invoke fever are referred to as pyrogens.

- Phagocytes rid the body of unwanted or harmful substances, such as dead cells, unused cellular secretions, dust, debris, and pathogens. After their recruitment to a particular site by chemotactic substances, they attach to, surround, ingest, and digest the unwanted or harmful substances.

- The four steps in phagocytosis are chemotaxis, attachment, ingestion, and digestion.

- Indications of inflammation include redness, heat, edema, and pain. Inflammation is often accompanied by pus formation, and sometimes there is a loss of function of the inflamed part of the body. The purposes of the inflammatory response are to localize an infection, prevent the spread of microbial invaders, neutralize toxins, and aid in the repair of damaged tissue.

- Lactoferrin and transferrin are host molecules that tie up iron, thereby preventing pathogens access to this essential mineral.

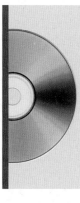

On the CD-ROM

- Increase Your Knowledge
- Microbiology—Hollywood Style
- Critical Thinking
- Additional Self-Assessment Exercises

Self-Assessment Exercises

After studying this chapter, answer the following multiple-choice questions.

1. Host defense mechanisms—ways in which the body protects itself from pathogens—can be thought of as an army consisting of how many lines of defense?
   a. 2
   b. 3
   c. 4
   d. 5

2. Which of the following is *not* part of the body's first line of defense?
   a. fever
   b. intact skin
   c. mucus
   d. pH of the stomach contents

3. Each of the following is considered a part of the body's second line of defense except:
   a. fever.
   b. inflammation.
   c. interferons.
   d. lysozyme.

4. Which of the following is *not* a consequence of activation of the complement system?
   a. attraction and activation of leukocytes
   b. increased phagocytosis by phagocytic cells (opsonization)
   c. lysis of bacteria and other foreign cells
   d. repair of damaged tissue

5. Each of the following is a primary purpose of the inflammatory response except:
   a. to localize the infection.
   b. to neutralize any toxins being produced at the site.
   c. to prevent the spread of microbial invaders.
   d. to stimulate the production of opsonins.

6. Which of the following cells is a granulocyte?
   a. eosinophil
   b. lymphocyte
   c. macrophage
   d. monocyte

7. All the following would be considered an aspect of microbial antagonism except:
   a. competition for nutrients.
   b. competition for space.
   c. production of bacteriocins.
   d. production of lysozyme.

8. Which of the following function as opsonins?
   a. antibodies
   b. antigens
   c. complement fragments
   d. both a and c

9. Which of the following statements about interferons is false?
   a. Interferons are virus-specific.
   b. Interferons have been used to treat hepatitis C and certain types of cancer.
   c. Interferons produced by a virus-infected cell will not save that cell from destruction.
   d. Interferons produced by virus-infected rabbit cells cannot be used to treat viral diseases in humans.

10. Which of the following is *not* one of the four cardinal signs or symptoms of inflammation?
   a. edema
   b. heat
   c. loss of function
   d. redness

16

SPECIFIC HOST DEFENSE MECHANISMS: AN INTRODUCTION TO IMMUNOLOGY

LEARNING OBJECTIVES

AFTER STUDYING THIS CHAPTER, YOU SHOULD BE ABLE TO:

- Define the following terms: immunology, immunity, antigenic determinant, immunoglobulins, primary response, secondary response, agammaglobulinemia, hypogammaglobulinemia, T cell, B cell, plasma cell, and immunosuppression
- Differentiate between humoral and cell-mediated immunity
- Distinguish between active acquired immunity and passive acquired immunity
- Distinguish between natural active acquired immunity and artificial active acquired immunity and cite an example of each

- Distinguish between natural passive acquired immunity and artificial passive acquired immunity and cite an example of each
- Outline the steps involved in the processing of T-independent antigens and T-dependent antigens
- Identify the two primary functions of the immune system
- Construct a diagram of a monomeric antibody molecule
- Identify and describe the five immunoglobulin classes (isotypes)
- List the types of cells that are killed by NK cells
- Name the four types of hypersensitivity reactions
- Outline the steps involved in allergic reactions, starting with the initial sensitization to an allergen and ending with the typical symptoms of an allergic reaction
- Cite six examples of allergens
- List five possible explanations for a positive TB skin test

INTRODUCTION

Immunology is the scientific study of the immune system and immune responses. Immune responses involve complex interactions among many different types of body cells and cellular secretions. Only certain basic fundamentals of immunology and immune responses are presented in this chapter. Topics briefly discussed here include active and passive acquired immunity to infectious agents, vaccines, antigens and antibodies, processes involved in antibody production, cell-mediated immune responses, allergies and other types of hypersensitivity reactions, autoimmune diseases, immunosuppression, and immunodiagnostic procedures.

According to accepted doctrine, the primary functions of the immune system are to (1) differentiate between "self" and "non-self" (something foreign), and (2) destroy that which is non-self.[a] As stated earlier, the immune system involves very complex interactions among many different types of cells and cellular secretions. Although it encompasses the whole body, the lymphatic system is the site and source of most immune activity. The cells involved in the immune responses originate in bone marrow, from which most blood cells develop. Three lines of lymphocytes—B lymphocytes (or B cells), T lymphocytes (or T cells), and natural killer (NK) cells—are derived from lymphoid stem cells of bone marrow.

There are two major types or categories of T cells; helper T cells and cytotoxic T cells. **Helper T cells** are also known as T helper cells, T_H cells, and CD4$^+$ T cells. The term CD4$^+$ cells refers to the fact that these cells possess on their surface an antigen designated as CD4. The primary function of

helper T cells is secretion of cytokines. T_H1 cells and T_H2 cells are subcategories of helper T cells. Cytokines secreted by T_H1 cells (referred to as type 1 cytokines) support cell-mediated immune responses (described below), involving macrophages, cytotoxic T cells, and NK cells. Cytokines secreted by T_H2 cells (referred to as type 2 cytokines) support humoral immune responses (described below) by inducing B-cell activation and differentiation of activated B cells into plasma cells.

Cytotoxic T cells are also known as T cytotoxic cells, T_C cells, and CD8$^+$ cells. The term CD8$^+$ cells refers to the fact that these cells possess on their surface an antigen designated as CD8. The primary function of cytotoxic T cells is destruction of virally infected host cells.

There are two major arms of the immune system: humoral immunity and cell-mediated immunity (Fig. 16-1).

---

[a] An Alternative Viewpoint. For more than 50 years, immunologists have relied on the self/non-self theory of immunity, which states that the immune system reacts to, or "does battle with," non-self (foreign molecules), but does not react to self (molecules that are part of the human body). However, there are certain immunologic events that are seemingly at odds with this theory. Recently, an alternative model of immunity has been proposed, called the Danger Model. This model "suggests that the immune system is more concerned with [tissue] damage than with foreignness, and is called into action by [danger or] alarm signals [emitted] from injured issues, rather than by the recognition of non-self....When distressed, [the tissues] stimulate immunity, and...they may also determine the [specific type] of [immune] response." The immune response "is tailored to the tissue in which the response occurs, rather than being tailored by the targeted pathogen." Thus, "immunity is controlled by an internal conversation between tissues and the cells of the immune system." (From Matzinger P. The danger model: a renewed sense of self. *Science* 2002;296:301–305.)

○ STUDY AID

The Key to Understanding Immunology

An understanding of immunology boils down to an understanding of two terms: *antigens* and *antibodies*. For the moment, think of antigens as molecules (usually proteins) that stimulate a person's immune system to produce antibodies. Think of antibodies as protein molecules that a person's immune system produces in response to antigens. Later in the chapter, antigens and antibodies will be discussed in more detail. Remember, if you understand antigens and antibodies, you are well on your way to understanding immunology.

○ STUDY AID

Sorting Out the *-Kines*

Various types of cells within the human body, including cells of the immune system, communicate with each other. They do so by means of chemical messages—proteins known as **cytokines.** If the cytokines are chemotactic agents, attracting leukocytes to areas where they are needed, they are referred to as **chemokines.**

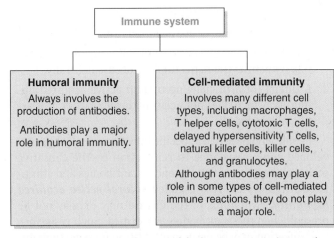

FIGURE 16-1. The two major arms of the immune system. (By permission of the Colorado Association for Continuing Medical Laboratory Education [CACMLE], Denver, CO.)

In *humoral immunity,* special glycoproteins (molecules composed of carbohydrate and protein) called *antibodies* are produced by B cells to recognize, bind with, inactivate, and destroy specific microbes. After their production, these humoral (circulating) antibodies remain in blood plasma, lymph, and other body secretions where they protect against the specific pathogens that stimulated their production. Thus, in humoral immunity, a person is immune to a particular pathogen because of the presence of specific protective antibodies that are effective against that pathogen. Because humoral immunity is mediated by antibodies, it is also known as *antibody-mediated immunity* (AMI).

The second major arm of the immune system—*cell-mediated immunity*—involves a variety of cell types, with antibodies only playing a minor role, if any. These immune responses are referred to as cell-mediated immune responses; they are briefly discussed later in this chapter.

Immunity

Immunity is the condition of being **immune** or resistant to a particular infectious disease. Humans are immune to certain infectious diseases simply because they are humans. For example, humans are not infected with some of the pathogens that infect their pets. One explanation for this is that human cells do not possess the appropriate cell surface receptors for some pathogens that cause diseases of pets. Other reasons for this natural or innate resistance are far more complex and, in some cases, not fully understood, and will not be addressed here.

What will be discussed in this section are the various immunities that humans acquire as life progresses, from conception onward—these types of immunity are collectively referred to as *acquired immunity.* Such immunity is often

HISTORICAL NOTE

Origins of Immunology

Some historians cite Edward Jenner's smallpox vaccine (first administered in 1796) or Louis Pasteur's vaccines against anthrax, cholera, and rabies (developed in the late 1800s) as the origin of the science of immunology. However, neither Jenner nor Pasteur understood how or why their vaccines worked. Most likely, immunology got its start in 1890, when Emil Behring and Kitasato Shibasaburo discovered antibodies while developing a diphtheria antitoxin. At about the same time, Elie Metchnikoff discovered phagocytes and introduced the cellular theory of immunity. By 1910, the main elements of clinical immunology (i.e., allergy, autoimmunity, and transplantation immunity) had been described, and immunochemistry had become a quantitative science. Major advances in immunology began to take shape in the late 1950s, when the focus shifted from serology (investigating antigens and antibodies in serum) to cells. Defining the role of lymphocytes signaled the start of the new era. The emphasis on immune cells and the emergence of the concepts and tools of molecular biology were the two most powerful influences on immunology since its inception. The roots of medical laboratory immunology are found in clinical microbiology—the very first immunologic procedures were designed to diagnose infectious diseases. In some medical facilities (primarily small ones), immunologic procedures are still performed in microbiology laboratories. In larger hospitals and medical centers, immunologic procedures are performed in an Immunology Laboratory, which is separate from the Microbiology Laboratory.

the result of the presence of protective antibodies that are directed against various pathogens.

Acquired Immunity

Immunity that results from the active production or receipt of antibodies during one's lifetime is called *acquired immunity.* If the antibodies are actually produced within the person's body, the immunity is called *active acquired immunity;* such protection is usually long-lasting. In *passive acquired immunity,* the person receives antibodies

Different Uses of the Term *Resistant*

As you have learned in previous chapters, bacteria can become resistant to certain antibiotics, meaning that they are no longer killed by those antibiotics. Such bacteria are said to be drug-resistant. Humans do not become resistant to antibiotics. Humans can become resistant (immune) to certain infectious diseases, however, in ways that are discussed in this chapter.

that were produced by another person or by more than one person, or, in some cases, by an animal; such protection is usually only temporary. In either case—active or passive—the immunity may result from either a natural or an artificial event. The four categories of acquired immunity are summarized in Table 16-1.

TABLE 16-1

Types of Acquired Immunity

Active acquired immunity

Natural active acquired immunity	Immunity that is acquired in response to the entry of a live pathogen into the body (i.e., in response to an actual infection)
Artificial active acquired immunity	Immunity that is acquired in response to vaccines

Passive acquired immunity

Natural passive acquired immunity	Immunity that is acquired by a fetus when it receives maternal antibodies in utero or by an infant when it receives maternal antibodies contained in colostrum
Artificial passive acquired immunity	Immunity that is acquired when a person receives antibodies contained in antisera or gamma globulin

Active Acquired Immunity

There are two types of active acquired immunity:

1. Natural (or naturally occurring) active acquired immunity, which, as the name implies, occurs naturally.
2. Artificial (or artificially occurring) active acquired immunity, which does not occur naturally; rather, it is artificially induced.

People who have had a specific infection usually have developed some resistance to reinfection by the causative pathogen because of the presence of antibodies and stimulated lymphocytes. This is called **natural active acquired immunity.** Symptoms of the disease may or may not be present when these antibodies are formed. Such resistance to reinfection may be permanent, lasting for a person's entire lifetime, or it may only be temporary. There is no immunity to reinfection after recovery from certain infectious diseases, even though antibodies are produced against the causative agents of these diseases. This is because the antibodies that are produced are not **protective antibodies** (i.e., the antibodies that are produced do not protect the person from being reinfected).

Artificial active acquired immunity is the second type of active acquired immunity. This type of immunity results when a person receives a vaccine. The administration of a vaccine (Fig. 16-2) stimulates a person's immune system to produce specific protective antibodies—antibodies that will protect the person should he or she become colonized with that particular pathogen in the future. Vaccines are discussed more fully in the following section.

Vaccines. The mere mention of the names of certain infectious diseases struck fear into the hearts of our ancestors. Today, thanks to childhood vaccines, residents of the United States rarely hear of those diseases, let alone live in fear of them. The Centers for Disease Control and Prevention (CDC) has stated that "Immunizations are one of the great public health success stories of the 20th century, having made once-common diseases such as diphtheria, measles, mumps, and pertussis diseases of the past. Vaccines are now available to protect children and adults against 15 life-threatening or debilitating diseases." (www.cdc.gov/programs/immun.htm)

A **vaccine** is defined as material that can artificially induce immunity to an infectious disease, usually after injection or, in some cases, ingestion of the material (e.g., oral polio vaccine). A person is deliberately exposed to a harmless version of a pathogen (or toxin), which will stimulate that person's immune system to produce protective antibodies and memory cells (described later), but will not cause disease in that person. In this manner, the person's immune system is primed to mount a strong protective response should the actual pathogen (or toxin) be encountered in the future. An ideal vaccine is one that:

- contains enough antigenic determinants to stimulate the immune system to produce protective antibodies

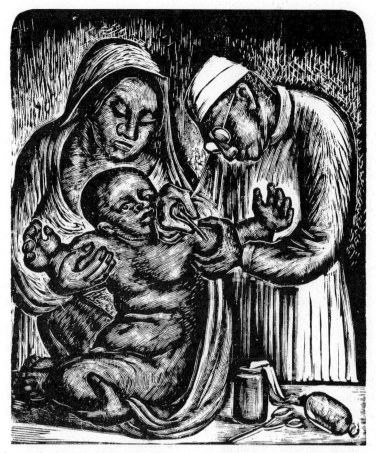

FIGURE 16-2. Vaccination. Wood engraving by Leopoldo Méndez, Mexico, 1935. (Zigrosser C. Medicine and the Artist [Ars Medica]. New York: Dover Publications, Inc., 1970. By permission of the Philadelphia Museum of Art.)

(i.e., antibodies that will protect individuals from infection by the pathogen)

- contains antigenic determinants from all the strains of the pathogen that cause that disease (e.g., the three strains of virus that cause polio); such vaccines are referred to as multivalent or polyvalent vaccines

- has few (preferably, no) side effects

- does not cause disease in the vaccinated person

Types of Vaccines. A variety of materials are used in vaccines (Table 16-2). Most vaccines are made from living or dead (inactivated) pathogens or from certain toxins they produce. The use of such vaccines illustrates a very important and practical application of the principles of microbiology and immunology. In general, vaccines made from living organisms are most effective, but they must be prepared from harmless organisms that are antigenically closely related to the pathogens or from weakened pathogens that have been genetically changed so that they are no longer pathogenic.

As microbiologists made further studies of the characteristics of vaccines, they found that it was practical to vaccinate against several diseases by combining specific vaccines in a single injection. Thus, the diphtheria-tetanus-pertussis (DTP) vaccine contains toxoids to prevent diphtheria and tetanus and portions of killed bacteria (*Bordetella pertussis*) to prevent whooping cough (pertussis). Another example is the measles-mumps-rubella (MMR) vaccine.

According to the CDC, U.S. children should receive the following vaccines between birth and entry into school:

- Hepatitis B (Hep B) vaccine

- Diphtheria toxoid-tetanus toxoid-acellular pertussis (DTaP) vaccine

- *Haemophilus influenzae* type b (HIB) conjugate vaccine

- Inactivated poliovirus (IPV) vaccine

- Measles-mumps-rubella (MMR) vaccine

- Varicella (chickenpox) vaccine

- Pneumococcal conjugate vaccine (PCV)

- Influenza vaccine

- Hepatitis A vaccine (recommended for children with certain risk factors)

(Reference: www.cdc.gov/nip/acip)

HISTORICAL NOTE

Vaccination

Since the time of the ancient Greeks, it has been observed that people who have recovered from certain infectious diseases, such as plague, smallpox, and yellow fever, rarely contract the same diseases again. The use of vaccines to prevent diseases may date as far back as the 11th century, when the Chinese used a powder prepared from dried smallpox scabs to immunize people, either by introducing the powder into a person's skin or by having the person inhale the powder. This method of preventing smallpox—using actual smallpox scabs—was known as the "Chinese method." One of those immunized in this manner was Edward Jenner, a British physician. Some years later, Jenner investigated the widespread belief that milkmaids, who usually had clear, unblemished skin, never developed smallpox. He hypothesized that having had cowpox (a much milder disease than smallpox and one that leaves no scars) protected the milkmaids from getting smallpox. Jenner prepared a smallpox vaccine, using material obtained from cowpox lesions. People injected with Jenner's vaccine were protected from smallpox. The words "vaccine" and "vaccination" come from *vacca,* the Latin word for cow. Because Jenner was the first person to publish (in 1798) the successful results of vaccination, he is generally given credit for originating the concept. During the late 19th century, Louis Pasteur developed successful vaccines to prevent cholera in chickens, anthrax in sheep and cattle, and rabies in dogs and humans. It was actually Pasteur who first used the terms *vaccine* and *vaccination.*

A successful vaccine for colds has not been developed, because so many different types of viruses cause colds. Maintaining a successful vaccine for influenza is also difficult because influenza viruses frequently change their surface antigens—a phenomenon known as *antigenic variation*.

How Vaccines Work. Vaccines stimulate the recipient's immune system to produce protective antibodies. The protective antibodies or memory cells produced in response to the vaccine then remain in the recipient's body to "do battle with" a particular pathogen, should that pathogen enter the recipient's body at some time in the future.

For example, when a person receives tetanus toxoid (an altered form of the toxin, tetanospasmin), protective antibodies referred to as antitoxins are produced. The antitoxins remain in the person's body. Should *Clostridium tetani* enter the person's body at some time in the future, and start to produce tetanospasmin, the antitoxins are there to latch onto and neutralize the toxin.

Some vaccines stimulate the body to produce protective antibodies that are directed against surface antigens. When the pathogen enters the person's body, the antibodies attach to the surface antigens. This prevents the pathogen from adhering to host cells.

In some cases, protective antibodies attached to surface antigens act as opsonins (discussed in Chapter 15), enabling phagocytes to attach to pathogens. Once attached to a pathogen, the phagocyte can ingest and digest it. In other cases, attachment of protective antibodies to surface antigens activates the complement cascade, with the end result being lysis of the pathogen.

Passive Acquired Immunity

Passive acquired immunity differs from active acquired immunity in that antibodies formed in one person are transferred to another to protect the latter from infection. Thus, in passive acquired immunity a person receives antibodies, rather than producing them. Because the person receiving the antibodies did not actively produce them, the immunity is temporary, lasting only about 3 to 6 weeks. The antibodies of passive acquired immunity may be transferred naturally or artificially.

In **natural passive acquired immunity,** small antibodies (like IgG, which is described later in this chapter) present in the mother's blood cross the placenta to reach the fetus while it is in the uterus (in utero). Also, colostrum, the thin, milky fluid secreted by mammary glands a few days before and after delivery, contains maternal antibodies to protect the infant during the first months of life.

Artificial passive acquired immunity is accomplished by transferring antibodies from an immune person to a susceptible person. After a patient has been exposed to a disease, the length of the incubation period usually does not allow sufficient time for postexposure vaccination to be an effective preventive measure. This is because a span of about 2 weeks is needed before sufficient antibodies are formed to protect the exposed person. To provide temporary protection in these situations, the patient is given human gamma globulin or "pooled" immune serum globulin (ISG); that is, antibodies taken from the blood of many immune people. In this manner, the patient receives some antibodies to all of the diseases to which the donors are immune. The ISG may be given to provide temporary protection against measles, mumps, polio, diphtheria, and hepatitis in people, especially infants, who are not immune and have been exposed to these diseases.

Hyperimmune serum globulin (or specific immune globulin) has been prepared from the serum of persons

TABLE 16-2

Types of Available Vaccines

TYPE OF VACCINE	EXAMPLES
Attenuated vaccines. The process of weakening pathogens is called attenuation, and the vaccines are referred to as *attenuated vaccines.* Most live vaccines are avirulent (nonpathogenic) mutant strains of pathogens that have been derived from the virulent (pathogenic) organisms; this is accomplished by growing them for many generations under various conditions or by exposing them to mutagenic chemicals or radiation. Attenuated vaccines should not be administered to immunsuppressed individuals, because even weakened pathogens could cause disease in these persons.	**Attenuated viral vaccines:** adenovirus, chicken pox (varicella), measles (rubeola), mumps, German measles (rubella), polio (oral Sabin vaccine), rotavirus, smallpox, yellow fever **Attenuated bacterial vaccines:** BCG (for protection against tuberculosis), cholera, tularemia, typhoid fever (oral vaccine)
Inactivated vaccines. Vaccines made from pathogens that have been killed by heat or chemicals—called *inactivated vaccines*—can be produced faster and more easily, but they are less effective than live vaccines. This is because the antigens on the dead cells are usually less effective and produce a shorter period of immunity.	**Inactivated viruses or viral antigens:** hepatitis A, influenza, Japanese encephalitis, other (EEE, WEE, Russian) encephalitis vaccines, polio (subcutaneous Salk vaccine), rabies **Inactivated bacterial vaccines:** anthrax, typhoid fever (subcutaneous vaccine), Q fever
Subunit vaccines. A *subunit vaccine* (or *acellular vaccine*) is one that uses antigenic (antibody-stimulating) portions of a pathogen, rather than using the whole pathogen. For example, a vaccine containing pili of *Neisseria gonorrhoeae* could theoretically stimulate the body to produce antibodies that would attach to *N. gonorrhoeae* pili, thus preventing the bacteria from adhering to cells. If *N. gonorrhoeae* cannot adhere to cells that line the urethra, they cannot cause urethritis. The material that is used to protect healthcare workers and others from hepatitis caused by hepatitis B virus (HBV) is being produced by genetically engineered yeasts. The genes that code for hepatitis B surface protein were introduced into yeast cells, which then produced large quantities of that protein. The proteins are then injected into people. Antibodies against the protein are produced in their bodies, and these antibodies serve to protect the people from HBV hepatitis.	Hepatitis B, Lyme disease, whooping cough
Conjugate vaccines. Successful conjugate vaccines have been made by conjugating bacterial capsular antigens (which by themselves are not very antigenic) to molecules that stimulate the immune system to produce antibodies against the less antigenic capsular antigens.	Hib (for protection against *Haemophilus influenzae* type b), meningococcal meningitis (*Neisseria meningitidis* serogroup C), pneumococcal pneumonia
Toxoid vaccines. A **toxoid** is an exotoxin that has been inactivated (made nontoxic) by heat or chemicals. Toxoids can be injected safely to stimulate the production of antibodies that are capable of neutralizing the exotoxins of pathogens, such as those that cause tetanus, botulism, and diphtheria. Antibodies that neutralize toxins are called **antitoxins,** and a serum containing such antitoxins is referred to as an **antiserum.**	Diphtheria, tetanus. Commercial antisera containing antitoxins are used to treat diseases such as tetanus and botulism. Such antisera are also used in certain types of laboratory tests, known as immunodiagnostic procedures.

TABLE 16-2

Types of Available Vaccines (continued)

TYPE OF VACCINE	EXAMPLES
DNA vaccines. Currently, *DNA vaccines* or *gene vaccines* are only experimental. A particular gene from a pathogen is inserted into plasmids, and the plasmids are then injected into skin or muscle tissue. Inside host cells, the genes direct the synthesis of a particular microbial protein (antigen). Once the cells start churning out copies of the protein, the body then produces antibodies directed against the protein, and these antibodies protect the person from infection with the pathogen.	Laboratory animals have been successfully protected using this technique, and reports of the induction of cellular immune responses in humans to a malarial parasite antigen, using DNA vaccines, have been published.
Autogenous vaccines. An *autogenous vaccine* is one that has been prepared from bacteria isolated from a localized infection, such as a staphylococcal boil. The pathogens are killed and then injected into the same person to induce production of more antibodies.	

with high antibody levels (titer) against certain diseases. For example, hepatitis B immune globulin (HBIG) is given to protect those who have been, or are apt to be, exposed to hepatitis B virus; tetanus immune globulin (TIG) is used to prevent tetanus in nonimmunized patients with deep, dirty wounds; and rabies immune globulin (RIG) may be given to

prevent rabies after a person is bitten by a rabid animal. Other examples include chickenpox immune globulin, measles immune globulin, pertussis immune globulin, poliomyelitis immune globulin, and zoster immune globulin. In potentially lethal cases of botulism, antitoxin antibodies are used to neutralize the toxic effects of the botulinal toxin. Remember that passive acquired immunity is always temporary because the antibodies are not actively produced by the B cells of the protected person.

Humoral Immunity

Antigens

Most **antigens** are foreign organic substances that are large enough to stimulate the production of antibodies; in other words, an antigen is an *anti*body-*gen*erating substance. Substances capable of stimulating the production of antibodies are said to be **antigenic.** Antigens may be proteins of more than 10,000 daltons[b] molecular weight, polysaccharides larger than 60,000 daltons, large molecules of DNA or RNA, or any combination of biochemical molecules (e.g., glycoproteins, lipoproteins, and nucleoproteins) that are cellular components of either microorganisms or macroorganisms (e.g., helminths). Foreign proteins are the best antigens.

A bacterial cell has many molecules on its surface capable of stimulating the production of antibodies; these individual molecules or antigenic sites are known as **antigenic**

CAUTIONARY NOTE

"In some surprising ways, we are in danger of becoming the victims of our own success. As our collective memory of infectious diseases like whooping cough and polio fades, the rare complications from vaccination loom large. Because of concerns about such complications, some parents are choosing not to have their children appropriately immunized. This poses a significant threat to the public health, since the microbes that cause the diseases are still very much with us. With the appearance of a large number of susceptible people again, we can expect to see the return of diseases we thought conquered." (From Needham C et al. *Intimate Strangers: Unseen Life on Earth.* Washington, DC: ASM Press, 2000.) The quote is as true today as when it was published.

[b] The term *dalton* is a unit of mass equal to 1/12 the mass of a carbon-12 atom. A dalton is equal to 1 in the atomic mass scale. Daltons are used to express molecular weight.

determinants (or *epitopes*). A bacterial cell could be described as a mosaic of antigenic determinants. The important point is that, in most cases, antigens must be *foreign* materials that the human body does not recognize as *self* antigens. Certainly, all invading microbes fall into this category. Some small molecules called **haptens** may act as antigens only if they are coupled with a large carrier molecule such as a protein. Then the antibodies formed against the antigenic determinant(s) of the hapten may combine with the hapten molecules when they are not coupled with the carrier protein. As an example, penicillin and other low-molecular-weight chemical molecules may act as haptens, causing some people to become allergic (or hypersensitive) to them.

Antibodies

Humoral immunity (or antibody-mediated immunity) involves the production of antibodies, as opposed to cell-mediated immunity (discussed later in this chapter), which does not involve antibody production. *Antibodies* are proteins produced by lymphocytes in response to the presence of an antigen. (As will be described later, the antibody-producing cells are a specific type of lymphocyte called B lymphocytes [or B cells], which usually work in coordination with T lymphocytes [T cells] and macrophages.) A bacterial cell has numerous antigenic determinants on its cell membrane, cell wall, capsule, and flagella that stimulate the production of *many different antibodies*. Usually, an antibody is specific in that it will recognize and bind to only the antigenic determinant that stimulated its production. **Example:** Antibodies produced against molecules located on bacterial pili can only recognize and bind to those particular molecules. Occasionally however, an antibody will bind to an antigenic determinant that is similar, but not identical, in structure to the antigenic determinant that stimulated its production; in this case, it is referred to as a cross-reacting antibody.

All antibodies are in a class of proteins called ***immunoglobulins***—globular glycoproteins in the blood that participate in immune reactions. The term *antibodies* is used to refer to immunoglobulins with particular specificity for an antigen. In addition to being found in blood, immunoglobulins are found in lymph, tears, saliva, and colostrum (Fig. 16-3). Antibodies found in the blood are called humoral or circulating antibodies. Those that provide protection against infectious diseases are called **protective antibodies.**

The amount and type of antibodies produced by a given antigenic stimulation depend on the nature of the antigen, the site of antigenic stimulus, the amount of antigen, and the number of times the person is exposed to the antigen. After the initial exposure to an antigen (such as a vaccine), there is a delayed primary response in the production of antibodies. During this lag phase, the antigen is processed by cells of the immune system.

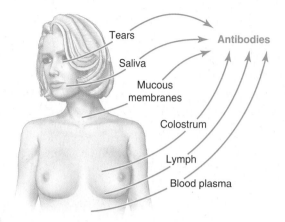

FIGURE 16-3. Body fluids and sites where antibodies are found.

For antibodies to be produced within the body, a complex series of events must occur, some of which are not completely understood. It is known that macrophages, T cells, and B cells often are involved in a cooperative effort. (The processing of antigens within the body is actually far more complex than the abbreviated explanation that follows.)

The majority of antigens are referred to as *T-dependent antigens,* because T cells (specifically, T_H cells) are involved in their processing. In other words, processing of these antigens is *dependent* on T cells. The processing of T-dependent antigens also involves macrophages and B cells. Other antigens are known as *T-independent antigens,* the processing of which requires only B cells. In other words, the processing occurs independently of T cells (see Fig. 16-4). T-independent antigens are large polymeric molecules (usually polysaccharides) containing repeating antigenic determinants; examples include the lipopolysaccharide (LPS) found in the cell walls of Gram-negative bacteria, bacterial flagella, and bacterial capsules. (Table 16-3 summarizes the processing of T-independent and T-dependent antigens.) Note that the processing of either category of antigen—T-independent or T-dependent—results in B cells developing into ***plasma cells*** that are capable of secreting antibodies.

The initial immune response to a particular antigen is called the ***primary response.*** In the primary response to an antigen, it takes about 10 to 14 days for antibodies to be produced. When the antigen is used up, the number of antibodies in the blood declines as the plasma cells die. Other antigen-stimulated B cells become memory cells, which are small lymphocytes that can be stimulated to rapidly produce large quantities of antibodies when later exposed to the same antigens. This increased production of antibodies after the second exposure to the antigen (e.g., a booster shot) is called the ***secondary response,*** *anamnestic response,* or *memory response.* A second booster shot of antigen many months later causes the antibody concentration to exceed the level of the secondary response. This is the reason why booster shots are given to protect against certain pathogens

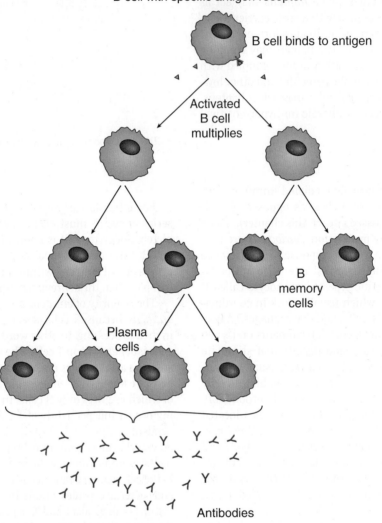

FIGURE 16-4. Processing of T-independent antigens (see text for details).

that one might encounter throughout life, such as the bacterium *C. tetani* (the cause of tetanus). In addition to memory B cells, memory T cells also contribute to immunologic memory.

Where Do Immune Responses Occur?

Immune responses to antigens in the blood are usually initiated in the spleen, whereas responses to microbes and other antigens in tissues are generated in lymph nodes located near the affected area. Antigens entering the body through mucosal surfaces (e.g., after inhalation or ingestion) activate immune responses in mucosa-associated lymphoid tissues. For example, immune responses to in-

tranasal and inhaled antigens occur in the tonsils and adenoids. Ingested antigens enter specialized epithelial cells called microfold or M cells, which then transport the antigens to Peyer's patches in the intestinal mucosa, where the immune responses are initiated. All of the various types of cells (macrophages, B cells, T cells, etc.) that collaborate to produce immune responses are present at these sites (spleen, lymph nodes, tonsils, adenoids, Peyer's patches).

Antibody Structure and Function

Antibodies belong to a class of glycoproteins called immunoglobulins. All antibodies are immunoglobulins, but not all immunoglobulins are antibodies. (However, in this

TABLE 16-3

Mechanisms by Which T-Dependent and T-Independent Antigens Are Processed by the Immune System

T-INDEPENDENT ANTIGEN	T-DEPENDENT ANTIGEN
Processing of T-independent antigens is initiated when an appropriate B cell makes physical contact with the free antigenic determinant (i.e., an antigenic determinant not bound to a major histocompatibility complex [MHC] molecule[a]).	After invasion of the body, an antigen (e.g., a bacterial cell) is ingested and digested by a macrophage
↓	↓
The activated B cell next undergoes extensive cell division, producing a clone of identical B cells	Within the macrophage, antigenic determinants of the bacterial cell (referred to as antigenic peptides or APs) attach to molecules called major histocompatibility complex (MHC) molecules
↓	↓
Some of the members of the newly formed clone mature into antibody-producing plasma cells, whereas others become memory cells (Fig. 16-4)	The combined AP-MHC molecules are then displayed on the surface of the macrophage; at this point, the macrophage is referred to as an **antigen-presenting cell** (APC).
	↓
	A T$_H$ cell attaches to one of the AP-MHC molecules, divides, and "sends out" (secretes) chemical signals (cytokines). (Note that T$_H$ cells assist in the production of antibodies, but do not manufacture antibodies themselves.)
	↓
	When the chemical signals reach a B cell that is capable of recognizing that particular signal, the activated B cell divides, producing a clone of identical B cells.
	↓
	Some of the members of the newly formed clone mature into antibody-producing plasma cells. Antibodies are expelled rapidly for several days until the plasma cell dies. Each plasma cell makes only one type of antibody; one that will bind with the antigenic determinant that activated the B cell and stimulated production of that antibody. Members of the clone that do not become plasma cells, and some of the activated T cells, remain in the body as memory cells, able to respond very quickly should the antigen enter the body again at a later date.

[a]Major histocompatibility complex (MHC) molecules are cell surface molecules that play roles in antigen presentation and rejection of foreign tissue transplants.

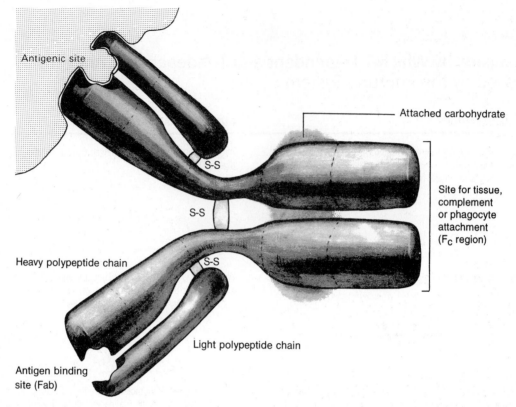

Antigenic site

Attached carbohydrate

S-S

Site for tissue, complement or phagocyte attachment (F$_C$ region)

S-S

Heavy polypeptide chain

S-S

Light polypeptide chain

Antigen binding site (Fab)

FIGURE 16-5. Basic structure of IgG.

book, the terms are used synonymously.) Antibodies are produced by plasma cells in response to stimulation of B cells by foreign antigens. Antibodies found in the blood are called humoral or circulating antibodies. Those that provide protection against infectious diseases are called *protective antibodies.*

The basic structure of an immunoglobulin molecule resembles the letter Y (Fig. 16-5). It consists of two identical light polypeptide chains, two identical heavy polypeptide chains, two antigen-binding sites, and an F$_C$ region. In this basic form, the molecule is referred to as a monomer. The light chains, which contain fewer amino acids than the heavy chains, are shorter and lighter in weight than the heavy chains. The chains are connected to each other by disulfide (—S—S—) bonds. The monomer is bivalent in the sense that it has two sites (called *antigen-binding sites*) that can bind specifically to the antigenic determinant that stimulated production of that antibody. The F$_C$ region enables the molecule to bind to cells (e.g., neutrophils, macrophages, basophils, mast cells) that possess surface receptors able to recognize the F$_C$ region.

Studies of the gamma globulin component of human blood have revealed that five classes (or *isotypes*) of immunoglobulins exist; they are designated IgA, IgD, IgE, IgG, and IgM (Ig stands for immunoglobulin). IgA and IgG have subclasses. Information about each of these classes is presented in Table 16-4.

Monoclonal Antibodies

Purified antibodies that are directed against specific antigens have been produced in laboratories by an innovative technique in which a single plasma cell that produces only one specific type of antibody is fused with a rapidly dividing tumor cell. The new long-lived, antibody-producing cell is called a **hybridoma.** These hybridomas are capable of producing large amounts of specific antibodies called **monoclonal antibodies.** The first monoclonal antibodies were produced in 1975; since then, many uses have been found for them. They are commonly used in **immunodiagnostic procedures (IDPs)**—immunologic procedures used in laboratories to diagnose diseases. The first diagnostic kit containing monoclonal antibodies was approved for use in the United States in 1981. Many other monoclonal antibody–based IDPs have been developed during the past 25 years. Monoclonal antibodies are also being evaluated for possible use in fighting diseases, killing tumor cells, boosting the immune system, and preventing organ rejection.

Antigen–Antibody Complexes

When an antibody combines with an antigen, an **antigen–antibody complex** (or *immune complex*) is formed. Antigen–antibody complexes are capable of activating the complement cascade (by the classical pathway),

TABLE 16-4

Immunoglobulin Classes

IG CLASS	MOLECULAR WEIGHT (IN DALTONS)	% OF TOTAL IG IN SERUM (APPROXIMATE)	FUNCTIONS
IgA	160,000 to 385,000; can exist as a monomer or as a dimer (two monomers held together by a short protein chain called a J-chain ["J" for joining])	10 to 20	The predominant immunoglobulin class in saliva, tears, seminal fluid, colostrum, breast milk, and mucous secretions of the nose, lungs, and gastrointestinal tract. In secretions, IgA is primarily present as secretory IgA (sIgA), a dimer that contains an additional protein called the secretory component. The secretory component apparently facilitates the transport of sIgA into secretions and may serve to protect the IgA molecule from enzymatic damage within the gastrointestinal tract. Protects external openings and mucous membranes from the attachment, colonization, and invasion of pathogens. IgA in colostrum and breast milk helps protect nursing newborns. In the intestine, IgA attaches to viruses, bacteria, and protozoal parasites, such as *Entamoeba histolytica,* and prevents the pathogens from adhering to mucosal surfaces, thus preventing invasion.
IgD	180,000 to 184,000 (a monomer)	<1	Found in large quantities on the surface of B cells. Its function is unknown, but it is possible that the IgD molecules on the B cell's surface serve as antigen receptors and determine which specific antigen that particular B cell is able to respond to.
IgE	188,000 to 200,000 (a monomer)	<1	In atopic individuals, IgE is produced in response to allergens. Found on the surfaces of basophils and mast cells. Plays a major role in allergic responses. (Basophils are granulocytes that circulate in the blood. Mast cells are morphologically very similar to basophils, but they are found in tissues—especially tissues that surround the eyes, nose, respiratory tract, and gastrointestinal tract.)
IgG	146,000 to 170,000 (a monomer; the lightest of the immunoglobulins)	70 to 85 (the most abundant immunoglobulin type in serum)	The only class of immunoglobulin that can cross the placenta. Maternal IgG antibodies that cross the placenta help protect the newborn during its first months of life. Antigen-bound IgG can bind to and activate complement, a process known as "complement fixation." IgG molecules can bind to a wide range of cellular receptors to promote phagocytosis and antibody-dependent cytotoxicity. As a result of memory cells, high levels of IgG are produced very rapidly (within 1 to 3 days) during the secondary response to antigens (described earlier). IgG antibodies are long-lived, sometimes persisting for the lifetime of the individual.
IgM	900,000 to 970,000 (a pentamer, consisting of five monomers held together by a J-chain; the largest of the immunoglobulins)	10	Because a pentamer has 10 antigen-binding sites, IgM can potentially bind to 10 identical antigenic determinants. Theoretically, an IgM molecule could bind to 10 separate virus particles, thus preventing the viruses from attaching to target cells. IgM antibodies are the first antibodies formed in the primary response to antigens (including pathogens), although IgG antibodies later become the most prevalent class. IgM antibodies are relatively short-lived, remaining in the bloodstream for only a few months. Because of its large size, IgM does not cross the placenta. Provides protection in the earliest stages of infection. Bactericidal to Gram-negative bacteria. IgM is the most efficient complement-fixing (complement-binding) immunoglobulin.

resulting in, among other effects, the activation of leukocytes, lysis of bacterial cells, and increased phagocytosis as a result of opsonization. Thus, acute extracellular bacterial infections are controlled almost entirely by antibody-mediated immunity (AMI). There is also a "dark side" to immune complexes, which will be discussed in a later section ("Type III Hypersensitivity Reactions").

How Antibodies Protect Us From Pathogens and Infectious Diseases

As previously mentioned, once they are produced, antibodies are very specific. Usually, a given antibody can only recognize and bind to the antigenic determinant that stimulated its production. Listed here are several examples that illustrate how antibodies protect us from pathogens and infectious diseases:

Example 1. A pathogen has entered a person's body and has started producing a toxin. That person's immune system responds by producing antibodies against the toxin; such antibodies are called **antitoxins.** Once produced, the antitoxins recognize, bind to, and neutralize the toxin molecules so that they can no longer cause harm (i.e., they are no longer toxic).

Example 2. Recall from Chapter 14 that viruses can only bind to host cells that bear the appropriate receptor on their surface. The molecule on the virus that recognizes and binds to the receptor is called an adhesin. A person has received a vaccine containing an attenuated virus (a virus that is no longer infectious). The vaccine stimulates that person's immune system to produce antibodies against the adhesin molecules. At some later date, should that same virus enter the person's body, those antibodies will adhere to the adhesin molecules, making it impossible for the virus to bind to host cells. If the virus is unable to bind to the appropriate host cell, it is unable to enter the cell, and the person is protected from infection with that virus.

Example 3. A person is infected with a piliated bacterium. (Recall that pili enable bacteria to attach to host cells, which, with certain bacterial pathogens, is necessary for the bacteria to cause disease.) That person's immune system responds by producing antibodies against the pili. The antibodies bind to the pili, making it impossible for the bacterial cells to bind to tissue. If the bacteria are unable to attach to tissue, they are unable to cause disease.

Example 4. A person is infected with an encapsulated bacterium. (Recall that bacterial capsules serve an antiphagocytic function, meaning that phagocytic white blood cells are unable to phagocytize encapsulated bacteria. The reason for this is that the phagocytes have no receptors on their surface that recognize the polysaccharide molecules. If the phagocyte is unable to attach to the encapsulated bacterium, it is unable to phagocytize it.) That person's immune system responds by producing antibodies against the capsular polysaccharide molecules. The antibodies attach to the capsule. This makes it possible for the phagocytes to bind to the encapsulated bacteria. Why?

Because the phagocytes have receptors on their surface that can recognize and bind to antibody molecules.

Cell-Mediated Immunity

Antibodies are unable to enter cells, including cells containing intracellular pathogens. Fortunately, there is an arm of the immune system capable of controlling chronic infections by intracellular pathogens (e.g., bacteria, protozoa, fungi, viruses). It is called **cell-mediated immunity** (CMI)—a complex system of interactions among many types of cells and cellular secretions (cytokines). (Only a brief overview of CMI can be provided here.) Included among the various cells that participate in CMI are macrophages, T_H cells, T_C cells, NK cells, and granulocytes. Although CMI does not involve the production of antibodies, antibodies produced during humoral immunity may play a minor role in some cell-mediated responses. A typical cell-mediated cytotoxic response would involve the following steps:

Step 1. A macrophage engulfs and partially digests a pathogen. Fragments (antigenic determinants) of the pathogen are then displayed on the surface of the macrophage (i.e., the macrophage acts as an antigen-presenting cell).

Step 2. A T_H cell binds to one of the antigenic determinants being displayed on the macrophage surface. The T_H cell produces cytokines, which reach an effector cell of the immune system (e.g., a T_C cell or NK cell).

Step 3. The effector cell binds to a target cell (i.e., a pathogen-infected host cell displaying the same antigenic determinant on its surface).

Step 4. Vesicular contents of the effector cell are discharged. These include perforin and other proteins and enzymes, which literally punch holes in the target cell membrane. Other cytokines released by effector cells are tumor necrosis factor (TNF) and NK cytotoxic factor.

Step 5. Toxins produced by the effector cells enter the target cell, causing disruption of DNA and organelles. The target cell dies.

Both humoral and cell-mediated immune responses play a role in the body's defense against viral infections. In cytolytic viral infections (e.g., herpes infections), the viruses can be neutralized and destroyed by antibodies and the complement system when they move in body fluids from a lysed cell to an intact cell. When the virus is established within body cells, the cell-mediated immune response can destroy the virus-infected cells, preventing viral multiplication. If the virus is not completely destroyed, however, it may become latent in nerve ganglion cells, as in herpes infections (e.g., shingles).

T_C cells and NK cells kill infected host cells when pathogens are established inside the cells. Thus, infected liver cells are destroyed in hepatitis infections during the body's battle against the disease. The AIDS virus (HIV) that targets T$_H$ cells is particularly destructive because it destroys the very cells that would have helped fight the infection. The lack of T$_H$ cells impairs both humoral and cell-mediated immunity, making AIDS patients very susceptible to many opportunistic infections and malignancies.

NK Cells

Natural killer (NK) cells are in a subpopulation of lymphocytes called large granular lymphocytes. Although they morphologically resemble lymphocytes, NK cells lack typical T or B cell surface markers. They also differ from T and B cells in other ways. For example, they do not proliferate in response to antigen and appear not to be involved in antigen-specific recognition. As the name implies, NK cells kill target cells, including foreign cells, host cells infected with viruses or bacteria, and tumor cells. Although NK cell activity is not dependent on antibodies, NK cells have receptors on their surface for the F$_C$ region of IgG antibodies. These receptors enable the cells to attach to and kill antibody-coated target cells; this is known as antibody-dependent cellular cytotoxicity. Once attached to an antibody-coated target cell, the NK cell inserts a molecule called perforin into the cell membrane of the target cell, creating an opening (pore), through which cytotoxic granules called granzymes are injected. Although firm evidence is lacking for an immune surveillance system within our bodies that monitors for and destroys malignant cells, NK cells may participate in such a system.

Hypersensitivity and Hypersensitivity Reactions

The term *hypersensitivity* refers to an overly sensitive immune system. In such situations, the immune system, in an attempt to protect the person, causes irritation or damage to certain cells and tissues in the body. This can be compared to a person who builds a fire in the living room to warm the house, and the fire burns down the house.

There are several different types of **hypersensitivity reactions.** Some types involve antibodies, whereas others do not. All types depend on the presence of antigen and T cells that are sensitized to that antigen. Hypersensitivity reactions are divided into two general categories, immediate-type and delayed-type, depending on the nature of the immune reaction and the time required for an observable reaction to occur (Table 16-5). *Immediate-type hypersensitivity reactions* occur from within a few minutes to 24 hours after contact with a particular antigen. There are three categories of immediate-type hypersensitivity reactions, referred to as type I, type II, and type III hypersensitivity reactions. A *delayed-type hypersensitivity reaction* usually takes more than 24 hours to manifest itself. Delayed-typed hypersensitivity reac-

---

TABLE 16-5

Types of Hypersensitivity Reactions

Immediate-type hypersensitivity reactions (occur from within a few minutes to 24 hours after contact with a particular antigen)

Type I hypersensitivity reactions	Anaphylactic reactions (allergic reactions)
Type II hypersensitivity reactions	Cytotoxic reactions (involve damage to or death of body cells)
Type III hypersensitivity reactions	Immune complex reactions (damage to tissues and organs is initiated by antigen–antibody complexes)

Delayed-type hypersensitivity (DTH) reactions (usually take 24 to 48 hours or longer to manifest themselves)

Type IV hypersensitivity reactions	Also known as cell-mediated reactions; antibodies play only a minor role, if any; an example is a positive TB skin test

---

tions are also known as type IV hypersensitivity reactions and cell-mediated reactions.

Type I Hypersensitivity Reactions

Type I hypersensitivity reactions (also known as anaphylactic reactions) include classic allergic responses such as hay fever symptoms, asthma, hives, and gastrointestinal symptoms that result from food allergies; allergic responses to insect stings and drugs; and anaphylactic shock. These reactions all involve IgE antibodies and the release of chemical mediators (especially histamine) from mast cells and basophils.

The Allergic Response

Type I immediate hypersensitivity is probably the most commonly observed type of hypersensitivity, because more than half the American population is allergic to something. People who are prone to allergies (*atopic persons*) produce IgE (sometimes called reagin) antibodies when they are exposed to *allergens* (antigens that cause allergic reactions). The IgE molecules bind to the

STUDY AID

Examples of Allergens.

Animal dander
Drugs (e.g., penicillin)
Foods (e.g., peanuts,
shellfish, dairy products)
House dust (dust-mite feces)

Insect venom
Latex
Mold spores
Pollens

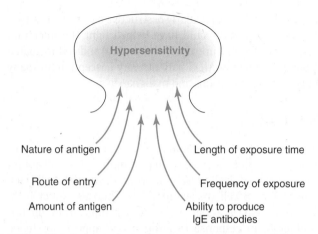

FIGURE 16-6. Factors in the development of type I hypersensitivity (allergies).

surface of basophils and mast cells by their F_C regions. The type and severity of an allergic reaction depend on a combination of factors, including the nature of the antigen, the amount of antigen entering the body, the route by which it enters, the length of time between exposures to the antigen, the person's ability to produce IgE antibodies, and the site of IgE attachment (Fig. 16-6).

The allergic reaction results from the presence of IgE antibodies bound to basophils in the blood or to mast cells in connective tissues—IgE antibodies that were produced in response to the person's first exposure to the allergen. When the allergen binds to cell-bound IgE during a subsequent exposure to the allergen, the sensitized cells respond by degranulation—the discharge and outpouring of irritating and damaging substances (chemical mediators) from the cytoplasmic granules (Figs. 16-7 through 16-9). These mediators of the allergic responses include histamine, prostaglandins, serotonin, bradykinin, slow-reacting substance of anaphylaxis (SRS-A), leukotrienes, and chemicals that attract eosinophils (eosinophilotactic agents).

Localized Anaphylaxis

Type I hypersensitivity reactions (*anaphylactic reactions*) may be localized or systemic. Localized reactions usually involve mast cell degranulation, whereas systemic reactions usually involve basophil degranulation. Hay fever, asthma, and hives are examples of localized anaphylaxis. The symptoms depend on how the allergen enters the body and the sites of IgE attachment. If the allergen (e.g., pollens, dust, fungal spores) is inhaled and deposits on the mucous membranes of the respiratory tract, the IgE antibodies that are produced attach to mast cells in that area. Subsequent exposure to those inhaled allergens allows them to bind to the attached IgE, causing mast cell degranulation. The released histamine initiates the classic symptoms of hay fever. Antihistamines function by binding to and thus blocking the sites where histamine binds. Antihistamines are not

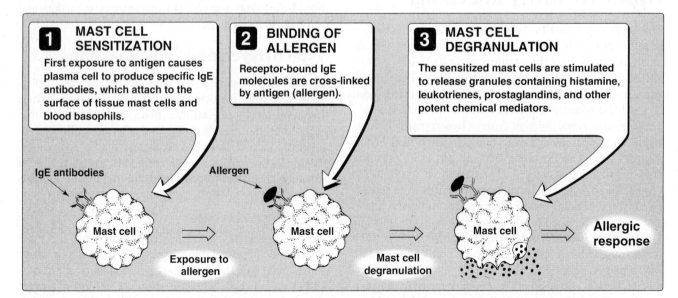

FIGURE 16-7. Events that occur in type I hypersensitivity reactions. (Harvey RA, Champe PA (eds.). Lippincott Illustrated Reviews: Microbiology. Philadelphia: Lippincott Williams & Wilkins, 2001.)

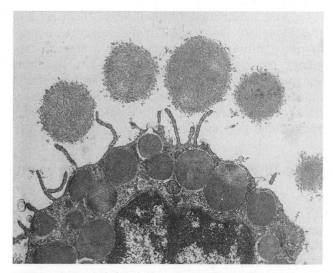

FIGURE 16-8. Transmission electron micrograph (TEM) showing degranulation of a rat mast cell. (TEM by P. Engelkirk.)

as effective in treating asthma, however, because the mediators of this lower respiratory allergy include chemical mediators in addition to histamine. Allergens (e.g., food and drugs) entering through the digestive tract can also sensitize the host, and subsequent exposure may result in the symptoms of food allergies (hives, vomiting, and diarrhea).

Systemic Anaphylaxis

Systemic *anaphylaxis* results from the release of chemical mediators from basophils in the bloodstream. It occurs throughout the body and thus tends to be a more serious condition than localized anaphylaxis. It may lead to a severe, potentially fatal condition known as *anaphylactic shock.* Most often, the allergens involved in systemic anaphylaxis are drugs or insect venom to which the host has been sensitized. Penicillin is an example of a hapten—a substance that must first bind to a host blood protein (a carrier protein) before IgE antibodies are produced.

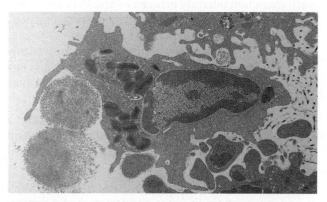

FIGURE 16-9. Transmission electron micrograph (TEM) showing phagocytosis of rat mast cell granules by a rat eosinophil. (TEM by P. Engelkirk.)

The IgE antibodies then bind to circulating basophils. Subsequent injections of penicillin into the sensitized host may cause degranulation of the basophils and release of large amounts of histamine and other chemical mediators into the circulatory system.

The shock reaction usually occurs immediately (within 20 minutes) after reexposure to the allergen. The first symptoms are flushing of the skin with itching, headache, facial swelling, and difficulty breathing; this is followed by falling blood pressure, nausea, vomiting, abdominal cramps, and urination (caused by smooth muscle contractions). In many cases, acute respiratory distress, unconsciousness, and death may follow shortly. Swift treatment with epinephrine (adrenaline) and antihistamine usually stops the reaction.

Healthcare professionals must take particular care to ask patients whether they have any allergies or sensitivities before administering drugs. In particular, those people with allergies to penicillin and other drugs and to insect stings should wear Medic-Alert tags so that they do not receive improper treatment during a medical crisis.

Latex Allergy

In 1997, the National Institute for Occupational Safety and Health (NIOSH) issued a warning that "workers exposed to latex gloves and other products containing natural rubber latex may develop allergic reactions, such as skin rashes; hives; nasal, eye, or sinus symptoms; asthma; and (rarely) shock" (www.cdc.gov/niosh/latexalt.html). One year later, it was estimated that as many as 17% of healthcare workers develop latex allergy, primarily as a result of wearing latex gloves. Latex can trigger any of three types of reactions:

- Irritant contact dermatitis (this is the most common type of reaction; dry, itchy, irritated areas on the skin; not a true allergy because the immune system is not involved).

- Allergic contact dermatitis (a type of delayed hypersensitivity or type IV allergy; skin reactions similar to those caused by poison ivy).

- Immediate type hypersensitivity (a systemic type I, IgE-mediated reaction that can be very serious, resulting in skin redness, hives, itching, respiratory symptoms, including asthma, and shock).

Once a person has become sensitized to latex, a reaction may occur even when the individual is not actually wearing latex gloves. Cornstarch is the powder most commonly used in latex gloves, and inhalation of allergen-laden cornstarch particles is sufficient to cause allergic symptoms. Latex-sensitive employees should avoid latex-containing items, but this is difficult to do in a hospital environment. It has been estimated that more than 20,000 medical products contain latex. Alternatives to powdered latex gloves are powder-free latex gloves and gloves made of materials other than latex.

Allergy Skin Testing and Allergy Shots

Anaphylactic reactions can be prevented by avoiding known allergens. In some cases, skin tests (scratch tests or intradermal injections of allergens) are used to identify the offending allergens. A skin test is considered positive if **cutaneous anaphylaxis** (i.e., swelling and redness at the scratch or injection site) occurs; this is referred to as a "wheal and flare" reaction.

Once the offending allergen is identified, immunotherapy may be accomplished by injecting small doses of allergen, repeatedly, several days apart. In hyposensitization, circulating IgG antibodies are produced rather than IgE antibodies. In theory, when the patient is later exposed in a natural manner to the allergen, the circulating IgG antibodies should bind with the allergen and block its attachment to the basophil- or mast cell–bound IgE. Such circulating IgG molecules, produced in response to allergy shots, are called **blocking antibodies.** Immunotherapy has been used in patients allergic to plant allergens, insect venoms, cat dander, and fire ant venom.

Type II Hypersensitivity Reactions

Type II hypersensitivity reactions are cytotoxic reactions, meaning that body cells are destroyed during these reactions. Type II hypersensitivity reactions include the cytotoxic reactions that occur in incompatible blood transfusions, Rh incompatibility reactions, and myasthenia gravis; all involve IgG or IgM antibodies and complement. A typical type II hypersensitivity reaction might follow this sequence:

Step 1. A particular drug binds to the surface of a cell.

Step 2. Anti-drug antibodies then bind to the drug.

Step 3. This initiates complement activation on the cell surface.

Step 4. The complement cascade leads to lysis of the cell.

Type III Hypersensitivity Reactions

Type III hypersensitivity reactions are immune complex reactions, such as those that occur in serum sickness and certain autoimmune diseases (e.g., systemic lupus erythematosus [SLE] and rheumatoid arthritis). They involve IgG or IgM antibodies, complement, and neutrophils. Serum sickness is a cross-reacting antibody immune reaction in which antibodies formed to globular proteins in horse serum may also bind with similar proteins in the patient's blood. The formation of these immune complexes (antigen + antibody + complement) causes the symptoms of hives, fever, kidney malfunction, and joint lesions of serum sickness. Horse serum containing antitoxins is used to treat botulism. About 10% of patients receiving this antiserum develop serum sickness.

Certain complications (sequelae) of untreated or inadequately treated strep throat and other *Streptococcus pyogenes* infections are the result of type III hypersensitivity reactions. IgG and IgM antibodies produced in response to *S. pyogenes* infection may bind with streptococcal antigens (e.g., M-protein). The resultant immune complexes become deposited in heart tissue, joints, or the glomeruli of the kidney. This causes inflammation at the site, leading to scarring, and, in some cases, abnormalities in or loss of function. Deposition of immune complexes in heart tissue leads to rheumatic heart, in joints leads to arthritis, and in kidneys leads to glomerulonephritis.

Type IV Hypersensitivity Reactions

Type IV hypersensitivity reactions are referred to as *delayed-type hypersensitivity* (DTH) or cell-mediated immune reactions and are part of cell-mediated immunity (CMI). (Recall that the immune system can be divided into humoral immunity and cell-mediated immunity.) Type IV hypersensitivity reactions are called delayed-type hypersensitivity reactions because they are usually observed 24 to 48 hours or longer after exposure or contact. They occur in tuberculin and fungal skin tests, contact dermatitis, and transplantation rejection. DTH is the prime mode of defense against intracellular bacteria and fungi. DTH involves a variety of cell types, including macrophages, cytotoxic T cells, and NK cells, but antibodies do not play a major role.

A classic example of a DTH reaction is a positive TB skin test. Purified protein derivative (PPD), a protein derived from *Mycobacterium tuberculosis,* is injected intradermally into a person. If an "immunologic memory" of that particular protein exists in the person's body, a DTH reaction will occur, producing the typical swelling and redness associated with a positive test result. The following events occur to produce the positive reaction:

Step 1. Within 2 to 3 hours after injection of the PPD, there is an influx of polymorphonuclear cells (PMNs) into the site.

Step 2. This is followed by an influx of lymphocytes and macrophages while the PMNs disperse.

Step 3. Within 12 to 18 hours, the area becomes red (*erythematous*) and swollen (*edematous*).

Step 4. The **erythema** (redness) and *edema* (swelling) reach maximum intensity between 24 and 48 hours.

Step 5. With time, as the swelling and redness disappear, the lymphocytes and macrophages disperse.

A positive TB skin test result does not necessarily mean that a person has tuberculosis, although that is one possibility. Actually, a positive TB skin test result may indicate any of five possibilities:

1. The person has active tuberculosis (in which case, a chest radiograph will show the disease, the person will probably be coughing, and the person's sputum will contain acid-fast bacilli).

2. The person had tuberculosis at some time in the past and recovered (in this case, the person should remember having had tuberculosis or the person's medical records will contain this information).

3. The person was infected with *M. tuberculosis* at some time in the past, but the organisms were killed by that person's host defense mechanisms (even though this person currently harbors no live *M. tuberculosis* cells, he or she will receive a 6-month course of isoniazid, because there is no way to differentiate possibility 3 from possibility 4).

4. The person currently harbors live *M. tuberculosis* organisms but does not actually have tuberculosis (in this case, a 6-month course of isoniazid will be initiated in an attempt to kill any *M. tuberculosis* cells in the person's body).

5. The person had received BCG vaccine at some time in the past (the person should remember having received BCG vaccine or he or she is from a country where BCG vaccine is routinely administered).

Many countries (excluding the United States) routinely immunize their citizens against tuberculosis using BCG vaccine. "BCG" stands for "bacillus Calmette-Guérin," a vaccine prepared from an attenuated strain of *Mycobacterium bovis*. Although this vaccine is only about 50% effective in preventing tuberculosis, it does cause recipients to have positive TB skin test results for variable periods after immunization.

A reaction that is similar to the positive TB skin test occurs in contact dermatitis (contact hypersensitivity), after contact with certain metals, the catechols of poison ivy, cosmetics, and topical medications. The rejection of transplanted tissues containing foreign histologic (tissue) antigens appears to occur in a similar manner, except that cytokines and antibodies cause the rejection of the transplant.

Autoimmune Diseases

An **autoimmune disease** results when a person's immune system no longer recognizes certain body tissues as self and attempts to destroy those tissues as if they were non-self or foreign. This may occur with certain tissues that are not exposed to the immune system during fetal development, so that they are not recognized as self. Such tissues may include the lens of the eye, the brain and spinal cord, and sperm. Subsequent exposure to this tissue (by surgery or injury) may allow antibodies (IgG or IgM) to be formed, which together with complement could cause destruction of these tissues, resulting in blindness, allergic encephalitis, or sterility. It is believed that certain drugs and viruses may alter the antigens on host cells, thus inducing the formation of autoantibodies or sensitized T cells to react against these altered tissue cells.

There are more than 80 recognized autoimmune diseases. It has been estimated that more than 10 million people in the United States suffer from these diseases.

Autoimmune diseases can be classified as organ-specific and non–organ-specific. Examples of organ-specific au-

toimmune diseases are Hashimoto's thyroiditis, Graves disease, and primary myxoedema thyrotoxicosis (all three of which affect the thyroid); pernicious anemia (affects the gastric mucosa); Addison's disease (affects the adrenal glands); and insulin-dependent diabetes mellitus (also known as type 1 diabetes; affects the pancreas). Non–organ-specific autoimmune diseases involve the skin, kidneys, joints, and muscles; examples include myasthenia gravis (affects muscle), dermatomyositis (affects skin), SLE (affects kidneys, lungs, skin, and brain), scleroderma (affects skin, lungs, kidneys, and the gastrointestinal tract), and rheumatoid arthritis (affects joints). Autoimmune diseases are the result of types II, III, or IV hypersensitivity reactions. For example, myasthenia gravis is the result of type II hypersensitivity, whereas rheumatoid arthritis and SLE are the result of type III hypersensitivity.

Immunosuppression

If a person's immune system is functioning properly, that person is said to be an ***immunocompetent person.*** If a person's immune system is not functioning properly, that person is said to be ***immunosuppressed,*** *immunodepressed,* or *immunocompromised.* The most common cause of immune deficiency worldwide is malnutrition. In addition, there are acquired and inherited immunodeficiencies.

Acquired immunodeficiencies may be caused by drugs (e.g., cancer chemotherapeutic agents and drugs given to transplant patients), irradiation, or certain infectious diseases (e.g., HIV infection). HIV infection leads to a decrease in T_H cells, which in turn prevents the production of antibodies against T-dependent antigens and, consequently, results in an inability to fight off certain pathogens. These pathogens overwhelm the patient's host defenses, eventually causing death. Persons with AIDS usually die of a variety of devastating infectious diseases, including viral, bacterial, fungal, and parasitic diseases. Immune responsiveness and the ability to produce antibodies also decline as the normal body ages, perhaps the result of a declining ability of T cells to regulate the immune response. This, in turn, results in greater susceptibility of the elderly to serious infectious diseases.

Inherited immunodeficiency diseases can be the result of deficiencies in antibody production, complement activity, phagocytic function, or NK cell function. Several inherited immunodeficiency diseases have already been mentioned: agammaglobulinemia, hypogammaglobulinemia, chronic granulomatous disease, and Chediak-Higashi syndrome. Others include severe combined immune deficiency (SCID), DiGeorge syndrome, and Wiskott-Aldrich syndrome. SCID patients have deficiencies of B cells or T cells or both, resulting in severe recurrent infections.

In DiGeorge syndrome, there is a congenital absence of the thymus and parathyroid glands; patients suffer frequent infections and delayed development. Wiskott-Aldrich syndrome patients have deficiencies in B cells, T cells, monocytes, and platelets; effects on the patient include bleeding, recurrent infections, and eczema. Bone marrow transplantation and gene therapy may be valuable in treating certain immunodeficiency diseases.

It is hoped that the increased knowledge of genetics that is being gained as a result of the Human Genome Project will lead to an increased understanding of these diseases and a variety of new methods by which they may be treated.

Some people are born lacking the ability to produce protective antibodies. Because they are unable to produce antibodies, they have no gamma globulins in their blood. This abnormality is called *agammaglobulinemia.* These persons are very susceptible to infections by even the least virulent microorganisms in their environment. One treatment for agammaglobulinemia that is often successful consists of a bone marrow transplant, which involves the transfer of precursor white blood cells from a closely related person. Some of these cells become lymphocytes. These lymphocytes may be implanted in the lymph nodes and become immunocompetent (i.e., capable of being stimulated by antigens to produce antibodies).

Persons who produce an insufficient amount of antibodies are said to have *hypogammaglobulinemia.* Their resistance to infection is lower than normal, so they usually do not recover from infectious diseases as readily as most other persons. One type, called Bruton's hypogammaglobulinemia, is a hereditary disease in which the numbers of circulating B cells are profoundly low or totally absent.

The Immunology Laboratory

As mentioned in Chapter 13, immunologic procedures may be performed in an Immunology Laboratory that is separate from the Clinical Microbiology Laboratory (CML), or within the Immunology Section of the CML, depending on the size of the medical facility. Immunologic procedures include tests to diagnose infectious diseases and immune system disorders, determine tissue compatibility for organ and tissue transplants, and detect and measure various serum components (immunochemical procedures). Only some of these procedures are discussed here.

Immunodiagnostic Procedures

Historically, the amount of time it takes to get laboratory results has been the most common criticism of the CML. Sometimes days or even weeks are necessary to isolate pathogens from clinical specimens, to get them growing in pure culture and large numbers, and to perform the tests necessary to identify them. With certain infectious diseases, it is impossible to isolate the pathogens, either because they are obligate intracellular pathogens or are extremely fastidious.

One solution to these problems has been the development of *immunodiagnostic procedures* (IDPs)—laboratory procedures that help to diagnose infectious diseases by detecting either antigens or antibodies in clinical specimens. The results of such procedures are often available on the same day that the clinical specimen is collected from the patient. IDPs performed on serum specimens are sometimes referred to as **serologic procedures.**

Some IDPs are designed to detect antigens, whereas others detect antibodies (Fig. 16-10). Detection of antigens in a clinical specimen is an indication that a particular pathogen is present in the patient, thus providing direct evidence that the patient is infected with that pathogen. Detection of antibodies directed against a particular pathogen is indirect evidence of infection with that pathogen. There are three possible explanations for the presence of antibodies to a particular pathogen:

- Present infection (i.e., the person is currently infected with the pathogen).

- Past infection (i.e., the person was infected with the pathogen in the past, and antibodies are still present in the person's body).

- Vaccination (i.e., the antibodies are the result of the person having been vaccinated against that particular pathogen at some time in the past; for example, a person's serum may contain antibodies against influenza viruses because the person received a flu shot last year).

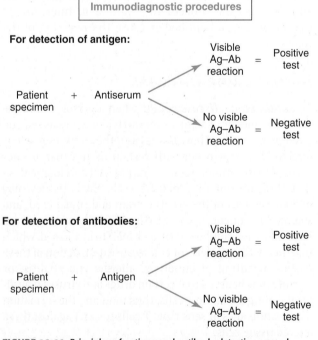

FIGURE 16-10. Principles of antigen and antibody detection procedures. Depending on the type of immunodiagnostic procedure being performed, the visible antigen–antibody (Ag–Ab) reaction might be agglutination (clumping) of cells or latex particles, formation of a precipitin line or band, fluorescence, or production of a color (as in enzyme immunoassays).

Because several explanations are possible for the presence of antibodies in a clinical specimen, the presence of antigens provides the best proof of current infection. Unfortunately, antigen detection procedures are not available for many infectious diseases. Another problem with antibody detection procedures is that it takes a person approximately 10 to 14 days to produce detectible antibodies; thus, even if the person is infected with a particular pathogen, antibodies will not be detectible for about 2 weeks.

Two ways to increase the value of antibody detection procedures to diagnose present infection are (1) to specifically test for IgM antibodies and (2) to use paired sera. Because IgM antibodies are the first antibodies to be produced during the initial exposure to an antigen (the primary response) and are relatively short-lived, the presence of IgM antibodies directed against a particular pathogen is evidence that the pathogen is currently infecting the individual. To test paired sera, one serum specimen (called the acute serum) is collected during the acute stage of the disease and another (called the convalescent serum) is collected 2 weeks later. A significant rise in antibody titer (concentration) between the acute and convalescent sera is evidence that the patient was actively producing antibodies against that pathogen during the 2-week period and, therefore, that pathogen is the cause of the patient's current infection.

Laboratories purchase the reagents used to detect either antigens or antibodies from commercial companies. The reagent used to detect antigens contains antibodies and is called an antiserum. An antiserum is usually prepared by inoculating a laboratory animal with the pathogen (usually dead pathogens are used), and then collecting blood from the animal several weeks later. The blood is allowed to clot, and the serum is drawn off. The reagent used to detect antibodies contains antigens. This is usually a suspension of the dead pathogen.

A variety of different laboratory tests have been designed so that a visible reaction will be observed if an antigen–antibody reaction takes place. Such tests, which include agglutination (involving the clumping of particles such as red blood cells or latex beads), precipitin (involving the production of a precipitate), immunofluorescence procedures, and enzyme-linked immunosorbent assays (ELISAs), are represented diagrammatically in Table 16-6. In the Blood Bank, agglutination tests are used to learn a person's blood type, which is determined by the types of antigens that are present on that person's red blood cells.

Antigen Detection Procedures

For detection of antigen, the clinical specimen is mixed with a particular antiserum (see Fig. 16-10). A visible reaction is the result of the formation of antigen–antibody complexes and indicates that the antigen is present in the clinical specimen; in such a case, the test result is considered positive. If the visible reaction is not observed, then the antigen is not present in the specimen and the test result is negative. **Example:** A drop of cerebrospinal fluid (CSF) from a patient with meningitis is mixed with a drop of antiserum containing antibodies against *H. influenzae*. A visible antigen–antibody reaction is evidence that the patient's CSF contained *H. influenzae* antigens, and the patient's condition is diagnosed as meningitis caused by *H. influenzae*.

Antibody Detection Procedures

For detection of antibodies, the clinical specimen is mixed with a suspension of a particular antigen (see Fig. 16-10). A visible reaction indicates that antibodies against that pathogen are present in the clinical specimen, and the test result is positive. If the visible reaction is not observed, then antibodies against that pathogen are not present in the specimen and the test result is negative. **Example:** A drop of serum from a patient suspected of having Lyme disease is mixed with a suspension of *Borrelia burgdorferi* (the causative agent of Lyme disease). A visible antigen–antibody reaction is evidence that the patient's serum contained antibodies against *B. burgdorferi*, and the patient's condition is diagnosed as Lyme disease.

The radioallergosorbent test (RAST) is used to detect and measure circulating IgE antibodies produced against allergens that individuals inhale, ingest, or otherwise come in contact with. RAST is used in place of or as an adjunct to intradermal skin testing (traditional allergy testing) to determine the allergen(s) to which a person is allergic.

Other IDPs

The Quellung Reaction

The Quellung reaction, another type of IDP, can be used to confirm the identity of *Streptococcus pneumoniae* in the laboratory. In this test, a loopful of *S. pneumoniae* antiserum is added to a drop of spinal fluid or sputum containing Gram-positive cocci, or to a drop of a suspension of Gram-positive cocci prepared from a colony. A drop of methylene blue dye is added, and the mixture is examined microscopically using the oil immersion lens and reduced light. If the cocci are *S. pneumoniae*, antibodies will have bound to the capsule, making the capsule appear swollen (Fig. 16-11); actually, the bound antibodies change the refractive index, making the capsule more visible, but it is not really swollen. This represents a positive Quellung reaction, and the organism can now be identified as *S. pneumoniae*. Using a variety of different commercially available antisera, the specific capsular serotype of this particular *S. pneumoniae* can also be determined.

Skin Testing

Skin testing is another type of IDP, but one that is performed in vivo (in the patient) rather than in vitro (in the

TABLE 16-6

Immunodiagnostic Procedures for Detection of Antibodies in a Patient's Serum

Reaction In Vitro	Reagents			Results	
	Antigen	Antibody	Other	Positive	Negative
Agglutination	Red blood cells or bacteria	Patient's serum		Clumping	No clumping
Precipitin	Toxins, hormones, proteins	Patient's serum	Agar or solution	Precipitate	No precipitate
Lysis by Complement	Cells, bacteria	Patient's serum	Complement	Lysis	No lysis
Fluorescent Antibody Technique	Pathogen	Patient's serum	Fluorescein - tagged rabbit anti - human antiserum	Fluorescent pathogen	No fluorescence
Capsular Swelling (Quellung Reaction)	Encapsulated bacteria	Patient's serum		Capsule appears to swell	No appearance of swelling
Enzyme-linked assay	Test microbe	Patient's serum	Enzyme linked antibody +Substrate	Color change	No color change

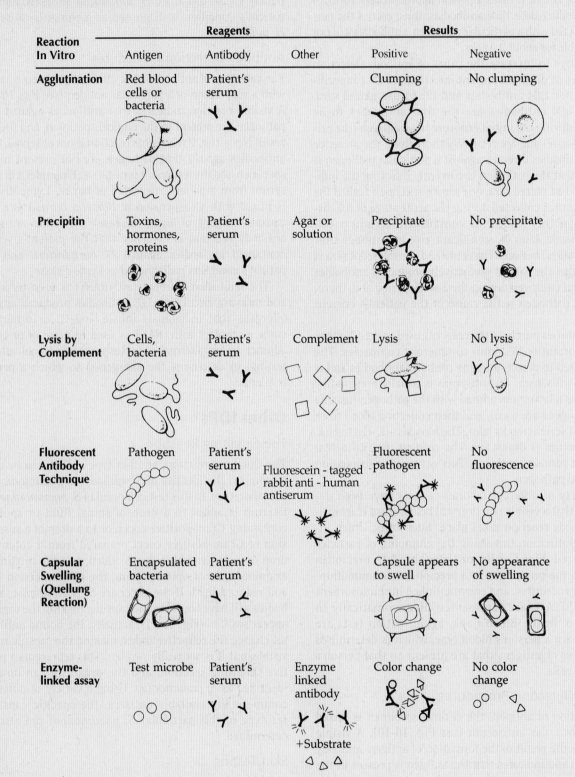

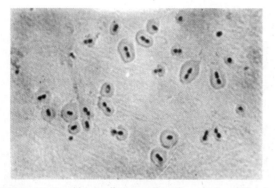

FIGURE 16-11. A positive Quellung reaction. The capsules of *Streptococcus pneumoniae* cells appear swollen as a result of a change in refractive index caused by the binding of antibodies to capsular polysaccharide. (See text for additional details.) (Volk WA, et al. Essentials of Medical Microbiology, 5th ed. Philadelphia: Lippincott-Raven, 1996.)

laboratory). In skin testing, antigens are injected within or beneath the skin (intradermally or subcutaneously, respectively). An example of a commonly used skin test is the tuberculosis skin test (previously described). Skin testing is also used to determine the allergens that an atopic individual is allergic to.

Procedures Used in the Diagnosis of Immunodeficiency Disorders

In addition to immunodiagnostic procedures, tests are performed in the Immunology Laboratory that enable the assessment of a patient's immune status and evaluation of immunodeficiency disorders. These include tests to diagnose B-cell deficiency states (humoral immunodeficiencies), cell-mediated immunodeficiencies, combined humoral and cell-mediated immunodeficiencies, phagocytic deficiency states, and complement deficiencies.

⊙ REVIEW OF KEY POINTS

- Immunology is the scientific study of the immune system and immune responses, including active and passive acquired immunity to infectious agents, antibody production, cell-mediated immune responses, allergic responses, other types of hypersensitivity reactions, autoimmune disorders, and immunodiagnostic procedures.

- The immune system is the third line of defense against pathogens; it is a specific host defense mechanism. Most immune responses involve the production of antibodies that recognize, bind to, and inactivate or destroy specific pathogens or their toxins. Immune responses involving the production of antibodies are known as humoral immunity or antibody-mediated immunity.

- There are also protective cell-mediated immune responses in which antibodies play only minor roles, if any. Cell-mediated immune responses involve a variety of cell types, including macrophages and various types of lymphocytes.

- Immunity to an infectious disease may be innate or acquired. If acquired, the immunity may have been acquired actively (in which case antibodies were actively produced by the person) or passively (in which case the person received antibodies that were produced by others). Active acquired immunity may occur naturally or artificially. Likewise, passive acquired immunity may occur naturally or artificially.

- The production of antibodies in response to a pathogen that has entered the body is an example of natural active acquired immunity. The production of antibodies in response to a vaccine is an example of artificial active acquired immunity. A fetus receiving antibodies that were produced by the mother is an example of natural passive acquired immunity. A soldier receiving antibodies contained in a shot of gamma globulin is an example of artificial passive acquired immunity.

- The various categories of vaccines include attenuated vaccines (weakened pathogens are injected), inactivated vaccines (killed pathogens are injected), subunit or acellular vaccines (only that part of the pathogen that stimulates the production of protective antibodies is injected), and toxoids (injection of toxins that have been modified so that they no longer cause disease).

- Antigens can be defined as substances that stimulate the immune system to produce antibodies. Proteins make the best antigens, but large polysaccharides can also serve as antigens. Individual antigenic molecules are referred to as antigenic determinants or epitopes.

- Antigens can be classified as being either T-independent or T-dependent, depending on the manner in which they are processed by the immune system. Only B cells are involved in the processing of T-independent antigens. A T-dependent antigen requires the interaction of a macrophage, a helper T cell, and a B cell. The end result is the same, in that antibodies are secreted by plasma cells.

- The amount and type of antibodies produced by a given antigenic stimulation depend on the nature of the antigen, the site of antigenic stimulus, the amount of antigen, and the number of times the person is exposed to the antigen.

- Immune responses involve complex interactions among different types of cells and cellular secretions, occurring mostly in the lymphatic system. Cells involved in immune responses originate in bone marrow (from which most blood cells develop); they include B cells (antibody producers), T cells (helper T cells, cytotoxic T cells, and natural killer (NK) cells.

- Antibodies are glycoproteins in a class of proteins known as immunoglobulins. There are five types of immunoglobulins, designated as IgA, IgD, IgE, IgG, and IgM. Three types—IgD, IgE, and IgG—are monomers, consisting of four protein chains (two light chains and two heavy chains), two antigen-binding sites, and an F_C region. Although IgA may be a monomer or a dimer, the dimer form is most important. IgM is a pentamer, having a total of 10 antigen-binding sites.

- Once produced, antibodies are capable of recognizing and binding to the antigenic determinant that stimulated their production. Antibodies function in several ways, including neutralization of toxins, preventing the attachment of pathogens to host cell receptors, serving as opsonins, and initiating the complement cascade.

- Hypersensitivity reactions may be immediate or delayed, depending on the nature of the immune reaction and the time required for an observable reaction. Type I hypersensitivity reactions (anaphylactic reactions) include the classic allergic responses of hay fever, asthma, and hives, resulting from allergies to pollen, mold spores, animal dander, foods, insect venom, drugs, and other allergens. Type I hypersensitivity reactions range from relatively mild, localized reactions to very severe, systemic reactions (e.g., anaphylactic shock).

- Type II hypersensitivity reactions are cytotoxic reactions. An example of a type II reaction is the massive destruction of red blood cells that occurs when a person receives a unit of incompatible blood (e.g., if a type A person receives a unit of type B blood). Type III reactions are immune complex reactions, resulting from the deposition of immune complexes beneath various membranes in the body; they can lead to rheumatic fever, rheumatoid arthritis, and glomerulonephritis. Type IV reactions are delayed-type hypersensitivity (cell-mediated) reactions, such as those that occur in positive TB and fungal skin tests, contact dermatitis, and transplant rejection. Autoimmune diseases may be the result of type II, type III, or type IV hypersensitivity reactions.

- Immunodiagnostic procedures (IDPs) are laboratory tests that are valuable in diagnosing infectious diseases by detecting either antigens or antibodies in clinical specimens. IDPs performed on serum specimens are called serologic procedures.

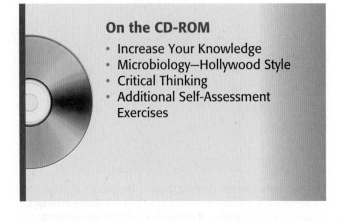

On the CD-ROM
- Increase Your Knowledge
- Microbiology—Hollywood Style
- Critical Thinking
- Additional Self-Assessment Exercises

Self-Assessment Exercises

After studying this chapter, answer the following multiple-choice questions.

1. Of the following, which is the *least* likely to be involved in cell-mediated immunity?
   a. antibodies
   b. cytokines
   c. macrophages
   d. T cells

2. Antibodies are secreted by:
   a. basophils.
   b. macrophages.
   c. plasma cells.
   d. T cells.

3. Humoral immunity involves all the following except:
   a. antibodies.
   b. antigens.
   c. NK cells.
   d. plasma cells.

4. Immunity that develops as a result of an actual infection is called:
   a. artificial active acquired immunity.
   b. artificial passive acquired immunity.
   c. natural active acquired immunity.
   d. natural passive acquired immunity.

5. Artificial passive acquired immunity would result from:
   a. having the measles.
   b. ingesting colostrum.
   c. receiving a gamma globulin injection.
   d. receiving a vaccine.

6. The vaccines that are used to protect people from diphtheria and tetanus are:
   a. antitoxins.
   b. attenuated vaccines.
   c. inactivated vaccines.
   d. toxoids.

7. Natural passive acquired immunity would result from:
   a. having the measles.
   b. ingesting colostrum.
   c. receiving a gamma globulin injection.
   d. receiving a vaccine.

8. Which of the following statements about IgM is *false?*
   a. IgM contains a J-chain.
   b. IgM has a total of 10 antigen-binding sites.
   c. IgM is a pentamer.
   d. IgM is a long-lived molecule.

9. Which of the following could be an effect of type III hypersensitivity?
   a. glomerulonephritis
   b. rheumatoid arthritis
   c. systemic lupus erythematosus (SLE)
   d. all of the above

10. Most likely, immunology got its start in 1890 when these scientists discovered antibodies while developing a diphtheria antitoxin.
    a. Edward Jenner and Louis Pasteur
    b. Elie Metchnikoff and Robert Koch
    c. Emil Behring and Kitasato Shibasaburo
    d. Jonas Salk and Albert Sabin

17

MAJOR VIRAL, BACTERIAL, AND FUNGAL DISEASES OF HUMANS

LEARNING OBJECTIVES

AFTER STUDYING THIS CHAPTER, YOU SHOULD BE
ABLE TO:
• Classify a particular infectious disease as a viral,
  bacterial, or fungal infection

• Categorize various infectious diseases by body system
  (e.g., respiratory system, circulatory system, etc.)
• Correlate a particular infectious disease with its major characteristics, causative agent, reservoir(s),
  mode(s) of transmission, and diagnostic laboratory
  procedures.

INTRODUCTION

Recall that pathogens cause two general categories of diseases: microbial intoxications and infectious diseases. **Microbial intoxications** follow ingestion of a toxin produced outside the body (in vitro) by a pathogen. Microbial intoxications are discussed in CD-ROM Appendix 1. **Infectious diseases,** on the other hand, follow colonization of the body by a pathogen. This chapter summarizes the major viral, bacterial, and fungal infectious diseases of humans. Protozoal and helminth infections of humans are discussed in Chapter 18.

This chapter is divided into sections that describe infectious diseases of various anatomic sites, including skin, ears, eyes, respiratory system, oral cavity (mouth), gastrointestinal tract, genitourinary system, circulatory system, and central nervous system. Although a particular disease may be described within one particular section of this chapter (e.g., in the section describing infectious diseases of the respiratory system), readers must keep in mind that some infectious diseases involve several body systems simultaneously, and that the pathogen may move from one body site to another.

Certain diseases described in this chapter are nationally notifiable infectious diseases, meaning that when a patient is diagnosed with one of these diseases in the United States, the information must be reported to the Centers for Disease Control and Prevention (CDC). As of 2005, there were approximately 60 nationally notifiable diseases. Most of them are described in this chapter, as are some diseases that are not nationally notifiable. (Refer to Chapter 11 for additional information about nationally notifiable diseases.)

STUDY AID

What to Learn?

As you will see, Chapters 17 and 18 contain an enormous amount of information. Of primary importance will be your ability to later recall the type and name of the pathogen that causes a particular infectious disease, and, if applicable, the vector that is involved in the transmission of the disease. For example, if your teacher says "plague," you should be able to state the name of the pathogen that causes plague (*Yersinia pestis*), the type of organism that it is (a Gram-negative bacillus), and the vector that is involved in the transmission of plague (the rat flea).

Infectious Diseases of the Skin

General Information

Terms relating to skin and infectious diseases of the skin are as follows:

- **Epidermis.** The superficial epithelial portion of the skin.
- **Dermis.** The layer of skin containing blood and lymphatic vessels, nerves, and nerve endings, glands, and hair follicles.
- **Dermatitis.** Inflammation of the skin.
- **Sebaceous glands.** Glands in the dermis that usually open into hair follicles and secrete an oily substance known as **sebum.**
- **Folliculitis.** Inflammation of a hair follicle, the sac that contains a hair shaft (Fig. 17-1).
- **Sty (stye).** Inflammation of a sebaceous gland that opens into a follicle of an eyelash.
- **Furuncle (boil).** A localized pyogenic (pus producing) infection of the skin, usually resulting from folliculitis.
- **Carbuncle.** A deep-seated pyogenic infection of the skin, usually arising from a coalescence of furuncles.

Viral Infections of the Skin

Table 17-1 contains information pertaining to viral infections of the skin.

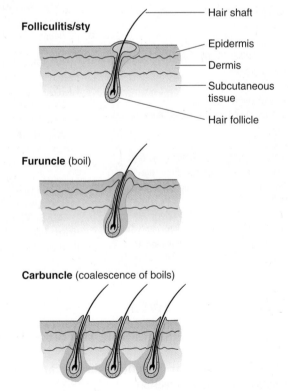

FIGURE 17-1. Infectious diseases of the skin: folliculitis/sty, furuncle, carbuncle. (See text for details.)

TABLE 17-1

Viral Infections of the Skin

DISEASE	ADDITIONAL INFORMATION

Chickenpox and Shingles. (1) Chickenpox (also known as varicella) is an acute, generalized viral infection, with fever, mild constitutional symptoms, and a skin rash. Vesicles also form in mucous membranes. Usually a mild, self-limiting disease, but can be severely damaging to a fetus. Serious complications include pneumonia, secondary bacterial infections, hemorrhagic complications, and encephalitis. Reye's (pronounced "rize") syndrome (a severe encephalomyelitis with liver damage) may follow clinical chickenpox if aspirin is given to children younger than 16 years of age. (2) Shingles (also known as herpes zoster) is a reactivation of the varicella virus, often the result of immunosuppression. Inflammation of sensory ganglia of cutaneous sensory nerves, producing fluid-filled blisters, pain, and paresthesia (numbness and tingling). Shingles may occur at any age, but is most common after age 50. Chickenpox is the leading cause of vaccine-preventable death in the U.S. A total of 26,659 new U.S. cases of chickenpox were reported to the CDC during 2004.

Patient Care. Airborne precautions for hospitalized patients.

Etiologic Agent. Varicella-zoster virus (VZV); a herpes virus (Family Herpesviridae) that is also known as human herpesvirus 3; a DNA virus.

Reservoirs and Mode of Transmission. Infected humans. Transmission is person to person by direct contact, droplet, or airborne spread of vesicle fluid or secretions of the respiratory system of persons with chickenpox.

Diagnosis. Usually made on clinical and epidemiologic grounds. Immunodiagnostic procedures are available.

German Measles, Rubella. A mild, febrile viral disease. A fine, pinkish, flat rash begins 1 or 2 days after the onset of symptoms; it starts on the face and neck and spreads to the trunk, arms, and legs. A milder disease than hard measles with fewer complications. During first trimester of pregnancy, may cause congenital rubella syndrome in fetus; this can lead to intrauterine death, spontaneous abortion, or congenital malformations of major organ systems. A total of 10 new U.S. cases were reported to the CDC in 2004.

Patient Care. Droplet precautions for hospitalized patients.

Etiologic Agent. Rubella virus; a RNA virus in the Family Togaviridae.

Reservoirs and Mode of Transmission. Infected humans. Transmission is by droplet spread or direct contact with nasopharyngeal secretions of infected people.

Diagnosis. Immunodiagnostic procedures.

Measles, Hard Measles, Rubeola. An acute, highly communicable viral disease with fever, conjunctivitis, cough, light sensitivity, Koplik spots in mouth, and red blotchy skin rash (Fig. 17-2). The rash begins on the face on the 3rd to 7th day and then becomes generalized. Complications include bronchitis, pneumonia, otitis media, and encephalitis. Rarely, autoimmune, subacute, sclerosing panencephalitis (SSPE) may follow a latent period of several years. A total of 37 new U.S. cases (11 indigenous, 26 imported) were reported to the CDC in 2004.

Patient Care. Airborne precautions for hospitalized patients.

Etiologic Agent. Measles (rubeola) virus; a RNA virus in the Family Paramyxoviridae.

Reservoirs and Mode of Transmission. Infected humans. Airborne transmission by droplet spread; direct contact with nasal or throat secretions of infected persons, or with articles freshly soiled with nose and throat secretions.

Diagnosis. Usually made on clinical and epidemiologic grounds. Immunodiagnostic procedures are available.

Monkeypox. A rare viral disease that causes fever, headache, muscle aches, backache, lymphadenitis, malaise (fatigue), and a rash. Monkeypox is a milder disease than smallpox. The disease occurs primarily in central and western Africa, although several people in the United States became ill in 2003 after handling infected prairie dogs. Unlike smallpox, the disease is rarely fatal.

Patient Care. Droplet precautions for hospitalized patients. Possibly contact precautions also.

Etiologic Agent. Monkeypox virus; in the same group of viruses (orthopoxviruses) as smallpox virus (variola), the virus used in the smallpox vaccine (vaccinia), and cowpox virus (varicella).

Reservoirs and Mode of Transmission. Infected animals. Transmission occurs via animal bite or contact with an infected animal's blood, body fluids, or rash. Human-to-human transmission occurs.

Diagnosis. Immunodiagnostic and molecular diagnostic procedures; virus isolation.

Smallpox. A systemic viral infection with fever, malaise, headache, prostration, severe backache, a characteristic skin rash, and occasional abdominal pain and vomiting. The rash is similar to, and must be distinguished from, the rash of chickenpox. The disease can become severe, with bleeding into the skin and mucous membranes, followed by death. The World Health Organization (WHO) was able to eradicate smallpox via a combination of isolation of infected persons and vaccination of others in the community. The last

Patient Care. Contact precautions for hospitalized patients. Droplet precautions may be indicated.

Etiologic Agent. Two strains of variola virus: variola minor (with a fatality rate of <1%), and variola major (with a fatality rate of 20 to 40% or higher); variola virus is a DNA virus in the Family Poxviridae.

(continues)

TABLE 17-1

Viral Infections of the Skin *(continued)*

DISEASE	ADDITIONAL INFORMATION
known case of naturally acquired smallpox in the world occurred in Somalia in October 1977. In May 1980, the WHO announced the global eradication of smallpox. Smallpox virus is currently stored in several laboratories, including the CDC and a comparable facility in Russia. Smallpox virus is a potential biologic warfare and bioterrorism agent.	**Reservoirs and Mode of Transmission.** Before smallpox was eradicated, infected humans were the only source of the virus. Transmission is person to person. Patients are most contagious before eruption of the rash, by aerosol droplets from oropharyngeal lesions. **Diagnosis.** Because of the potential danger of the use of smallpox virus as a bioterrorism agent, physicians must become familiar with the clinical and epidemiologic features of smallpox and how to distinguish smallpox from chickenpox. Laboratory diagnosis is by tissue culture, immunodiagnostic procedures, and molecular diagnostic procedures.
Warts. Many varieties of skin and mucous membrane lesions, including common warts (verrucae vulgaris), venereal warts, and plantar warts. Most are harmless, but some can become cancerous.	**Etiologic Agent.** At least 70 different types of human papillomaviruses (HPV); Genus Papillomavirus in the Family Papovaviridae; they are DNA viruses. **Reservoirs and Mode of Transmission.** Infected humans. Transmission is usually by direct contact. Genital warts are sexually transmitted. Easily spread from one area of the body to another, but most are not very contagious from person to person (genital warts are an exception). **Diagnosis.** Clinical grounds.

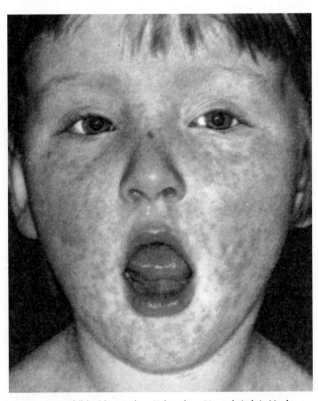

FIGURE 17-2. Child with measles. (Schaechter M, et al. (eds.). Mechanisms of Microbial Disease, 3rd ed. Philadelphia:Lippincott Williams & Wilkins, 1999.)

Bacterial Infections of the Skin

Information pertaining to bacterial infections of the skin is contained in Table 17-2.

Wound Infections

When the protective skin barrier is broken as a result of burns, puncture wounds, surgical procedures, or bites, opportunistic indigenous microflora and environmental bacteria can invade and cause local or deep

○ STUDY AID

Beware of Similar Sounding Names

Do not confuse varicella, variola, and vaccinia viruses. **Varicella virus** (which is a type of herpes virus) is the cause of chickenpox. **Variola virus** is the cause of smallpox and is often referred to as smallpox virus. **Vaccinia virus** is the cause of cowpox; it is used to make the vaccine that protects against smallpox. The words *vaccine* and *vaccination* are derived from *vacca*, Latin for cow.

TABLE 17-2

Bacterial Infections of the Skin

DISEASE	ADDITIONAL INFORMATION
Acne. A common condition in which pores become clogged with dried sebum, flaked skin, and bacteria; leads to the formation of blackheads and whiteheads (collectively known as acne pimples) and inflamed, infected abscesses; more common among teenagers; not a nationally notifiable disease in the U.S.	**Etiologic Agent.** *Propionibacterium acnes* and other *Propionibacterium* spp. (all are anaerobic, Gram-positive bacilli). **Reservoirs and Mode of Transmission.** Infected humans. Probably not transmissible. **Diagnosis.** Clinical grounds.
Anthrax, Woolsorter's Disease. Anthrax can affect the skin (cutaneous anthrax), the lungs (inhalation or pulmonary anthrax), or the GI tract (gastrointestinal anthrax), depending on the portal of entry of the causative agent. In cutaneous anthrax, depressed blackened lesions called eschars occur, caused by a necrotoxin (a toxin that kills cells). Inhalation and gastrointestinal anthrax are often fatal, but cutaneous anthrax usually is not. Ordinarily, human cases in the U.S. are quite rare. However, 18 U.S. cases occurred in the fall of 2001 as a result of the mailing of letters that had purposely been contaminated with *B. anthracis* spores. The 18 cases included 11 cases of inhalation anthrax (5 fatal) and 7 cases of cutaneous anthrax (0 fatal). (See Chapter 11 for more information.) No new U.S. cases were reported to the CDC in 2004.	**Patient Care.** Standard precautions for hospitalized patients. **Etiologic Agent.** *Bacillus anthracis,* a spore-forming, Gram-positive bacillus (Fig. 17-3). **Reservoirs and Mode of Transmission.** Anthrax-infected animals; spores may be present in soil, animal hair, wool, animal skins and hides, and products made from them. Transmission is by entry of endospores through breaks in skin, inhalation of spores, or ingestion of bacteria in contaminated meat. Person-to-person transmission is very rare. **Diagnosis.** Isolation of *B. anthracis* from blood, lesions, or discharges and identification using biochemical- or enzyme-based tests. Immunodiagnostic procedures are available.
Gas Gangrene, Myonecrosis. *Necrosis* (tissue death) caused by *ischemia* (lack of oxygen) is called *gangrene.* Gangrene may or may not involve pathogens. However, one type of gangrene, called *gas gangrene* (also known as myonecrosis) *always* involves pathogens. Gases released from the infecting pathogens cause pockets of gas to develop in the infected tissue. Rapid and extensive tissue damage may necessitate amputation of the infected extremity. Gas gangrene is not a communicable disease and is not a nationally notifiable disease in the U.S.	**Patient Care.** Standard precautions for hospitalized patients. **Etiologic Agent.** Various anaerobic bacteria in the genus *Clostridium,* especially *Clostridium perfringens.* After the *Clostridium* spores germinate in the wound, the vegetative pathogens produce necrotizing enzymes and toxins, which rapidly destroy tissue, especially muscle tissue. **Reservoirs and Mode of Transmission.** Soil. Humans become infected when soil containing clostridial spores enters an open wound. **Diagnosis.** The presence of Gram-positive or Gram-variable bacilli in Gram-stained smears of wound specimens should lead one to suspect gas gangrene. Often, no leukocytes are observed, as they have been killed by toxins produced by the clostridia. Once isolated on culture media, the species can be determined using biochemical- or enzyme-based tests.
Leprosy, Hansen or Hansen's Disease. (1) Lepromatous leprosy. Numerous nodules in skin; there may be involvement of the nasal mucosa and eyes. (2) Tuberculoid leprosy. Relatively few skin lesions; peripheral nerve involvement tends to be severe, with loss of sensation. Hansen's disease is named for G.A. Hansen who, in 1873, discovered the bacillus that causes leprosy. Occurs primarily in warm, wet areas of the tropics and subtropics. The worldwide prevalence of leprosy was estimated to be about 1.5 million cases in 1997; 105 new U.S. cases were reported to the CDC in 2004. Most U.S. cases involve people who emigrated from developing countries.	**Patient Care.** Contact precautions for hospitalized patients with lepromatous leprosy. Standard precautions for patients with tuberculoid leprosy. **Etiologic Agent.** *Mycobacterium leprae;* an acid-fast bacillus. **Reservoirs and Mode of Transmission.** Infected humans (in nasal discharges and shed from cutaneous lesions); armadillos in Texas and Louisiana have a naturally occurring disease that is identical to experimental leprosy in this animal, suggesting that transmission from armadillos to humans is possible. The exact mode of transmission has not been clearly established. The organisms may gain entrance through the respiratory system or broken skin. Does not appear to be easily transmitted from person to person. Prolonged, close contact with an infected individual appears to be necessary. The tuberculoid form of leprosy is not contagious. **Diagnosis.** *M. leprae* cannot be grown on artificial culture media; can be cultured only in laboratory animals (nine-banded armadillos or mouse foot pads). Demonstration of acid-fast bacilli in skin smears or skin biopsy specimens.

(continues)

TABLE 17-2

Bacterial Infections of the Skin *(continued)*

DISEASE	ADDITIONAL INFORMATION
Staphylococcal Skin Infections (Folliculitis, Furuncles, Carbuncles, Abscesses, Impetigo, Impetigo of the Newborn, Scalded Skin Syndrome). Virtually all infected hair follicles, boils (furuncles), carbuncles, and styes involve *Staphylococcus aureus*. The majority of common skin lesions are localized, discrete, and uncomplicated. However, seeding of the bloodstream may lead to pneumonia, lung abscess, osteomyelitis, sepsis, endocarditis, meningitis, or brain abscess. With impetigo (Fig. 17-4), which occurs mainly in children, pus-filled blisters (*pustules*) may appear anywhere on the body. Impetigo of the newborn (impetigo neonatorum) and staphylococcal scalded skin syndrome (SSSS) may occur as epidemics in hospital nurseries. None of these staphylococcal diseases are nationally notifiable diseases in the U.S.	**Patient Care.** Contact precautions for hospitalized patients with major staphylococcal skin, wound, or burn infections. **Etiologic Agent.** *Staphylococcus aureus,* a Gram-positive coccus. Impetigo may also be caused by *Streptococcus pyogenes,* another Gram-positive coccus. *S. aureus* spreads through skin by producing hyaluronidase. SSSS is produced by strains of *S. aureus* that produce exfoliative (or epidermolytic) toxin, which causes the top layer of skin (epidermis) to split from the rest of the skin. **Reservoirs and Mode of Transmission.** Infected humans. Persons with a draining lesion or any purulent discharge are the most common sources of epidemic spread. Transmission is via direct contact with a person having a purulent lesion or is an asymptomatic carrier. In hospitals, spread by hands of healthcare workers. **Diagnosis.** The infecting strain must be isolated on culture media and identified using biochemical- or enzyme-based tests. Susceptibility testing must be performed because many strains of *S. aureus* are multidrug-resistant.
Streptococcal Skin Infections (Scarlet Fever, Erysipelas, Necrotizing Fasciitis). (1) Streptococcal impetigo. Usually superficial; may proceed through vesicular, pustular, and encrusted stages. (2) Scarlet fever (scarlatina). Widespread, pink-red rash, most obvious on the abdomen, sides of the chest, and in skin folds; severe cases may be accompanied by high fever, nausea, and vomiting. (3) Erysipelas. An acute cellulitis, with fever, constitutional symptoms, and hot, tender, red eruptions (sometimes referred to as St. Anthony's fire). (4) Necrotizing fasciitis is the name of the disease caused by the so-called flesh-eating bacteria. *Fasciitis* is inflammation of the *fascia* (fibrous tissue that envelops the body beneath the skin; also encloses muscles and groups of muscles). A total of 2,590 new U.S. cases of invasive streptococcal group A disease and 132 new U.S. cases of streptococcal toxic shock syndrome were reported to the CDC during 2004.	**Patient Care.** Contact precautions for hospitalized patients with major group A streptococcal skin, wound, or burn infections. **Etiologic Agent.** *Streptococcus pyogenes;* a Gram-positive coccus, also known as group A β-hemolytic streptococcus, GAS, and "Strep A." Scarlet fever is caused by erythrogenic toxin, produced by some strains of *S. pyogenes.* It can be a complication (sequela) of untreated strep throat (streptococcal pharyngitis). **Reservoirs and Mode of Transmission.** Infected humans. Transmission is person to person via large respiratory droplets or direct contact with patients or carriers; rarely by indirect contact through objects. **Diagnosis.** The infecting strain must be isolated on culture media and identified using biochemical- or enzyme-based tests. Immunodiagnostic procedures are available, some of which are referred to as "rapid strep tests." Currently, susceptibility testing is not routinely performed because *S. pyogenes* has not yet developed resistance to penicillin. Some strains have become resistant to other antimicrobial agents, however.

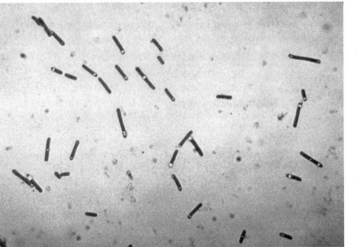

FIGURE 17-3. *Bacillus anthracis.* Gram-stain of bacteria from culture. The clear areas are unstained endospores. (Photo courtesy of the Centers for Disease Control and Prevention and Dr. William A. Clark.)

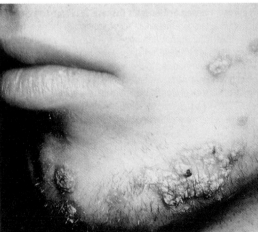

FIGURE 17-4. Impetigo. (Schaechter M, et al. (eds.). Mechanisms of Microbial Disease, 3rd ed. Philadelphia: Lippincott Williams & Wilkins, 1999.)

A Closer Look at *Staphylococcus aureus*

Staphylococcus aureus is a catalase-positive (meaning that it produces the enzyme, catalase), Gram-positive coccus, usually arranged in clusters. In the laboratory, *S. aureus* can be differentiated from other *Staphylococcus* species of human origin by using the coagulase test; *S. aureus* is coagulase-positive (meaning that it produces the enzyme, coagulase), whereas the other staphylococci are coagulase-negative. *S. aureus* is a facultative anaerobe and opportunistic pathogen that is often found in low numbers as indigenous microflora of the skin. Approximately 20 to 30% of the general population are "staph carriers," their nasal passages being colonized with *S. aureus*. Infections caused by *S. aureus* are often referred to as staph infections. It is a major cause of skin, soft tissue, respiratory, bone, joint, endovascular, and wound infections. Most pimples, boils, carbuncles, and styes involve *S. aureus*. It is a less common cause of pneumonia and urinary tract infections. *S. aureus* is one of the four most common causes of nosocomial infections, often causing postsurgical wound infections. Strains of *S. aureus* produce a variety of exotoxins, including cytotoxins, exfoliative toxin, and leukocidin. Some strains produce toxic shock syndrome-1 (TSS-1) toxin, the cause of toxic shock syndrome. Some strains (those that produce an enterotoxin) are the cause of staphylococcal food poisoning, one of the most common types of food poisoning. Strains of *S. aureus* produce a variety of exoenzymes, including protease, lipase, and hyaluronidase that destroy tissues; coagulase that causes clot formation; and staphylokinase that dissolves clots. Especially troublesome strains of *S. aureus* are methicillin-resistant *S. aureus* (MRSA) strains (which are resistant to most of the drugs used to treat staph infections) and vancomycin-intermediate *S. aureus* (VISA) strains (which are resistant to the dosages of vancomycin usually used to treat staph infections).

A Closer Look at *Streptococcus pyogenes*

Streptococcus pyogenes is also known as group A strep, GAS, and Strep A. It is a β-hemolytic, catalase-negative, Gram-positive coccus, usually arranged in chains. In the laboratory, *S. pyogenes* can be differentiated from other β-hemolytic *Streptococcus* species of human origin by using the A-disk (bacitracin sensitivity) test; *S. pyogenes* is bacitracin-sensitive (killed by bacitracin), whereas the other β-hemolytic streptococci are bacitracin-resistant. It is a facultative anaerobe and opportunistic pathogen that is infrequently found in low numbers as indigenous microflora of the upper respiratory tract. *S. pyogenes* is the cause of streptococcal **pharyngitis** (strep throat) and a frequent cause of skin infections (e.g., impetigo and erysipelas) and wound infections. Untreated strep throat or other *S. pyogenes* infections can lead to a variety of sequelae (complications), including scarlet fever, toxic shock syndrome (TSS), rheumatic fever (sometimes referred to as rheumatic heart disease because it includes myocarditis and endocarditis), rheumatoid arthritis, and glomerulonephritis. Scarlet fever is caused by strains that produce erythrogenic toxin. Some strains of *S. pyogenes* produce a toxin that causes TSS, although most cases of TSS are caused by *S. aureus*. Some strains of *S. pyogenes* (referred to as the "flesh-eating bacteria") produce necrotizing enzymes that cause rapid and extensive destruction of tissue (a condition known as necrotizing fasciitis). Necrotizing fasciitis has a mortality rate of approximately 20 to 30%.

TABLE 17-3

Fungal Infections of the Skin

DISEASE	ADDITIONAL INFORMATION
Dermatophytosis, Tinea ("Ringworm") Infections, Dermatomycosis. The dermatophytoses (**tinea infections** or "ringworm" infections) are named in accordance with the site of infection: fungal lesions of the scalp (tinea capitis), beard area (tinea barbae), groin area (tinea cruris or jock itch), trunk of the body (tinea corporis), foot (tinea pedis or athlete's foot), and nails (tinea unguium or onychomycosis). Some fungal infections cause only limited irritation, scaling, and redness. Others cause itching, swelling, blisters, and severe scaling. Tinea infections are not nationally notifiable diseases in the U.S.	*Etiologic Agent.* Various species of filamentous fungi, including *Microsporum, Epidermophyton,* and *Trichophyton* spp.; they are collectively referred to as **dermatophytes.** Reservoirs and Mode of Transmission. Infected humans, animals, and soil. Transmission is by direct or indirect contact with lesions of infected humans or animals; contaminated floors, shower stalls, locker room benches, barber clippers, combs, hairbrushes, clothing. Spores enter through breaks in skin and moist areas and germinate into filamentous growths. Diagnosis. Microscopic examination of potassium hydroxide (KOH) preparations of skin scrapings can reveal the presence of fungal hyphae (Fig. 17-5). (The KOH preparation is described in CD-ROM Appendix 5.) Dermatophytes can be cultured on various media including Sabouraud dextrose agar. Molds are identified using a combination of macroscopic and microscopic observations (see Chapter 13).

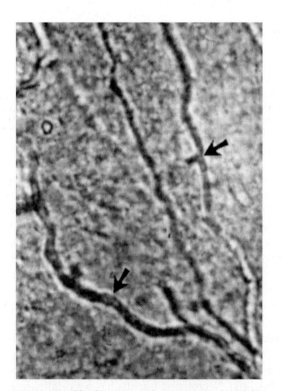

FIGURE 17-5. Fungal hyphae (arrows) in KOH preparation of skin scrapings from a patient with tinea corporis. (Schaechter M, et al. (eds.). Mechanisms of Microbial Disease, 3rd ed. Philadelphia: Lippincott Williams & Wilkins, 1999.)

tissue infections. The pathogens may spread through blood or lymph, causing serious systemic infections.

Fungal Infections of the Skin

Table 17-3 contains information pertaining to fungal infections of the skin.

Infectious Diseases of the Ears

General Information

There are three pathways for pathogens to enter the ear: (1) through the eustachian (auditory) tube, from the throat and nasopharynx; (2) from the external ear; and (3) by the blood or lymph. Usually, bacteria are trapped in the middle ear when a bacterial infection in the throat and nasopharynx causes the eustachian tube to close. The result is an anaerobic condition in the middle ear, allowing obligate and facultative anaerobes to grow and cause pressure on the tympanic membrane (eardrum). Swollen lymphoid (adenoid) tissues, viral infections, and allergies may also close the eustachian tube, especially in young children. Infection of the middle ear is known as **otitis media,** whereas infection of the outer ear canal is known as **otitis externa** (Fig. 17-6).

Viral and Bacterial Ear Infections

Information pertaining to viral and bacterial ear infections is contained in Table 17-4.

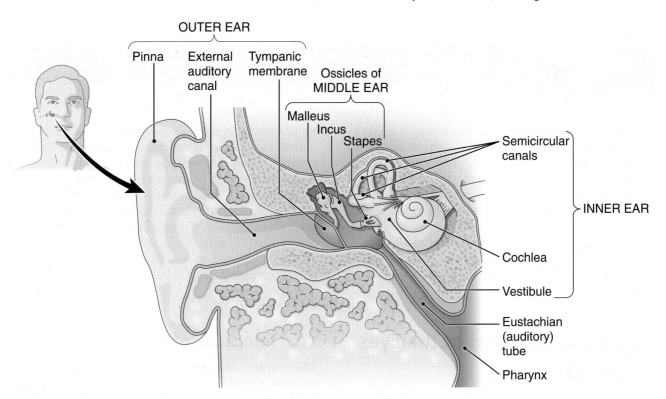

FIGURE 17-6. Anatomy of the ear. (Cohen BJ, Taylor JJ. Memmler's The Human Body in Health and Disease, 10th Ed. Philadelphia: Lippincott Williams & Wilkins, 2005.)

TABLE 17-4

Viral and Bacterial Ear Infections

DISEASE	ADDITIONAL INFORMATION
Otitis Externa, External Otitis, Ear Canal Infection, Swimmer's Ear. Infection of the ear canal with itching, pain, a malodorous discharge, tenderness, redness, swelling, and impaired hearing; most common during the summer swimming season; trapped water in the external ear canal can lead to wet, softened skin, which is more easily infected by bacteria or fungi; otitis externa is often referred to as "swimmer's ear," because it often results from swimming in water contaminated with *Pseudomonas aeruginosa.* Not a nationally notifiable disease in the U.S.	**Etiologic Agent.** *Escherichia coli, Pseudomonas aeruginosa, Proteus vulgaris, Staphylococcus aureus;* rarely by a fungus, such as *Aspergillus.* **Reservoirs and Mode of Transmission.** Contaminated swimming pool water; sometimes indigenous microflora; articles inserted in ear canal for cleaning out debris and wax. **Diagnosis.** Material from the infected ear canal should be sent to the microbiology laboratory for culture and susceptibility (C&S). Most strains of *P. aeruginosa* are multidrug-resistant.
Otitis Media, Middle Ear Infection. Often develops as a complication of the common cold. Persistent and severe earache; temporary hearing loss; pressure in middle ear; bulging of the eardrum (tympanic membrane); nausea, vomiting, diarrhea, and fever in young children; may lead to rupture of the eardrum, bloody discharge, and then pus from the ear. Severe complications, including bone infection, permanent hearing loss, and meningitis, may occur. It is most common in young children, particularly those between 3 months and 3 years of age. Otitis media is not a nationally notifiable disease in the U.S.	**Etiologic Agent.** Otitis media may be caused by bacteria or viruses. The three most common bacterial causes are *Streptococcus pneumoniae* (a Gram-positive diplococcus), *Haemophilus influenzae* (a Gram-negative bacillus), and *Moraxella catarrhalis* (a Gram-negative diplococcus). Less common bacterial causes include *Streptococcus pyogenes* and *Staphylococcus aureus.* Viral causes include measles virus, parainfluenza virus, and respiratory syncytial virus (RSV). **Reservoirs and Mode of Transmission.** Probably not communicable. **Diagnosis.** If there is a discharge from the ear, a sample should be sent to the microbiology laboratory for C&S. β-Lactamase testing should be performed on isolates of *H. influenzae* and *S. pneumoniae.*

A Closer Look at *Streptococcus pneumoniae*

Streptococcus pneumoniae is also known as pneumo-coccus (pl., pneumococci). It is an encapsulated, α-hemolytic, catalase-negative, Gram-positive coccus, usually arranged in pairs (diplococci). In the laboratory, *S. pneumoniae* can be differentiated from other α-hemolytic *Streptococcus* species of human origin by using the P-disk (Optochin sensitivity) test; *S. pneumoniae* is Optochin-sensitive (killed by Optochin), whereas the other α-hemolytic streptococci are Optochin-resist-ant. *S. pneumoniae* is a facultative anaerobe and oppor-tunistic pathogen, found in low numbers as indigenous microflora of the upper respiratory tract. It is the most common cause of bacterial pneumonia in the world; the pneumonia it causes is often referred to as pneumococ-cal pneumonia. *S. pneumoniae* is also a common cause of meningitis (especially in the elderly) and causes about one third of U.S. cases of otitis media. Many strains of *S. pneumoniae* are penicillin-resistant and some strains are multidrug-resistant. A vaccine is available to prevent pneumococcal infections in the elderly.

Infectious Diseases of the Eyes

General Information

Terms relating to the eye and infectious diseases of the eye include the following:

- **Conjunctiva.** The thin, tough lining that covers the inner wall of the eyelid and the sclera (the white of the eye)
- **Conjunctivitis.** An infection or inflammation of the con-junctiva (see Fig. 17-7).
- **Keratitis.** An infection or inflammation of the cornea—the domed covering over the iris and lens.
- **Keratoconjunctivitis.** An infection that involves both the cornea and conjunctiva.

Viral Infections of the Eyes

Adenoviruses, enteroviruses, and herpes simplex viruses can cause conjunctivitis, keratitis, and keratoconjunctivitis. People with viral infections (e.g., cold sores) should wash their hands thoroughly before inserting or removing contact lenses or otherwise touching their eyes. Antiviral agents may be prescribed for herpes simplex infections, ei-ther as an ointment or eye drops. Contact precautions should be instituted for hospitalized patients.

Bacterial Infections of the Eyes

Table 17-5 contains information pertaining to bacterial in-fections of the eyes.

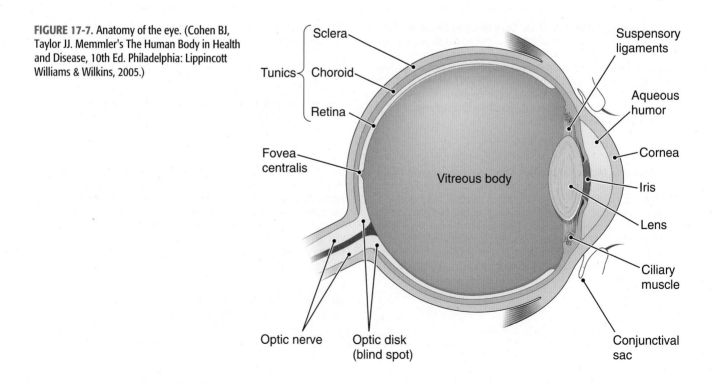

FIGURE 17-7. Anatomy of the eye. (Cohen BJ, Taylor JJ. Memmler's The Human Body in Health and Disease, 10th Ed. Philadelphia: Lippincott Williams & Wilkins, 2005.)

TABLE 17-5

Bacterial Infections of the Eyes

DISEASE	ADDITIONAL INFORMATION
Bacterial Conjunctivitis, "Pinkeye." Irritation, reddening of conjunctiva, edema of eyelids, mucopurulent discharge, sensitivity to light; highly contagious. Not a nationally notifiable disease in the U.S.	**Patient Care.** Contact precautions for hospitalized patients. **Etiologic Agent.** *Haemophilus influenzae* biogroup *aegyptius* and *Streptococcus pneumoniae* are the most common causes, although many other bacteria can cause pinkeye. **Reservoirs and Mode of Transmission.** Infected humans. Human-to-human transmission via contact with eye and respiratory discharges; contaminated fingers, facial tissues, clothing, eye makeup, eye medications, ophthalmic instruments, and contact lens-wetting and lens-cleaning agents. **Diagnosis.** Infections of the eye caused by bacteria (including chlamydias) and viruses should be differentiated from allergic manifestations and irritation by microscopic examination of the *exudate* (oozing pus), culture of pathogens, and/or immunodiagnostic procedures.
Chlamydial Conjunctivitis, Inclusion Conjunctivitis, Paratrachoma. In neonates, acute conjunctivitis with mucopurulent discharge; may result in mild scarring of conjunctivae and cornea; may be concurrent with chlamydial nasopharyngitis or pneumonia; in adults, may be concurrent with nongonococcal urethritis or cervicitis. Not a nationally notifiable disease in the U.S.	**Patient Care.** Contact precautions for hospitalized patients. **Etiologic Agent.** Certain serotypes (serovars) of *Chlamydia trachomatis.* **Reservoirs and Mode of Transmission.** Infected humans. Transmission is by contact with genital discharges of infected people; contaminated fingers to eye; infection in newborns via infected birth canal; nonchlorinated swimming pools ("swimming pool conjunctivitis"). **Diagnosis.** Chlamydias do not grow on artificial media; diagnosis by cell culture or immunodiagnostic procedures.
Trachoma, Chlamydia Keratoconjunctivitis. Highly contagious, acute or chronic conjunctival inflammation, resulting in scarring of cornea and conjunctiva, deformation of eyelids, and blindness. Trachoma is most common in poverty-stricken areas of the hot, dry Mediterranean countries and the Far East. It is the leading cause of blindness in the world. Trachoma occurs only rarely in the United States; it is not a nationally notifiable disease in the U.S.	**Patient Care.** Contact precautions for hospitalized patients. **Etiologic Agent.** Certain serotypes (serovars) of *Chlamydia trachomatis.* **Reservoirs and Mode of Transmission.** Infected humans. Transmission is by direct contact with infectious ocular or nasal secretions or contaminated articles; also spread by flies. **Diagnosis.** Microscopic observation of intracellular chlamydial elementary bodies in epithelial cells of Giemsa-stained conjunctival scrapings or by an immunofluorescent procedure; alternatively, the chlamydias can be isolated from specimens using cell culture techniques.
Gonococcal Conjunctivitis, Gonorrheal Ophthalmia Neonatorum. Acute redness and swelling of conjunctiva, purulent discharge (Fig. 17-8); corneal ulcers, perforation, and blindness, if untreated. Gonorrhea (to be discussed later), in any form, is a nationally notifiable disease in the U.S.	**Patient Care.** Contact precautions for hospitalized patients. **Etiologic Agent.** *Neisseria gonorrhoeae;* Gram-negative, kidney-bean–shaped diplococci; also known as gonococcus (pl., gonococci) or GC. **Reservoirs and Mode of Transmission.** Infected humans (the maternal cervix). Transmission is via contact with the infected birth canal during delivery; adult infection can result from finger-to-eye contact with infectious genital secretions. **Diagnosis.** Microscopic observation of Gram-negative cocci in smears of purulent material; isolation of *N. gonorrhoeae* on appropriate culture media (e.g., chocolate agar or modified chocolate agar, such as Thayer-Martin agar, Martin-Lewis agar, or Transgrow).

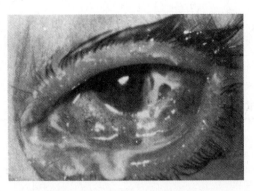

FIGURE 17-8. Purulent conjunctivitis caused by *Neisseria gonorrhoeae.* (Moffett HL. Clinical Microbiology, 2nd ed. Philadelphia: JB Lippincott, 1980.)

Infectious Diseases of the Respiratory System

General Information

For purposes of discussion, the respiratory system can be divided into the upper respiratory tract (URT) and the lower respiratory tract (LRT). The URT includes the paranasal sinuses, nasopharynx, oropharynx, epiglottis, and larynx (voice box). The LRT includes the trachea (windpipe), bronchial tubes, and alveoli of the lungs.

Microflora of the URT may cause opportunistic infections of the respiratory system. Infectious diseases of the URT (e.g., colds and sore throats) are more common than infectious diseases of the LRT; they may predispose the patient to more serious infections, such as sinusitis, otitis media, bronchitis, and pneumonia. LRT infections are the most common cause of death from infectious diseases.

Terms relating to infectious diseases of the respiratory system are as follows:

- **Bronchitis.** Inflammation of the mucous membrane lining of the bronchial tubes; most commonly caused by respiratory viruses (Fig. 17-9).
- **Bronchopneumonia.** Combination of bronchitis and pneumonia.
- **Epiglottitis.** Inflammation of the epiglottis (the mouth of the windpipe); may cause respiratory obstruction, especially in children; frequently caused by *Haemophilus influenzae* type b.
- **Laryngitis.** Inflammation of the mucous membrane of the larynx (voice box).
- **Pharyngitis.** Inflammation of the mucous membrane and underlying tissue of the pharynx; commonly referred to as sore throat. Most cases of pharyngitis are caused by viruses.
- **Pneumonia.** Inflammation of one or both lungs. Alveolar sacs become filled with exudate, inflammatory cells, and fibrin. Most cases of pneumonia are caused by bac-

teria or viruses, but pneumonia can also be caused by fungi and protozoa.
- **Sinusitis.** Inflammation of the lining of one or more of the paranasal sinuses. The most common causes are *S. pneumoniae* and *H. influenzae.* Less common causes are *S. pyogenes, Moraxella catarrhalis,* and *S. aureus.*

Viral Infections of the Upper Respiratory Tract

Information pertaining to viral infections of the upper respiratory tract is contained in Table 17-6.

Bacterial Infections of the Upper Respiratory Tract

Table 17-7 contains information pertaining to bacterial infections of the upper respiratory tract.

Infections of the Lower Respiratory Tract Having Multiple Causes

Information pertaining to infections of the lower respiratory tract having multiple causes is contained in Table 17-8.

Viral Infections of the Lower Respiratory Tract

Table 17-9 contains information pertaining to viral infections of the lower respiratory tract.

Bacterial Infections of the Lower Respiratory Tract

Information pertaining to bacterial infections of the lower respiratory tract is contained in Table 17-10.

Fungal Infections of the Lower Respiratory Tract

Table 17-11 contains information pertaining to fungal infections of the lower respiratory tract.

Infectious Diseases of the Oral Region

General Information

As discussed in Chapter 10, the oral cavity (mouth) is a complex ecosystem suitable for growth and interrelationships of many types of microorganisms (Fig. 17-13). Although the actual indigenous microflora of the mouth varies greatly from one person to the next, studies have shown that it includes about 300 identified species of bacteria, both aerobes and

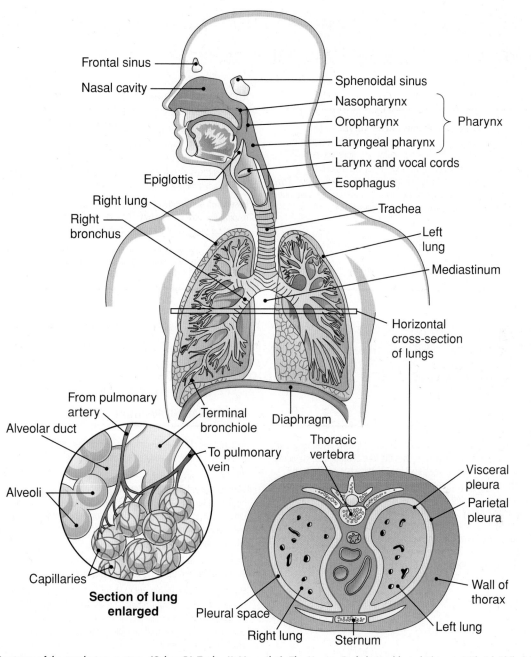

FIGURE 17-9. Anatomy of the respiratory system. (Cohen BJ, Taylor JJ. Memmler's The Human Body in Health and Disease, 10th Ed. Philadelphia: Lippincott Williams & Wilkins, 2005.)

anaerobes. Many additional, as yet unclassified bacteria also live there. Some members of the oral microflora are beneficial—they produce secretions that are antagonistic to other bacteria. Although several species of *Streptococcus* (*S. salivarius, S. mitis, S. sanguis,* and *S. mutans*) and *Actinomyces* species often interact to protect the oral surfaces, in other circumstances they are involved in oral disease.

In the healthy mouth, saliva secreted by salivary and mucous glands helps control the growth of opportunistic oral flora. Saliva contains enzymes (including lysozyme), immunoglobulins (IgA), and buffers to control the near-neutral pH and continually flushes microbes and food particles

through the mouth. Other antimicrobial secretions and phagocytes are found in the mucus that coats the oral surfaces. The hard, complex, calcium tooth enamel, bathed in protective saliva, usually resists damage by oral microbes; however, if the ecologic balance is upset or is not properly maintained, oral disease may result.

Viral Infections of the Oral Region

Cold Sores, Fever Blisters, Herpes Labialis

Fever blisters are superficial clear vesicles on an erythematous (reddened) base, which may appear on the face or

TABLE 17-6

Viral Infections of the Upper Respiratory Tract

DISEASE	ADDITIONAL INFORMATION
The Common Cold, Acute Viral Rhinitis, Acute Coryza. A viral infection of the lining of the nose, sinuses, throat, and large airways. Produces coryza (profuse discharge from nostrils), sneezing, runny eyes, sore throat, chills, malaise; may be accompanied by laryngitis, tracheitis, or bronchitis; secondary bacterial infections, including sinusitis and otitis media, may follow. Most common in fall, winter, and spring. On average, most people have one to six colds annually. Not a nationally notifiable disease in the U.S.	**Patient Care.** Droplet precautions for hospitalized patients. **Etiologic Agent.** Many different viruses cause colds; rhinoviruses (of which there are more than 100 serotypes) are the major cause in adults; other cold-causing viruses include coronaviruses, parainfluenza viruses, RSV, influenza viruses, adenoviruses, and enteroviruses. **Reservoirs and Mode of Transmission.** Infected humans. Transmission is via respiratory secretions by way of hands and fomites; direct contact with or inhalation of airborne droplets. **Diagnosis.** Laboratory diagnosis is usually not required, but cell culture techniques can often demonstrate the specific cause.

TABLE 17-7

Bacterial Infections of the Upper Respiratory Tract

DISEASE	ADDITIONAL INFORMATION
Diphtheria. An acute, contagious bacterial disease primarily involving tonsils, pharynx, larynx, and nose. A cytotoxin causes the formation of a tough, adherent, grayish-white membrane in the throat, which may cause difficulty in breathing. Sore throat, swollen and tender cervical lymph nodes, tonsillitis, swelling of the neck; CNS and heart may be affected; sometimes fatal. There is also a cutaneous form of diphtheria, which is more common in the tropics. At one time, diphtheria was a major killer of children in the U.S. However, as a result of widespread vaccination with diphtheria toxoid (an altered form of diphtheria toxin), no new U.S. cases were reported to the CDC in 2004. Unfortunately, diphtheria continues to be a major killer of children in developing countries, where epidemics are occurring.	**Patient Care.** Droplet precautions for hospitalized patients with pharyngeal diphtheria. Contact precautions for hospitalized patients with cutaneous diphtheria. **Etiologic Agent.** *Corynebacterium diphtheriae;* pleomorphic, Gram-positive bacilli that form characteristic V-, L-, and Y-shaped arrangements of bacilli. Only strains infected with a particular corynebacteriophage (called β-phage) are toxigenic (toxin producing); the exotoxin (diphtheria toxin) is coded for by a bacteriophage gene. **Reservoirs and Mode of Transmission.** Infected humans. Transmission is via airborne droplets, direct contact, contaminated fomites, and raw milk. **Diagnosis.** A nasopharyngeal swab and a throat swab, preferably containing a sample of the membrane, should be sent to the microbiology laboratory for culture. Special media called Loeffler serum medium and cystine-tellurite or Tinsdale medium are used for culture and identification of *C. diphtheriae.* Toxigenicity is determined using laboratory animals (rabbits or guinea pigs).
Streptococcal Pharyngitis, Strep Throat. An acute bacterial infection of the throat with sore throat, chills, fever, headache; beefy red throat; white patches of pus on pharyngeal epithelium; enlarged tonsils; enlarged and tender cervical lymph nodes. The infection may spread to the middle ear, sinuses, or the organs of hearing. Untreated strep throat can lead to complications (sequelae) such as scarlet fever (caused by erythrogenic toxin), rheumatic fever, and glomerulonephritis. The latter two conditions result from the deposition of immune complexes beneath heart and kidney tissue, respectively. Some strains produce a pyrogenic exotoxin that causes toxic shock syndrome and some strains (the so-called flesh-eating bacteria) can cause necrotizing fasciitis. More than 200,000 cases/year in the U.S., mostly among children (3 to 15 years of age). Not a nationally notifiable disease in the U.S.	**Patient Care.** Contact precautions for hospitalized patients. **Etiologic Agent.** *Streptococcus pyogenes;* β-hemolytic, catalase-negative, Gram-positive cocci in chains; also known as group A streptococcus, GAS, or Strep A. **Reservoirs and Mode of Transmission.** Infected humans. Transmission is human to human by direct contact, usually hands; aerosol droplets; secretions from patients and nasal carriers; and contaminated dust, lint, or handkerchiefs; contaminated milk and milk products have been associated with foodborne outbreaks of streptococcal pharyngitis. **Diagnosis.** The sole purpose of a routine throat culture is to determine whether a patient does or does not have strep throat. If β-hemolytic streptococci are isolated, they are tested to determine whether they are group A streptococci. Rapid strep tests (based on detection of antigen) can be performed on throat swabs, but if the test is negative, a more traditional test (such as a throat culture and bacitracin susceptibility) should be performed.

TABLE 17-8

Infections of the Lower Respiratory Tract Having Multiple Causes

DISEASE	ADDITIONAL INFORMATION

DISEASE

Pneumonia. An acute nonspecific infection of the small air sacs (alveoli) and tissues of the lung, with fever, productive cough (meaning that sputum is coughed up), acute chest pain, chills, and shortness of breath; clinically diagnosed by abnormal chest sounds and chest radiographs. Pneumonia is often a secondary infection that follows a primary viral respiratory infection. About 2 million people have pneumonia in the U.S. per year. Of those, approximately 40,000 to 70,000 die. In developing countries, pneumonia and dehydration from severe diarrhea are the leading causes of death. Certain specific types of pneumonia are nationally notifiable diseases in the U.S. For example, 2,093 new U.S. cases of legionellosis and 12 new U.S. cases of psittacosis were reported to the CDC during 2004.

ADDITIONAL INFORMATION

Patient Care. Droplet precautions for hospitalized patients.

Etiologic Agent. Pneumonia may be caused by Gram-positive or Gram-negative bacteria, mycoplasmas, chlamydias, viruses, fungi, or protozoa. Community-acquired bacterial pneumonia is most frequently caused by *Streptococcus pneumoniae* (pneumococcal pneumonia). *S. pneumoniae* is the most common cause of pneumonia in the world (Fig. 17-10). Other bacterial pathogens include *Haemophilus influenzae, Staphylococcus aureus, Klebsiella pneumoniae,* and occasionally other Gram-negative bacilli and anaerobic members of the oral flora. Atypical pathogens include *Legionella pneumonophila* (legionellosis), *Mycoplasma pneumoniae* (mycoplasmal pneumonia; primary atypical pneumonia), *Chlamydophila pneumoniae* (chlamydial pneumonia). Psittacosis (ornithosis; parrot fever), a type of pneumonia caused by *Chlamydophila psittaci,* is normally acquired by inhalation of respiratory secretions and desiccated droppings of infected birds (e.g., parrots, parakeets). Fungi such as *Histoplasma capsulatum* (histoplasmosis), *Coccidioides immitis* (coccidioidomycosis), *Candida albicans* (candidiasis), *Cryptococcus neoformans* (cryptococcosis), *Blastomyces* (blastomycosis), *Aspergillus* (aspergillosis; Fig. 17-11), and *Pneumocystis jiroveci* (previously considered to be a protozoan) may be causative agents of pneumonia, especially in immunocompromised individuals. Various species of bread molds can cause pneumonia in immunosuppressed patients; a condition known as *mucormycosis (zygomycosis).* Viral pneumonia may be caused by adenoviruses, respiratory syncytial virus (RSV), parainfluenza viruses, cytomegalovirus, measles virus, chickenpox virus, and other viruses. Hospital-acquired bacterial pneumonia is most often caused by Gram-negative bacilli, especially *Klebsiella, Enterobacter, Serratia,* and *Acinetobacter* species. *Pseudomonas aeruginosa* and *S. aureus* are also frequent causes of nosocomial pneumonias. Pneumonia is the most common fatal infection acquired in hospitals.

Reservoirs and Mode of Transmission. In most cases, infected humans; other reservoirs include infected psittacine birds (parrots and parakeets) in psittacosis, soil and bird droppings in histoplasmosis and cryptococcosis. Depending on the pathogen involved, transmission is by droplet inhalation, direct oral contact, contact with contaminated hands and fomites, or inhalation of yeasts and fungal spores.

Diagnosis. A good-quality sputum specimen (coughed up from the patient's lungs) must be sent to the microbiology laboratory for C&S. It must be sputum—*not* saliva. A laboratory workup of saliva will not provide clinically relevant information. Laboratory personnel can differentiate between saliva and sputum by preparing and examining a Gram-stained smear of the specimen. Sputum will contain numerous white blood cells (WBCs) and few epithelial cells, whereas saliva will contain few (if any) WBCs and numerous epithelial cells.

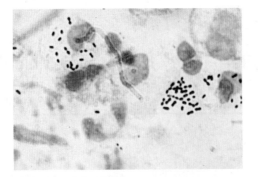

FIGURE 17-10. Gram-positive *Streptococcus pneumoniae* in a Gram-stained smear of a purulent (pus-containing) sputum. Note the diplococci. Several pink-stained polymorphonuclear leukocytes (PMNs) can also be seen. PMNs stain pink in the Gram-staining procedure. (Koneman's Color Atlas and Textbook of Diagnostic Microbiology, 6th ed. Philadelphia: Lippincott Williams & Wilkins, 2006.)

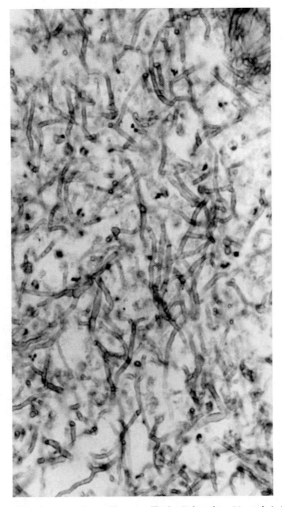

FIGURE 17-11. *Aspergillus fumigatus* in lung tissue from a patient with aspergillosis. (Schaechter M, et al. (eds.). Mechanisms of Microbial Disease, 3rd ed. Philadelphia: Lippincott Williams & Wilkins, 1999.)

TABLE 17-9

Viral Infections of the Lower Respiratory Tract

DISEASE	ADDITIONAL INFORMATION
Acute, Febrile, Viral Respiratory Disease. Characterized by fever and one or more of the following systemic reactions: chills, headache, general aching, malaise, anorexia, and sometimes GI disturbances in infants. May include one or more of the following: rhinitis, pharyngitis, tonsillitis, laryngitis, bronchitis, pneumonia, conjunctivitis, otitis media, sinusitis. Acute, febrile, viral respiratory diseases are not nationally notifiable diseases in the U.S.	**Patient Care.** Contact precautions for hospitalized patients. **Etiologic Agent.** Parainfluenza viruses, respiratory syncytial virus (RSV), adenovirus, rhinoviruses, certain coronaviruses, coxsackieviruses, and echoviruses. RSV is the major viral respiratory tract pathogen of early infancy; it may cause pneumonia, croup, bronchitis, otitis media, and death. **Reservoirs and Mode of Transmission.** Infected humans. Transmission is via direct oral contact or by droplets; indirectly via handkerchiefs, eating utensils, other fomites; some viruses are transmitted via the fecal–oral route. **Diagnosis.** Isolation of the causative agent from respiratory secretions, using cell cultures. Immunodiagnostic procedures are available.
Avian Influenza (Bird Flu). Bird flu is primarily a disease of birds, but can cause human disease. In humans, the virus causes a respiratory infection with symptoms ranging from flulike symptoms (fever, cough, sore throat, muscle aches) to eye infections, pneumonia, acute and severe respiratory distress, and other severe and life-threatening complications.	**Patient care.** Droplet precautions. **Etiologic Agent.** Avian influenza viruses; three prominent subtypes, designated H5, H7, and H9. **Reservoirs and Mode of Transmission.** Infected wild and domesticated birds. Bird-to-human transmission occurs via contact with infected poultry or surfaces that have been contaminated with excretions from infected birds. As of Spring, 2006, very few human-to-human transmissions had occurred. However, influenza viruses commonly mutate, and increased instances of human-to-human transmission are likely to occur in the future. **Diagnosis.** Immunodiagnostic and molecular diagnostic procedures; cell culture. **Note:** See box entitled "A Closer Look at Bird Flu."
Hantavirus Pulmonary Syndrome (HPS). Acute viral disease characterized by fever, myalgias (muscular pain), GI complaints, cough, difficulty breathing, and hypotension (decreased blood pressure). The Sin Nombre hantavirus (meaning the hantavirus with no name) was the cause of the "mystery illness" that occurred in the Four Corners area of the United States in the spring and summer of 1993. Since then, sporadic cases have been reported in many states; sporadic cases and outbreaks have occurred in South America. Only 24 new U.S. cases were reported to the CDC in 2004.	**Patient Care.** Standard precautions for hospitalized patients. **Etiologic Agent.** At least five different hantaviruses (Sin Nombre, Bayou, Black Creek Canal, New York-1, Monongahela) have caused HPS in the U.S.; other strains have caused HPS in South America. **Reservoirs and Mode of Transmission.** Rodents, including the deer mouse, pack rats, and chipmunks. Transmission is via inhalation of aerosolized rodent feces, urine, and saliva. Person-to-person transmission is rare. **Diagnosis.** Immunodiagnostic procedures.
Influenza, Flu. An acute, viral respiratory infection with fever, chills, headache, aches and pains throughout the body (most pronounced in the back and legs), sore throat, cough, nasal drainage; sometimes causing bronchitis, pneumonia, and death in severe cases; nausea, vomiting, and diarrhea may occur, particularly in children. Although the term *stomach flu* is often heard, influenza viruses rarely cause GI symptoms. Stomach flu (also known as the 24-hour flu) is caused by different viruses. The 1918–1919 Spanish flu pandemic (also known as the swine flu epidemic) killed between 20 and 50 million people, worldwide. The 1957–1958 Asian flu and 1968–1969 Hong Kong flu pandemics killed about 70,000 and 34,000 U.S. citizens, respectively. Flu epidemics occur in the U.S. almost every year, affecting 10 to 20% of the general population. Influenza is not a nationally notifiable disease in the U.S.	**Patient Care.** Droplet precautions for hospitalized patients. **Etiologic Agent.** Influenza viruses, types A, B, and C, are RNA viruses in the Orthomyxovirus family (see Fig. 17-12). Influenza A viruses cause severe symptoms and are associated with pandemics and widespread epidemics. Influenza B viruses cause less severe disease and more localized outbreaks. Influenza C viruses usually do not cause epidemics or significant disease. **Reservoirs and Mode of Transmission.** Infected humans are the primary reservoir; pigs and birds also serve as reservoirs. Because pig cells have receptors for both avian and human strains of influenza virus, pigs serve as "mixing bowls," resulting in new strains containing RNA segments from both avian and human strains. It is thought that the 1918 pandemic was caused by an avian influenza virus that jumped directly from birds to humans. Transmission is via airborne spread; direct contact.

(continues)

TABLE 17-9

Viral Infections of the Lower Respiratory Tract *(continued)*

DISEASE	ADDITIONAL INFORMATION
	Diagnosis. Isolation of influenza virus from pharyngeal or nasal secretions, using cell culture techniques; immunodiagnostic procedures; demonstration of a rise in antibody titer (concentration) between acute and convalescent sera (see Chapter 16).
Severe Acute Respiratory Syndrome (SARS). A viral respiratory illness, with high fever, chills, headache, a general feeling of discomfort, and body aches; sometimes diarrhea. Most patients develop a dry cough, followed by pneumonia. SARS was first reported in southern China in late 2002. During 2002–2003, 8,098 people developed SARS, 774 of whom died. Several additional cases in China were reported in 2004, but no U.S. cases of SARS were reported to the CDC in that year.	Patient Care. Droplet precautions for hospitalized patients. Possibly contact precautions also. Etiologic Agent. SARS-associated coronavirus (SARS-CoV). Reservoirs and Mode of Transmission. Infected individuals. Transmission is by respiratory droplets, or by touching the mouth, nose, or eye after touching a contaminated surface or object. Scientists traced the 2002 outbreak to raccoonlike animals called Himalayan palm civets, which are sold for food in live animal markets in China. There is some evidence to indicate that the civets could have been infected by Chinese horseshoe bats. It is not known how the bats became infected. Diagnosis. Immunodiagnostic and molecular diagnostic procedures; cell culture.

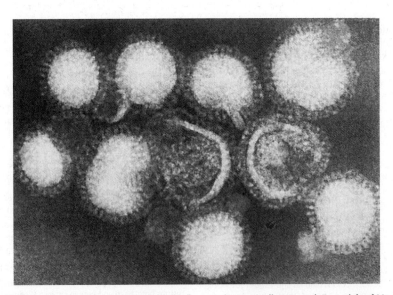

FIGURE 17-12. Transmission electron micrograph of negatively stained influenza viruses. (Volk WA, et al. Essentials of Medical Microbiology, 5th ed. Philadelphia: Lippincott-Raven, 1996.)

A Closer Look at Bird Flu

Avian influenza A/H5N1, or bird flu, is primarily a viral disease of birds. Wild birds carry the virus in their intestines, but they do not become ill. Domesticated birds, such as chickens, ducks, and turkeys, become infected by contact with contaminated nasal, respiratory, or fecal material from infected birds. Fecal–oral transmission is the most common mode of spread between birds. Domesticated birds can become very sick and die, and contact with these birds can cause human illness. The first documented human outbreak of avian influenza occurred in Hong Kong in 1997; 18 people were hospitalized, 6 of whom died. At that time, about 1.5 million chickens were slaughtered to remove the source of the virus. Since then, additional human cases have occurred in many countries, including Cambodia, China, Indonesia, Iraq, Thailand, Turkey, and Vietnam. The disease has affected birds in these and many additional countries. As of June 2006, approximately 225 human cases had occurred worldwide, with about 128 deaths (greater than 50% mortality rate), and the world was bracing and preparing itself for a worldwide pandemic of bird flu. The CDC has estimated that a medium-level influenza pandemic could cause between 89,000 and 207,000 deaths in the United States. The CDC was advising that travelers to endemic areas of Asia avoid poultry farms, contact with animals in live food markets, and any surfaces that appear to be contaminated with feces from poultry or other animals.

TABLE 17-10

Bacterial Infections of the Lower Respiratory Tract

DISEASE	ADDITIONAL INFORMATION
Legionellosis, Legionnaire's Disease, Pontiac Fever. An acute bacterial pneumonia with anorexia, malaise, myalgia, headache, high fever, chills, dry cough followed by a productive cough, shortness of breath, diarrhea, pleural and abdominal pain; there is about a 40% fatality rate. Pontiac fever is not associated with pneumonia or death. Legionnaire's disease was first recognized as a disease after an outbreak in a Philadelphia hotel in 1976, but evidence exists that prior epidemics and deaths were caused by *Legionella* spp. Epidemics continue to occur, often associated with hotels, cruise ships, hospitals, and supermarkets. It usually affects the elderly; people with preexisting respiratory disease, diabetes mellitus, renal disease, or malignancy; people who are immunocompromised; heavy smokers; and heavy drinkers. A total of 2,093 new U.S. cases were reported to the CDC in 2004.	**Patient Care.** Standard precautions for hospitalized patients. **Etiologic Agent.** *Legionella pneumophila,* a poorly staining, Gram-negative bacillus; additional *Legionella* spp. can also cause the disease; as of 2000, there were 35 known species of *Legionella.* **Reservoirs and Mode of Transmission.** Environmental water sources; ponds, lakes, creeks, hot water and air-conditioning systems, cooling towers, evaporative condensers, whirlpool spas, hot tubs, shower heads, humidifiers, tap water and water distillation systems, decorative fountains, perhaps soil and dust; aerosols have been produced by vegetable misting devices in supermarkets. Airborne transmission from water and perhaps dust; probably not person-to-person. **Diagnosis.** Sputum, blood, and urine specimens should be sent to the microbiology laboratory for C&S. *Legionella* spp. stain poorly and require cysteine and other nutrients to grow. The recommended culture medium is buffered charcoal yeast extract agar. Immunodiagnostic procedures are available.
Mycoplasmal Pneumonia, Primary Atypical Pneumonia. Gradual onset with headache, malaise, dry cough, sore throat, and, less often, chest discomfort. Scant sputum at first, which may increase as the disease progresses. Illness may last from a few days to a month or more. Most common in people 5 to 35 years of age. Pneumonias produced by mycoplasmas and chlamydias are the most common types of atypical pneumonias (i.e., pneumonias that are caused by organisms other than those that are the typical causes of pneumonia). Not a nationally notifiable disease in the U.S.	**Patient Care.** Droplet precautions for hospitalized patients. **Etiologic Agent.** *Mycoplasma pneumoniae;* tiny, Gram-negative bacteria, lacking cell walls. **Reservoirs and Mode of Transmission.** Infected humans. Transmission is via droplet inhalation; direct contact with an infected person or articles contaminated with nasal secretions or sputum from an ill, coughing patient. **Diagnosis.** Demonstration of a rise in antibody titer between acute and convalescent sera. On artificial media, *M. pneumoniae* produces tiny "fried egg" colonies, having a dense central area and a less dense periphery.

(continues)

TABLE 17-10

Bacterial Infections of the Lower Respiratory Tract *(continued)*

DISEASE	ADDITIONAL INFORMATION
Tuberculosis, TB. An acute or chronic mycobacterial infection of the lower respiratory tract; malaise, fever, night sweats, weight loss, productive cough; shortness of breath, chest pain; hemoptysis (coughing up blood) and hoarseness in advanced stages. May invade lymph nodes to cause systemic disease; tuberculosis may affect many areas of the body including the kidney, urinary bladder, and bones. A resurgence of tuberculosis in the U.S. occurred during the late 1980s and early 1990s, primarily as a result of the HIV/AIDS epidemic and the emergence of multidrug-resistant strains of *M. tuberculosis.* During 2004, a total of 14,517 new U.S. cases of tuberculosis were reported to the CDC. Other *Mycobacterium* spp. also commonly cause infections in AIDS patients. (See Chapter 11 for additional information regarding the current TB pandemic.)	**Patient Care.** Airborne precautions for hospitalized patients. Wear a type N95 respirator when working with hospitalized tuberculosis patients. **Etiologic Agent.** Primarily *Mycobacterium tuberculosis* (a slow-growing, acid-fast, Gram-positive to Gram-variable bacillus); occasionally other *Mycobacterium* spp. (e.g., *M. africanum* or *M. bovis* from cattle); *M. tuberculosis* is sometimes referred to as the tubercle bacillus. **Reservoirs and Mode of Transmission.** Primarily, infected humans; rarely, primates, cattle, other infected mammals. Transmission is via airborne droplets produced by infected people during coughing, sneezing, and even singing; prolonged direct contact with infected individuals. Bovine tuberculosis may result from exposure to infected cattle or ingestion of unpasteurized, contaminated milk or other dairy products. **Diagnosis.** Demonstration of acid-fast bacilli (AFB) in sputum specimens provides a rapid, presumptive diagnosis of tuberculosis. Isolation of *M. tuberculosis* on Löwenstein-Jensen or Middlebrook culture media takes about 3 to 6 weeks, owing to the organism's long generation time (about 18 to 24 hours). A variety of more rapid techniques are available for isolation and identification of *M. tuberculosis,* including automated and semi-automated instruments, DNA probes, polymerase chain reaction, and gas-liquid chromatography. Susceptibility testing should be performed as soon as possible because many strains of *M. tuberculosis* are multidrug-resistant. Infected patients show a positive delayed hypersensitivity skin test (the Mantoux purified protein derivative [PPD] tuberculin skin test), and pulmonary tubercles may be seen on chest radiographs. Recall from Chapter 16 that a positive TB skin test result may indicate any of five possibilities, including past infection, present infection, or receipt of BCG vaccine.
Whooping Cough, Pertussis. A highly contagious, acute bacterial childhood (usually) infection. The first stage (the prodromal or catarrhal stage) of the disease involves mild, coldlike symptoms. The second stage (the paroxysmal stage) produces severe, uncontrollable coughing fits. The coughing often ends in a prolonged, high-pitched, deeply indrawn breath (the "whoop," from which whooping cough gets its name). The coughing fits produce a clear, tenacious mucus and vomiting; they may be so severe as to cause lung rupture, bleeding in the eyes and brain, broken ribs, rectal prolapse, or hernia. The third stage (the recovery or convalescent stage) usually begins within 4 weeks of onset. Parapertussis is a similar but milder disease. A total of 25,827 new U.S. cases of whooping cough were reported to the CDC in 2004.	**Patient Care.** Droplet precautions for hospitalized patients. **Etiologic Agent.** Pertussis is caused by *Bordetella pertussis,* a small, encapsulated, nonmotile, Gram-negative coccobacillus that produces endotoxin and exotoxins. Parapertussis is caused by *Bordetella parapertussis.* A related organism, *Bordetella bronchiseptica,* causes respiratory infections in animals, including kennel cough in dogs. **Reservoirs and Mode of Transmission.** Infected humans. Transmission is via droplets produced by coughing. **Diagnosis.** Nasopharyngeal aspirates or swabs should be sent to the microbiology laboratory. Special media, such as Bordet-Gengou agar (a potato-based medium) or Regan-Lowe agar (a charcoal/horse blood medium), are used to isolate *B. pertussis.* Nucleic acid and immunodiagnostic procedures are also available.

TABLE 17-11

Fungal Infections of the Lower Respiratory Tract

DISEASE	ADDITIONAL INFORMATION
Coccidioidomycosis. Starts as a respiratory infection, with fever, chills, cough, and (rarely) pain. May progress to the disseminated form of the disease, which is frequently fatal; lung lesions, abscesses throughout the body, especially in subcutaneous tissues, skin, bone, and CNS. A total of 6,449 new U.S. cases were reported to the CDC during 2004.	**Patient Care.** Standard precautions for hospitalized patients. **Etiologic Agent.** *Coccidioides immitis,* a dimorphic fungus; exists as a mold in soil and on culture media (25°C), where it produces arthrospores (arthroconidia); appears as spherical yeast cells, called spherules, in tissues; *C. immitis* arthrospores have potential use as a bioterrorist agent. **Reservoirs and Mode of Transmission.** Soil in arid and semiarid areas of the Western Hemisphere; in U.S., from California to southern Texas. Transmission is via inhalation of arthrospores, especially during wind and dust storms; not directly transmissible person to person. **Diagnosis.** Direct examination and culturing of sputum, pus, urine, cerebrospinal fluid (CSF), or biopsy materials. The mold form is highly infectious. All work must be performed in a BSL-2 or BSL-3 facility (refer to CD-ROM Appendix 4). Skin tests and immunodiagnostic procedures are also available.
Cryptococcosis. A deep mycosis, usually presenting as a meningitis, although infection of the lungs, kidneys, prostate, skin, and bone also occur; a common infection in AIDS patients. Not a nationally notifiable disease in the U.S., where an estimated 300 cases occur each year.	**Patient Care.** Standard precautions for hospitalized patients. **Etiologic Agent.** Two subspecies of *Cryptococcus neoformans;* an encapsulated yeast. **Reservoirs and Mode of Transmission.** Pigeon nests, pigeon droppings, other bird droppings, soil. Transmission is via inhalation of yeasts; not transmitted person to person. **Diagnosis.** Pulmonary infection and meningitis can be presumptively diagnosed by observing encapsulated budding yeasts in an India ink preparation (see CD-ROM Appendix 5) of sputum or spinal fluid, respectively. Culture and identification using biochemical tests are required for definitive diagnosis. Immunodiagnostic procedures are available.
Histoplasmosis. A systemic mycosis of varying severity, ranging from asymptomatic to acute to chronic; the primary lesion is usually in the lungs. The acute disease involves malaise, fever, chills, headache. Although not a nationally notifiable disease, histoplasmosis is the most common systemic fungal disease in the U.S., occurring primarily in the Ohio, Mississippi, and Missouri River valleys.	**Patient Care.** Standard precautions for hospitalized patients. **Etiologic Agent.** *Histoplasma capsulatum* var. *capsulatum,* a dimorphic fungus that grows as a mold in soil and as a yeast in animal and human hosts. **Reservoirs and Mode of Transmission.** Soil containing bird droppings, especially chicken droppings; bat droppings in caves; around starling, blackbird, and pigeon roosts. Transmission is via inhalation of conidia (asexual spores) from soil. **Diagnosis.** Observation of yeast form in stained smears of clinical specimens. Culture and identification by biochemical tests. Produces mold colonies when incubated at room temperature and yeast colonies when incubated at body temperature. Conversion from the mold form to the yeast form can sometimes be accomplished in the laboratory. Skin tests and immunodiagnostic procedures are available.
Pneumocystis Pneumonia (PCP), Interstitial Plasma-Cell Pneumonia. An acute to subacute pulmonary disease found in malnourished, chronically ill children; premature infants; and immunosuppressed patients (patients whose immune systems are not functioning properly), such as AIDS patients. A common, contributory cause of death in AIDS patients. *Pneumocystis* causes an asymptomatic infection in immunocompetent people (people whose immune systems are functioning properly). Patients have fever, difficulty in breathing, rapid breathing, dry cough, and cyanosis; pulmonary infiltration of alveoli with frothy exudate; usually fatal in untreated patients. PCP is not a nationally notifiable disease in the U.S.	**Patient Care.** Standard precautions for hospitalized patients. **Etiologic Agent.** *Pneumocystis jiroveci* (previously called *Pneumocystis carinii*); has both protozoal and fungal properties; was classified as a protozoan for many years; currently classified as a fungus. **Reservoirs and Mode of Transmission.** Infected humans. The mode of transmission is unknown; perhaps direct contact, perhaps transfer of pulmonary secretions from infected to susceptible persons, or perhaps airborne. **Diagnosis.** Demonstration of *Pneumocystis* in material from bronchial brushings, open lung biopsy, lung aspirates, or smears of tracheobronchial mucus by various staining methods. *P. jiroveci* cannot be cultured.

Porphyromonas, Fusobacterium, Prevotella, Actinomyces, and *Treponema* spp.) to become involved in the production of oral diseases. The coating that forms on unclean teeth, called *dental plaque,* is a coaggregation of bacteria and their products. Many of these microorganisms produce a slime layer or glycocalyx that enables them to attach firmly and cause damage to the tooth enamel. Certain carbohydrates, especially sucrose, are metabolized by streptococci (especially *S. mutans*), lactobacilli, and *Actinomyces* spp., producing lactic acid, which rapidly dissolves the tooth enamel. When plaque remains on teeth for more than 72 hours, it hardens into tartar or calculus, which cannot be completely removed by brushing and flossing.

lips. They crust and heal within a few days. Reactivation may be caused by trauma, fever (hence the name), physiologic changes, or disease. The infection may be severe and extensive in immunosuppressed individuals. Cold sores are usually caused by herpes simplex virus type 1 (HSV 1), although they can also be caused by herpes simplex type 2 (HSV 2). HSV 1 and HSV 2 are also known as human herpesvirus 1 and human herpesvirus 2, respectively. They are DNA viruses in the Family Herpesviridae. Either of these viruses may also infect the genital tract, although genital herpes infections are usually caused by HSV 2.

Bacterial Infections of the Oral Cavity

The anaerobic environment produced by oxidation–reduction reactions of the oral flora organisms allows certain genera of anaerobic bacteria (e.g., *Bacteroides,*

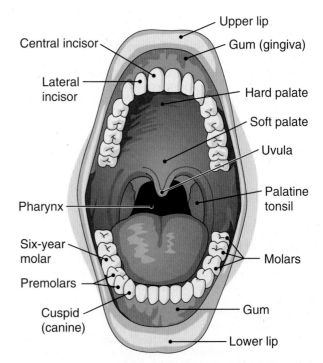

FIGURE 17-13. Anatomy of the mouth. (Cohen BJ, Taylor JJ. Memmler's *The Human Body in Health and Disease,* 10th Ed. Philadelphia: Lippincott Williams & Wilkins, 2005.)

Terms relating to infectious diseases of the oral cavity are as follows:

- **Dental caries.** Tooth decay or cavities. Starts when the external surface (the enamel) of a tooth is dissolved by organic acids, which are produced by masses of microorganisms attached to the tooth (dental plaque); followed by enzymatic destruction of the protein matrix, cavitation, and bacterial invasion. The most common cause of tooth decay is *S. mutans,* which produces lactic acid as an end product in the fermentation of glucose.
- **Gingivitis.** Inflammation of the gingiva (gums).
- **Periodontitis.** Inflammation of the periodontium (tissues that surround and support the teeth, including the gingiva and supporting bone); in severe cases, teeth loosen and fall out.

Oral infections result from the unique microbial population, reduced host defenses, improper diet, and poor dental hygiene. These diseases are the consequence of at least four microbial activities, including (1) formation of dextran (a polysaccharide) from sugars by streptococci, (2) acid production by lactobacilli, (3) deposition of calculus by *Actinomyces* species, and (4) secretion of inflammatory substances (endotoxin) by *Bacteroides* species. This combination of circumstances damages the teeth, soft tissues (gingiva), alveolar bone, and the periodontal fibers attaching teeth to bone. Diseases such as gingivitis, periodontitis, and trench mouth are collectively known as *periodontal diseases*.

Periodontal diseases can be prevented by maintaining good health, proper oral hygiene (tooth brushing, using tartar-control toothpaste, and flossing), an adequate diet without sugars, and regular fluoride treatments to help control the microbial population and to prevent damaging bacterial interactions. Severe gingivitis and periodontitis require professional care by a specially trained dentist called a periodontist. Using techniques known as scaling and planing, periodontists remove tartar that has accumulated on tooth surfaces up to one fifth of an inch below the gum line—areas where tooth brushing and flossing cannot reach. After dental surgery, periodontists often prescribe a chlorhexidine mouth rinse as a temporary substitute for brushing and flossing.

Acute Necrotizing Ulcerative Gingivitis (ANUG), Vincent's Angina, Trench Mouth

Disease Characteristics. The term "trench mouth" originated in World War I, where soldiers developed the infection while fighting in trenches. It is usually the result of a combination of poor oral hygiene, physical or emotional stress, and poor diet. It involves painful, bleeding gums and tonsils, erosion of gum tissue, and swollen lymph nodes beneath the jaw. It causes extremely bad breath.

Pathogens. Trench mouth is a synergistic infection involving two or more species of anaerobic bacteria of the indigenous oral microflora. The most commonly involved bacteria are *Fusobacterium nucleatum (*an anaerobic, Gram-negative bacillus) and *Treponema vincentii* (a spirochete). Other commonly involved anaerobic Gram-negative bacilli are *Bacteroides* spp., *Prevotella intermedius,* and *Prevotella melaninogenica.*

Prevention and Control. As is true for other periodontal diseases, trench mouth can be prevented by good oral hygiene. Trench mouth is thought to be noncontagious. Standard precautions are sufficient for hospitalized patients.

Fungal Infections of the Oral Cavity

Thrush

Disease Characteristics. Thrush is a yeast infection of the oral cavity. It is common in infants, elderly patients, and immunosuppressed individuals. White, creamy patches occur on the tongue, mucous membranes, and the corners of the mouth. Thrush can be a manifestation of disseminated *Candida* infection (candidiasis).

Pathogens. The yeast, *Candida albicans,* and related species.

Diagnosis. Observation of yeast cells and pseudohyphae (strings of elongated buds) in microscopic examination of wet mounts, and culture confirmation.

Infectious Diseases of the Gastrointestinal (GI) Tract

General Information

The digestive tract consists of a long tube with many expanded areas designed for digestion of food, absorption of nutrients, and elimination of undigested materials (Fig. 17-14). Transient and resident microbes continuously enter and leave the GI tract. Most of the microorganisms ingested with food are destroyed in the stomach and duodenum by the low pH (gastric contents have a pH of approximately 1.5), and are inhibited from growing in the lower intestines by the resident microflora (microbial antagonism). They are then flushed from the colon during defecation, along with large numbers of indigenous microbes. The indigenous microflora of the GI tract was discussed in Chapter 10.

Terms relating to infectious diseases of the GI tract include the following:

- **Colitis.** Inflammation of the colon (the large intestine).
- **Diarrhea.** An abnormally frequent discharge of semisolid or fluid fecal matter. Some laboratory workers define diarrheal specimens as "stool specimens that conform to the shape of the container."
- **Dysentery.** Frequent watery stools, accompanied by abdominal pain, fever, and dehydration. The stool specimens may contain blood or mucus.
- **Enteritis.** Inflammation of the intestines, usually referring to the small intestine.

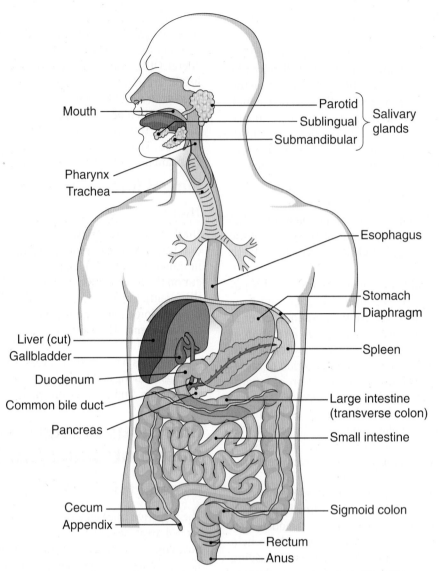

FIGURE 17-14. Anatomy of the gastrointestinal tract. (Cohen BJ, Taylor JJ. Memmler's The Human Body in Health and Disease, 10th Ed. Philadelphia: Lippincott Williams & Wilkins, 2005.)

- **Gastritis.** Inflammation of the mucosal lining of the stomach.
- **Gastroenteritis.** Inflammation of the mucosal linings of the stomach and intestines.
- **Hepatitis.** Inflammation of the liver; usually the result of viral infection, but can be caused by toxic agents.

Infections of the GI Tract Having Multiple Causes

Diarrhea can have many causes. It is a symptom in a wide variety of conditions and diseases; it can be caused by certain foods or drugs; or it may be the result of an infectious disease. If the diarrhea is the result of an infectious disease, the pathogen may be a virus, a bacterium, a protozoan, or a helminth. Dysentery may also be caused by a variety of pathogens, including bacteria (e.g., *Shigella* spp.

cause bacillary dysentery) and protozoa (e.g., amebiasis and balantidiasis; Chapter 18).

Viral Infections of the GI Tract

Information pertaining to viral infections of the GI tract is contained in Table 17-12.

Viral Hepatitis

Hepatitis, or inflammation of the liver, can have many causes, including alcohol, drugs, and viruses. Viral hepatitis refers to hepatitis caused by any one of about a dozen different viruses, including hepatitis A virus (HAV), hepatitis B virus (HBV), hepatitis C virus (HCV), hepatitis D virus (HDV), hepatitis E virus (HEV), hepatitis G virus (HGV), hepatitis GB virus A (HGBV-A), hepatitis GB virus B (HGBV-B), and hepatitis GB virus C (HGBV-C). Hepatitis can also occur as a result of viral diseases such as infectious

TABLE 17-12

Viral Infections of the GI Tract

DISEASE	ADDITIONAL INFORMATION
Viral Gastroenteritis, Viral Enteritis, Viral Diarrhea. Viral gastroenteritis may be an endemic or epidemic illness in infants, children, and adults. Symptoms include nausea, vomiting, diarrhea, abdominal pain, myalgia, headache, malaise, and low-grade fever. Although most often a self-limiting disease lasting 24 to 48 hours, viral gastroenteritis (especially caused by rotaviruses) can be fatal in infants and young children. In developing countries, rotavirus infections are responsible for more than 800,000 diarrheal deaths per year. Although viral gastroenteritis is sometimes referred to as stomach flu or 24-hour flu, keep in mind that *flu* is an abbreviated form of influenza, which is a respiratory disease. Viral gastroenteritis is not a nationally notifiable disease in the U.S.	**Patient Care.** Contact precautions for hospitalized patients. **Etiologic Agent.** The most common viruses infecting children in their first years of life are enteric adenoviruses, astroviruses, caliciviruses (including Norwalk-like viruses), and rotaviruses. Those infecting children and adults include Norwalk virus, certain Norwalk-like viruses, and rotaviruses. **Reservoirs and Mode of Transmission.** Infected humans; possibly contaminated water and shellfish. Transmission is most often via the fecal–oral route. Airborne transmission and contact with contaminated fomites may cause hospital epidemics. Foodborne, waterborne, and shellfish transmission have been reported. **Diagnosis.** By electron microscopic examination of stool specimens or by immunodiagnostic procedures.

mononucleosis, yellow fever, and cytomegalovirus infection. See Table 17-13 for information about viral types, modes of transmission, and types of disease. A variety of immunodiagnostic procedures are available for diagnosis of viral hepatitis.

In 2004, the number of new U.S. cases of acute hepatitis A, hepatitis B, and hepatitis C reported to the CDC were 5,970, 6,741, and 713, respectively. The number of actual cases is thought to be much higher. The World Health Organization (WHO) estimates that 350 million people are chronically infected with HBV worldwide, that about 1 million people die each year as a result of HBV infections, and that more than 2 million new acute clinical cases occur annually.

Vaccines are available for HAV and HBV. The HAV vaccine, which contains inactivated virus grown in cell culture, is recommended for people at increased risk of acquiring hepatitis A (including military personnel and others traveling to regions where HAV is endemic, homosexual and bisexual males, and users of illicit drugs). The HBV vaccine is a subunit vaccine, produced by genetically engineered *Saccharomyces cerevisiae* (common baker's yeast). At first, only recommended for persons at high risk of acquiring HBV infection (such as infants born to HBV antigen-positive mothers, household contacts of HBV carriers, homosexual and bisexual males, and users of illicit drugs), it is now also routinely administered to U.S. children. It is required for healthcare workers exposed to blood.

In addition to vaccination against HBV, healthcare personnel practice standard precautions (Chapter 12), which are designed to reduce the risk of transmission of bloodborne and other pathogens in hospitals. Hepatitis B immune

globulin can be given to unvaccinated people who have been exposed to HBV, perhaps by accidental needlestick injury.

Bacterial Infections of the GI Tract

Table 17-14 contains information pertaining to bacterial infections of the GI tract.

Enterovirulent *Escherichia coli*

Escherichia coli is a Gram-negative bacillus that is found in the GI tract of all humans. The strains and serotypes of *E. coli* that are part of the indigenous microflora of the GI tract are opportunistic pathogens. They usually cause no harm while in the GI tract, but have the potential to cause serious infections if they gain access to the bloodstream, the urinary bladder, or a wound. *E. coli* is the major cause of septicemia, urinary tract infections, and nosocomial infections. There are other strains and serotypes of *E. coli* in nature that are not indigenous microflora of the human colon and always cause disease when they are ingested. Collectively, these strains and serotypes are referred to as enterovirulent *E. coli*. Information pertaining to two general types, the enterohemorrhagic *E. coli* and the enterotoxigenic *E. coli*, is contained in Table 17-15.

Bacterial Foodborne Intoxications, Foodborne Infections, Food Poisoning

The term *food poisoning* is broad and may include diseases resulting from the ingestion of chemical contaminants as well as bacteria or bacterial toxins, phycotoxins, mycotoxins, viruses, or protozoa. Technically, diseases resulting from the ingestion of toxin-producing microorganisms are called *infectious diseases,* whereas diseases resulting from the ingestion of preformed microbial toxins are called

TABLE 17-13

Most Common Types of Viral Hepatitis

DISEASE NAME	NAME/TYPE OF VIRUS	MODE OF TRANSMISSION	TYPE OF DISEASE
Type A Hepatitis; HAV Infection; Infectious Hepatitis; Epidemic Hepatitis.	Hepatitis A virus; HAV; a nonenveloped, linear ssRNA virus in the Genus Hepatovirus, Family Picornaviridae	Fecal–oral transmission; person to person; infected food handlers; fecally contaminated foods and water.	Abrupt onset; varies in clinical severity from a mild illness lasting 1 to 2 weeks to a severe disabling disease lasting several months; no chronic infection.
Type B Hepatitis; HBV Infection; Serum Hepatitis.	Hepatitis B virus; HBV; an enveloped, circular dsDNA virus in the Genus Ortho-hepadnavirus, Family Hepadnaviridae; the only DNA virus that causes hepatitis.	Sexual or household contact with an infected person; mother to infant before or during birth; injected drug use; tattooing; needlesticks and other types of nosoco-mial transmission.	Usually an insidious (gradual) onset; severity ranges from inapparent cases to fulminating, fatal cases; chronic infections occur; may lead to cirrhosis or hepatocellular carcinoma.
Type C Hepatitis; HCV Infection; Non-A Non-B Hepatitis.	Hepatitis C virus; HCV; non A non B hepatitis virus; an enveloped, linear ssRNA virus in the Genus Hepacivirus, Family Flaviviridae.	Primarily parenterally transmitted (e.g., via blood transfusion); rarely, sexually.	Usually an insidious onset; 50 to 80% of patients develop a chronic infection; may lead to cirrhosis or hepatocellular carcinoma.
Type D Hepatitis; Delta Hepatitis.	Hepatitis D virus; HDV; delta virus; an enveloped, circular ssRNA viral satellite (a defec-tive RNA virus) in the Genus Deltavirus.	Exposure to infected blood and body fluids; contami-nated needles; sexual trans-mission; coinfection with HBV is necessary.	Usually an abrupt onset; may progress to a chronic and severe disease.
Type E Hepatitis.	Hepatitis E virus; HEV; a spherical, nonenveloped, ssRNA virus in the Genus Calicivirus, Family Caliciviri-dae.	Fecal–oral transmission; primarily via fecally contami-nated drinking water; also person to person.	Similar to Type A hepatitis; no evidence of a chronic form.
Type G Hepatitis.	Hepatitis G virus; HGV; a lin-ear ssRNA virus in the Genus Hepacivirus, Family Flaviviridae.	Parenteral	Can cause chronic hepatitis.

ds, double stranded; *ss,* single-stranded.

TABLE 17-14

Bacterial Infections of the GI Tract

DISEASE	ADDITIONAL INFORMATION
Bacterial Gastritis and Ulcers. Infection with *Helicobacter pylori* can cause chronic bacterial gastritis and duodenal ulcers. Gastritis is suspected when a person has upper abdominal pain with nausea or heartburn. People with duodenal ulcers may experience gnawing, burning, aching, mild to moderate pain just below the breastbone, an empty feeling, and hunger. The pain usually occurs when the stomach is empty. Drinking milk, eating, or taking antacids generally relieves the pain, but it usually returns 2 or 3 hours later. Gastric ulcers and gastric adenocarcinoma are also epidemiologically associated with *H. pylori* infection. Gastric ulcers can cause swelling of the tissues leading into the small intestine, which prevents food from easily passing out of the stomach. This, in turn, can cause pain, bloating, nausea, or vomiting after eating. Gastric ulcers and duodenal ulcers are types of peptic ulcers. Complications of peptic ulcers include penetration, perforation, bleeding, and obstruction. Gastritis and ulcers are not nationally notifiable diseases in the U.S.	**Etiologic Agent.** *Helicobacter pylori* is a curved, microaerophilic, capnophilic, Gram-negative bacillus that is found on the mucus-secreting epithelial cells of the stomach. No other bacteria are known to grow in the extremely acidic stomach. **Reservoirs and Mode of Transmission.** Infected humans. Transmission is probably via ingestion; presumed to be either oral–oral or fecal–oral transmission. **Diagnosis.** Diagnostic techniques include staining and culturing of gastric and duodenal biopsy specimens, the urea breath test, the NH_4 excretion test, DNA probes, and immunodiagnostic procedures. In the urea breath test, the patient ingests radioactively labeled urea and his or her breath is analyzed 60 minutes later for radioactively labeled CO_2. The enzyme urease, produced by *H. pylori*, splits the urea into ammonia and CO_2; hence, the presence of radioactively labeled CO_2 indicates the presence of *H. pylori*. In the NH_4 excretion test, the patient consumes urea containing radioactively labeled nitrogen. The ammonia produced in the stomach by *H. pylori* is absorbed into the blood and excreted in the urine, and the amount of radioactively labeled NH_4 in the urine is measured.
Campylobacter Enteritis. An acute bacterial enteric disease ranging from asymptomatic to severe, with diarrhea, nausea, vomiting, fever, malaise, abdominal pain; usually self-limiting, lasting 2 to 5 days. Stools may contain gross or occult (hidden) blood, mucus, and WBCs. Although *Campylobacter* enteritis is not a nationally notifiable disease, *Campylobacter* spp. are the major cause of bacterial diarrhea in the U.S.	**Patient Care.** Contact precautions for hospitalized patients. **Etiologic Agent.** *Campylobacter jejuni* and less commonly, *Campylobacter coli*; curved, S-shaped, or spiral-shaped Gram-negative bacilli; often having a "gull-winged" morphology after cell division (a pair of curved bacilli); microaerophilic and capnophilic; optimal growth temperature of 42°C. **Reservoirs and Mode of Transmission.** Animals, including poultry, cattle, sheep, swine, rodents, birds, kittens, puppies, and other pets. Most raw poultry is contaminated with *C. jejuni*, thus necessitating proper methods of cleaning and disinfecting in the kitchen (see Chapter 8). Transmission is via ingestion of contaminated food (e.g., chicken, pork), raw milk, water; contact with infected pets, farm animals; contaminated cutting boards. **Diagnosis.** Recovery of *Campylobacter* from stool specimens, using selective medium (Campy blood agar, containing several antimicrobial agents to suppress growth of other bacteria), a Campy gas mixture (5% O_2, 10% CO_2, 85% N_2), and 42°C incubation.
Cholera. An acute, bacterial, diarrheal disease with profuse watery stools, occasional vomiting, rapid dehydration; if untreated, circulatory collapse, renal failure, and death may occur. More than 50% of untreated people with severe cholera die. Occurs worldwide, with periodic epidemics and pandemics. A recent Western Hemisphere cholera pandemic started in Peru in 1991; by 1994, more than 950,000 cases had been reported in 21 countries in the Western Hemisphere. Only 5 new U.S. cases were reported to the CDC in 2004. Most U.S. cases involve the ingestion of raw or undercooked seafood (e.g., oysters) from the coastal waters of Louisiana and Texas.	**Patient Care.** Contact precautions for hospitalized patients. **Etiologic Agent.** Certain biotypes of *Vibrio cholerae* serogroup 01; curved (comma-shaped), Gram-negative bacilli that secrete an *enterotoxin* (a toxin that adversely affects cells in the intestinal tract) called *choleragen*. Other *Vibrio* spp. (*Vibrio parahaemolyticus, Vibrio vulnificus*) also cause diarrheal diseases. Vibrios are halophilic (salt-loving) and are thus found in marine environments. **Reservoirs and Mode of Transmission.** Infected humans and aquatic reservoirs (copepods and other zooplankton). Transmission is via the fecal–oral route; contact with feces or vomitus of infected people; ingestion of fecally contaminated water and foods (especially raw or undercooked shellfish and other seafood); flies. **Diagnosis.** Rectal swabs or stool specimens should be inoculated onto thiosulfate-citrate-bile-sucrose (TCBS) agar; different *Vibrio* spp. produce different reactions on this medium. Biochemical tests are used to identify the various species. Biotyping is accomplished using commercially available antisera.

(continues)

TABLE 17-14

Bacterial Infections of the GI Tract (continued)

DISEASE	ADDITIONAL INFORMATION

Salmonellosis. Gastroenteritis with sudden onset of headache, abdominal pain, diarrhea, nausea, and sometimes vomiting. Dehydration may be severe. May develop into septicemia or localized infection in any tissue of the body. A total of 41,660 new U.S. cases of salmonellosis were reported to the CDC in 2004.

Patient Care. Standard precautions for most hospitalized patients. Contact precautions for diapered or incontinent patients.

Etiologic Agent. Gastrointestinal salmonellosis is caused by members of the family *Enterobacteriaceae* that some microbiologists call *Salmonella typhimurium* and *Salmonella enteritidis* (of which there are more than 2,000 serotypes), and other microbiologists call *Salmonella* serotype typhimurium and *Salmonella* serotype enteritidis. They are Gram-negative bacilli that invade intestinal cells, release endotoxin, and produce cytotoxins and enterotoxins. About 200 of the *S. enteritidis* serotypes cause gastrointestinal salmonellosis in the U.S.

Reservoirs and Mode of Transmission. A wide range of domestic and wild animals, including poultry, swine, cattle, rodents, reptiles (e.g., pet iguanas and turtles), pet chicks, dogs and cats; also infected humans (e.g., patients, carriers). Transmission is via ingestion of contaminated food (e.g., eggs, unpasteurized milk, meat, poultry, raw fruits and vegetables); fecal–oral transmission from person to person; food handlers; contaminated water supplies.

Diagnosis. Stool specimens should be submitted to the microbiology laboratory for C&S. *Salmonella* spp. are non–lactose-fermenters and thus produce colorless colonies on MacConkey agar. Biochemical tests are used for identification, and commercially available antisera are used for serotyping.

Typhoid Fever, Enteric Fever. A systemic bacterial disease with fever, severe headache, malaise, anorexia, a rash on the trunk in about 25% of patients, nonproductive cough, and constipation. Bacteremia; pneumonia; gallbladder, liver, bone infection; endocarditis; meningitis, and other complications may occur. About 10% of untreated patients die. Worldwide, an estimated 17 million cases per year with approximately 600,000 deaths. A total of 322 new U.S. cases were reported to the CDC in 2004.

Patient Care. Standard precautions for most hospitalized patients. Contact precautions for diapered or incontinent patients.

Etiologic Agent. *Salmonella typhi* (the typhoid bacillus); Gram-negative bacilli that release endotoxin and produce exotoxins. A similar, but less severe, infection is caused by *Salmonella paratyphi.*

Reservoirs and Mode of Transmission. Infected humans for typhoid and paratyphoid; rarely, domestic animals for paratyphoid. Some people become carriers after infection, shedding the pathogens in their feces or urine. (Refer to Chapter 11 for the "Typhoid Mary" story.) Transmission is via the fecal–oral route; food or water contaminated by feces or urine of patients or carriers; oysters harvested from fecally contaminated waters; fecally contaminated fruits and raw vegetables; from feces to food by flies.

Diagnosis. Isolation of *S. typhi* from blood, urine, feces, or bone marrow. Identification by biochemical tests. Immunodiagnostic procedures are available.

Shigellosis, Bacillary Dysentery. An acute bacterial infection of the lining of the small and large intestine; diarrhea with blood, mucus, and pus; nausea, vomiting, cramps, fever, and as many as 20 bowel movements a day; sometimes *toxemia* (toxins in the blood) and convulsions (in children); other serious complications (e.g., hemolytic uremic syndrome) may occur. Worldwide, shigellosis is estimated to cause approximately 600,000 deaths per year, with about two thirds of the cases and most of the deaths occurring in children younger than 10 years of age. A total of 13,987 new U.S. cases were reported to the CDC in 2004.

Patient Care. Standard precautions for most hospitalized patients. Contact precautions for diapered or incontinent patients.

Etiologic Agent. *Shigella dysenteriae, Shigella flexneri, Shigella boydii,* and *Shigella sonnei;* nonmotile, Gram-negative bacilli; members of the family *Enterobacteriaceae;* plasmid associated with toxin production and virulence; relatively few (10 to 100) organisms are required to cause disease.

Reservoirs and Mode of Transmission. Infected humans. Direct or indirect fecal–oral transmission from patients or carriers; fecally contaminated hands and fingernails; fecally contaminated food, milk, drinking water; flies can transfer organisms from latrines to food.

Diagnosis. Presence of leukocytes in stool specimens. Immediate inoculation of Gram-negative (GN) enrichment broth and solid media (such as MacConkey, xylose-lysine-deoxycholate [XLD], and Hektoen enteric [HE] agar) with fresh feces or rectal swab. *Shigella* spp. produce colorless colonies on MacConkey agar because they are non–lactose-fermenters. Identification by culture, biochemical, and immunodiagnostic procedures.

TABLE 17-15

Enterovirulent *Escherichia coli*

DISEASE	ADDITIONAL INFORMATION
Enterohemorrhagic *Escherichia coli* (EHEC) Diarrhea. Hemorrhagic, watery diarrhea; abdominal cramping. Usually there is no fever or only a slight fever. About 5% of infected people (especially children younger than age 5 and the elderly) develop hemolytic-uremic syndrome (HUS), with anemia, low platelet count, and kidney failure. The first recognized outbreak of diarrhea caused by enterohemorrhagic *E. coli* (O157:H7) occurred in 1982, involving contaminated hamburger meat (i.e., hamburger meat contaminated with cattle feces). Since then, there have been several well-publicized epidemics involving the same serotype. Not all of the outbreaks have involved meat; some have involved unpasteurized milk and apple juice, lettuce, and other raw vegetables. It has been estimated that *E. coli* O157:H7 infection accounts for as many as 73,000 cases of illness and 60 deaths in the U.S. per year. A total of 2,544 new U.S. cases of *E. coli* O157:H7 infection and 200 new U.S. cases of HUS were reported to the CDC in 2004.	**Patient Care.** Standard precautions for most hospitalized patients. Contact precautions for diapered or incontinent patients. **Etiologic Agent.** *Escherichia coli* O157:H7 (a serotype that possesses a cell wall antigen designated "O157" and a flagellar antigen designated "H7") is the most commonly involved EHEC serotype; others include O26:H11, O111:H8, and O104:H21; these are Gram-negative bacilli that produce potent cytotoxins called Shiga-like toxins (so-named because of their close resemblance to Shiga toxin, produced by *Shigella dysenteriae*). **Reservoirs and Mode of Transmission.** Cattle; also infected humans. Transmission is via the fecal–oral route; inadequately cooked, fecally contaminated beef; unpasteurized milk; person to person; fecally contaminated water. **Diagnosis.** *E. coli* O157:H7 infection should be suspected in any patient with bloody diarrhea. Stool specimens should be inoculated onto sorbitol-MacConkey (SMAC) agar. Colorless, sorbitol-negative colonies should then be assayed for O157 antigen using commercially available antiserum. Other immunodiagnostic procedures are available.
Enterotoxigenic *E. coli* (ETEC) Diarrhea, Traveler's Diarrhea. Profuse, watery diarrhea with or without mucus or blood, vomiting, abdominal cramping; dehydration and low-grade fever may occur. ETEC diarrhea is not a nationally notifiable disease in the U.S. Enterotoxigenic strains of *E. coli* are the most common cause of traveler's diarrhea worldwide and a common cause of diarrheal disease in young children in developing countries.	**Patient Care.** Standard precautions for most hospitalized patients. Contact precautions for diapered or incontinent patients. **Etiologic Agent.** Many different serotypes of enterotoxigenic *E. coli* that produce either a heat-labile toxin, a heat-stable toxin, or both. **Reservoirs and Mode of Transmission.** Infected humans. Transmission is via the fecal–oral route; ingestion of fecally contaminated food or water. **Diagnosis.** Isolation of the organism from stool specimens, followed by demonstration of enterotoxin production, DNA probe techniques, or immunodiagnostic procedures.

microbial intoxications. The distinction is based on where the toxin is actually produced—in the body (in vivo) or in the food (in vitro). The incubation time (the time that elapses between ingestion and onset of symptoms) is usually shorter in microbial intoxications. If toxin-producing bacteria are ingested, the incubation time will depend on the number of bacteria ingested, their generation time, and the amount of time it takes them to produce enough toxin to produce symptoms. According to the CDC, approximately 76 million cases of foodborne illness occur each year in the United States, resulting in more than 5,000 deaths and 325,000 hospitalizations. CD-ROM Appendix 1 contains information pertaining to microbial intoxications.

Infectious Diseases of the Genitourinary (GU) System

The genitourinary (or urogenital) system consists of the urinary tract and the genital tract. Infectious diseases of the urinary tract are described first.

Urinary Tract Infections (UTIs)

For purposes of discussion, urinary tract infections (UTIs) can be divided into upper UTIs and lower UTIs. Upper UTIs include infections of the kidneys (nephritis or **pyelonephritis**) and ureters (ureteritis). Lower UTIs include infections of the urinary bladder (cystitis), the urethra (urethritis), and, in males, the prostate (prostatitis).

UTIs may be caused by any of a variety of microorganisms introduced by poor personal hygiene, sexual intercourse, the insertion of catheters, and other means. The urinary tract is usually protected from pathogens by the frequent flushing action of urination. The acidity of normal urine also discourages growth of many microorganisms. Indigenous microflora are found at and near the outer opening (meatus) of the urethra of both males and females.

Terms relating to infectious diseases of the urinary tract include the following:

- **Cystitis.** Inflammation of the urinary bladder (Fig. 17-15); the most common type of UTI. The most common cause of cystitis is *E. coli* (Fig. 17-16). Other common

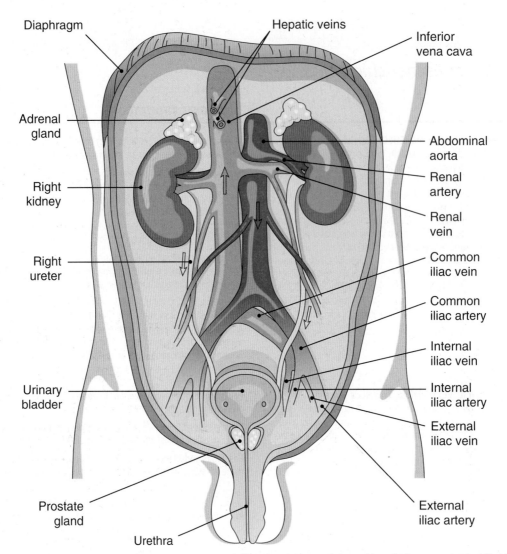

FIGURE 17-15. Anatomy of the urinary tract. (Cohen BJ, Taylor JJ. Memmler's The Human Body in Health and Disease, 10th Ed. Philadelphia: Lippincott Williams & Wilkins, 2005.)

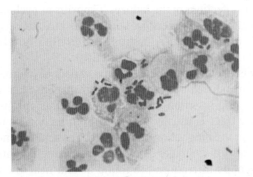

FIGURE 17-16. Many Gram-negative bacilli and many pink-staining PMNs can be seen in this Gram-stained urine sediment from a patient with cystitis (urinary bladder infection). (Koneman's Color Atlas and Textbook of Diagnostic Microbiology, 6th ed. Philadelphia: Lippincott Williams & Wilkins, 2006.)

causes of cystitis are species of *Klebsiella, Proteus, Enterobacter, Pseudomonas,* and *Enterococcus* as well as *Staphylococcus saprophyticus, Staphylococcus epidermidis,* and *C. albicans.*

- **Nephritis.** General term referring to inflammation of the kidneys. *Pyelonephritis* is inflammation of the renal parenchyma. *E. coli* is the most common cause of nephritis and pyelonephritis. Most often, nephritis is preceded by cystitis; the bacteria migrate up the ureters, from the urinary bladder to the kidneys. Bacteria may also gain access to the kidneys through the bloodstream.

- **Ureteritis.** Inflammation of one or both ureters. Usually caused by the spreading of infection upward from the urinary bladder or downward from the kidneys.

- **Urethritis.** Inflammation of the urethra. Pathogens are usually transmitted sexually. The most common causes of urethritis are *Chlamydia trachomatis, Neisseria gonorrhoeae,* ureaplasmas, and mycoplasmas. Urethritis that is not caused by *N. gonorrhoeae* is often referred to as nonspecific urethritis (NSU) or nongonococcal urethritis (NGU).

- **Prostatitis.** Inflammation of the prostate gland. Most often, prostatitis is not an infectious disease. If it is caused by a pathogen, the pathogen may be a bacterium, a virus, a fungus, or a protozoan.

Infections of the Genital Tract

As previously mentioned, indigenous microflora are found at and near the outer opening of the urethra and within the distal urethra of both males and females. Additionally, the female genital region supports the growth of many other microorganisms. In the adult vaginal microflora, there are many species of *Lactobacillus, Staphylococcus, Streptococcus, Enterococcus, Neisseria, Clostridium, Actinomyces, Prevotella,* diphtheroids, enteric bacilli, and *Candida.* The balance among these microbes depends on the estrogen levels and pH of the site. Should any of these or other microorganisms invade further into the GU system, a variety of nonspecific infections may occur. The male and female reproductive systems are shown in Figure 17-17.

Terms relating to infectious diseases of the genital tract are as follows:

- **Bartholinitis.** Inflammation of the Bartholin's ducts in females.

- **Cervicitis.** Inflammation of the cervix (that part of the uterus that opens into the vagina).

- **Endometritis.** Inflammation of the endometrium (the inner layer of the uterine wall).

- **Epididymitis.** Inflammation of the epididymis (an elongated structure connected to the testis).

- **Pelvic inflammatory disease (PID).** Inflammation of the fallopian tubes; also known as *salpingitis.*

- **Vaginitis.** Inflammation of the vagina. The three most common causes of vaginitis in the United States, each causing about one third of the cases, are *C. albicans* (a yeast), *Trichomonas vaginalis* (a protozoan), and a mixture of bacteria (including bacteria in the genera *Mobiluncus* and *Gardnerella*). When caused by a mixture of bacteria, the infection is referred to as *bacterial vaginosis (BV).* In general, infections that result from the actions of two or more bacteria are called synergistic or polymicrobial infections. A wet mount preparation is usually used to diagnose vaginitis (see CD-ROM Appendix 5).

- **Vulvovaginitis.** Inflammation of the vulva (the external genitalia of females) and the vagina.

Sexually Transmitted Diseases of the Genital Tract

The term *sexually transmitted disease* (STD), formerly called venereal disease (VD), includes any of the infections transmitted by sexual activities. They are diseases of not only the genital and urinary tracts, but also of the skin, mucous membranes, blood, lymphatic and digestive systems, and many other body areas. Epidemic STDs include acquired immunodeficiency syndrome (AIDS), chlamydial and herpes infections, gonorrhea, and syphilis. Because the AIDS virus (HIV) primarily causes damage to helper T cells and, thus, inhibits antibody production, it is discussed later with diseases of the circulatory system. Diseases such as hepatitis B, amebiasis, and giardiasis can also be transmitted by sexual activities, as can many other diseases.

Viral STDs

Information pertaining to viral STDs is contained in Table 17-16.

Bacterial STDs

Table 17-17 contains information pertaining to bacterial STDs.

Other Bacterial STDs

Other bacterial pathogens may also be sexually transmitted. Three bacterial STDs seen more often in parts of the world other than in the United States are chancroid, granuloma inguinale, and lymphogranuloma venereum (LGV). Chancroid is caused by the Gram-negative bacterium *Haemophilus ducreyi.* Granuloma inguinale is a chronic infection caused by a Gram-negative bacterium named *Calymmatobacterium granulomatis (Donovania granulomatis).* LGV is a chlamydial infection involving the lymph nodes, rectum, and reproductive tract. It is caused by certain serotypes of *C. trachomatis.* It should be noted that many sexually transmitted diseases are transmitted simultaneously; thus, when a patient is diagnosed with one STD, others should be sought. A total of 30 new U.S. cases of chancroid were reported to the CDC during 2004. Neither granuloma inguinale nor LGV are nationally notifiable diseases in the United States.

Infectious Diseases of the Circulatory System

General Information

The circulatory system consists of the cardiovascular system and the lymphatic system. The cardiovascular (*cardio* for heart, and *vascular* for the various types of blood ves-

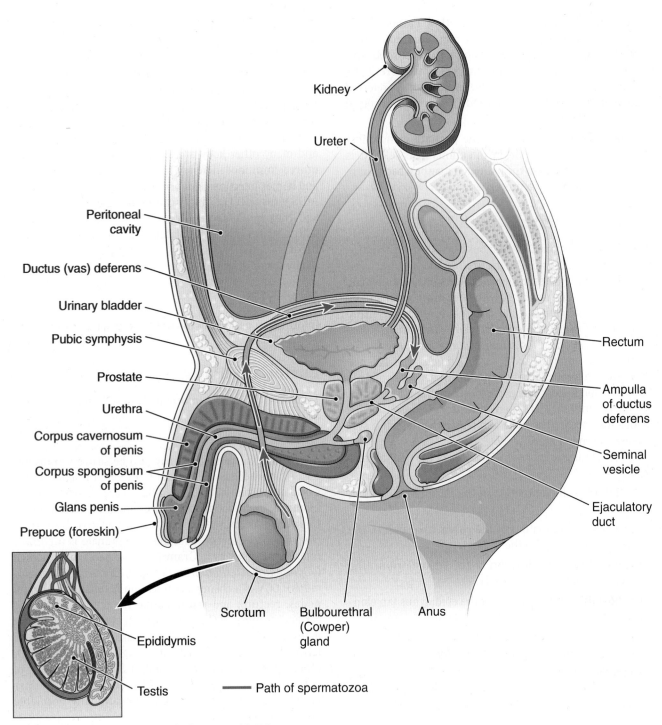

Kidney

Ureter

Peritoneal cavity

Ductus (vas) deferens

Urinary bladder

Pubic symphysis

Prostate

Urethra

Corpus cavernosum of penis

Corpus spongiosum of penis

Glans penis

Prepuce (foreskin)

Rectum

Ampulla of ductus deferens

Seminal vesicle

Ejaculatory duct

Scrotum

Bulbourethral (Cowper) gland

Anus

Epididymis

Testis

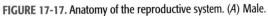 Path of spermatozoa

FIGURE 17-17. Anatomy of the reproductive system. (*A*) Male.

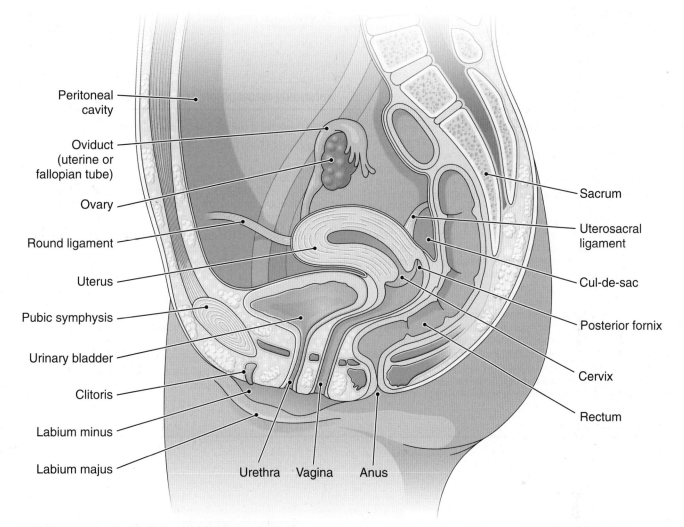

Peritoneal cavity

Oviduct (uterine or fallopian tube)

Ovary

Round ligament

Uterus

Pubic symphysis

Urinary bladder

Clitoris

Labium minus

Labium majus

Sacrum

Uterosacral ligament

Cul-de-sac

Posterior fornix

Cervix

Rectum

Urethra   Vagina   Anus

FIGURE 17-17. *(continued)* *(B)* Female. (Cohen BJ, Taylor JJ. Memmler's The Human Body in Health and Disease, 10th Ed. Philadelphia: Lippincott Williams & Wilkins, 2005.)

sels) system includes the heart, arteries, capillaries, veins, and blood. Blood is composed of plasma (the liquid portion) plus the various cellular elements. (The cellular elements of blood are discussed in Chapter 15).

Terms relating to infectious diseases of the cardiovascular system are as follows:

- **Endocarditis.** Inflammation of the endocardium—the endothelial membrane that lines the cavities of the heart (Fig. 17-20).

- **Myocarditis.** Inflammation of the myocardium—the muscular walls of the heart.

- **Pericarditis.** Inflammation of the pericardium—the membranous sac around the heart.

Normally, the blood is sterile; it contains no resident microflora. ***Transient bacteremia*** (the temporary presence of bacteria in the blood) often results from dental extractions, wounds, bites, and damage to the intestinal, respiratory, or reproductive tract mucosa. Even aggressive tooth brushing can lead to transient bacteremia. However, when pathogenic organisms are capable of resisting or overwhelming the phagocytes and other body defenses—or when an individual is immunosuppressed or is otherwise more susceptible than normal—a systemic disease called *septicemia* may occur. A patient with septicemia experiences chills, fever, and prostration (extreme exhaustion) and has bacteria or their toxins in the bloodstream.

Although dozens of infectious diseases can be transmitted by donated blood, in the United States donor blood is currently only tested for evidence of the following nine pathogens: cytomegalovirus, hepatitis B virus, hepatitis C virus, human immunodeficiency virus types 1 and 2, human T-cell lymphotrophic viruses I and II, *Treponema pallidum*, and West Nile virus.

The lymphatic system consists of lymphatic vessels,

TABLE 17-16

Viral STDs

DISEASE	ADDITIONAL INFORMATION
Anogenital Herpes Viral Infections, Genital Herpes. In general, herpes simplex infections are characterized by a localized primary lesion, latency, and a tendency to localized recurrence. In women, the principal sites of primary anogenital herpes virus infection are the cervix and vulva, with recurrent disease affecting the vulva, perineal skin, legs, and buttocks. In men, lesions appear on the penis, and in the anus and rectum of persons engaging in anal sex (Fig. 17-18). The initial symptoms are usually itching, tingling, and soreness, followed by a small patch of redness and then a group of small, painful blisters. The blisters break and fuse to form painful, circular sores, which become crusted after a few days. The sores heal in about 10 days but may leave scars. The initial outbreak is more painful, prolonged, and widespread than subsequent outbreaks and may be associated with fever. Not a nationally notifiable disease in the U.S.	Patient Care. Contact precautions for hospitalized patients. Etiologic Agent. Usually herpes simplex virus, type 2 (HSV 2); occasionally HSV-1. Reservoirs and Mode of Transmission. Infected humans. Transmission is via direct sexual contact; oral–genital, oral–anal, or anal–genital contact during presence of lesions; mother-to-fetus or mother-to-neonate transmission occurs during pregnancy and birth. Diagnosis. Observation of characteristic cytologic changes in tissue scrapings or biopsy specimens; immunodiagnostic procedures.
Genital Warts, Genital Papillomatosis, Condyloma Acuminatum. Genital warts start as tiny, soft, moist, pink or red swellings, which grow rapidly and may develop stalks. Their rough surfaces give them the appearance of small cauliflowers. Multiple warts often grow in the same area, most often on the penis in males and the vulva, vaginal wall, cervix, and skin surrounding the vaginal area in women. Genital warts also develop around the anus and in the rectum in males or females who engage in anal sex.	Etiologic Agent. Human papillomaviruses (HPV) of the papovavirus group of DNA viruses (human wart viruses); HPV genotypes 16 and 18 have been associated with cervical cancer. Reservoirs and Mode of Transmission. Infected humans. Transmission is via direct contact, usually sexual; through breaks in skin or mucous membranes; from mother to neonate during birth. Diagnosis. Clinical grounds.

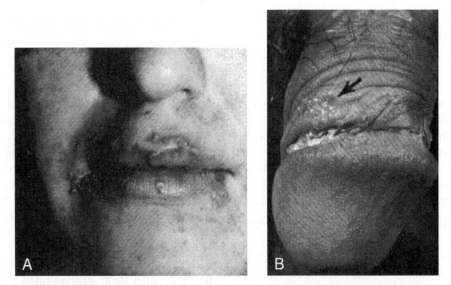

FIGURE 17-18. Herpes simplex infections. (*A*) Cold sores. (*B*) Genital herpes. (Dobson RL, Abele DC. The Practice of Dermatology. Philadelphia: JB Lippincott, 1985.)

TABLE 17-17

Bacterial STDs

DISEASE	ADDITIONAL INFORMATION
Genital Chlamydial Infections, Genital Chlamydiasis. The most frequent cause of nongonococcal urethritis (NGU), causing mucopurulent urethral discharge, urethral itching, and burning on urination; may also cause epididymitis, infertility, and proctitis in men. Most commonly causes endocervical and urethral infections, salpingitis, infertility, and chronic pelvic pain in women. Infection during pregnancy may result in premature rupture of membranes and preterm delivery as well as conjunctivitis and pneumonia in neonates. May be concurrent with gonorrhea. Genital chlamydial infections were the most common notifiable infectious diseases in the U.S. in 2004 (929,462 new cases reported to the CDC that year). The number of new U.S. genital chlamydia infections reported to CDC in 2004 exceeded the number of new U.S. gonorrhea cases by 599,330.	Patient Care. Standard precautions for hospitalized patients. Etiologic Agent. Certain serotypes of *Chlamydia trachomatis;* tiny, obligately intracellular, Gram-negative bacteria. Less common causes of NGU are *Ureaplasma urealyticum* (closely related to mycoplasmas), herpes simplex viruses, and *Trichomonas vaginalis.* Reservoirs and Mode of Transmission. Infected humans. Transmission is via direct sexual contact or mother-to-neonate during birth. Diagnosis. Identification of *C. trachomatis* by cell culture, staining, and immunodiagnostic procedures.
Gonorrhea. Gonorrhea can be manifested in a multitude of ways, some of which involve the GU tract (described below) and some of which do not (e.g., conjunctivitis [see Fig. 17-8], rash, pharyngitis, proctitis, arthritis). Gonococcal infections of the GU tract include urethritis and epididymitis in males and cervicitis, Bartholinitis, pelvic inflammatory disease (PID), salpingitis, endometritis, and vulvovaginitis in females. Urethral discharge and painful urination are common in infected males, usually starting 2 to 7 days after infection. Infected women may be asymptomatic for weeks or months, during which time severe damage to the reproductive system may occur. Gonorrhea is the second most common nationally notifiable infectious disease in the U.S. During 2004, a total of 330,132 new U.S. cases were reported to the CDC.	Patient Care. Standard precautions for most hospitalized patients. Contact precautions for newborn infants and children with gonococcal infection. Etiologic Agent. *Neisseria gonorrhoeae,* also known as gonococcus or GC; Gram-negative diplococci; some strains (called penicillinase-producing *N. gonorrhoeae* or PPNG) possess plasmids containing the gene for penicillinase production; some strains are multidrug-resistant. Reservoirs and Mode of Transmission. Infected humans. Transmission is via direct mucous membrane-to-mucous membrane contact, usually sexual contact; adult-to-child (may indicate sexual abuse); mother-to-neonate during birth. Diagnosis. Typical appearance of Gram-stained urethral discharge from male patients, with numerous white blood cells and numerous intracellular and extracellular Gram-negative diplococci. Culture on chocolate agar or a modified chocolate agar (such as Thayer-Martin medium, Martin-Lewis medium, New York City agar, or Transgrow). β-Lactamase testing of isolates, followed by antimicrobial susceptibility testing if β-lactamase–positive. Isolates are identified using biochemical tests. Immunodiagnostic procedures are available.
Syphilis. A treponemal disease that occurs in three stages: primary syphilis—a painless lesion known as a chancre (Fig. 17-19A); secondary syphilis—a skin rash (especially on the palms and soles) about 4 to 6 weeks later, with fever and mucous membrane lesions (Fig. 17-19B), and a long latent period (as long as 5 to 20 years); and then tertiary syphilis—with damage to the CNS, cardiovascular system, visceral organs, bones, sense organs, and other sites. Damage to the CNS or heart is usually not reversible. During 1986–1990, an epidemic of syphilis occurred throughout the United States, but since then, syphilis rates have declined each year. A total of 33,401 new U.S. cases were reported to the CDC in 2004.	Patient Care. Standard precautions for hospitalized patients. Etiologic Agent. *Treponema pallidum;* a Gram-variable, tightly coiled spirochete that is too thin to be seen with brightfield microscopy (see Figs. 2-5 and 2-10). Reservoirs and Mode of Transmission. Infected humans. Transmission is via direct contact with lesions, body secretions, mucous membranes, blood, semen, saliva, and vaginal discharges of infected people, usually during sexual contact; blood transfusions; transplacentally from mother to fetus. Diagnosis. Primary syphilis can be diagnosed by darkfield microscopy (see Fig. 2–5) of material scraped from the margin of chancres. Many immunodiagnostic procedures are available, such as the RPR, VDRL, and FTA-Abs tests for detecting antibodies in serum or spinal fluid specimens and fluorescent antibody procedures for detecting antigen in material obtained from lesions or lymph nodes.

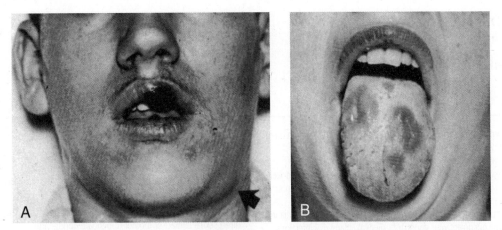

FIGURE 17-19. Syphilis. (*A*) Primary syphilis, showing a chancre of the lip and unilateral adenopathy (arrow). (*B*) Secondary syphilis, with mucous patches on the tongue. (Dobson RL, Abele DC. The Practice of Dermatology. Philadelphia: JB Lippincott, 1985.)

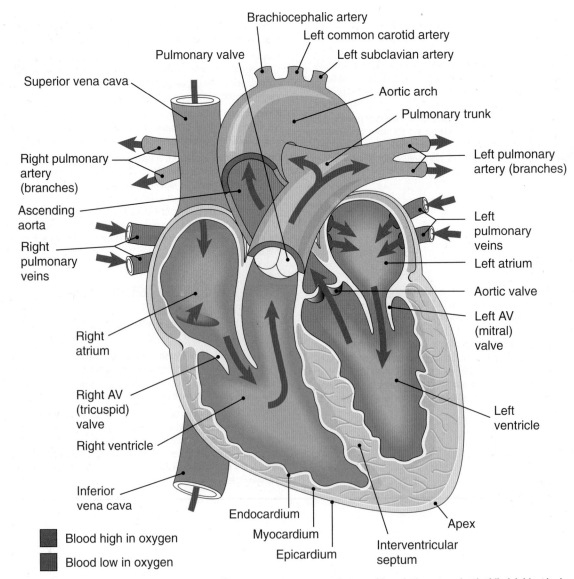

FIGURE 17-20. Anatomy of the heart. (Cohen BJ, Taylor JJ. Memmler's The Human Body in Health and Disease, 10th Ed. Philadelphia: Lippincott Williams & Wilkins, 2005.)

lymphoid tissue (including lymph nodes, tonsils, thymus, and spleen), and lymph (the liquid that circulates through the lymphatic system). Lymph occasionally picks up microorganisms from the intestine, lungs, and other areas, but these transient organisms are usually quickly engulfed by phagocytic cells in the liver and lymph nodes. The lymphatic system contains many lymphocytes (discussed in Chapter 16).

Terms relating to infectious diseases of the lymphatic system:

- **Lymphadenitis.** Inflamed and swollen lymph nodes.
- **Lymphadenopathy.** Diseased lymph nodes.
- **Lymphangitis.** Inflamed lymphatic vessels.

Viral Infections of the Circulatory System

Information pertaining to viral infections of the circulatory system is contained in Table 17-18.

Viral Hemorrhagic Fevers

Hemorrhagic fevers are caused by many different viruses, including dengue virus, yellow fever virus, Crimean-Congo hemorrhagic fever virus, Lassa virus, Ebola virus, and Marburg virus. Diseases caused by the latter two are described in Table 17-19.

Rickettsial and Ehrlichial Infections of the Cardiovascular System

Table 17-20 contains information pertaining to rickettsial and ehrlichial diseases of the cardiovascular system.

Other Bacterial Infections of the Cardiovascular System

Infective Endocarditis

Infective (or infectious) endocarditis is usually caused by a bacterium or a fungus. It is characterized by the presence of vegetations (bacteria and blood clots) on or within the endocardium, most commonly involving a heart valve. Abnormal or damaged valves are most susceptible to infection, although valves can become contaminated during open heart surgery. The vegetations can break loose and be transported to vital organs, where they can block arterial blood flow. Obviously, such obstructions are very serious, possibly leading to strokes, heart attacks, and death.

The two most common types of infective endocarditis are acute bacterial endocarditis and subacute bacterial endocarditis. Acute bacterial endocarditis is usually caused by colonization of heart valves by virulent bacteria such as *S. aureus* (the most common cause), *S. pneumoniae, N. gon-*orrhoeae, *S. pyogenes,* and *Enterococcus faecalis.* In subacute bacterial endocarditis (SBE), heart valves are infected by less virulent organisms such as α-hemolytic streptococci of oral origin (viridans streptococci), *S. epidermidis, Enterococcus* spp., and *Haemophilus* spp. Fungal endocarditis is rare, but cases of *Candida* and *Aspergillus* endocarditis do occur.

Oral streptococci can enter the bloodstream after minor or major dental procedures, oral surgery, and aggressive tooth brushing. Phlebotomy procedures and insertion of intravenous catheters sometimes force organisms from the skin into the bloodstream. Intravenous drug users are at high risk of developing infective endocarditis as a result of contaminated needles, syringes, and drug solutions.

Blood cultures are required for diagnosis of infective endocarditis. Treatment will depend on the specific pathogen involved and the antimicrobial susceptibility results.

Additional information pertaining to bacterial infections of the cardiovascular system is contained in Table 17-21.

Infectious Diseases of the Central Nervous System (CNS)

General Information

The nervous system is composed of the central nervous system (CNS) and the peripheral nervous system (Fig. 17-22). The CNS consists of the brain, the spinal cord, and the three membranes (or **meninges [sing., meninx]**) that cover the brain and spinal cord (Fig. 17-23). The CNS is well protected and remarkably resistant to infection; it is encased in bone, bathed and cushioned in cerebrospinal fluid (CSF), and nourished by capillaries. These capillaries make up the blood–brain barrier, supplying nutrients but not allowing larger particles, such as macromolecules (e.g., antibodies and most antibiotics), cells of the immune system, and microorganisms, to pass from the blood into the brain. The peripheral nervous system consists of nerves that branch from the brain and spinal cord.

There are no indigenous microflora of the nervous system. Microbes must gain access to the CNS through trauma (fracture or medical procedure), by the blood and lymph to the CSF, or along the peripheral nerves.

Terms relating to infectious diseases of the CNS include the following:

- **Encephalitis.** Inflammation of the brain.
- **Encephalomyelitis.** Inflammation of the brain and spinal cord.

TABLE 17-18

Viral Infections of the Circulatory System

DISEASE	ADDITIONAL INFORMATION
Human Immunodeficiency Virus (HIV) Infection, Acquired Immune Deficiency Syndrome (AIDS). Signs and symptoms of acute HIV infection (i.e., infection with the AIDS virus) usually occur within several weeks to several months after infection with HIV. Initial symptoms include an acute, self-limited mononucleosis-like illness lasting a week or two. Unfortunately, acute HIV infection is often undiagnosed or misdiagnosed because anti-HIV antibodies are not usually detected during this early phase of infection. Other signs and symptoms of acute HIV infection include fever, rash, headache, lymphadenopathy, pharyngitis, myalgia, arthralgia (joint pain), aseptic meningitis, retroorbital pain, weight loss, depression, GI distress, night sweats, and oral or genital ulcers. In the absence of anti-HIV treatment, approximately 90% of HIV-infected individuals ultimately develop AIDS. AIDS is a severe, life-threatening syndrome that represents the late clinical stage of infection with HIV. Invasion and destruction of helper T cells (Chapter 16) leads to suppression of the patient's immune system (immunosuppression). Because the immune system of HIV-infected people is unable to produce antibodies in response to T-dependent antigens (Chapter 16), secondary infections caused by viruses (e.g., Cytomegalovirus, herpes simplex), protozoa (e.g., *Cryptosporidium, Toxoplasma*), bacteria (e.g., mycobacteria), and fungi (e.g., *Candida, Cryptococcus, Pneumocystis*) become systemic and cause death. Persons with AIDS die as a result of overwhelming infections caused by a variety of pathogens, often opportunistic pathogens. Kaposi's sarcoma (a previously rare type of cancer) is a frequent complication of AIDS; it is thought to be caused by a type of herpesvirus called human herpesvirus 8. Previously considered to be a universally fatal disease, certain combinations of drugs, referred to as cocktails, are extending the life of some HIV-positive patients. In the absence of effective anti-HIV treatment, the AIDS case-fatality rate is very high (approaching 100%). A total of 44,108 new U.S. cases were reported to the CDC during 2004. (See Chapter 11 to learn more about the current AIDS pandemic.)	**Patient Care.** Standard precautions for hospitalized patients. Additional transmission-based precautions for specific infections that occur in AIDS patients. **Etiologic Agent.** Human immunodeficiency virus (HIV) (see Fig. 4-7 in Chapter 4); two types have been identified—type 1 (HIV-1; more common in the U.S.) and type 2 (HIV-2); RNA viruses in the Family Retroviridae (retroviruses). Most likely, HIV-1 first invades dendritic cells in the genital and oral mucosa; these cells then fuse with CD4+ lymphocytes (helper T cells) and spread to deeper tissues. HIV-1 can be cultured from plasma about 5 days after infection. **Reservoirs and Mode of Transmission.** Infected humans. Transmission is via direct sexual contact, homosexual or heterosexual; sharing of contaminated needles and syringes by intravenous drug abusers; transfusion of contaminated blood and blood products; transplacental transfer from mother to child; breast-feeding by HIV-infected mothers; transplantation of HIV-infected tissues or organs; and needlestick, scalpel, and broken glass injuries. There is no evidence of HIV transmission via biting insects. **Diagnosis.** Immunodiagnostic procedures for detection of antigen and antibodies. Most HIV-infected individuals develop detectable antibodies within 1 to 3 months after infection. However, there may be a more prolonged interval of up to 6 months, or even longer in some cases. Antigen detection procedures detect an HIV antigen known as p24. PCR tests are also available.
Infectious Mononucleosis, "Mono," "Kissing Disease." An acute viral disease; may be asymptomatic or may be characterized by fever, sore throat, lymphadenopathy (especially posterior cervical lymph nodes), *splenomegaly* (enlarged spleen), and fatigue; usually a self-limited disease of one to several weeks' duration; rarely fatal. Not a nationally notifiable disease in the U.S.	**Patient Care.** Standard precautions for hospitalized patients. **Etiologic Agent.** Epstein-Barr virus (EBV); also known as human herpesvirus 4; a DNA virus in the Family Herpesviridae; infects and transforms B cells, although it also infects other types of cells; known to be *oncogenic* (cancer causing); causes or is associated with various types of cancer, including lymphomas (e.g., Hodgkin's disease and Burkitt's lymphoma), carcinomas (e.g., nasopharyngeal carcinoma and gastric carcinoma), and sarcomas. **Reservoirs and Mode of Transmission.** Infected humans. Transmission is person to person, by direct contact with saliva; kissing facilitates spread among adolescents; can be transmitted via blood transfusion. **Diagnosis.** Immunodiagnostic procedures.
Mumps, Infectious Parotitis. An acute viral infection characterized by fever, swelling and tenderness of the salivary glands; complications can include *orchitis* (inflammation of the testes), *oophoritis* (inflammation of the ovaries), meningitis, encephalitis, deafness, pancreatitis, arthritis, mastitis, nephritis, thyroiditis, and pericarditis. A total of 258 new U.S. cases were reported to the CDC in 2004.	**Patient Care.** Droplet precautions for hospitalized patients. **Etiologic Agent.** Mumps virus; an RNA virus in the Family Paramyxoviridae. **Reservoirs and Mode of Transmission.** Infected humans. Transmission is via droplet spread and direct contact with the saliva of an infected person. **Diagnosis.** Immunodiagnostic procedures, cell culture.

TABLE 17-19

Viral Hemorrhagic Fevers

DISEASE	ADDITIONAL INFORMATION
Viral Hemorrhagic Diseases. Extremely serious, acute viral illnesses. Sudden onset of fever, malaise, myalgia, and headache, followed by pharyngitis, vomiting, diarrhea, rash, and internal hemorrhaging. Case-fatality rates for Marburg virus infection and Ebola virus infection have been 25% and 50 to 90%, respectively. All known cases of both diseases occurred in or could be traced to Africa.	**Patient Care.** Contact precautions for hospitalized patients. **Etiologic Agent.** Ebola virus and Marburg virus; filamentous viruses in the Family Filoviridae. Ebola virus is about 80 nm in width and up to 1 mm in length. Marburg virus is about 80 nm in width and 790 nm in length. **Reservoirs and Mode of Transmission.** Infected humans; infected African green monkeys in Marburg infection. Transmission is person to person via direct contact with infected blood, secretions, internal organs, or semen; also by needlestick. Risk is highest when the patient is vomiting, having diarrhea, or hemorrhaging. **Diagnosis.** Immunodiagnostic procedures, PCR, and cell culture. Laboratory studies of viral hemorrhagic fevers represent an extreme biohazard and should be conducted only in BSL-4 containment facilities.

- **Meningitis.** Inflammation of the membranes (meninges) that surround the brain and spinal cord.
- **Meningoencephalitis.** Inflammation of the brain and meninges.
- **Myelitis.** Inflammation of the spinal cord.

Infections of the CNS Having Multiple Causes

Meningitis

Meningitis—inflammation of the meninges—can have many causes, including the ingestion of poisons, the ingestion or injection of drugs, a reaction to a vaccine, or a pathogen. If caused by a pathogen, the culprit might be a virus, a bacterium, a fungus, or a protozoan.

Viral meningitis may be caused by a virus that specifically infects the meninges, or may be the result of an immune reaction to a virus that does not specifically infect the brain (e.g., chickenpox, measles, and rubella viruses). Viral meningitis is sometimes referred to as aseptic meningitis, because in about 50% of the cases, the pathogen cannot be identified. The various types of viruses that cause meningitis include enteroviruses (the major cause in the U.S.), coxsackieviruses, echoviruses, mumps virus, **arboviruses** (arthropod-borne viruses), poliovirus, adenoviruses, measles virus, herpes simplex, and varicella virus. Viral meningitis tends to be less serious than bacterial meningitis.

Historically, the three major causes of bacterial meningitis have been *H. influenzae* (the primary cause in children), *Neisseria meningitidis* (the primary cause in

adolescents), and *S. pneumoniae* (the primary cause in the elderly). The vaccination of children with the Hib vaccine has drastically reduced the incidence of *H. influenzae* meningitis in children in the United States. The major causes of bacterial meningitis in neonates are *Streptococcus agalactiae* (Group B, β-hemolytic streptococci), *E. coli* and other members of the family *Enterobacteriaceae*, and *Listeria monocytogenes*. Less common causes of bacterial meningitis are *S. aureus, Pseudomonas aeruginosa, Salmonella,* and *Klebsiella*.

Early symptoms of bacterial meningitis include fever, headache, stiff neck, sore throat, and vomiting. Then neurologic symptoms of dizziness, convulsions, minor paralysis, and coma occur; death may result within a few hours. Meningitis is a medical emergency, and steps must be taken immediately to determine the cause. Diagnosis is usually made by a combination of patient symptoms, physical examination, and Gram-staining and culture of the CSF.

Free-living amebae that may cause *meningoencephalitis* are in the genera *Naegleria* and *Acanthamoeba*. Other protozoa that may invade the meninges are *Toxoplasma* and *Trypanosoma*. Occasionally, fungal pathogens, especially *C. neoformans* (an encapsulated yeast), cause meningitis.

Several CNS diseases are caused by toxins. Examples of bacterial neurotoxins are botulinal toxin (the exotoxin that causes botulism) and **tetanospasmin** (the cause of tetanus). Diseases caused by fungal toxins (mycotoxins) include ergot from grain molds and mushroom poisoning. *Gonyaulax*, an alga found in algal blooms, produces neurotoxins, which may concentrate in bivalve shellfish and cause paralytic symptoms

TABLE 17-20

Rickettsial and Ehrlichial Diseases of the Cardiovascular System

DISEASE	ADDITIONAL INFORMATION
Rocky Mountain Spotted Fever, Tickborne Typhus Fever. A tickborne rickettsial disease characterized by sudden onset of moderate to high fever, extreme exhaustion (prostration), muscle pain, severe headache, chills, conjunctival infection, and maculopapular rash on extremities on about the third day, which spreads to the palms, soles, and much of the body; in about 4 days, small purplish areas (petechiae) develop as a result of bleeding in the skin; although death is uncommon, it can occur. Occurs in the Western Hemisphere, including all parts of the U.S., especially the Atlantic seaboard. A total of 1,713 new U.S. cases were reported to the CDC in 2004.	**Patient Care.** Standard precautions for hospitalized patients. **Etiologic Agent.** *Rickettsia rickettsii;* a Gram-negative bacterium; an obligate intracellular pathogen that invades endothelial cells (cells that line blood vessels). **Reservoirs and Mode of Transmission.** Infected ticks on dogs, rodents, and other animals. Transmission is via the bite of an infected tick. **Diagnosis.** Immunodiagnostic procedures.
Endemic Typhus Fever, Murine Typhus Fever, Fleaborne Typhus. An acute febrile disease (similar to, but milder than, epidemic typhus, which is described next) with shaking chills, headache, fever, and a faint, pink rash. Worldwide occurrence, but rare in the U.S. (fewer than 80 cases reported annually). Not a nationally notifiable disease in the U.S.	**Patient Care.** Standard precautions for hospitalized patients. **Etiologic Agent.** *Rickettsia typhi;* a Gram-negative bacterium; an obligate intracellular pathogen. **Reservoirs and Mode of Transmission.** Rats, mice, possibly other mammals, infected rat fleas. Transmission is rat → flea → human; infected fleas defecate while feeding and the rickettsiae in the feces are rubbed into the bite wound or other superficial abrasions. **Diagnosis.** Immunodiagnostic procedures.
Epidemic Typhus Fever, Louseborne Typhus. An acute rickettsial disease, often with sudden onset of headache, chills, prostration, fever, and general pains. A rash appears on the fifth or sixth day, initially on the upper trunk, followed by spread to the entire body, but usually not to the face, palms, or soles. May be fatal if untreated. Occurs in colder climates, where people may live under unhygienic conditions and are louse-infested; in World War I, body lice were referred to as "cooties" by soldiers. Not a nationally notifiable disease in the U.S.	**Patient Care.** Standard precautions for hospitalized patients. **Etiologic Agent.** *Rickettsia prowazekii;* a Gram-negative bacterium; an obligate intracellular pathogen. **Reservoirs and Mode of Transmission.** Infected humans and body lice (*Pediculus humanus;* see Fig. 18–5 in Chapter 18). Transmission is human → louse → human; infected lice defecate while feeding and the rickettsiae in the feces are rubbed into the bite wound or other superficial abrasions. **Diagnosis.** Immunodiagnostic procedures.
Ehrlichiosis. An acute, febrile illness ranging from asymptomatic to mild to severe and life-threatening. Patients usually present with acute influenza-like illness with fever, headache, and generalized malaise. Reminiscent of Rocky Mountain spotted fever, without the rash. The estimated fatality rate is about 5%. The first human U.S. case of ehrlichiosis (a person with HME) occurred in 1991. Cases of HME are more common than HGE cases. Most HME cases have occurred in the southeast and mid-Atlantic states, whereas most HGE cases have occurred in states with high rates of Lyme disease (particularly Connecticut, Minnesota, New York, and Wisconsin). In these states, the tick that transmits the HGE agent is the same tick that transmits *Borrelia burgdorferi,* the causative agent of Lyme disease. The two different types of ehrlichiosis seem to be transmitted by different species of ticks. A total of 537 new U.S. cases of HGE and 338 new U.S. cases of HME were reported to the CDC in 2004.	**Patient Care.** Standard precautions for hospitalized patients. **Etiologic Agent.** Gram-negative coccobacilli that are closely related to rickettsias; obligate intraleukocytic pathogens. *Ehrlichia chaffeensis* invades human monocytes, causing human monocytic ehrlichiosis (HME). *Anaplasma phagocytophilum* invades human granulocytes, causing human granulocytic ehrlichiosis (HGE). A canine species, *Ehrlichia ewingii,* has caused a small number of human cases. **Reservoirs and Mode of Transmission.** Reservoir unknown. Transmission is via tick bite. **Diagnosis.** Immunodiagnostic procedures and nucleic acid assays.

TABLE 17-21

Bacterial Infections of the Cardiovascular System

DISEASE	ADDITIONAL INFORMATION

Lyme Disease, Lyme Borreliosis. A tickborne disease characterized by three stages: (1) an early, distinctive, targetlike, red skin lesion (usually at the site of the tick bite), expanding to a diameter of 6 inches (15 cm), often with a central clearing; (2) early systemic manifestations that may include fatigue, chills, fever, headache, stiff neck, muscle pain, joint aches, with or without lymphadenopathy; and (3) neurologic abnormalities (e.g., aseptic meningitis, facial paralysis, myelitis, and encephalitis) and cardiac abnormalities (e.g., arrhythmias, pericarditis) several weeks or months after the initial symptoms appear. The first U.S. cases occurred in 1975 in Lyme, Connecticut. Since then, Lyme disease has been reported in 45 states (mainly the mid-Atlantic, Northeast, and North Central states) and it occurs in many other areas of the world. A total of 19,804 new U.S. cases were reported to the CDC in 2004. Lyme disease is the most common arthropodborne disease in the U.S.

Patient Care. Standard precautions for hospitalized patients.

Etiologic Agent. *Borrelia burgdorferi;* a Gram-negative, loosely coiled spirochete (Fig. 17-21).

Reservoirs and Mode of Transmission. Ticks, rodents (especially deer mice), and mammals (especially deer). Transmission is via tick bite.

Diagnosis. Observation of the characteristic targetlike skin lesion, plus immunodiagnostic procedures and PCR. *B. burgdorferi* can be grown in the laboratory on a special medium (Barbour-Stoenner-Kelley [BSK] medium at 33°C).

Plague, "Black Death," Bubonic Plague, Pneumonic Plague, Septicemic Plague. An acute, often severe zoonosis. Initial signs and symptoms may include fever, chills, malaise, myalgia, nausea, prostration, sore throat, and headache. (1) Bubonic plague is named for the swollen, inflamed, and tender lymph nodes (buboes) that develop, usually lymph nodes receiving drainage from the site of the flea bite. In about 90% of cases, the inguinal (groin area) lymph nodes are involved. (2) Pneumonic plague, which is highly communicable, involves the lungs; it can result in localized outbreaks or devastating epidemics. (3) Septicemic plague, septic shock, meningitis, and death may occur. During the Middle Ages, plague was referred to as the "black death" because of the darkened, bruised appearance of the corpses. The blackened skin and foul smell were the result of cell necrosis and hemorrhaging into the skin. Plague probably dates back a thousand or more years BC. In the past 2,000 years, the disease has killed millions of people, perhaps hundreds of millions. Huge plague epidemics occurred in Asia and Europe, including the European plague epidemic of 1348–1350, which killed about 44% of the population (40 million of 90 million people). The last major plague epidemic in Europe occurred in 1721. Plague still occurs, but the availability of insecticides and antibiotics have greatly reduced the incidence of this dreadful disease. Only 3 new U.S. cases were reported to the CDC in 2004.

Patient Care. Standard precautions for hospitalized patients with bubonic and septicemic plague. Droplet precautions for hospitalized pneumonic plague patients.

Etiologic Agent. *Yersinia pestis;* a nonmotile, bipolar-staining, Gram-negative coccobacillus; sometimes referred to as the plague bacillus.

Reservoirs and Mode of Transmission. Wild rodents (especially ground squirrels in the U.S.) and their fleas; rarely, rabbits, wild carnivores, and domestic cats. Transmission is usually via flea bite (rodent → flea → human). Also, handling of tissues of infected rodents, rabbits, and other animals as well as droplet transmission from person to person (in pneumonic plague).

Diagnosis. Observation of typical appearance (bipolar-staining bacilli that resemble safety pins) in Gram-stained or Wright-Giemsa–stained sputum, CSF, or material aspirated from a bubo. Culture, biochemical tests, immunodiagnostic tests.

Tularemia, Rabbit Fever. An acute zoonosis with a variety of clinical manifestations depending on portal of entry into the body. Most often presents as a skin ulcer and regional lymphadenitis. Ingestion results in pharyngitis, abdominal pain, diarrhea, and vomiting. Inhalation results in pneumonia and septicemia, with a 30 to 60% fatality rate. A total of 134 new U.S. cases were reported to the CDC in 2004.

Patient Care. Contact precautions for hospitalized patients with open lesions; otherwise standard precautions only.

Etiologic Agent. *Francisella tularensis;* a small, pleomorphic, Gram-negative coccobacillus; some strains are more virulent than others.

Reservoirs and Mode of Transmission. Wild animals, especially rabbits, muskrats, beavers; some domestic animals; hard ticks. Transmission is via tick bite; ingestion of contaminated meat or drinking water; entry of organisms into wound while skinning infected animals; inhalation of dust; animal bites. Not transmitted person to person.

Diagnosis. Culture, biochemical tests, and immunodiagnostic procedures.

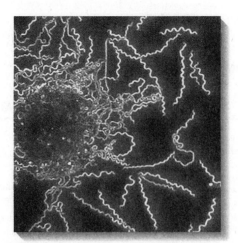

FIGURE 17-21. *Borrelia burgdorferi* as seen by darkfield microscopy. (Strohl WA, et al. Lippincott's Illustrated Reviews: Microbiology. Philadelphia: Lippincott Williams & Wilkins, 2001.)

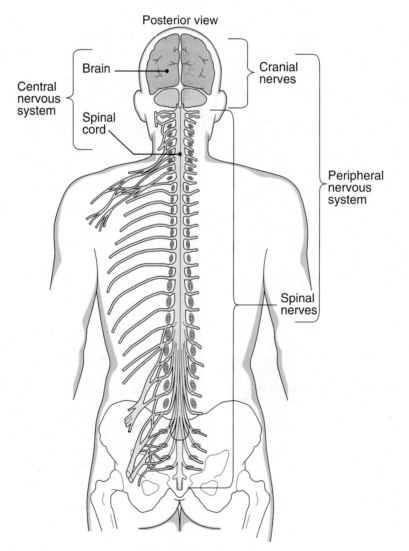

FIGURE 17-22. Anatomy of the central nervous system. (Cohen BJ, Taylor JJ. Memmler's The Human Body in Health and Disease, 10th Ed. Philadelphia: Lippincott Williams & Wilkins, 2005.)

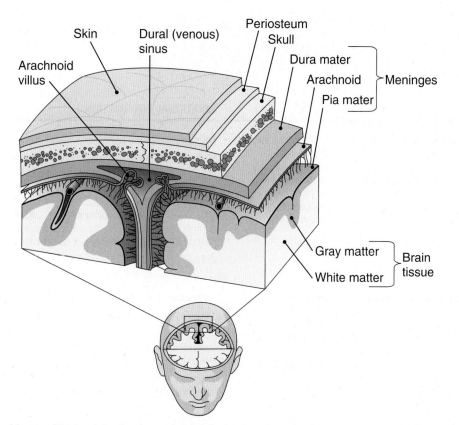

FIGURE 17-23. Section of the top of the head showing the meninges and related structures. (Cohen BJ, Taylor JJ. Memmler's The Human Body in Health and Disease, 10th Ed. Philadelphia: Lippincott Williams & Wilkins, 2005.)

after ingestion of the contaminated shellfish. A variety of other algae also produce neurotoxins (refer to Chapter 5).

Viral Infections of the CNS

Table 17-22 contains information pertaining to viral infections of the CNS.

Bacterial Infections of the CNS

Information pertaining to bacterial infections of the CNS is contained in Table 17-24.

Fungal Infections of the CNS

See "cryptococcosis," which was previously described under "Fungal Infections of the Lower Respiratory Tract." Also see information about the India ink preparation in CD-ROM Appendix 5.

Appropriate Therapy for Viral, Bacterial, and Fungal Infections

Recommendations for the treatment of infectious diseases change frequently. The infectious diseases described in this chapter must be treated using the antiviral, antibacterial, or antifungal drugs—whichever are appropriate—as recommended in recent issues of *The Medical Letter* (www.medicalletter.com), the most recent edition of the *Physician's Desk Reference* (PDR; www.pdr.net), or other reliable, up-to-date sources of such information. For certain diseases, antisera (e.g., for botulism and tetanus) or serum immune globulins (e.g., varicella-zoster immune globulin) are available for treatment. Additional information about antimicrobial agents can be found in Chapter 9.

TABLE 17-22

Viral Infections of the CNS

DISEASE	ADDITIONAL INFORMATION
Lymphocytic Choriomeningitis. A rodentborne viral disease that presents as aseptic meningitis, encephalitis, or meningoencephalitis. Asymptomatic or mild febrile disease also occurs. Some patients develop fever, malaise, lack of appetite, muscle aches, headache, nausea, vomiting, sore throat, coughing, joint pain, chest pain, and salivary gland pain. Possible complications of CNS involvement include deafness and temporary or permanent neurologic damage. An association between LCMV infection and myocarditis has been suggested.	**Patient Care.** Standard precautions for hospitalized patients. **Etiologic Agent.** The lymphocytic choriomeningitis virus (LCMV), a member of the Family Arenaviridae. **Reservoirs and Mode of Transmission.** Infected rodents, primarily the common house mouse. Humans become infected after exposure to mouse urine, droppings, saliva, or nesting materials. The virus can enter broken skin, the nose, the eyes, or the mouth, or via the bite of an infected rodent. Organ transplantation is a possible means of transmission. **Diagnosis.** Immunodiagnostic procedures or virus isolation.
Poliomyelitis, Polio, Infantile Paralysis. In most patients, a minor illness with fever, malaise, headache, nausea, and vomiting. In about 1% of patients, the disease progresses to severe muscle pain, stiffness of the neck and back, with or without flaccid paralysis. Major illness is more likely to occur in older children and adults. Although once a major health problem in the U.S., vaccines became available in the 1950s. The World Health Organization (WHO) is attempting to eradicate polio worldwide. No new U.S. cases were reported to the CDC in 2004.	**Patient Care.** Contact precautions for hospitalized patients. **Etiologic Agent.** Polioviruses; RNA viruses in the Family Picornaviridae (small RNA viruses). **Reservoirs and Mode of Transmission.** Infected humans. Transmission is person to person, primarily via the fecal–oral route; also by throat secretions. **Diagnosis.** Isolation of poliovirus from stool samples, CSF, or oropharyngeal secretions using cell culture techniques; immunodiagnostic procedures.
Rabies. A usually fatal, acute viral encephalomyelitis of mammals, with mental depression, restlessness, headache, fever, malaise, paralysis (which usually starts in the lower legs and moves upward through the body), salivation, spasms of throat muscles induced by a slight breeze or drinking water, convulsions, and death caused by respiratory failure. Rabies is endemic in every country of the world except Antarctica and in every state except Hawaii. Worldwide, an estimated 35,000 to 40,000 people die of rabies annually. Seven new human cases and 6,345 new animal cases were reported to the CDC in 2004.	**Patient Care.** Standard precautions for hospitalized patients. **Etiologic Agent.** Rabies virus; a bullet-shaped, enveloped RNA virus in the Family Rhabdoviridae. **Reservoirs and Mode of Transmission.** Many wild and domestic mammals, including dogs, foxes, coyotes, wolves, jackals, skunks, raccoons, mongooses, and bats. Transmission is usually via the bite of a rabid animal, which introduces virus-laden saliva; airborne transmission from bats in caves; person to person by saliva is theoretically possible but has never been documented. **Diagnosis.** Virus isolation using cell culture techniques or immunodiagnostic procedures; observation of Negri bodies in animal brain tissue. Negri bodies are viral RNA-nucleoprotein complexes found in the cytoplasm of virus-infected cells (i.e., they are intracytoplasmic inclusions).
Viral Encephalitis, Arthropodborne Viral Encephalitis. An acute inflammatory viral disease. Infections range from asymptomatic to mild fever and headache to severe. Severe infections may involve headache, high fever, stupor, disorientation, coma, tremors, occasional convulsions, spastic paralysis, and death. Over the years, St. Louis encephalitis virus has been the most common mosquito-transmitted pathogen in the United States. The situation changed in 2002, when West Nile virus took over the No. 1 spot. During 2004, a total of 1,273 new U.S. cases of viral encephalitis were reported to the CDC (1,142 cases of West Nile virus encephalitis, 112 cases of California serogroup viral encephalitis, 12 cases of St. Louis encephalitis, 6 cases of Eastern equine encephalitis [EEE], and 1 case of Powassan virus encephalitis). The California serogroup includes California encephalitis virus and LaCrosse encephalitis virus. The term *arboviruses* is sometimes used in reference to viruses that are transmitted by arthropods.	**Patient Care.** Standard precautions for hospitalized patients. **Etiologic Agent.** See Table 17-23. **Reservoirs and Mode of Transmission.** See Table 17-23. **Diagnosis.** Immunodiagnostic procedures and cell culture. **Note:** See box entitled "A Closer Look at West Nile Virus."

TABLE 17-23

Selected Arthropodborne Viral Encephalitides of the United States

DISEASE	PATHOGEN	RESERVOIRS	VECTORS
Eastern Equine Encephalitis (EEE)	EEE virus; an RNA virus in the Family Togaviridae	Birds, horses	*Aedes, Coquilletidia, Culex,* and *Culiseta* mosquitoes
California Encephalitis	California encephalitis virus; an RNA virus in the Family Bunyaviridae	Rodents, rabbits	*Aedes* and *Cules* mosquitoes
LaCrosse Encephalitis	LaCrosse encephalitis virus; an RNA virus in the Family Bunyaviridae	Chipmunks, squirrels	*Aedes* mosquitoes
St. Louis Encephalitis	St. Louis encephalitis virus; an RNA virus in the Family Flaviviridae	Birds	*Culex* mosquitoes
West Nile Virus Encephalitis	West Nile virus; an RNA virus in the Family Flaviviridae	Birds, perhaps horses	*Culex* mosquitoes
Western Equine Encephalitis (WEE)	WEE virus; an RNA virus in the Family Togaviridae	Birds, horses	*Aedes* and *Culex* mosquitoes

A Closer Look at West Nile Virus

West Nile virus (WNV) is a flavivirus that is commonly found in Africa, West Asia, and the Middle East. It is closely related to St. Louis encephalitis virus. WNV can infect humans, birds, mosquitoes, horses, and some other mammals. Humans become infected primarily by mosquitoes, but WNV transmission has also been reported through blood transfusion, organ transplantation, transplacental transfer, and breast-feeding. WNV can cause very severe CNS infections, referred to as West Nile encephalitis, West Nile meningitis, and West Nile meningoencephalitis. West Nile fever is another manifestation of WNV disease, characterized by fever, headache, tiredness, aches, and sometimes rash. The first human and equine cases of West Nile encephalitis in North America occurred in the United States in 1999. The number of human cases of WNV disease in the United States in recent years are as follows: 2001, 66 cases, 9 deaths; 2002, 4,156 cases, 284 deaths; 2003, 9,862 cases, 264 deaths; 2004, 2,539 cases, 100 deaths. According to the CDC, 1 of every 5 infected people develops symptoms of illness, and 1 in 150 infected people develops CNS disease. During 2003, 12,066 WNV-infected dead birds, 5,145 WNV-infected horses, and 106 other WNV-infected animals were reported to the CDC.

TABLE 17-24

Bacterial Infections of the CNS

DISEASE	ADDITIONAL INFORMATION
Botulism (see CD-ROM Appendix 1: "Microbial Intoxications").	
Listeriosis. Generally, only a mild febrile illness in healthy, immunocompetent individuals. Can be manifested as meningoencephalitis or septicemia in newborns and elderly or immunosuppressed adults, with fever, intense headache, nausea, vomiting, delirium, coma, occasionally collapse, shock, and death. Causes fever and spontaneous abortion in pregnant women. A total of 753 new U.S. cases of listeriosis were reported to the CDC during 2004.	**Patient Care.** Contact precautions for hospitalized patients. **Etiologic Agent.** *Listeria monocytogenes;* a Gram-positive coccobacillus. **Reservoirs and Mode of Transmission.** Soil, water, mud, silage, infected mammals and humans; soft cheeses *(Listeria* multiplies in contaminated refrigerated foods.)* Transmission is via ingestion of raw or contaminated milk, soft cheeses, and vegetables; transmitted from mother to fetus in utero or during passage through an infected birth canal. **Diagnosis.** Isolation and identification of the pathogen from CSF, blood, amniotic fluid, placenta, and other specimens. Gram-positive coccobacilli in Gram-stained smears of neonatal CSF.
Tetanus, Lockjaw. An acute neuromuscular disease induced by a bacterial exotoxin (tetanospasmin), with painful muscular contractions, primarily of the masseter (the muscle that closes the jaw) and neck muscles; spasms, rigid paralysis, respiratory failure, and death may result. A total of 34 new U.S. cases were reported to the CDC in 2004.	**Patient Care.** Standard precautions for hospitalized patients. **Etiologic Agent.** *Clostridium tetani* (Fig. 17-24); a motile, Gram-positive, anaerobic, spore-forming bacillus that produces a potent neurotoxin called tetanospasmin. **Reservoirs and Mode of Transmission.** Soil contaminated with human, horse, or other animal feces (*C. tetani* is a member of the indigenous intestinal flora of humans and animals.) Spores of *C. tetani* are introduced into a puncture wound, burn, or needlestick by contamination with soil, dust, or feces. Under anaerobic conditions in the wound, spores germinate into vegetative *C. tetani* cells, which produce the exotoxin in vivo. **Diagnosis.** Usually made on clinical and epidemiologic grounds. Attempts to isolate *C. tetani* from wounds or demonstrate antibody production are rarely successful.

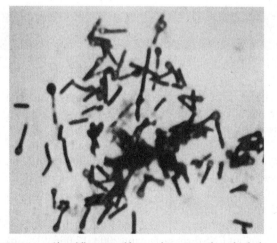

FIGURE 17-24. *Clostridium tetani* from culture. Note the spherical terminal endospores giving the bacilli a drumstick or tennis racket appearance. (Volk WA, et al. Essentials of Medical Microbiology, 5th ed. Philadelphia: Lippincott-Raven, 1996.)

◎ REVIEW OF KEY POINTS

Because of the large quantity of information contained in this chapter, a "Review of Key Points" has been omitted. As a minimum, students should learn the type and name of the pathogen that causes each of the infectious diseases described in this chapter and the manner in which the disease is transmitted. Whenever applicable, students should know the type of arthropod vector that is involved in the transmission of the disease.

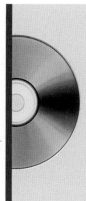

On the CD-ROM

- Increase Your Knowledge
- Critical Thinking
- Case Studies
- Additional Self-Assessment Exercises

Self-Assesssment Exercises

After studying this chapter, answer the following multiple-choice questions.

1. The most common sexually transmitted disease in the United States is caused by:
   a. *Candida albicans.*
   b. *Chlamydia trachomatis.*
   c. *Neisseria gonorrhoeae.*
   d. *Trichomonas vaginalis.*

2. Infectious hepatitis is caused by:
   a. HAV.
   b. HBV.
   c. HCV.
   d. HDV.

3. *Streptococcus pneumoniae* is a common cause of:
   a. meningitis.
   b. otitis media.
   c. pneumonia.
   d. all of the above.

4. *Staphylococcus aureus* is a common cause of:
   a. food poisoning.
   b. nosocomial infections.
   c. skin and wound infections.
   d. all of the above

5. Which of the following diseases may be caused by *Streptococcus pyogenes*?
   a. impetigo
   b. necrotizing fasciitis
   c. strep throat
   d. all of the above

6. Which of the following diseases may be caused by *Chlamydia trachomatis*?
   a. inclusion conjunctivitis
   b. nongonococcal urethritis (NGU)
   c. trachoma
   d. all of the above

7. An infection of the urinary bladder is known as:
   a. cystitis.
   b. pyelonephritis.
   c. ureteritis.
   d. urethritis.

8. Which of the following organisms is the most common cause of urethritis?
   a. *Candida albicans*
   b. *Chlamydia trachomatis*
   c. *Neisseria gonorrhoeae*
   d. *Trichomonas vaginalis*

9. Which of the following organisms is the most common cause of cystitis?
   a. *Chlamydia trachomatis*
   b. *Escherichia coli*
   c. *Neisseria gonorrhoeae*
   d. *Trichomonas vaginalis*

10. Which of the following associations is *incorrect*?
    a. cryptococcosis. . .parrots and parakeets
    b. plague. . .rat flea
    c. Rocky Mountain spotted fever. . .tick
    d. West Nile virus encephalitis. . .mosquito

18

MAJOR PARASITIC DISEASES OF HUMANS: AN INTRODUCTION TO MEDICAL PARASITOLOGY

So, naturalists observe, a flea
Hath smaller fleas that on him prey
And these have smaller still to bite 'em;
And so proceed ad infinitum.

from Poetry, a Rhapsody, 1733
by Jonathan Swift (1667–1745)

LEARNING OBJECTIVES

AFTER STUDYING THIS CHAPTER, YOU SHOULD BE ABLE TO:

- Differentiate between the following: ectoparasites versus endoparasites; definitive hosts versus intermediate hosts; facultative parasites versus obligate parasites; and mechanical vectors versus biologic vectors
- Classify a particular parasitic infection as a protozoal or helminth disease
- Categorize various parasitic infections by body system (e.g., respiratory system, gastrointestinal tract, circulatory system)
- Correlate a particular parasitic infection (e.g., giardiasis) with its major characteristics, causative agent, reservoir(s), mode(s) of transmission, and diagnostic laboratory procedures

INTRODUCTION

Although parasitology is a branch of microbiology, not all organisms studied in a parasitology course are microorganisms. In fact, of the three categories of organisms (parasitic protozoa, helminths, and arthropods) that are studied in a parasitology course, only one category (parasitic protozoa) contains microorganisms. Thus, in this chapter, parasitic protozoa are discussed in greater detail than helminths and arthropods.

Parasitism is a symbiotic relationship that is of benefit to one party or symbiont (the parasite) and usually detrimental to the other party (the **host**). This does not mean that the parasite necessarily causes disease in the host, although disease does occur in certain parasitic relationships. In virtually all parasitic relationships, the parasite deprives the host of nutrients.

Parasites are defined as organisms that live *on* or *in* other living organisms (hosts), at whose expense they gain some advantage. There are many types of plant parasites (i.e., parasites of plants) and many types of animal parasites (i.e., parasites of animals); this discussion will be limited to animal parasites.

Parasites that live on the outside of the host's body are referred to as ***ectoparasites,*** whereas those that live inside are called *endoparasites.* Arthropods such as mites, ticks, and lice are examples of ectoparasites. Parasitic protozoa and helminths are examples of endoparasites.

The life cycle of a particular parasite may involve one or more hosts. If more than one host is involved, the *definitive host* is defined as the host that harbors the adult or sexual stage of the parasite or the sexual phase of the life cycle. The *intermediate host* is the host that harbors the larval or asexual stage of the parasite or the asexual phase of the life cycle. Parasite life cycles range from simple to complex. There are one-host parasites, two-host parasites, and three-host parasites. Knowing the life cycle of a particular parasite enables public health workers and clinicians to control and diagnose the infection.

An *accidental host* is a living organism that can serve as a host in a particular parasite's life cycle, but is not a usual host in that life cycle. Some accidental hosts are dead-end hosts. A *dead-end host* is a host from which the parasite cannot continue its life cycle.

A *facultative parasite* is an organism that can be parasitic but does not have to live as a parasite. It is capable of living an independent life (apart from a host). The free-living amebae that can cause keratoconjunctivitis and primary amebic meningoencephalitis are examples of facultative parasites. An *obligate parasite,* on the other hand, has no choice. To survive, it must be a parasite. Most parasites that infect humans are obligate parasites.

Parasitology is the study of parasites, and a *parasitologist* is someone who studies parasites. As previously stated, if you were to take an upper-division or graduate-level parasitology course, it would be divided into three areas of study: the study of parasitic protozoa, the study of helminths, and the study of arthropods.

Parasitic Protozoa

Protozoa are in the Kingdom Protista. Most are unicellular. Protozoa are classified taxonomically by their mode of locomotion. Protozoa in the category known as *Amoebozoa* (amebae) move by means of pseudopodia (false feet). Protozoa classified in four phyla (*Metamonada, Parabasalia, Percolozoa,* and *Euglenozoa*) move by means of flagella (flagellates). Protozoa in the category *Ciliophora* (ciliates) move by means of cilia. Protozoa classified as *Sporozoa* have no pseudopodia, flagella, or cilia, and therefore do not move.

Not all protozoa are parasitic. For example, many of the pond water protozoa (e.g., *Paramecium* and *Stentor* spp.) studied in introductory biology and microbiology courses are not parasites. Some protozoa are facultative parasites, capable of a free-living existence but also capable of becoming parasites when they accidentally gain entrance to the

body. *Acanthamoeba* spp. and *Naegleria fowleri* are examples of facultative parasites. These free-living amebae normally reside in soil or water, but can cause serious diseases when they gain entrance to the eyes or central nervous system.

Because protozoa are tiny, protozoal infections are most often diagnosed by microscopic examination of body fluids, tissue specimens, or feces. Peripheral blood smears are usually stained with Giemsa stain, whereas fecal specimens are stained with trichrome, iron-hematoxylin, or acid-fast stains. Most parasitic protozoal infections are diagnosed by observing either trophozoites or cysts in the specimen. The *trophozoite* is the motile, feeding, dividing stage in a protozoan's life cycle, whereas the *cyst* is the dormant stage (in some ways, cysts are much like bacterial spores).

Protozoal Infections of Humans

Protozoal Infections of the Skin

Table 18-1 contains information about protozoal infections of the skin.

Protozoal Infections of the Eyes

Protozoal infections of the eyes include conjunctivitis and keratoconjunctivitis (inflammation of the cornea and conjunctiva), caused by amebae in the genus *Acanthamoeba*, and toxoplasmosis, caused by a sporozoan named *Toxoplasma gondii*. Although toxoplasmosis is described here under protozoal infections of the eyes, there are many manifestations of toxoplasmosis in addition to ocular disease. Ocular manifestations of toxoplasmosis occur primarily in immunosuppressed patients, in whom the infection can lead to enucleation (removal of the infected eyeball). Amebic conjunctivitis and keratoconjunctivitis can also result in enucleation.

Table 18-2 contains information about these diseases.

Protozoal Infections of the Gastrointestinal Tract

Of the many protozoal infections of the gastrointestinal (GI) tract, only amebiasis, balantidiasis, cryptosporidiosis, cyclosporiasis, and giardiasis are discussed here. Three of these diseases (cryptosporidiosis, cyclosporiasis, and giardiasis) are nationally notifiable infectious diseases in the United States. Recall from Chapter 11 that cases of nationally notifiable infectious diseases must be reported to the Centers for Disease Control and Prevention (CDC). Table 18-3 contains information about protozoal infections of the gastrointestinal tract.

TABLE 18-1

Protozoal Infections of the Skin

DISEASE	ADDITIONAL INFORMATION
Leishmaniasis. There are three forms: cutaneous, mucosal, and visceral leishmaniasis. The cutaneous form starts with a papule that enlarges into a craterlike ulcer. Individual ulcers may coalesce. **Geographic Occurrence.** Leishmaniasis occurs in many regions of the world, including Pakistan, India, China, the Middle East, Africa, South and Central America, and Mexico; cases have also occurred in south central Texas. It is estimated that between 1.5 and 2 million people have leishmaniasis and that about 57,000 people die each year of the disease.	**Etiologic Agent.** Various species of flagellated protozoa in the genus *Leishmania;* the motile, extracellular form is called a promastigote; the nonmotile, intracellular form is called an amastigote. **Reservoirs and Mode of Transmission.** Infected humans, domestic dogs, a variety of wild animals. Leishmaniasis is principally a zoonosis and is usually transmitted via the bite of an infected sand fly. Transmission by blood transfusion and person-to-person contact has been reported. **Diagnosis.** Microscopic identification of the amastigote form in stained preparations from aspirates and biopsies of ulcers; seen within macrophages and close to disrupted cells. The promastigote form can be cultured on suitable media. An intradermal test (called the Montenegro test) and immunodiagnostic tests are also available.

TABLE 18-2

Protozoal Infections of the Eyes

DISEASE	ADDITIONAL INFORMATION
Amebic Conjunctivitis and Keratoconjunctivitis. An amebic infection causing inflammation of the conjunctiva, corneal ulcers, pus formation, and severe pain; can lead to loss of vision. **Geographic Occurrence.** Worldwide; amebic eye infections occur in many countries on all continents.	**Etiologic Agent.** Several species of amebae in the genus *Acanthamoeba.* **Reservoirs and Mode of Transmission.** Ameba-contaminated water. Infections have occurred primarily in soft contact lens wearers who have used nonsterile, homemade cleaning or wetting solutions, or have become infected in ameba-contaminated spas or hot tubs. **Diagnosis.** By microscopic examination of scrapings, swabs, or aspirates of the eye, or by culture on media seeded with *Escherichia coli* or another member of the Family *Enterobacteriaceae.* The bacteria on the media serve as "food" for the amebae.
Toxoplasmosis. A systemic sporozoal infection that, in immunocompetent persons, may be asymptomatic or may resemble infectious mononucleosis. Serious disease, even death, may occur in immunodeficient persons, involving the CNS, lungs, muscles, and heart. Cerebral toxoplasmosis is common in AIDS patients. Infection during early pregnancy may lead to fetal infection, causing death of the fetus or serious birth defects (e.g., brain damage). **Geographic Occurrence.** Worldwide.	**Etiologic Agent.** *Toxoplasma gondii;* an intracellular sporozoan. **Reservoirs and Mode of Transmission.** Definitive hosts include cats and other felines that usually acquire infection by eating infected rodents or birds. Intermediate hosts include rodents, birds, sheep, goats, swine, and cattle. Humans usually become infected by eating infected raw or undercooked meat (usually pork or mutton) containing the cyst form of the parasite or by ingesting oocysts shed in the feces of infected cats. Oocysts may be present in food or water contaminated by feline feces. Children may ingest oocysts from sand boxes containing cat feces. Infection can also be acquired transplacentally, by blood transfusion, or by organ transplantation. **Diagnosis.** Immunodiagnostic procedures; demonstration of the pathogen in body tissues or fluids by biopsy or necropsy; or isolation of the pathogen in animals or cell culture.

TABLE 18-3

Protozoal Infections of the Gastrointestinal Tract

DISEASE	ADDITIONAL INFORMATION
Amebiasis, Amebic Dysentery, Amebic Abscesses, Amebomas. A protozoal gastrointestinal infection that may be asymptomatic, mild, or severe; often with dysentery, fever, chills, bloody or mucoid diarrhea or constipation, and colitis. Amebae may invade mucous membranes of the colon, forming abscesses and granulomas (called amebomas), which are sometimes mistaken for carcinoma. Amebae may also be disseminated via the bloodstream to extraintestinal sites, leading to abscesses of the liver, lung, brain, and other organs. Depending on their location, untreated extraintestinal amebic abscesses can be fatal. **Geographic Occurrence.** Worldwide.	**Etiologic Agent.** *Entamoeba histolytica;* an ameba in the subphylum Sarcodina; occurs in two stages: the cyst stage (the dormant, infective stage), and the motile, metabolically active, reproducing trophozoite stage (the actual amebae). **Reservoirs and Mode of Transmission.** Symptomatic or asymptomatic humans; fecally contaminated food or water. Transmission is by ingestion of fecally contaminated food or water containing cysts, flies transporting cysts from feces to food, soiled hands of infected food handlers, and oral–anal sexual contact. **Diagnosis.** Microscopic observation of *E. histolytica* trophozoites or cysts in stained smears of fecal specimens. Physical features of *E. histolytica* trophozoites and cysts enable differentiation from most other pathogenic and nonpathogenic amebae found in stool specimens. The presence of red blood cells within trophozoites indicates invasive amebiasis.
Balantidiasis. A protozoal gastrointestinal infection of the colon causing diarrhea or dysentery, colic, nausea, and vomiting. **Geographic Occurrence.** Worldwide.	**Etiologic Agent.** *Balantidium coli,* a ciliated protozoan. (**Note:** *B. coli* is the only ciliate that causes disease in humans.) It is primarily a parasite of pigs. **Reservoirs and Mode of Transmission.** Pigs and anything that might be contaminated with pig feces (e.g., drinking water). Transmission is by ingestion of *B. coli* cysts in fecally contaminated food or water. **Diagnosis.** Identifying trophozoites or cysts of *B. coli* in fecal specimens, which may also contain blood and mucus. *B. coli* is the largest of the protozoa that infect humans.
Cryptosporidiosis. A coccidial infection that may be asymptomatic or may cause diarrhea, cramping, and abdominal pain; may be prolonged, fulminant, and fatal in immunosuppressed patients; may also be a respiratory disease. **Geographic Occurrence.** Worldwide. The largest waterborne outbreak that has ever occurred in the United States was the 1993 cryptosporidiosis outbreak in Milwaukee, WI, which affected more than 400,000 people. A total of 3,577 new U.S. cases of cryptosporidiosis were reported to the CDC during 2004.	**Etiologic Agent.** *Cryptosporidium parvum,* a coccidian (Coccidia are classified in the subphylum Sporozoa. Other coccidial parasites of humans are in the genera *Cyclospora, Isospora,* and *Sarcocystis.*) **Reservoirs and Mode of Transmission.** Infected humans, cattle and other domestic animals. Fecal–oral transmission; person-to-person, animal-to-person, contaminated water or food. **Diagnosis.** Microscopic observation of small (4–6 μm), acid-fast oocysts in stained smears of fecal specimens. Immunodiagnostic procedures are available.
Cyclosporiasis. A coccidial gastrointestinal infection, causing watery diarrhea (6 or more stools per day), nausea, anorexia, abdominal cramping, fatigue, and weight loss. The diarrhea lasts between 9 and 43 days in immunocompetent patients, and months in immunocompromised patients. **Geographic Occurrence.** Cyclosporiasis has been diagnosed in Asia, the Caribbean, Mexico, Peru, and the United States. A total of 171 new U.S. cases of cyclosporiasis were reported to the CDC during 2004.	**Etiologic Agent.** *Cyclospora cayetanensis,* a coccidian. **Reservoirs and Mode of Transmission.** Fecally contaminated water sources and produce that has been rinsed with fecally contaminated water. Transmission is primarily waterborne, but outbreaks have involved contaminated raspberries, basil, and lettuce. **Diagnosis.** Microscopic observation of the 8- to 9-μm diameter, acid-fast oocysts, about twice the size of *Cryptosporidium* oocysts. Oocysts autofluoresce a bright green to intense blue under ultraviolet fluorescence.

(continues)

TABLE 18-3

Protozoal Infections of the Gastrointestinal Tract (continued)

DISEASE	ADDITIONAL INFORMATION
Giardiasis. A protozoal infection of the duodenum (the uppermost portion of the small intestine); may be asymptomatic, mild, or severe; with diarrhea, steatorrhea (loose, pale, malodorous, fatty stools), abdominal cramps, bloating, abdominal gas, fatigue, and possibly weight loss. **Geographic Occurrence.** Worldwide.	**Etiologic Agent.** *Giardia lamblia* (also called *Giardia intestinalis*), a flagellated protozoan. Trophozoites attach by means of a ventral sucker to the mucosal lining of the duodenum. Trophozoites or cysts are expelled in feces. **Reservoirs and Mode of Transmission.** Infected humans; possibly beaver and other wild and domestic animals that have consumed water containing *Giardia* cysts; fecally contaminated drinking water and recreational water; day care centers. Transmission is by the fecal–oral route; ingestion of cysts in fecally contaminated water or foods; person-to-person by soiled hands to mouth (as occurs in day care centers). Large community outbreaks have resulted from drinking treated but unfiltered water. Filtration is necessary because the concentrations of chlorine used in routine water treatment do not kill *Giardia* cysts, especially in cold water. Smaller outbreaks have involved contaminated food, person-to-person transmission in day care centers, and fecally contaminated recreational water (e.g., swimming and wading pools). **Diagnosis.** Microscopic observation of trophozoites or cysts in stained smears of fecal specimens. The characteristic trophozoite contains two nuclei, giving it the appearance of a face (Fig. 18-1). It appears to be looking up at the person observing it microscopically. The *Giardia* trophozoite has been described as resembling an owl face, a clown face, or an old man with glasses. Immunodiagnostic procedures are also available.

Protozoal Infections of the Genitourinary Tract

Table 18-4 contains information about protozoal infections of the genitourinary tract.

Protozoal Infections of the Circulatory System

Table 18-5 contains information about protozoal infections of the circulatory system.

Protozoal Infections of the Central Nervous System

Protozoal infections of the central nervous system (CNS) include African trypanosomiasis, amebic abscesses, primary amebic meningoencephalitis (PAM), and toxoplasmosis. Each of these diseases, except PAM, was discussed earlier in this chapter. Table 18-6 contains information about PAM.

Helminths

The word **helminth** means parasitic worm. Although helminths are not microorganisms, the various procedures used to diagnose helminth infections are performed in the Clinical Microbiology Laboratory. These procedures often involve the observation of microscopic stages in the life cycles of these parasites. Helminths infect humans, other animals, and plants, but only helminth infections of humans are discussed here. The helminths that infect humans are always endoparasites.

Helminths are multicellular, eucaryotic organisms in the Kingdom Animalia. The two major divisions of helminths are roundworms (*Nematoda* or **nematodes**) and flatworms (*Platyhelminthes*). The flatworms are further divided into tapeworms (**cestodes**) and flukes (**trematodes**).

The typical helminth life cycle includes three stages: the *egg,* the *larva,* and the *adult worm.* Adults produce eggs, from which larvae emerge, and the larvae mature into adult worms. The host that harbors the larval stage is called the *intermediate host,* whereas the host that harbors the adult worm is called the *definitive host.* Sometimes helminths have more than one intermediate host or more than one definitive host. The fish tapeworm, for example, is what is known as a three-host parasite, having one definitive host (human) and two intermediate hosts (a freshwater crustacean called a *Cyclops* and a freshwater fish) in its life cycle. Dogs, cats, or humans can serve as definitive hosts for the dog tapeworm.

Helminth infections are primarily acquired by ingesting the larval stage, although some larvae are injected into the body via the bite of infected insects, and others enter the body by penetrating skin.

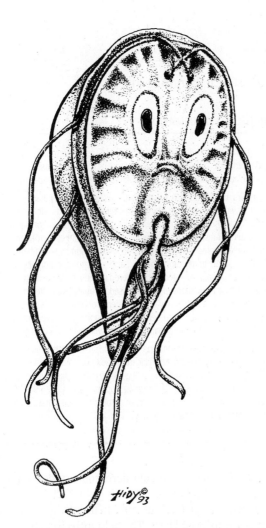

FIGURE 18-1. *Giardia lamblia* trophozoite, 10 to 20 μm long by 5 to 15 μm wide. *G. lamblia* trophozoites are easy to recognize in microscopically examined fecal specimens. Their two oval nuclei resemble eyes. As you observe a *Giardia* trophozoite through the microscope, it appears to be looking up at you.

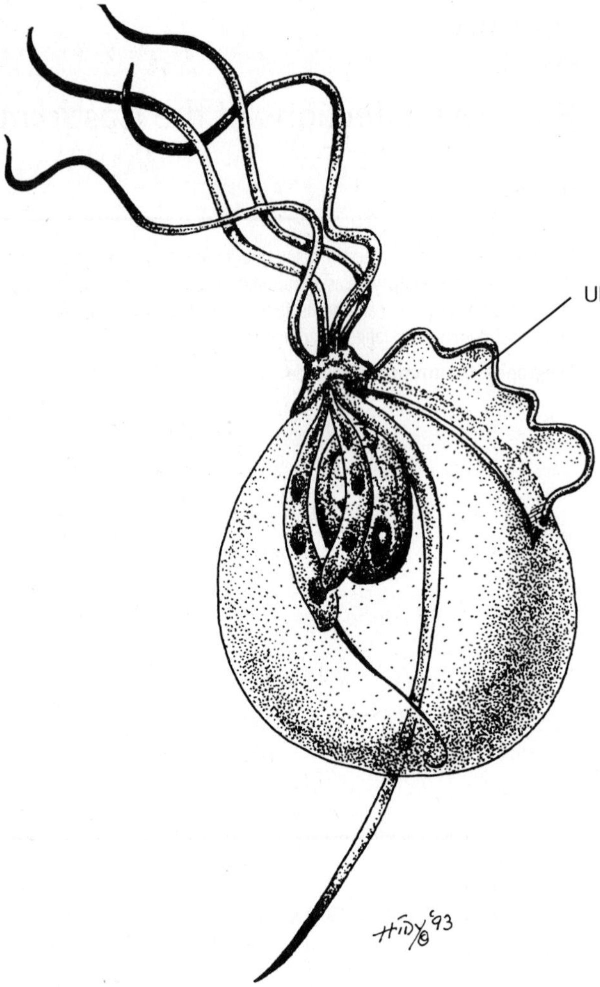

UM

FIGURE 18-2. *Trichomonas vaginalis* trophozoite, 7 to 23 μm long by 5 to 15 μm wide. *T. vaginalis* trophozoites are easy to recognize in a wet mount preparation of a freshly collected clinical specimen. Their flagella and undulating membrane (UM) cause them to be constantly in motion. When they die, however, they become spherical and cannot be distinguished from white blood cells.

TABLE 18-4

Protozoal Infections of the Genitourinary Tract

DISEASE

Trichomoniasis. A sexually transmitted protozoal disease causing vaginitis in women, with a profuse, thin, foamy, malodorous, greenish-yellowish discharge; may cause urethritis or cystitis; often asymptomatic; rarely symptomatic in men, but may cause prostatitis, urethritis, or infection of the seminal vesicles. It has been estimated that approximately one third of the U.S. cases of vaginitis are caused by *T. vaginalis* (another third are caused by *Candida albicans,* and another third by bacteria). Persons with trichomoniasis often also have gonorrhea (up to 40% of trichomoniasis cases in some studies).

Geographic Occurrence. Worldwide.

ADDITIONAL INFORMATION

Etiologic Agent. *Trichomonas vaginalis;* a flagellate.

Reservoirs and Mode of Transmission. Infected humans; transmission is by direct contact with vaginal and urethral discharges of infected people during sexual intercourse. Because this organism exists only in the fragile trophozoite stage (there is no cyst stage), it cannot survive very long outside the human body.

Diagnosis. Vaginitis caused by *T. vaginalis* can be diagnosed by performing a wet mount examination (described in CD-ROM Appendix 5) of freshly collected vaginal discharge material and observing the motile trophozoites (Fig. 18-2). Culture procedures are also available. Sometimes *T. vaginalis* trophozoites are seen in urine and Papanicolaou (Pap) smears.

TABLE 18-5

Protozoal Infections of the Circulatory System

DISEASE	ADDITIONAL INFORMATION
African trypanosomiasis, African sleeping sickness. A systemic disease caused by hemoflagellates (flagellated protozoa in the bloodstream). Early stages include a painful chancre at the site of a tsetse fly bite, fever, intense headache, insomnia, lymphadenitis, anemia, local edema, and rash. Later stages of the disease include body wasting, falling asleep (sleeping sickness), coma, and death if untreated. **Geographic Occurrence.** African trypanosomiasis is transmitted by the tsetse fly (Genus *Glossina*), so the disease only occurs in tropical Africa, where tsetse flies are found. It is estimated that more than 300,000 people have African trypanosomiasis and that about 66,000 people die each year of the disease.	**Etiologic Agent.** Two different subspecies of *Trypanosoma brucei* cause African trypanosomiasis. *T. brucei* ssp. *gambiense,* in west and central Africa, causes most cases of sleeping sickness; the disease may last several years. *T. brucei* ssp. *rhodesiense,* in east Africa, causes a more rapidly fatal form of African trypanosomiasis; usually lethal within weeks or a few months without treatment. **Reservoirs and Mode of Transmission.** Infected humans (*T. brucei* ssp. *gambiense*); wild animals, cattle (*T. brucei* ssp. *rhodesiense*). Transmission is by the bite of an infected tsetse fly. **Diagnosis.** Observation of the trypomastigote form of the parasite in blood, lymph, or CSF (Fig. 18-3). Immunodiagnostic procedures are also available.
American Trypanosomiasis, Chagas' Disease. An acute disease in children, with an inflammatory response at the site of the reduviid bug bite, fever, malaise, lymphadenopathy, **hepatomegaly** (enlarged liver), and **splenomegaly** (enlarged spleen). May be asymptomatic. Chronic irreversible complications include heart damage, arrhythmias, enlarged esophagus (megaesophagus), and enlarged colon (megacolon). Life-threatening meningoencephalitis may occur. **Geographical Occurrence.** Chagas' disease is primarily a disease of South America, Central America, and Mexico, although a few cases have occurred in the U.S. (by bug bite or blood transfusion). As increasing numbers of infected people enter the U.S. from endemic areas, there is a growing concern about the safety of the blood supply. Currently, donor blood is not routinely screened in the U.S. for the presence of *T. cruzi.* It is estimated that between 16 and 18 million people have Chagas' disease and that about 50,000 people die each year of the disease.	**Etiologic Agent.** *Trypanosoma cruzi;* occurs as a hemoflagellate (the trypomastigote form) and as a nonmotile, intracellular parasite (the amastigote form). **Reservoirs and Mode of Transmission.** Infected humans and more than 150 different species of domestic and wild animals, including dogs, cats, rodents, carnivores, and primates. The vectors of American trypanosomiasis are rather large insects known as reduviid bugs (also called triatome bugs, kissing bugs, and cone-nosed bugs). The bugs become infected when they take blood meals from infected animals. The bugs defecate as they take a blood meal or feed at the corner of a sleeping person's eye. The person becomes infected when they rub the feces (containing the parasite) into the bite wound or eye. Transmission by blood transfusion and organ transplantation also occurs. **Diagnosis.** Observation of trypomastigotes in blood or amastigotes in tissue or lymph node biopsy specimens (Fig. 18-4). Immunodiagnostic procedures are available. Xenodiagnosis is performed in endemic countries. In this procedure, sterile (noninfected) reduviid bugs are allowed to take blood meals from persons suspected of having Chagas' disease. (The bite is painless.) The bugs are then taken to a laboratory, where their feces are periodically checked microscopically for the presence of the parasite.
Babesiosis. A sporozoal disease that may include fever, chills, myalgia, fatigue, jaundice, and anemia; potentially severe, sometimes fatal, especially in splenectomized and elderly people. Patients may be simultaneously infected with *Borrelia burgdorferi* (the causative agent of Lyme disease), which is transmitted by the same species of tick. **Geographic Occurrence.** Babesiosis is an endemic disease in many parts of the world, including Europe, Mexico, and the United States. Most U.S. cases occur in New York and New England.	**Etiologic Agent.** *Babesia microti* and other *Babesia* spp., including *Babesia divergens* in Europe; intraerythrocytic sporozoan parasites. **Reservoirs and Mode of Transmission.** Rodents for *B. microti;* cattle for *B. divergens.* Transmission is by tick bite; rarely by blood transfusion. **Diagnosis.** Observation and identification of the parasites within red blood cells in Giemsa-stained blood smears; differentiation from malarial parasites is necessary; immunodiagnostic procedures are also available.

(continues)

TABLE 18-5

Protozoal Infections of the Circulatory System *(continued)*

DISEASE	ADDITIONAL INFORMATION
Malaria. A systemic sporozoal infection with malaise, fever, chills, sweating, headache, and nausea. The frequency with which the cycle of chills, fever, and sweating is repeated is referred to as periodicity and depends on the particular species of malarial parasite that is causing the infection. In addition to these symptoms, falciparum malaria may be accompanied by cough, diarrhea, respiratory distress, shock, renal and liver failure, pulmonary and cerebral edema, coma, and death. **Geographic Occurrence.** Malaria is a major health problem in many tropical and subtropical countries, with an estimated 300 to 500 million cases and 1.5 to 2.7 million deaths annually. About 90% of all malaria cases occur in Africa, where approximately 1 million children die of malaria each year. Malaria is a nationally notifiable infectious disease in the United States. A total of 1,458 new U.S. cases of malaria were reported to the CDC in 2004, most of which were imported cases. A few nonimported, mosquito-transmitted cases of malaria occur in the U.S. each year. (Refer to Chapter 11 for additional information regarding the current malaria pandemic.)	**Etiologic Agent.** Four different species of *Plasmodium* cause human malaria: *Plasmodium vivax* (the most common species), *Plasmodium falciparum* (the most deadly), *Plasmodium malariae,* and *Plasmodium ovale. P. vivax* and *P. ovale* cause chills and fever every 48 hours (referred to as tertian malaria), whereas *P. malariae* causes chills and fever every 72 hours (referred to as quartan malaria). *P. falciparum* periodicity varies from 36 to 48 hours. Mixed infections (infections involving more than one *Plasmodium* species) occur in certain geographic areas. Drug-resistant strains of *P. vivax* and *P. falciparum* are common. These sporozoan protozoa have a complex life cycle involving a female *Anopheles* mosquito, the liver and erythrocytes of an infected human, and many life cycle stages. The life cycle of malarial parasites is depicted in Figure 18-5. **Reservoirs and Mode of Transmission.** Infected humans and infected mosquitoes. Transmission is by injection of sporozoites into the human bloodstream by an infected female *Anopheles* mosquito while taking a blood meal; also by blood transfusion or contaminated needles and syringes. **Diagnosis.** Observation and identification of intraerythrocytic *Plasmodium* parasites in Giemsa-stained blood smears (Fig. 18-6). Several types of immunodiagnostic procedures are being tested.

TABLE 18-6

Protozoal Infections of the Central Nervous System

DISEASE	ADDITIONAL INFORMATION
Primary Amebic Meningoencephalitis (PAM). An amebic disease causing inflammation of the brain and meninges, sore throat, headache, hallucinations, nausea, vomiting, high fever, stiff neck; death occurs within 10 days, usually on the 5th or 6th day. **Geographic Occurrence.** Worldwide.	**Etiologic Agent.** *Naegleria fowleri,* a free-living ameba (amebae in the genera *Acanthamoeba* and *Balamuthia* can cause similar conditions). **Reservoirs and Mode of Transmission.** Water and soil. The amebae usually enter the nasal passages while diving or swimming in ameba-contaminated water (e.g., ponds, lakes, swimming hole, thermal springs, hot tubs, spas, public swimming pools). After the amebae colonize the nasal tissues, they invade the brain and meninges by traveling along the olfactory nerves. **Diagnosis.** By microscopic examination of wet mount preparations of fresh CSF. Because they are colorless and transparent, amebae are difficult to see in wet mounts, unless the microscope light is turned very low. Phase-contrast microscopy is helpful. Smears of CSF sediment can be stained with Wright or Giemsa stain. Leukocytes and amebae are similar in appearance. Unfortunately, most cases of PAM are diagnosed after the patient's death by observing amebae in stained sections of brain tissue.

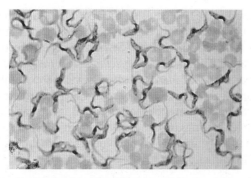

FIGURE 18-3. A stained peripheral blood smear from a patient with African trypanosomiasis. Many trypomastigotes of *Trypanosoma brucei* can be seen among the red blood cells. *T. brucei* trypomastigotes are 14 to 33 μm long by 1.5 to 3.5 μm wide. (Koneman EW, et al. Color Atlas and Textbook of Diagnostic Microbiology, 5th ed. Philadelphia: Lippincott-Raven, 1997.)

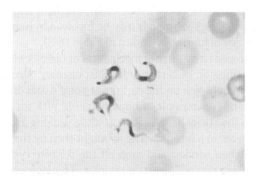

FIGURE 18-4. A stained peripheral blood smear from a patient with American trypanosomiasis (Chagas' disease). Several trypomastigotes of *Trypanosoma cruzi*, with their typical "C" shape, can be seen among the red blood cells. (Koneman's Color Atlas and Textbook of Diagnostic Microbiology, 6th ed. Philadelphia: Lippincott-Raven, 2006.)

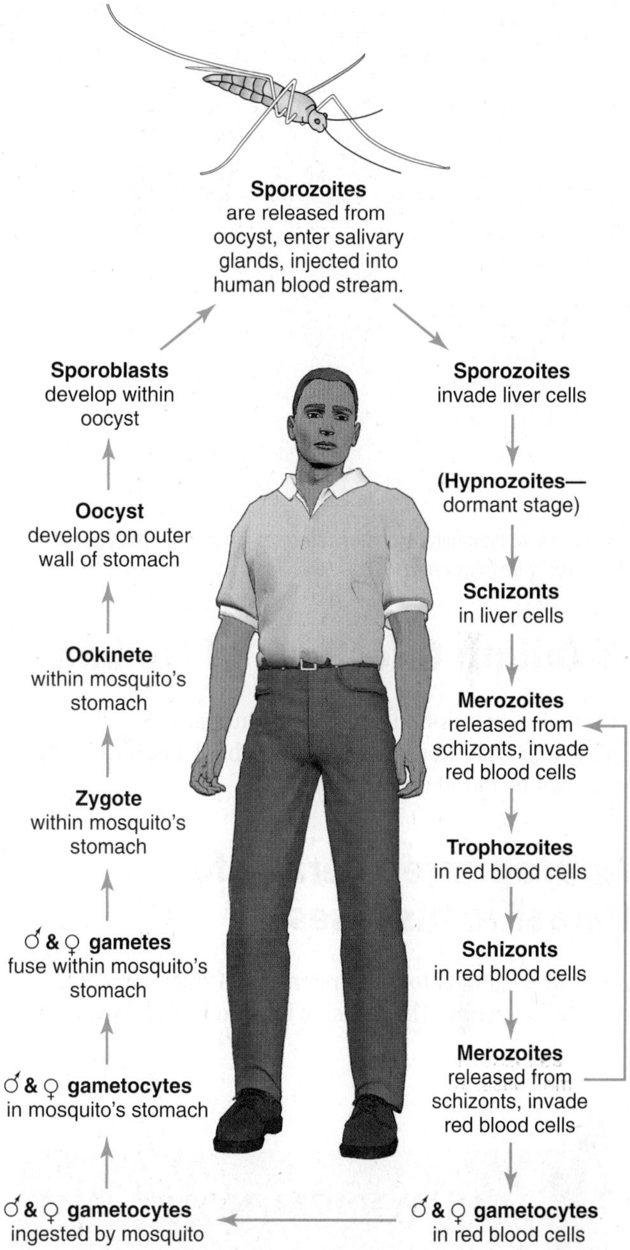

Sporozoites
are released from oocyst, enter salivary glands, injected into human blood stream.

Sporoblasts
develop within oocyst

Sporozoites
invade liver cells

Oocyst
develops on outer wall of stomach

(Hypnozoites—
dormant stage)

Schizonts
in liver cells

Ookinete
within mosquito's stomach

Merozoites
released from schizonts, invade red blood cells

Zygote
within mosquito's stomach

Trophozoites
in red blood cells

♂ & ♀ **gametes**
fuse within mosquito's stomach

Schizonts
in red blood cells

♂ & ♀ **gametocytes**
in mosquito's stomach

Merozoites
released from schizonts, invade red blood cells

♂ & ♀ **gametocytes**
ingested by mosquito

♂ & ♀ **gametocytes**
in red blood cells

FIGURE 18-5. Life cycle of malarial parasites. Malarial parasites have a complex life cycle, involving many different life cycle stages. Humans become infected when an infected, female *Anopheles* mosquito injects sporozoites while taking a blood meal. The sporozoites enter the human bloodstream, are transported to the liver, and invade liver cells (hepatocytes), where schizonts (liver cells containing numerous merozoites) develop. Merozoites are released when the schizont ruptures. Each merozoite can invade another liver cell, leading to schizont development, and the release of more merozoites. With *Plasmodium vivax* and *Plasmodium ovale*, dormant forms (hypnozoites) may remain in hepatocytes, causing relapses months to years later. Eventually, merozoites enter the peripheral bloodstream where they invade erythrocytes. Within an erythrocyte, the merozoite transforms into a trophozoite. The trophozoite may mature into any of three life cycle stages: a schizont (an erythrocyte containing numerous merozoites), a male gametocyte, or a female gametocyte. When the schizonts rupture, merozoites are released and they invade other erythrocytes.

For the parasite life cycle to continue, at least one male and one female gametocyte must be ingested by a female *Anopheles* mosquito while taking a blood meal from the infected person. Within the mosquito's stomach, the female gametocyte matures into a female gamete, and the male gametocyte produces several male gametes. A male gamete fuses with a female gamete, producing a zygote. Because the sexual phase of the life cycle occurs in the mosquito, the mosquito is considered to be the definitive host. The zygote matures into a motile form called an ookinete. The ookinete escapes from the stomach by squeezing between cells in the stomach wall and encysts on the outer wall of the mosquito's stomach, becoming an oocyst. Within the oocyst, sporoblasts develop and mature into sporozoites. When the oocyst bursts open, the sporozoites are released, some of which enter the mosquito's salivary glands. The portion of the life cycle that occurs within the mosquito takes 8 to 35 days, depending on the particular *Plasmodium* species and temperature.

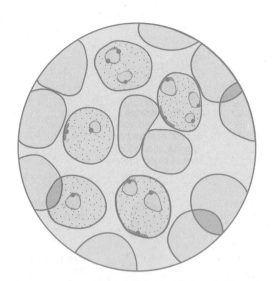

FIGURE 18-6. Peripheral blood erythrocytes infected with trophozoites of *Plasmodium falciparum*.

Helminth Infections of Humans

The major helminth infections of humans are shown in Table 18-7. Additional information about helminth infections can be found on the CD-ROM.

Appropriate Therapy for Parasitic Diseases

Recommendations for the treatment of infectious diseases change frequently. The parasitic infections described in this

chapter must be treated using the appropriate antiprotozoal drug(s) or antihelminth drug(s), as recommended in recent issues of *The Medical Letter* (www.medicalletter.com), the most recent edition of the *Physician's Desk Reference* (PDR; www.pdr.net), *The Merck Manual* (www.merck.com/pubs), or other reliable, up-to-date sources of such information. Additional information about antiprotozoal agents can be found in Chapter 9. Drugs used to treat helminth infections are also known as anthelmintics, anthelminthics, antihelmintics, and antihelminthics.

Arthropods

There are many different classes of arthropods, but only three are studied in a parasitology course: *insects* (Class Insecta), *arachnids* (Class Arachnida), and certain *crustaceans* (Class Crustacea). The insects that are studied include lice, fleas, flies, mosquitoes, and reduviid bugs. Arachnids include mites and ticks. Crustaceans include crabs, crayfish, and certain *Cyclops* species. Arthropods may be involved in human diseases in any of four ways (shown in Table 18-8).

Arthropods may serve as mechanical or biologic vectors in the transmission of certain infectious diseases. ***Mechanical vectors*** merely pick up the parasite at point A and drop it off at point B. For example, a housefly could pick up parasite cysts on the sticky hairs of its legs while walking around on animal feces in a meadow. The fly might then fly through an open kitchen window and drop off the parasite cysts while walking on a pie cooling on the counter. A ***biologic vector,*** on the other hand, is an arthropod in whose body the pathogen multiplies or matures (or both). Many arthropod vectors of human diseases are biologic vectors. A particular arthropod may serve as both a host and a biologic vector. Refer back to Table 11-3 in Chapter 11 for a list of arthropods that serve as vectors of human infectious diseases. Several arthropods that serve as vectors of human diseases are shown in Figure 18-7.

⊙ REVIEW OF KEY POINTS

- Parasites are defined as organisms that live *on* or *in* other living organisms (hosts), at whose expense they gain some advantage (usually by depriving the host of nutrients). Of the three categories of organisms (parasitic protozoa, helminths, and arthropods) that are studied in a parasitology course, only one category (parasitic protozoa) contains microorganisms.

- Parasites that live on the outside of the host's body are referred to as *ectoparasites,* whereas those that live inside are called *endoparasites.*

- The *definitive host* is defined as the host that harbors the adult or sexual stage of the parasite or the sexual phase of the life cycle. The *intermediate host* is the host that harbors the larval or asexual stage of the parasite or the asexual phase of the life cycle.

TABLE 18-7

Helminth Infections of Humans

ANATOMIC LOCATION	HELMINTH DISEASE	HELMINTH THAT CAUSES THE DISEASE
Skin	Onchocerciasis (also known as "river blindness")	*Onchocerca volvulus* (N); microfilariae (tiny prelarval stages) of these helminths are found in the skin
Muscle and Subcutaneous Tissues	Trichinosis Dracunculiasis	*Trichinella spiralis* (N) *Dracunculus medinensis* (N); also known as the guinea worm
Eyes	Onchocerciasis Loiasis	*Onchocerca volvulus* (N); microfilariae enter the eyes, causing an intense inflammatory reaction *Loa loa* (N); also known as the African eyeworm
Respiratory System	Paragonimiasis	*Paragonimus westermani* (T); the lung fluke
Gastrointestinal Tract	Ascariasis infection Hookworm infection Pinworm infection (enterobiasis) Whipworm infection (trichuriasis) Strongyloidiasis Beef tapeworm infection Dog tapeworm infection Dwarf tapeworm infection Fish tapeworm infection Pork tapeworm infection Rat tapeworm infection Fasciolopsiasis Fascioliasis Clonorchiasis	*Ascaris lumbricoides* (N); the large intestinal roundworm of humans *Ancylostoma duodenale* (N) or *Necator americanus* (N) *Enterobius vermicularis* (N) *Trichuris trichiura* (N) *Strongyloides stercoralis* (N) *Taenia saginata* (C) *Dipylidium caninum* (C) *Hymenolepis nana* (C) *Diphyllobothrium latum* (C) *Taenia solium* (C) *Hymenolepis diminuta* (C) *Fasciolopsis buski* (T); an intestinal fluke *Fasciola hepatica* (T); a liver fluke *Clonorchis sinensis* (T); also known as the Chinese or Oriental liver fluke
Circulatory System	Filariasis Schistosomiasis (also known as bilharzia)	*Wuchereria bancrofti* (N) and *Brugia malayi* (N); microfilariae of these helminths are found in the bloodstream Trematodes in the genus *Schistosoma*
Central Nervous System	Cysticercosis Hydatid cyst disease	Cysts (the larval stage) of the pork tapeworm (*Taenia solium*) are found in the brain *Echinococcus granulosis* (C) or *Echinococcus multilocularis* (C); in addition to the brain, hydatid cysts (the larval form of these helminths) can form in many other locations in the body

N, nematode; *C*, cestode; *T*, trematode.

TABLE 18-8

Ways in Which Arthropods May Be Involved in Human Diseases

TYPE OF INVOLVEMENT	EXAMPLE(S)
The arthropod may actually be the *cause* of the disease.	Scabies, a disease in which microscopic mites live in subcutaneous tunnels and cause intense itching.
The arthropod may serve as the *intermediate host* in the life cycle of a parasite.	Flea in the life cycle of the dog tapeworm. Beetle in the life cycle of the rat tapeworm. *Cyclops* sp. in the life cycle of the fish tapeworm. Tsetse fly in the life cycle of African trypanosomiasis. *Simulium* black fly in the life cycle of onchocerciasis. Mosquito in the life cycle of filariasis.
The arthropod may serve as the *definitive host* in the life cycle of a parasite.	Female *Anopheles* mosquito in the life cycle of malarial parasites.
The arthropod may serve as a *vector* in the transmission of an infectious disease.	Oriental rat flea in the transmission of plague. Tick in the transmission of Rocky Mountain spotted fever and Lyme disease. Louse in the transmission of epidemic typhus.

- A *facultative parasite* is an organism that can be parasitic but does not have to live as a parasite. It is capable of living an independent life (apart from a host). An *obligate parasite* has no choice. To survive, it must be a parasite.

- Students should learn the type and name of the protozoal parasite that causes each of the diseases described in the section entitled "Protozoal Infections of Humans," as well as the manner in which each of those diseases is transmitted.

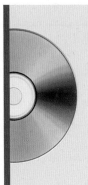

On the CD-ROM

- Increase Your Knowledge
- A Closer Look at Helminth Infections
- Critical Thinking
- Case Studies
- Additional Self-Assessment Exercises

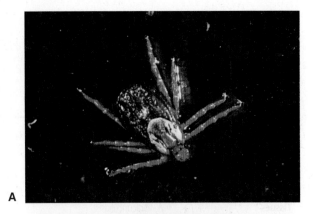

A

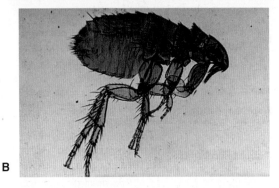

B

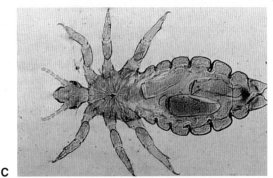

C

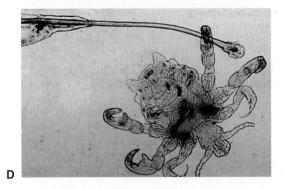

D

FIGURE 18-7. Arthropod ectoparasites and vectors of human infectious diseases. (*A*) *Dermacentor andersoni,* the wood tick; one of the tick vectors of Rocky Mountain spotted fever. (*B*) *Xenopsylla cheopis,* the oriental rat flea; the vector of plague and endemic typhus. (*C*) *Pediculus humanus,* the human body louse; a vector of epidemic typhus. (*D*) *Phthirus pubis,* the pubic louse; because of its appearance, it is also known as the crab louse. (Koneman's Color Atlas and Textbook of Diagnostic Microbiology, 5th ed. Philadelphia: Lippincott-Raven, 1997.)

Self-Assessment Exercises

After studying this chapter, answer the following multiple-choice questions.

1. Humans develop malaria after the injection of *Plasmodium* _____ into the bloodstream by an infected female *Anopheles* mosquito when she takes a blood meal.
   a. male and female gametocytes
   b. schizonts
   c. sporozoites
   d. trophozoites

2. These *Plasmodium* life cycle stages must be ingested by a female *Anopheles* mosquito for the *Plasmodium* life cycle to continue in the mosquito.
   a. male and female gametocytes
   b. schizonts
   c. sporozoites
   d. trophozoites

3. Which of the following protozoal diseases is *not* transmitted via an arthropod vector?
   a. African trypanosomiasis
   b. American trypanosomiasis
   c. babesiosis
   d. giardiasis

4. Which of the following protozoal diseases is *least* likely to be transmitted via blood transfusion?
   a. American trypanosomiasis
   b. babesiosis
   c. malaria
   d. trichomoniasis

5. Which of the following protozoal diseases is *least* likely to be transmitted via an infected food handler who fails to wash his or her hands after using the bathroom?
   a. amebiasis
   b. cryptosporidiosis
   c. giardiasis
   d. toxoplasmosis

6. You are visiting a friend whose parents raise pigs. Which of the following diseases are you *most* likely to acquire by drinking well water at their farm?
   a. amebiasis
   b. balantidiasis
   c. cryptosporidiosis
   d. giardiasis

7. You are working on a cattle ranch. Which of the following diseases are you *most* apt to acquire as you perform your duties at the ranch?
   a. amebiasis
   b. balantidiasis
   c. cryptosporidiosis
   d. giardiasis

8. Which of the following protozoal diseases are you *most* likely to acquire by eating a rare hamburger?
   a. amebiasis
   b. balantidiasis
   c. giardiasis
   d. toxoplasmosis

9. Which of the following associations is incorrect?
   a. African trypanosomiasis. . .tsetse fly
   b. amebiasis. . .fecally contaminated water
   c. Chagas' disease. . .mosquito
   d. toxoplasmosis. . .cats

10. Which of the following is an example of an infectious disease that is caused by a facultative parasite?
    a. African trypanosomiasis
    b. giardiasis
    c. malaria
    d. primary amebic meningoencephalitis

A

ANSWERS TO SELF-ASSESSMENT EXERCISES

Chapter 1

1. A
2. B
3. D
4. D
5. B
6. B
7. D
8. B
9. B
10. B

Chapter 2

1. D
2. B
3. A
4. D
5. D
6. B
7. A
8. D
9. B
10. B

Chapter 3

1. C
2. C
3. B
4. C
5. C
6. C
7. B
8. C
9. A
10. C

Chapter 4

1. D
2. A
3. A
4. C
5. A
6. B
7. C
8. A
9. D
10. A

Chapter 5

1. D
2. D
3. B
4. C
5. D
6. C
7. D
8. A
9. D
10. D

Chapter 6

1. A
2. A
3. C
4. A
5. A
6. D
7. D
8. D
9. D
10. C

Chapter 7

1. C
2. A
3. D
4. A
5. C
6. D
7. D
8. B
9. C
10. A

Chapter 8

1. B
2. B
3. B
4. D
5. C
6. C
7. A
8. D
9. B
10. A

Chapter 9

1. C
2. D
3. B
4. D
5. B
6. C
7. A
8. B
9. B
10. C

Chapter 10

1. D
2. A
3. D
4. A
5. A
6. B
7. C
8. A
9. D
10. C

Chapter 11

1. B
2. D
3. A
4. D
5. A
6. B
7. A
8. C
9. C
10. D

Chapter 12

1. A
2. D
3. B
4. B
5. B
6. B
7. A
8. D
9. A
10. D

Chapter 13

1. D
2. C
3. C
4. D
5. A
6. D
7. C
8. D
9. D
10. D

Chapter 14

1. D
2. A
3. D
4. B
5. C
6. B
7. C
8. B
9. A
10. D

Chapter 15

1. B
2. A
3. D
4. D
5. D
6. A
7. D
8. D
9. A
10. C

Chapter 16

1. A
2. C
3. C
4. C
5. C
6. D
7. B
8. D
9. D
10. C

Chapter 17

1. B
2. A
3. D
4. D
5. D
6. D
7. A
8. B
9. B
10. A

Chapter 18

1. C
2. A
3. D
4. D
5. D
6. B
7. C
8. D
9. C
10. D

B

COMPENDIUM OF IMPORTANT BACTERIAL PATHOGENS OF HUMANS

Bacillus anthracis (Buh-sil-us an-thray-sis). An aerobic, spore-forming, Gram-positive bacillus; the causative agent of anthrax in humans, cattle, swine, sheep, rabbits, guinea pigs, and mice; causes a cutaneous, respiratory, or gastrointestinal disease, depending on the portal of entry.

Bacteroides (Bak-ter-oy-dez) species. Anaerobic, Gram-negative bacilli; common members of the indigenous microflora of the oral cavity, gastrointestinal tract, and vagina; opportunistic pathogens that cause a variety of infections, including appendicitis, peritonitis, abscesses, and postsurgical wound infections.

Bordetella pertussis (Bor-duh-tel-uh per-tus-sis). A fastidious, Gram-negative coccobacillus; the causative agent of whooping cough, which is also called pertussis.

Borrelia burgdorferi (Boh-ree-lee-uh burg-door-fur-eye). A Gram-negative, loosely coiled spirochete; the causative agent of Lyme disease; transmitted from infected deer and mice to humans by tick bite.

Campylobacter jejuni (Kam-pih-low-bak-ter juh-ju-nee). A curved, Gram-negative bacillus, having a characteristic corkscrew-like motility; often seen in pairs (described as a gull-wing morphology because a pair of curved bacilli resembles a bird); microaerophilic and capnophilic; a common cause of gastroenteritis with malaise, myalgia, arthralgia, headache, and cramping abdominal pain.

Chlamydia (Kluh-mid-ee-uh) species. Pleomorphic, Gram-negative bacteria that are obligate intracellular pathogens; unable to grow on artificial media; etiologic agents of nongonococcal urethritis (NGU), trachoma, inclusion conjunc-tivitis, lymphogranuloma venereum, pneumonia, and psittacosis (ornithosis); different serotypes cause different diseases.

Clostridium botulinum (Klos-trid-ee-um bot-yu-ly-num). An anaerobic, spore-forming, Gram-positive bacillus; common in soil; produces a neurotoxin called botulinum toxin, which causes botulism, a very serious and sometimes fatal type of food poisoning.

Clostridium difficile (Klos-trid-ee-um dif-fuh-seal). An anaerobic, spore-forming, Gram-positive bacillus; it can colonize the intestinal tract, where overgrowth (superinfection) commonly occurs after ingestion of oral antibiotics; this organism produces two toxins—an enterotoxin that causes antibiotic-associated diarrhea (AAD) and a cytotoxin that causes pseudomembranous colitis (PMC); a common cause of nosocomial infections.

Clostridium perfringens (Klos-trid-ee-um purr-frin-jens). An anaerobic, spore-forming, Gram-positive bacillus; common in feces and soil; the most common cause of gas gangrene (myonecrosis); produces an enterotoxin that produces a relatively mild type of food poisoning.

Clostridium tetani (Klos-trid-ee-um tet-an-eye). An anaerobic, spore-forming, Gram-positive bacillus; common in soil; produces a neurotoxin called tetanospasmin, which causes tetanus.

Corynebacterium diphtheriae (Kuh-ry-nee-bak-teer-ee-um dif-thee-ree-ee). A pleomorphic, Gram-positive bacillus; toxigenic (toxin-producing) strains cause diphtheria, whereas nontoxigenic strains do not.

Enterococcus (En-ter-oh-kok-us) species. Gram-positive cocci; common members of the indigenous microflora of the gastrointestinal tract; opportunistic pathogens; a fairly common cause of cystitis and nosocomial infections; some strains, called vancomycin-resistant enterococci (VRE), are multidrug-resistant.

Escherichia coli (Esh-er-ick-ee-uh koh-ly). A member of the family *Enterobacteriaceae;* a Gram-negative bacillus; a facultative anaerobe; a very common member of the indigenous microflora of the colon; an opportunistic pathogen; the most common cause of septicemia and urinary tract and nosocomial infections; some serotypes (called the enterovirulent *E. coli*) are always pathogens.

Francisella tularensis (Fran-suh-sel-luh tool-uh-ren-sis). A Gram-negative bacillus; the causative agent of tularemia; may enter the body by inhalation, ingestion, tick bite, or penetration of broken or unbroken skin; tularemia frequently follows contact with infected animals (e.g., rabbits).

Fusobacterium (Few-zoh-bak-teer-ee-um) species. Anaerobic, Gram-negative bacilli; common members of the indigenous microflora of the oral cavity, gastrointestinal tract, and vagina; opportunistic pathogens that cause a variety of infections, including oral and respiratory infections.

Haemophilus influenzae (He-mof-uh-lus in-flu-en-zee). A fastidious, Gram-negative bacillus; a facultative anaerobe; encapsulated; found in low numbers as indigenous microflora of the upper respiratory tract; an opportunistic pathogen; a cause of bacterial meningitis, ear infections, and respiratory infections, but is *not* the cause of influenza (which is caused by influenza viruses); some strains are ampicillin-resistant.

Helicobacter pylori (Hee-luh-ko-bak-ter py-lor-ee). A curved, Gram-negative bacillus; capable of colonizing the stomach; a common cause of stomach and duodenal ulcers.

Klebsiella pneumoniae (Kleb-see-el-uh new-moh-nee-ee). A member of the family *Enterobacteriaceae;* a Gram-negative bacillus; a facultative anaerobe; a common member of the indigenous microflora of the colon; an opportunistic pathogen; a fairly common cause of pneumonia and cystitis.

Lactobacillus (Lak-toh-buh-sil-us) species. Gram-positive bacilli; some species are found in foods (e.g., yogurt, cheese); other species are common members of the indigenous microflora of the vagina and gastrointestinal tract; rarely pathogenic.

Legionella pneumophila (Lee-juh-nel-luh new-mah-fill-uh). An aerobic, Gram-negative bacillus; common in soil and water; the causative agent of legionellosis (a type of pneumonia); can contaminate water tanks and pipes; has caused epidemics in hotels, hospitals, and cruise ships.

Listeria monocytogenes (Lis-teer-ee-uh mon-oh-sigh-toj-uh-nees). A Gram-positive bacillus; the causative agent of listeriosis; can cause meningitis, encephalitis, septicemia, endocarditis, abortion, and abscesses; enters the body via ingestion of contaminated foods (e.g., cheese).

Mycobacterium leprae (My-koh-bak-teer-ee-um lep-ree). An aerobic, acid-fast, Gram-variable bacillus; referred to as the leprosy bacillus or Hansen's bacillus; the causative agent of leprosy (Hansen's disease); transmitted from person to person; has been found in wild armadillos, which are now used as laboratory animals to propagate this organism.

Mycobacterium tuberculosis (My-koh-bak-teer-ee-um tuber-kyu-loh-sis). An acid-fast, Gram-variable bacillus; causes tuberculosis; many strains are multidrug-resistant.

Mycoplasma pneumoniae (My-koh-plaz-muh new-moh-nee-ee). A small, pleomorphic, Gram-negative bacterium; lacks a cell wall; the causative agent of atypical pneumonia.

Neisseria gonorrhoeae (Ny-see-ree-uh gon-or-ree-ee). Also known as gonococcus or GC; a fastidious, Gram-negative diplococcus; microaerophilic and capnophilic; always a pathogen; causes gonorrhea; many strains are penicillin-resistant.

Neisseria meningitidis (Ny-see-ree-uh men-in-jih-tid-is). Also known as meningococcus; an aerobic, Gram-negative diplococcus; found as indigenous microflora of the upper respiratory tract of some people (referred to as carriers); a common cause of bacterial meningitis; also causes respiratory infections.

Nocardia (No-kar-dee-uh) species. Aerobic, acid-fast, Gram-positive bacilli; the causative agents of nocardiosis (a respiratory disease) and mycetoma (a tumorlike disease, most often involving the feet).

Peptostreptococcus (Pep-toh-strep-toh-kok-us) species. Anaerobic, Gram-positive cocci; common members of the indigenous microflora of the gastrointestinal tract, vagina, and oral cavity; opportunistic pathogens that cause a variety of infections, including abscesses, oral infections, and appendicitis.

Porphyromonas (Porf-uh-row-mow-nus) species. Anaerobic, Gram-negative bacilli; common members of the indigenous microflora of the oral cavity and gastrointestinal tract; opportunistic pathogens that cause a variety of infections, including abscesses, oral infections, and bite wound infections.

Prevotella (Pree-voh-tel-luh) species. Anaerobic, Gram-negative bacilli; common members of the indigenous microflora of the vagina and gastrointestinal tract; opportunistic pathogens that cause a variety of infections, including abscesses.

Proteus (Pro-tee-us) species. Members of the family *Enterobacteriaceae;* Gram-negative bacilli; facultative anaerobes; common members of the indigenous microflora of the colon; opportunistic pathogens; a fairly common cause of cystitis.

Pseudomonas aeruginosa (Su-doh-moh-nas air-uj-in-oh-suh). An aerobic, Gram-negative bacillus; produces a characteristic blue-green pigment (pyocyanin); has a characteristic fruity odor; causes burn wound, ear, urinary tract, and respiratory infections; one of the major causes of nosocomial infections; most strains are multidrug-resistant and resistant to some disinfectants.

Rickettsia (Rih-ket-see-uh) species. Gram-negative bacilli that are obligate intracellular pathogens; unable to grow on artificial media; the causative agents of typhus and typhus-like diseases (e.g., Rocky Mountain spotted fever); all rickettsial diseases are transmitted by arthropods (ticks, fleas, mites, lice).

Salmonella (Sal-moh-nel-uh) species. Members of the family *Enterobacteriaceae;* Gram-negative bacilli; facultative anaerobes; a fairly common cause of food poisoning, especially cases caused by contaminated poultry; *Salmonella typhi* is the causative agent of typhoid fever.

Shigella (She-gel-uh) species. Members of the family *Enterobacteriaceae;* Gram-negative bacilli; facultative anaerobes; a major cause of gastroenteritis and childhood mortality in the developing nations of the world.

Staphylococcus aureus (Staf-ih-low-kok-us aw-ree-us). (See the shaded box in Chapter 17 entitled, "A Closer Look at *Staphylococcus aureus*.")

Streptococcus agalactiae (Strep-toh-kok-us ay-guh-lak-tee-ee). Also known as group B streptococcus; a β-hemolytic, Gram-positive coccus; often colonizes the vagina; a frequent cause of neonatal meningitis.

Streptococcus pneumoniae (Strep-toh-kok-us new-moh-nee-ee). (See the shaded box in Chapter 17 entitled, "A Closer Look at *Streptococcus pneumoniae*.")

Streptococcus pyogenes (Strep-toh-kok-us py-oj-uh-nees). (See the shaded box in Chapter 17 entitled, "A Closer Look at *Streptococcus pyogenes*.")

Treponema pallidum (Trep-oh-nee-muh pal-luh-dum). A very thin, tightly coiled spirochete; the causative agent of syphilis.

Vibrio cholerae (Vib-ree-oh khol-er-ee). An aerobic, curved (comma-shaped), Gram-negative bacillus; halophilic; lives in salt water; the causative agent of cholera.

Yersinia pestis (Yer-sin-ee-uh pes-tis). A Gram-negative bacillus; the causative agent of plague in humans, rodents, and other mammals; transmitted from rat to rat and rat to human by the rat flea.

C

USEFUL CONVERSIONS

Length Conversions

To convert inches into centimeters, multiply by 2.54.
To convert centimeters into inches, multiply by 0.39.
To convert yards into meters, multiply by 0.91.
To convert meters into yards, multiply by 1.09.

1 mile (mi) = 1.609 kilometers
1 yard (yd) = 0.914 meter
1 foot (ft) = 30.48 centimeters
1 inch (in) = 2.54 centimeters
1 kilometer (km) = 0.62 mile
1 meter (m) = 39.37 inches
1 centimeter (cm) = 0.39 inch
1 millimeter (mm) = 0.039 inch

Note: Information about micrometers and nanometers can be found in Figure 2-1 in Chapter 2.

Volume Conversions

To convert gallons into liters, multiply by 3.78.
To convert liters into gallons, multiply by 0.26.
To convert fluid ounces into milliliters, multiply by 29.6.
To convert milliliters into fluid ounces, multiply by 0.034.

1 gallon (gal) = 3.785 liters
1 quart (qt) = 0.946 liter
1 pint (pt) = 0.473 liter
1 fluid ounce (fl oz) = 29.573 milliliters
1 liter (L) = 1.057 quarts
1 milliliter (mL) = 0.0338 fluid ounce

Weight Conversions

To convert ounces into grams, multiply by 28.4.
To convert grams into ounces, multiply by 0.035.
To convert pounds into kilograms, multiply by 0.45.
To convert kilograms into pounds, multiply by 2.2.

1 pound (lb) = 0.454 kilogram
1 ounce (oz) = 28.35 grams
1 kilogram (kg) = 2.2 pounds
1 gram (g) = 0.035 ounce
1 gram = 1,000 milligrams (mg)
1 gram = 1,000,000 micrograms (μg)

Temperature Conversions

To convert Celsius (°C) into Fahrenheit (°F), use °F = (°C × 1.8) + 32.
To convert Fahrenheit (°F) into Celsius (°C), use °C = (°F − 32) × 0.556.

ADDITIONAL RESOURCES

ASM Press
1752 N Street NW
Washington, DC 20036-2904
800-546-2416
http://estore.asm.org

Cambridge Educational
P.O. Box 2053
Princeton, NJ 08543-2053
800-257-5126
http://www.cambridgeeducational.com

Carolina Biological Supply Company
2700 York Road
Burlington, NC 27215
800-334-5551
http://www.carolina.com

Films for the Humanities & Sciences
P.O. Box 2053
Princeton, NJ 08543-2053
800-257-5126
http://www.films.com

Insight Media
2162 Broadway
New York, NY 10024-0621
800-233-9910
http://www.insight-media.com

Scientific Device Laboratory (SDL)
411 E. Jarvis Avenue
Des Plaines, IL 60018
847-803-9495
http://www.scientificdevice.com

Teacher's Media Company
c/o Global Video, LLC
P.O. Box 4455-PS
Scottsdale, AZ 85261
800-262-8837
http://www.teachersvideo.com

Ward's Natural Science
P.O. Box 92912
Rochester, NY 14692-9012
800-962-2660
http://www.wardsci.com

Glossary

A

Abiogenesis (ab'-ee-oh-jen-uh-sis). The theory that life can arise from nonliving matter; also known as *spontaneous generation* (Chap. 1)

Acid-fast stain. A differential staining procedure that differentiates acid-fast bacteria from non–acid-fast bacteria; primarily used in the presumptive diagnosis of tuberculosis (Chap. 4)

Acidophile (uh-sid'-oh-file). An organism that prefers acidic environments; such an organism is said to be *acidophilic* (Chap. 8)

Acquired immunodeficiency syndrome (AIDS). A disease characterized by a variety of opportunistic infections and malignancies; caused by human immunodeficiency virus (HIV) (Chap. 17)

Acquired immunity. Immunity or resistance acquired at some point in an individual's lifetime (Chap. 16)

Acquired resistance. When bacteria become resistant to a drug that they were once susceptible to (Chap. 9)

Active acquired immunity. Immunity or resistance acquired as a result of the active production of antibodies (Chap. 16)

Active carrier. A person who has recovered from an infectious disease but continues to harbor and transmit the causative agent of that disease (Chap. 11)

Acute disease. A disease having a sudden onset and short duration (Chap. 14)

Adenosine triphosphate (uh-den'-oh-seen try-fos'-fate). The major energy-carrying (energy-storing) molecule in a cell (Chap. 7)

Adhesins (ad-hee'-zinz). Molecules on the surface of a pathogen that enable the pathogen to recognize and bind to a particular receptor on the surface of a host cell; also known as *ligands* (Chap. 14)

Aerial hyphae (high'-fee). Mycelial hyphae extending above the surface (of the soil, agar, skin, or wherever the mycelium is growing); where spores are produced; also called *reproductive hyphae* (Chap. 5)

Aerotolerant anaerobe (air-oh-tol'-er-ant an'-air-obe). An organism that can live in the presence of oxygen but grows best in an anaerobic environment (an environment containing no oxygen) (Chap. 4)

Agammaglobulinemia (ay-gam'-uh-glob'-yu-luh-nee'-me-uh). Absence of, or extremely low levels of, the gamma fraction of serum globulin; the absence of immunoglobulins in the bloodstream (Chap. 16)

AIDS. See *acquired immunodeficiency syndrome*

Airborne precautions. Standardized safety precautions that are practiced in a healthcare setting to prevent infections transmitted by the airborne route (Chap. 12)

Algae (al'-gee), sing. *alga*. Eucaryotic, photosynthetic organisms that range in size from unicellular to multicellular; includes many seaweeds (Chap. 5)

Algicidal (al'-juh-side-ul) **agent.** A disinfectant or chemical that specifically kills algae (Chap. 8)

Alkaliphile (al'-kuh-luh-file). An organism that prefers alkaline (basic) environments; such an organism is said to be *alkaliphilic* (Chap.8)

Allergen (al'-ur-jin). An antigen to which some people become allergic (Chap. 16)

Ameba (uh-me'-bah), pl. *amebae*. A type of protozoan that moves by means of pseudopodia; in the phylum Sarcodina (which is a subphylum in some classification schemes) (Chap. 5)

Ames test. A method of testing compounds to determine whether they are mutagenic (i.e., to see whether they cause mutations in bacteria); uses a mutant strain of *Salmonella* (Chap. 7)

Amino (uh-me'-no) **acids.** The basic units or building blocks of proteins (Chap. 6)

Ammonification (uh-mon'-uh-fuh-kay'-shun). Conversion of nitrogenous compounds (e.g., proteins) into ammonia (Chap. 10)

Amphitrichous (am-fit'-ri-kus) **bacterium.** A bacterium that possesses one flagellum or more than one flagellum at each end (pole) of the cell (Chap. 3)

Anabolic reactions. Metabolic reactions that require energy for the creation of chemical bonds; also known as *biosynthetic reactions* (Chap. 7)

Anabolism (uh-nab'-oh-lizm). Term referring to all of the anabolic reactions that occur within a cell (Chap. 7)

Anaerobe (an'-air-obe). An organism that does not require oxygen for survival; can exist in the absence of oxygen (Chap. 4)

Anaphylactic (an-uh-fuh-lak'-tick) reactions. Allergic reactions; may be localized or systemic; also known as type I hypersensitivity reactions (Chap. 16)

Anaphylactic (an-uh-fuh-lak'-tick) shock. Shock after anaphylaxis; may lead to death (Chap. 16)

Anaphylaxis (an-uh-fuh-lak'-sis). An immediate, severe, sometimes fatal, systemic allergic reaction (Chap. 16)

Anoxygenic photosynthesis (an'-ox-uh-gen'-ik foe-toe-sin'-thuh-sis). A type of photosynthesis in which oxygen is not produced (Chap. 4)

Antagonism (an-tag'-ohn-izm). As the term relates to the use of drugs, the use of two drugs that work against each other; also see *microbial antagonism* (Chap. 9)

Antibacterial agents. Technically, any physical or chemical agents that kill or inhibit the growth of bacteria; in this book, the term is reserved for drugs that are used to treat bacterial diseases (Chap. 9)

Antibiogram (an-tee-by'-oh-gram). The pattern of susceptible (S) and resistant (R) results obtained when antimicrobial susceptibility testing is performed on a particular microorganism (Chap. 12)

Antibiotic (an'-tee-by-ot'-tik). A substance produced by a microorganism that kills or inhibits the growth of other microorganisms (Chap. 1)

Antibody (an'-tee-bod-ee). A glycoprotein produced by lymphocytes in response to an antigen; if it protects the host in some manner, it is referred to as a *protective antibody* (Chap. 15)

Anticodon (an-tee-ko'-don). A trinucleotide sequence that is complementary to a codon; found on a transfer RNA molecule (Chap. 6)

Antifungal agents. Technically, any physical or chemical agents that kill or inhibit the growth of fungi; in this book, the term is reserved for drugs that are used to treat fungal diseases (Chap. 9)

Antigen (an'-tuh-jen). A substance, usually foreign, that stimulates the production of antibodies; an *anti*body *gen*erating substance; also known as an *immunogen* (Chap. 15)

Antigen–antibody complex. The structure produced as a result of the binding of an antibody to an antigen; also known as an *immune complex* (Chap. 16)

Antigen-presenting cell (APC). A macrophage that is displaying antigenic determinants on its surface (Chap. 16)

Antigenic (an-tuh-jen'-ick). If a molecule is antigenic, it stimulates the immune system to produce antibodies; such a molecule is also said to be *immunogenic* (Chap. 16)

Antigenic determinant. The smallest part of an antigen capable of stimulating the production of antibodies; an antigenic molecule; also known as an *epitope* (Chap. 16)

Antigenic variation. The ability of a microorganism to change its surface antigens (Chap. 16)

Antimicrobial (an'-tee-my-kro'-be-ul) agents. Technically, any physical or chemical agents that kill or inhibit the growth of microorganisms; in this book, the term is reserved for drugs that are used to treat infectious diseases (Chap. 9)

Antiprotozoal agents. Technically, any physical or chemical agents that kill or inhibit the growth of protozoa; in this book, the term is reserved for drugs that are used to treat protozoal diseases (Chap. 9)

Antisepsis (an-tee-sep'-sis). Prevention of infection by inhibiting the growth of pathogens (Chap. 8)

Antiseptic (an-tee-sep'-tick). An agent or substance capable of effecting antisepsis; usually refers to a chemical disinfectant that is safe to use on skin and other living tissues (Chap. 8)

Antiseptic technique. Procedures followed to effect antisepsis; the use of antiseptics (Chap. 8)

Antiserum (an-tee-see'-rum). A serum containing specific antibodies; also known as an *immune serum* (Chap. 16)

Antitoxins (an-tee-tok'-sinz). Antibodies produced in response to a toxin; often capable of neutralizing the toxin that stimulated their production (Chap. 16)

Antiviral agents. Technically, any physical or chemical agents that inactivate viruses; in this book, the term is reserved for drugs that are used to treat viral diseases (Chap. 9)

Apoenzyme. A protein that cannot function as an enzyme (i.e., cannot catalyze a chemical reaction) until it attaches to a cofactor (Chap. 6)

Arbovirus (are'-boh-vy'-rus). A virus that is transmitted by an arthropod; an arthropodborne virus (Chap. 17)

Archaea (are-key'-uh). One of the three domains in the Three-Domain System of classification; members of this domain (archaeans or archaeons) are procaryotes; the other two domains are *Bacteria* and *Eucarya* (Chap. 3)

Archaeans (are-key'-ans). Members of the Domain *Archaea*; also called *archaeons* (Chap. 3)

Artificial active acquired immunity. Active acquired immunity that is induced artificially (e.g., by injecting a vaccine into an individual) (Chap. 16)

Artificial media. Culture media that are prepared in the laboratory; they do not occur naturally; also known as *synthetic media* (Chap. 8)

Artificial passive acquired immunity. Passive acquired immunity that is induced artificially (e.g., by injecting antibodies into an individual) (Chap. 16)

Asepsis (a-sep'-sis). Literally, "without infection"; a condition in which living pathogens are absent (Chap. 8)

Aseptate hyphae. Fungal hyphae that do not contain septa (cross-walls) (Chap. 5)

Aseptic (ay-sep'-tick) techniques. Measures taken to ensure that living pathogens are absent (Chap. 8)

Asexual reproduction. A type of reproduction in which a single organism is the sole parent; it passes copies of its entire genome to its offspring (Chap. 3)

Asymptomatic (ay'-simp-tow-mat'-ick) disease. A disease having no symptoms; also referred to as a *subclinical disease* (Chap. 14)

Asymptomatic infection. The presence of a pathogen in or on the body, without any clinical symptoms of disease; also referred to as a *subclinical infection* (Chap. 14)

Atopic (ay-tope'-ick) person. Allergic person; one who suffers from allergies (Chap. 16)

Attenuated (uh-ten'-yu-ay-ted). An adjective meaning weakened, less pathogenic; used to describe certain microorganisms (Chap. 16)

Attenuated vaccine. A vaccine prepared from an attenuated microorganism (Chap. 16)

Attenuation (uh-ten-yu-ay-'shun). The process by which microorganisms are attenuated (Chap. 16)

Autoclave (aw'-toe-klav). An apparatus used for sterilization by steam under pressure (Chap. 8)

Autogenous (aw-toj'-uh-nus) vaccine. A vaccine prepared from microorganisms or cells obtained from the person's own body (Chap. 16)

Autoimmune (aw-toh-uh-myun') disease. A disease in which the body produces antibodies directed against its own tissues (Chap. 16)

Autolysis (aw-tol'-uh-sis). Autodigestion; self-digestion (Chap. 3)

Autotroph (aw'-toe-trof). An organism that uses carbon dioxide as its sole carbon source (Chap. 7)

Avirulent (ay-veer'-yu-lent) strains. Strains that are not virulent; not pathogenic; not capable of causing disease (Chap. 14)

B

B cells (B lymphocytes). The leukocytes that produce antibodies (Chap. 16)

Bacillus (bah-sil'-us), pl. *bacilli*. A rod-shaped bacterium; there is also a bacterial genus named *Bacillus,* made up of aerobic, Gram-positive, spore-forming bacilli (Chap. 2)

Bacteremia (bak-ter-ee'-me-uh). The presence of bacteria in the bloodstream (Chap. 13)

Bacteria (back-teer'-ee-uh). Microorganisms in the Domain *Bacteria* (Chap. 3)

Bacteria (back-teer'-ee-uh). One of the three domains in the Three-Domain System of classification; members of this domain (bacteria) are procaryotes; the other two domains are *Archaea* and *Eucarya* (Chap. 3)

Bacterial vaginosis (BV). A vaginal infection caused by a variety of bacteria; an example of a *synergistic infection* (Chap. 17)

Bactericidal (bak-tear'-eh-sigh'-dull) agent. A chemical agent or drug that kills bacteria; a *bactericide* (Chap. 8)

Bacteriocins (bak-teer'-ee-oh-sinz). Proteins produced by certain bacteria (those possessing bacteriocinogenic plasmids) that can kill other bacteria (Chap. 10)

Bacteriologist (back'-tier-ee-ol'-oh-jist). One who specializes in the science of bacteriology (Chap. 1)

Bacteriology (back'-tier-ee-ol'-oh-gee). The study of bacteria (Chap. 1)

Bacteriophage (back-tier'-ee-oh-faj). A virus that infects a bacterium; also known simply as a *phage* (Chap. 4)

Bacteriostatic (bak-tear'-ee-oh-stat'-ick) agent. A chemical agent or drug that inhibits the growth of bacteria (Chap. 8)

Bacteriuria (bak-ter-ee'-yu'-ree-uh). The presence of bacteria in the urine (Chap. 13)

Barophile (bar'-oh-file). An organism that thrives under high environmental pressure; such an organism is said to be *barophilic* (Chap. 8)

Bartholinitis (bar-toe-lin-eye'-tis). Inflammation of the Bartholin's gland in females (Chap. 17)

Basophil (bay'-so-fil). A type of granulocyte found in blood; its granules contain acidic substances (e.g., histamine) that attract basic dyes (Chap. 15)

Beneficial mutation. A mutation that is of benefit to the mutant organism (Chap. 7)

β-Lactam ring. One of the two double-ringed structures found in penicillin and cephalosporin molecules (Chap. 9)

β-Lactamases. Enzymes that destroy the β-lactam ring in antibiotics such as penicillin and cephalosporins (Chap. 9)

Binary (by'-nare-ee) fission. A method of reproduction whereby one cell divides to become two cells; the method by which bacteria reproduce (Chap. 3)

Biochemistry (by-oh-kem'-is-tree). The chemistry of living organisms; the chemistry of life (Chap. 6)

Biocidal (by-o-sigh'-dull) agent. A chemical agent that destroys living organisms, especially microorganisms (Chap. 8)

Biofilms. Complex and tenacious communities of assorted microorganisms (Chap. 10)

Biogenesis (by-oh-gen'-uh-sis). The theory that life originates only from preexisting life and never from nonliving matter (Chap. 1)

Biologic catalysts. Enzymes; biologic molecules that catalyze chemical reactions (Chap. 6)

Biologic vector. An arthropod vector (such as a flea or tick) within which a pathogen multiplies or matures (Chap. 18)

Biologic warfare (bw) agents. Pathogens used as weapons in warfare (Chap. 11)

Biology. The study of living organisms; the study of life (Chap. 1)

Bioremediation (by'-oh-ruh-meed'-ee-a-shun). The use of microorganisms to clean up industrial and toxic wastes (Chap. 1)

Biotechnology (by'-oh-tek-nol'-oh-gee). The use of microorganisms in industry to produce chemicals, antibiotics, foods, beverages, and other products (Chap. 1)

Bioterrorist agents. Pathogens used by terrorists (Chap. 11)

Biotherapeutic (by'-oh-ther-uh-pu'-tik) agents. Microorganisms used for therapeutic purposes (to treat various diseases or conditions) (Chap. 10)

Biotype. The pattern of positive and negative biochemical test results obtained when a particular microorganism is tested; in some biochemical test systems (e.g., minisystems), biotype refers to the specific code number generated by the test results (Chap. 12)

Blocking antibodies. IgG antibodies produced by the body in response to allergy shots; they combine with allergens, thus preventing the allergens from attaching to IgE antibodies on the surface of basophils and mast cells (Chap. 16)

Botulinal (bot'-you-ly-nal) **toxin.** The neurotoxin produced by *Clostridium botulinum*; causes botulism; known by various other names such as botulin and botulinum toxin (Chap. 14)

Brightfield microscope. Alternate name for a compound light microscope; refers to the fact that objects are observed against a bright background (or bright field) (Chap. 2)

Broad-spectrum antibiotics. Antibiotics that are effective against a wide range of bacteria; they are effective against both Gram-positive and Gram-negative bacteria (Chap. 9)

Bronchitis (brong-ky'-tis). Inflammation of the mucous membrane lining of the bronchial tubes (Chap. 17)

Bronchopneumonia (brong'-ko-new-mow'-nee-uh). Combination of bronchitis and pneumonia (Chap. 17)

C

Calibrated loop. A bacteriologic loop manufactured to contain a precise volume of liquid (usually 0.01 mL or 0.001 mL) (Chap. 13)

Candidiasis (kan-duh-dy'-uh-sis). Infection with, or disease caused by, a yeast in the genus *Candida*—usually *Candida albicans*; also known as *moniliasis* (Chap. 10)

Capnophile (cap'-no-file). An organism that grows best in the presence of increased concentrations of carbon dioxide; such an organism is said to be *capnophilic* (Chap. 4)

Capsid (kap'-syd). The external protein coat or covering of a virion (Chap. 4)

Capsomeres (kap'-so-meers). The individual protein subunits that make up the capsid of some virions (Chap. 4)

Capsule (kap'-sool). An organized layer of glycocalyx, firmly attached to the outer surface of a bacterial cell wall; some yeasts are also encapsulated (Chap. 3)

Carbohydrates (kar-boh-high'-drates). Organic compounds containing carbon, hydrogen, and oxygen in a ratio of 1:2:1; also known as *saccharides* (Chap. 6)

Carbuncle (kar'-bung-kul). A deep-seated pyogenic (pus-producing) infection of the skin, usually arising from a coalescence of furuncles (Chap. 17)

Carrier (keh'-ree-er). An individual having an asymptomatic infection that can be transmitted to other susceptible individuals (Chap. 10)

Catabolic (cat-uh-bohl'-ik) **reactions.** Metabolic reactions that involve the breaking of chemical bonds and the release of energy; also known as *degradative reactions* (Chap. 7)

Catabolism (kuh-tab'-oh-lizm). Term referring to all the catabolic reactions that occur within a cell (Chap. 7)

Catalyst (kat'-uh-list). A substance (usually an enzyme) that speeds up a chemical reaction but is not itself consumed or permanently changed in the process (Chap. 6)

Catalyze (cat'-uh-lyz). To act as a catalyst; to speed up a reaction (Chap. 6)

Cell (sell). The smallest unit of living structure capable of independent existence (Chap. 3)

Cell-mediated immunity. A type of immunity involving many different cell types (e.g., macrophages, various types of lymphocytes), but where antibodies play only a minor role, if any; also known as *delayed hypersensitivity* (Chap. 16)

Cell membrane (sell mem'-brain). The protoplasmic boundary of all cells; provides selective permeability and serves other important functions (Chap. 3)

Cell theory. The theory stating that all living organisms are composed of cells (Chap. 3)

Cell wall. The outermost layer of many types of cells (e.g., algal, bacterial, fungal, and plant cells); it serves to protect the cell (Chap. 3)

Cellulose (sell'-you-los). A polysaccharide found in the cell walls of algae and plants (Chap. 3)

Centimeter (sen'-tuh-me-ter). One hundredth of a meter (Chap. 2)

Central Dogma. The flow of genetic information within a cell; from DNA to a mRNA molecule to a protein molecule (Chap. 6)

Cephalosporinase (sef'-uh-low-spore'-uh-nase). An enzyme that destroys the β-lactam ring in cephalosporin antibiotics; a type of β-lactamase (Chap. 9)

Cerebrospinal (sir-ee'-broh-spy'-nul) **fluid (CSF).** The fluid within the spinal cord and the ventricles and cavities of the brain; also referred to simply as *spinal fluid* (Chap. 13)

Cervicitis (sir-vuh-sigh'-tis). Inflammation of the cervix (the part of the uterus that opens into the vagina) (Chap. 17)

Cestodes (sess'-toadz). A subcategory of flatworms; includes tapeworms (Chap. 18)

Chemically defined media. Types of culture media where the exact chemical composition is known (Chap. 8)

Chemoautotroph (keem'-oh-awe'-toe-trof). An organism that uses chemicals as an energy source and carbon dioxide as a carbon source; a type of autotroph (Chap. 7)

Chemoheterotroph (keem'-oh-het'-er-oh-trof). An organism that uses chemicals as an energy source and organic chemicals as a carbon source; a type of heterotroph (Chap. 7)

Chemokines. Chemotactic agents produced by various types of cells in the body (Chap. 15)

Chemolithotroph (keem'-oh-lith'-oh-trof). A type of chemotroph that uses inorganic compounds as a source of energy; also referred to as a *lithotroph* (Chap. 7)

Chemoorganotroph (keem'-oh-or-gan'-oh-trof). A type of chemotroph that uses organic compounds as a source of energy; also referred to as an *organotroph* (Chap. 7)

Chemosynthesis (keem'-oh-syn'-thuh-sis). The process of obtaining energy and synthesizing organic compounds from simple inorganic reactions; carried out by some chemoautotrophic bacteria (Chap. 7)

Chemotactic (keem'-oh-tack'-tick) agents. Chemical substances that attract leukocytes; also referred to as *chemotactic factors, chemotactic substances,* and *chemoattractants* (Chap. 15)

Chemotaxis (keem'-oh-tack'-sis). The movement of cells in response to a chemical (e.g., the attraction of phagocytes to an area of injury) (Chap. 15)

Chemotherapeutic (keem'-oh-ther-uh-pyu'-tik) agent. Any chemical used to treat any disease or medical condition (Chap. 9)

Chemotherapy (keem'-oh-ther'-uh-pee). The treatment of a disease (including an infectious disease) using chemical substances or drugs (Chap. 9)

Chemotroph (keem'-oh-trof). An organism that uses chemicals as an energy source (Chap. 7)

Chitin (ky'-tin). A polysaccharide found in fungal cell walls but not found in the cell walls of other microorganisms; also found in the exoskeleton of beetles and crabs (Chap. 3)

Chloroplast (klor'-oh-plast). A membrane-bound organelle found in the cytoplasm of algal and plant cells; a *plastid* that contains chlorophyll (Chap. 3)

Choleragin (kol'-er-uh-jen). The enterotoxin that causes cholera; produced by *Vibrio cholerae* (Chap. 17)

Chromosomes (kro'-mow-soamz). Cellular structures where most (sometimes all) of the cell's genes are located; eucaryotic chromosomes consist of linear double-stranded DNA molecules and proteins (histones and nonhistone proteins); a procaryotic chromosome usually consists of a single, long, supercoiled, circular, double-stranded DNA molecule (Chap. 3)

Chronic disease. A disease having an insidious (slow) onset and a long duration (Chap. 14)

Ciliates (sil'-ee-itz), sing. *ciliate.* Ciliated protozoa (Chap. 5)

Ciliophora (sil'-ee-auf'-oh-rah). The phylum of protozoa containing the ciliates; sometimes referred to as *Ciliata* (Chap. 5)

Cilium (sil'-ee-um), pl. *cilia.* A thin, usually short, hairlike organelle of motility (Chap. 3)

Clean-catch, midstream urine (CCMS urine). A urine specimen that has been collected in a manner that minimizes contamination with indigenous microflora; the proper type of specimen for a urine culture (Chap. 13)

Clinical laboratory scientists. Laboratory professionals possessing a baccalaureate degree in clinical laboratory science (medical technology); also known as *medical technologists* or *MTs* (Chap. 13)

Clinical laboratory technicians. Laboratory professionals possessing an associate degree in clinical laboratory tech-

nology (medical laboratory technology); also known as *medical laboratory technicians* or *MLTs* (Chap. 13).

Clinical specimens. Various types of specimens (e.g., blood, urine, cerebrospinal fluid) collected from patients (Chap. 13)

Clinically relevant laboratory results. Laboratory results that provide the physician with useful, accurate information about a patient's disease (Chap. 13)

Coagulase (ko-ag'-yu-lace). A bacterial enzyme that causes plasma to clot; converts fibrinogen (a plasma protein) to fibrin (Chap. 14)

Coccobacillus (kok'-ko-buh-sil'-us), pl. *coccobacilli.* A very short bacillus (Chap. 4)

Coccus (kok'-us), pl. *cocci.* A spherical bacterium (Chap. 2)

Codon (koh'-don). A sequence of three consecutive nucleotides in a strand of mRNA that provides the genetic information (code) for a certain amino acid to be incorporated into a growing protein chain (Chap. 6)

Coenzyme (koh'-en-zym). A type of cofactor; several vitamins are coenzymes (Chap. 6)

Cofactor (koh'-fak'-tor). An ion or molecule essential for the enzymatic action of certain proteins (called apoenzymes) (Chap. 6)

Colicin (kol'-uh-sin). A type of bacteriocin produced by *Escherichia coli* and other closely related bacteria (Chap. 10)

Coliforms (ko'-lee-forms). *Escherichia coli* and other lactose-fermenting members of the Family *Enterobacteriaceae* (Chap. 11)

Colitis (ko-ly'-tis). Inflammation of the colon (the large intestine) (Chap. 17)

Collagen (kol'-luh-jen). The major protein in the white fibers of connective tissue, cartilage, and bone (Chap. 14)

Collagenase (kol'-uh-juh-nace). A bacterial enzyme that causes the breakdown of collagen (Chap. 14)

Commensalism (ko-men'-sul-izm). A symbiotic relationship in which one party derives benefit and the other party is unaffected; many members of the indigenous microflora are commensals (Chap. 10)

Communicable (kuh-myun'-uh-kuh-bul) disease. A disease capable of being transmitted person-to-person (Chap. 11)

Community-acquired infection. Any infection acquired outside a healthcare setting (Chap. 12)

Competence (kom'-puh-tense). As used in this book, the ability of a bacterial cell to take up (absorb) free (naked) DNA from the environment; may lead to transformation (Chap. 7)

Competent bacteria. Bacteria capable of taking up (absorbing) free (naked) DNA from the environment (Chap. 7)

Complement (kom'-pluh-ment). A protein complex of 25–30 components (including proteins designated C1 through C9) found in blood; involved in inflammation, chemotaxis, phagocytosis, and lysis of bacteria (Chap. 15)

Complement cascade. The stepwise manner in which proteins of the complement system (complement components) interact with each other (Chap. 15)

Complex media. Culture media, the exact chemical composition of which is unknown; often contain ground-up animal organs (e.g., brain, heart, liver) or yeast extract (Chap. 8)

Compound light microscope. A compound microscope that uses visible light as its source of illumination (Chap. 2)

Compound microscope. A microscope containing more than one magnifying lens (Chap. 2)

Conidium (ko-nid'-ee-um), pl. *conidia*. An asexual fungal spore (Chap. 5)

Conjugate (kon'-ju-git) vaccine. A vaccine prepared by linking a weakly antigenic molecule (e.g., bacterial capsule material) to a powerful antigen (Chap. 16)

Conjugation (kon-ju-gay'-shun). As used in this book, the union of two bacterial cells for the purpose of genetic transfer; *not* a reproductive process (Chap. 3)

Conjunctiva (kon-junk-ty'vuh). The mucous membrane that lines the eyelids and covers the anterior portion of the eyeball (Chap. 17)

Conjunctivitis (kon-junk'-tuh-vi'-tis). Inflammation of the conjunctiva (Chap. 17)

Constitutive genes. Genes that are expressed at all times (Chap. 6)

Contact precautions. Standardized safety precautions that are practiced in a healthcare setting to prevent infections transmitted by contact (Chap. 12)

Contagious disease. A disease easily transmitted from one person to another; a type of communicable disease (Chap. 11)

Contamination (kon-tam-uh-nay'-shun). As used in this book, a condition indicating the presence of undesirable or accidentally introduced microorganisms (which would be referred to as *contaminants*) (Chap. 8)

Contractile vacuole. An organelle that pumps water out of a protozoal cell (Chap. 5)

Convalescent (kon-vuh-less'-ent) carrier. A person who no longer shows the signs or symptoms of a particular infectious disease but continues to harbor and transmit the causative agent during the convalescence period (Chap. 11)

Covalent (koh-vayl'-ent) bond. A type of chemical bond in which two atoms share a pair of electrons (Chap. 6)

Crenated (kree'-nay-ted). Wrinkled, shriveled; e.g., the appearance of erythrocytes placed into a hypertonic solution (Chap. 8)

Crenation (kree-nay'-shun). The process of becoming, or state of being, crenated (Chap. 8)

Cutaneous anaphylaxis. Swelling and redness at the site where an antigen is injected intradermally or subcutaneously; also known as a wheal-and-flare reaction (Chap. 16)

Cyanobacteria (sigh'-an-oh-bak-tier'-ee-uh). A group of photosynthetic bacteria (Chap. 4)

Cyst. As the term applies to parasitology, the dormant, survival stage in a protozoan's life cycle; its tough wall enables the cyst to resist desiccation and temperature extremes (Chap. 5)

Cystitis (sis-ty'-tis). Inflammation or infection of the urinary bladder (Chap. 18)

Cytokines (sigh'-toe-kynz). Soluble chemical messages released by cells of the body; the manner in which different types of cells communicate with each other; examples include *lymphokines* (produced by lymphocytes) and *monokines* (produced by monocytes) (Chap. 16)

Cytokinesis (sigh'-toe-kuh-knee'-sis). Division of the cytoplasm, resulting in two daughter cells; follows mitosis (Chap. 3)

Cytology (sigh-tol'-oh-gee). The study of cells (Chap. 3)

Cytoplasm (sigh'-toe-plazm). A type of protoplasm; lies outside the nucleus of a eucaryotic cell (Chap. 3)

Cytoskeleton. A system of fibers (microtubules, microfilaments, and intermediate filaments) running throughout the cytoplasm of eucaryotic cells (Chap. 3)

Cytostome (sigh'-toe-stoam). A primitive mouth possessed by some protozoa (Chap. 5)

Cytotoxins (sigh'-tow-tok'-sinz). Toxic substances that inhibit or destroy cells (Chap. 14)

D

Darkfield microscope. A compound light microscope that has been fitted with a darkfield condenser; refers to the fact that objects are observed against a dark background (or dark field) (Chap. 2)

Death phase. The part of a bacterial growth curve during which no multiplication occurs and organisms are dying; the fourth and final phase in a bacterial growth curve (Chap. 8)

Decimeter (des'-uh-me-ter). One tenth of a meter (Chap. 2)

Decomposers. Microorganisms that decompose or break down substances (Chap. 1)

Definitive host. In a parasitic relationship, the host that harbors the adult or sexual stage of a parasite, or the sexual phase of the parasite's life cycle (Chap. 18)

Dehydration synthesis reaction. An anabolic reaction in which two molecules are bonded together as a result of the loss of a water molecule; also called a dehydrolysis reaction (Chap. 6)

Dehydrogenation (dee-hy'-drah-jen-ay'-shun) reactions. Chemical reactions in which a pair of hydrogen atoms is removed from a compound, usually by the action of enzymes called dehydrogenases (Chap. 7)

Delayed-type hypersensitivity (DTH) reactions. Hypersensitivity reactions that usually take more than 24 hours to manifest themselves; also known as *cell-mediated immune reactions* and *type IV hypersensitivity reactions* (Chap. 16)

Denitrifying (dee'-ni-truh-fy-ing) bacteria. Bacteria capable of converting nitrates into nitrogen gas; the process is known as *denitrification* (Chap. 10)

Dental caries (kay'-reez). Tooth decay (Chap. 17)

Deoxyribonucleic (dee-ox'-ee-ry'-bow-new-clay'-ick) **acid (DNA).** A macromolecule containing the genetic code in the form of genes (Chap. 3)

Dermatitis (der-muh-ty'-tis). Inflammation of the skin (Chap. 17)

Dermatophytes (der-mah'-toh-fytes). Fungi that cause superficial mycoses of the skin, hair, and nails; the cause of tinea infections (ringworm infections) (Chap. 17)

Dermis (der'-mis). The layer of skin containing blood and lymphatic vessels, nerves and nerve endings, glands, and hair follicles (Chap. 17)

Desiccation (des-uh-kay'-shun). The process of being desiccated (thoroughly dried) (Chap. 8)

Diarrhea (die-uh-ree'-uh). An abnormally frequent discharge of semisolid or fluid fecal matter (Chap. 17)

Differential (dif-er-en'-shul) **media.** Culture media that enable microbiologists to readily differentiate one organism or group of organisms from another (Chap. 8)

Differential staining procedures. Bacterial staining procedures that enable differentiation of two groups of bacteria; e.g., the Gram stain enables differentiation of Gram-positive bacteria from Gram-negative bacteria (Chap. 4)

Dimorphism (dy-more'-fizm). A phenomenon whereby an organism can exist in two shapes or forms; e.g., dimorphic fungi can exist either as yeasts or molds (Chap. 5)

Dipeptide (dy-pep'-tide). A protein consisting of two amino acids held together by a peptide bond (Chap. 6)

Diplobacilli (dip'-low-bah-sill'-eye). Bacilli arranged in pairs (Chap. 4)

Diplococci (dip'-low-kok'-sigh). Cocci arranged in pairs (Chap. 4)

Diploid (dip'-loyd) **cells.** Eucaryotic cells containing two sets of chromosomes (Chap. 3)

Disaccharide (die-sack'-uh-ride). A carbohydrate consisting of two monosaccharides; examples include sucrose (table sugar), lactose (milk sugar), and maltose (malt sugar) (Chap. 6)

Disinfectant (dis-in-fek'-tent). A chemical agent used to destroy pathogens or inhibit their growth and vital activity; usually refers to a chemical agent used on nonliving materials (Chap. 8)

Disinfection (dis-in-fek'-shun). The process of destroying pathogens and their toxins (Chap. 8)

DNA nucleotides. The building blocks of DNA; each DNA nucleotide consists of a nitrogenous base, deoxyribose, and a phosphate group (Chap. 6)

DNA polymerase (poh-lim'-er-ace). The most important enzyme required in DNA replication (Chap. 6)

DNA replication (rep-luh-kay'-shun). Production of two new DNA molecules (called daughter molecules) from one parent DNA molecule (Chap. 6)

DNA vaccine. An experimental type of vaccine that stimulates host cells to produce numerous copies of a harmless microbial protein (antigen); the host's immune system then produces antibodies directed against the protein, and these antibodies protect the person from infection with the pathogen that possesses the protein; also known as a *gene vaccine* (Chap. 16)

Double bond. A type of chemical bond, containing two pairs of shared electrons (Chap. 6)

Droplet precautions. Standardized safety precautions that are practiced in a healthcare setting to prevent infections transmitted by droplets (Chap. 12)

Drug-binding site. A specific molecule on the surface of a cell that a particular drug attaches to (Chap. 9)

Dysentery (dis'-en-tay-ree). Frequent watery stools, accompanied by abdominal pain, fever, and dehydration; the stool specimens may contain blood or mucus (Chap. 17)

E

Ecology (ee-kol'-oh-jee). The branch of biology concerned with the total complex of interrelationships among living organisms; encompassing the relationships of organisms to each other, to the environment, and to the entire energy balance within a given ecosystem (Chap. 7)

Ecosystem (ee'-koh-sis-tem). An ecologic system that includes all the organisms and the environment within which they occur naturally (Chap. 7)

Ectoparasite (ek'-toh-par'-uh-site). A parasite that lives on the external surface of its host (Chap. 18)

Edema (uh-dee'-muh). Swelling caused by an accumulation of watery fluid in cells, tissues, or body cavities; swollen areas are described as being *edematous* (Chap. 15)

Electron (ee-lek'-tron) **micrograph.** Photograph taken through the lens system of an electron microscope (Chap. 2)

Electron microscope. A type of microscope that uses electrons as a source of illumination (Chap. 2)

Electron transport chain. A series of biochemical reactions by which energy is transferred in a stepwise manner; a major source of energy in some cells (Chap. 7)

Empiric (em-peer'-uh-kul) **therapy.** Treatment or therapy that is initiated by a physician (or other healthcare professional) before receipt of test results (Chap. 9)

Empty magnification. Microscopy term meaning an increase in magnification without any concurrent increase in resolving power (Chap. 2)

Encephalitis (en-sef-uh-ly'-tis). Inflammation or infection of the brain (Chap. 13)

Encephalomyelitis (en-sef-uh-low-my'-uh-ly'-tis). Inflammation or infection of the brain and spinal cord (Chap. 17)

Endemic (en-dem'-ick) **disease.** A disease that is always present in a community or geographic area (Chap. 11)

Endocarditis (en'-doh-kar-dy'-tis). Inflammation of the endocardium (the innermost lining of the heart) (Chap. 17)

Endoenzyme (en'-doh-en'-zym). An enzyme produced by a cell that remains within the cell; an intracellular enzyme (Chap. 7)

Endometritis (en'-dough-me-try'-tis). Inflammation of the endometrium (the inner layer of the uterine wall) (Chap. 17)

Endoparasite (en-doh-par'-uh-site). A parasite that lives within the body of its host (Chap. 18)

Endoplasmic reticulum (end-oh-plaz'-mick re-tick'-you-lum) (ER). A network of membranous tubules and flattened sacs in the cytoplasm of a eucaryotic cell; ER with attached ribosomes is called rough ER (RER) or granular ER; ER having no attached ribosomes is called smooth ER (SER) (Chap. 3)

Endospore (en'-dough-spore). Thick-walled, resistant body formed within a bacterial cell for the purpose of survival; a bacterial cell produces only one endospore, and from that endospore emerges (a process known as germination) one bacterial cell; also referred to as a *bacterial spore* (Chap. 3)

Endosymbiont (en'-doh-sym'-be-ont). The party in a symbiotic relationship that lives within the body of the other symbiont (Chap. 10)

Endotoxin (en-doh-tok'-sin). The lipid portion of the lipopolysaccharide found in the cell walls of Gram-negative bacteria; intracellular toxin (Chap. 14)

Enriched media. Culture media that enable microbiologists to isolate fastidious organisms from samples or specimens and grow them in the laboratory (Chap. 8)

Enteric (en-tare'-ik) bacilli. Gram-negative bacilli in the Family *Enterobacteriaceae* (Chap. 10)

Enteritis (en-ter-eye'-tis). Inflammation of the intestines, usually referring to the small intestine (Chap. 17)

Enterotoxin (en-ter-oh-tok'-sin). A bacterial exotoxin specific for cells of the intestinal mucosa (Chap. 14)

Enzyme (en'-zyme). A protein molecule that catalyzes (causes or speeds up) a chemical reaction; remains unchanged in the process; a biologic catalyst (Chap. 6)

Eosinophil (ee-oh-sin'-oh-fil). A type of granulocyte found in blood; its granules contain basic substances (e.g., major basic protein) that attract acidic dyes (Chap. 15)

Eosinophilia (ee'-oh-sin-oh-fil'-ee-uh). An abnormally high number of eosinophils in the bloodstream (Chap. 15)

Epidemic (ep-uh-dem'-ick) disease. A disease occurring in a higher than usual number of cases in a population during a given time interval (Chap. 11)

Epidemiology (ep-uh-dee-me-ol'-oh-jee). The study of relationships between the various factors that determine the frequency and distribution of diseases (Chap. 11)

Epidermis (ep-ee-derm'-is). The superficial epithelial portion of the skin (Chap. 17)

Epididymitis (ep-uh-did-uh-my'-tis). Inflammation of the epididymis (a tubular structure within the testis) (Chap. 17)

Epiglottitis (ep-ee-glot-eye-tis). Inflammation of the epiglottis (the mouth of the windpipe) (Chap. 17)

Episome (ep'-eh-som). An extrachromosomal element (plasmid) that may either integrate into the host bacterium's chromosome or replicate and function stably when physically separated from the chromosome (Chap. 7)

Erythema (air-uh-thee'-muh). Redness of the skin; a reddened area of skin is described as being *erythematous* (Chap. 16)

Erythrocytes (ee-rith'-roh-sites). Red blood cells (Chap. 13)

Erythrogenic (ee-rith-roh-jen'-ick) toxin. The exotoxin produced by *Streptococcus pyogenes* that causes scarlet fever; *erythrogenic* means "produces redness," referring to the red rash of scarlet fever (Chap. 14)

Essential amino acids. Amino acids that must be provided to an organism because the organism is unable to synthesize them (Chap. 6)

Essential fatty acids. Fatty acids that must be provided to an organism because the organism is unable to synthesize them (Chap. 6)

Essential nutrients. Any nutrients that must be provided to an organism because the organism is unable to synthesize them (Chap. 7)

Etiologic (e'-tee-oh-loj'-ik) agent. The causative agent of an infectious disease (i.e., the pathogen that causes the disease) (Chap. 1)

Etiology. Cause; as in the etiology of a disease (Chap. 1)

Eucarya (you-ker'-ee-uh). One of the three domains in the Three-Domain System of classification; alternate spelling = *Eukarya*; members of this domain are eucaryotes; the other two domains are *Archaea* and *Bacteria* (Chap. 3)

Eucaryotic (you'-kar-ee-ah'-tick) cells. Cells containing a true nucleus; organisms possessing such cells are referred to as *eucaryotes;* can also be spelled eukaryotic (Chap. 3)

Exfoliative (eks-foh'-lee-uh-tiv) toxin. The exotoxin produced by *Staphylococcus aureus* that causes staphylococcal scalded skin syndrome (SSSS); also known as *epidermolytic toxin* (Chap. 14)

Exoenzyme (ek-soh-en'-zyme). An enzyme produced by a cell that is released from the cell; an extracellular enzyme (Chap. 7)

Exotoxin (ek-soh-tok'-sin). A toxin that is released from the cell; an extracellular toxin (Chap. 14)

Exudate (eks'-yu-date). Any fluid (e.g., pus) that exudes (oozes) from tissue, often as a result of injury, infection, or inflammation (Chap. 17)

F

Facultative (fak'-ul-tay-tive) anaerobe. An organism that can live either in the presence or absence of oxygen (Chap. 4)

Facultative intracellular pathogen. A pathogen that can live either intracellularly or extracellularly (Chap. 14)

Facultative parasite. An organism that is capable of being a parasite but is also capable of a free-living existence (Chap. 18)

Fascia (fash'-ee-uh). A sheet of fibrous tissue that envelops the body beneath the skin; also encloses muscles and groups of muscles (Chap. 17)

Fasciitis (fas-ee-eye'-tis). Inflammation in fascia (Chap. 17)

Fastidious (fas-tid'-ee-us) microorganisms. Microorganisms that are difficult to isolate from specimens and grow in the laboratory, owing to their complex nutritional requirements (Chap. 1)

Fatty acid. Any acid derived from fats by hydrolysis; fatty acids are the building blocks of lipids (Chap. 6)

Fermentation (fer-men-tay'-shun). An anaerobic biochemical pathway in which substances are broken down, and energy and reduced compounds are produced; oxygen does not participate in the process (Chap. 7)

Fermentative pathways. Metabolic pathways in which oxygen does not participate (Chap. 7)

Fimbriae (fim'-bree-ee), sing. fimbria (fim'-bree-uh). See pili (Chap. 3)

Fixed macrophages. Macrophages that remain localized within certain organs and tissues; also known as histocytes or histiocytes (Chap. 15)

Flagella (fluh-jel'-uh), sing. flagellum. Whiplike organelles of motility; procaryotic and eucaryotic flagella differ in structure; procaryotic flagella are composed of a protein called flagellin; eucaryotic flagella are composed of nine doublet microtubules arranged around two central microtubules (a 9 + 2 arrangement) (Chap. 3)

Flagellates (flaj'-eh-letz). Flagellated protozoa (Chap. 5)

Flagellin (flaj'-eh-lin). The protein of which bacterial flagella are composed (Chap. 3)

Fluorescence (floor'-es-ence) microscope. A type of compound light microscope that uses an ultraviolet (UV) light source (Chap. 2)

Folliculitis (foh-lick-you-ly'-tis). Inflammation of a hair follicle, the sac that contains a hair shaft (Chap. 17)

Fomites (foh'-mitz). Inanimate objects or substances capable of absorbing and transmitting a pathogen (e.g., clothing, bed linens, towels, eating utensils) (Chap. 11)

Fungemia (fun-gee'-me-uh)). The presence of fungi in the bloodstream (Chap. 13)

Fungi (fun'-ji), sing. fungus. Eucaryotic, nonphotosynthetic microorganisms that are saprophytic or parasitic (Chap. 5)

Fungicidal (fun-juh-sigh'-dull) agent. A chemical agent or drug that kills fungi; a fungicide or mycocide (Chap. 8)

Furuncle (few'-rung-kul). A localized pyogenic (pus-producing) infection of the skin, usually resulting from folliculitis; often referred to as a boil (Chap. 17)

G

Gangrene (gang'-green). Necrosis (cell death) as a result of ischemia (lack of blood flow) (Chap. 17)

Gas gangrene. Gangrene caused by Clostridium spp.; the gas that forms in the necrotic tissue is the result of bacterial fermentations; also known as myonecrosis (Chap. 17)

Gastritis (gas-try'-tis). Inflammation of the mucosal lining of the stomach (Chap. 17)

Gastroenteritis (gas'-tro-en-ter-eye'-tis). Inflammation of the mucosal linings of the stomach and intestines (Chap. 17)

Gene (jeen). A functional unit of heredity that occupies a specific space (locus) on a chromosome; contains the genetic information that will enable a cell to produce a protein (usually), an rRNA molecule, or a tRNA molecule (Chap. 3)

Gene product. The molecule (usually a protein) that is coded for by a gene (Chap. 3)

Gene therapy. The insertion of normally functioning genes into a cell to correct problems associated with abnormally functioning genes (Chap. 7)

Generation time. The time required for a cell to split into two cells; also called the doubling time (Chap. 3)

Genetic (juh-net'-ick) code. The sequence of nucleotide bases on a DNA molecule that provides the information necessary for cells to produce gene products (Chap. 6)

Genetic engineering. The insertion of foreign genes into microorganisms to enable the microorganisms to produce specific gene products or to enable them to be used for other purposes (Chap. 1)

Genetics (juh-net'-iks). The branch of science concerned with heredity (Chap. 7)

Genotype (jeen'-oh-type). The complete genetic constitution of an individual (i.e., all of that individual's genes); also known as the genome (Chap. 3)

Genus (jee'-nus), pl. genera. The first name in binomial nomenclature; a genus contains closely related species (Chap. 3)

Germ. Slang term for pathogen (Chap. 1)

Germicidal (jer-muh-sigh'-dull) agent. A chemical agent or drug that kills pathogens; a germicide (Chap. 8)

Gingivitis (jin-juh-vy'-tis). Inflammation or infection of the gingiva (gums) (Chap. 17)

Glucose (glue'-kohs). A biologically important, six-carbon monosaccharide; a hexose; $C_6H_{12}O_6$; also called dextrose; the product of complete hydrolysis of polysaccharides such as cellulose, starch, and glycogen (Chap. 6)

Glycocalyx (gly-ko-kay'-licks). Extracellular material that may or may not be firmly attached to the outer surface of the cell wall; capsules and slime layers are examples (Chap. 3)

Glycogen (gly'-koh-jen). A polysaccharide stored by animal cells as a food reserve; composed of numerous glucose molecules (Chap. 6)

Glycolysis (gly-kol'-eh-sis). The anaerobic, energy-producing breakdown of glucose into two molecules of pyruvic acid via a series of chemical reactions; an example of a biochemical pathway; also called anaerobic glycolysis (Chap. 7)

Glycosidic (gly'-ko-sid'-ik) bond. The covalent bond that holds monosaccharides together in carbohydrate molecules (Chap. 6)

Golgi (goal'-jee) complex. A membranous system located within the cytoplasm of a eucaryotic cell; associated with the transport and packaging of secretory proteins; also known as Golgi apparatus or Golgi body (Chap. 3)

Gonococcus (gon'-oh-kok-us), pl. gonococci. A slang term for Neisseria gonorrhoeae; abbreviated GC (Chap. 13)

Gram stain. A differential staining procedure named for its developer, Hans Christian Gram, a Danish bacteriologist; differentiates bacteria into those that stain blue-to-purple (called Gram-positive bacteria) and those that stain pink-to-red (called Gram-negative bacteria) (Chap. 4)

Granulocytes (gran'-yu-loh-sites). A category of leukocytes having prominent cytoplasmic granules; neutrophils, eosinophils, and basophils are examples (Chap. 15)

Growth curve. As used in this book, a graphic representation of the change in size of a bacterial population over a period of time; includes a lag phase, a log phase, a stationary phase, and a death phase (Chap. 8)

H

Haloduric (hail-oh-dur'-ick) **organisms.** Organisms capable of surviving in a salty environment (Chap. 8)

Halophiles (hail'-oh-file). Organisms whose growth is enhanced by a high salt concentration; such an organism is said to be *halophilic* (Chap. 8)

Haploid (hap'-loyd) **cells.** Eucaryotic cells containing only one set of chromosomes (Chap. 3)

Hapten (hap'-ten). A small, nonantigenic molecule that becomes antigenic when combined with a larger molecule (e.g., a carrier protein) (Chap. 16)

Harmful mutation. A mutation that causes harm to the mutant organism (Chap. 7)

HBV. Hepatitis B virus; the causative agent of serum hepatitis (Chap. 17)

Helminth (hel'-minth). A parasitic worm (Chap. 18)

Hemolysin (he-moll'-uh-sin). A bacterial enzyme capable of lysing erythrocytes (Chap. 14)

Hemolysis (he-moll'-uh-sis). Destruction of erythrocytes in such a manner that hemoglobin is liberated into the surrounding environment (Chap. 8)

Hepatitis (hep-uh-ty'-tis). Inflammation of the liver (Chap. 17)

Heptose. A monosaccharide containing seven carbon atoms (Chap. 6)

Heterotroph (het'-er-oh-trof). An organism that uses organic chemicals as a source of carbon (Chap. 7)

Hexose. A monosaccharide containing six carbon atoms (Chap. 6)

Histamine (his'-tuh-meen). Potent chemical released from basophils and mast cells during allergic reactions; causes constriction of bronchial smooth muscles and vasodilation (Chap. 16)

HIV. Human immunodeficiency virus; the causative agent of AIDS (Chap. 4)

Holoenzyme. Apoenzyme plus cofactor; a whole (functional) enzyme (Chap. 6)

Hospital-acquired infection. See *nosocomial infection*

Host. In a parasitic relationship, the organism on or in which a parasite lives (Chap. 10)

Host defense mechanisms. Mechanisms that serve to protect the body from pathogens and the infections they cause (Chap. 15)

Humoral immunity. A type of immunity in which antibodies play a major role; also known as *antibody-mediated immunity (AMI)* (Chap. 16)

Hyaluronic (high'-uh-lu-ron'-ick) **acid.** A gelatinous mucopolysaccharide that acts as an intracellular cement in body tissue (Chap. 14)

Hyaluronidase (high'-uh-lu-ron'-uh-dase). A bacterial enzyme that breaks down hyaluronic acid; sometimes called diffusing or spreading factor, because it enables bacteria to invade deeper into tissue (Chap. 14)

Hybridoma (high-brid-oh'-muh). A tumor produced in vitro by fusion of mouse tumor cells and specific antibody-producing cells; used in the production of monoclonal antibodies (Chap. 16)

Hydrocarbon (high-droh-kar'-bun). An organic compound consisting of only hydrogen and carbon atoms (Chap. 6)

Hydrolysis (hi-drol'-eh-sis) **reaction.** A chemical process whereby a compound is cleaved into two or more simpler compounds with the uptake of the H and OH parts of a water molecule on either side of the chemical bond that is cleaved (Chap. 6)

Hypersensitivity (high'-per-sen-suh-tiv'-uh-tee) **reactions.** Exaggerated immunologic reactions that result from an overly sensitive immune system (Chap. 16)

Hypertonic (hi-per-tahn'-ick) **solution.** A solution having a greater osmotic pressure than cells placed into that solution; a higher concentration of solutes exists outside the cell (Chap. 8)

Hyphae (hy'-fee), sing. *hypha.* Long, thin, intertwined, cytoplasmic filaments that make up a mold colony (*mycelium*) (Chap. 5)

Hypogammaglobulinemia (high'-poh-gam'-uh-glob-yu-luh-nee'-me-uh). Decreased quantity of the gamma fraction of serum globulin, including a decreased quantity of immunoglobulins (Chap. 16)

Hypotonic (hi-poh-tahn'-ick) **solution.** A solution having a lower osmotic pressure than cells placed into that solution; a lower concentration of solutes exists outside the cell (Chap. 8)

I

Iatrogenic (eye-at-roh-jen'-ick) **infection.** An infection caused by medical treatment; literally, "physician-induced," but could be caused by any healthcare professional (Chap. 12)

Immediate-type hypersensitivity reactions. Hypersensitivity reactions that occur from within a few minutes to 24 hours after contact with a particular antigen (Chap. 16)

Immune (im-myun'). To be free from the possibility of acquiring a particular infectious disease; to be resistant to an infectious disease (Chap. 16)

Immunity (im-myu'-nuh-tee). The status of being immune or resistant to an infectious disease (Chap. 16)

Immunocompetent (im'-you-no-kom'-puh-tent) **person.** A person who is able to mount a normal immune response;

a person whose immune system is functioning properly (Chap. 16)

Immunodiagnostic (im'-yu-noh-dy-ag-nos'-tick) procedures. Laboratory procedures used to diagnose infectious diseases by using the principles of immunology; used to detect either antigen or antibody in patients' specimens (Chap. 16)

Immunoglobulins (im'-yu-noh-glob'-yu-lin). A class of glycoproteins, which contains antibodies (Chap. 16)

Immunohematology laboratory. The laboratory where donor blood is collected, tested, and stored; often referred to as the *Blood Bank* (Chap. 13)

Immunologist (im-you-nol'-oh-jist). One who specializes in the science of immunology (Chap. 16)

Immunology (im-you-nol'-oh-je). The study of immunity and the immune system (Chap. 16)

Immunosuppressed (im'-you-no-sue-pressed) person. A person whose immune system is not functioning properly; such persons are also said to be *immunodepressed* or *immunocompromised* (Chap. 16)

In vitro (in vee'-trow). In an artificial environment, as in a laboratory setting; used in reference to what occurs *outside* an organism (Chap. 1)

In vivo (in vee'-voh). Used in reference to what occurs *within* a living organism (Chap. 1)

Inactivated vaccine. A vaccine prepared from inactivated (killed) microorganisms (Chap. 16)

Incidence. The number of new cases of a particular disease in a defined population during a specific period of time (Chap. 11)

Inclusion bodies. Distinctive clusters of virions, frequently formed in the nucleus or cytoplasm of cells infected with certain viruses (Chap. 4)

Incubation. In microbiology, refers to holding a culture at a particular temperature for a certain length of time (Chap. 8)

Incubator. In microbiology, the chamber within which cultures are held at a particular temperature for a certain length of time (Chap. 8)

Incubatory (in'-kyu-buh-tor'-ee) carrier. A person capable of transmitting a pathogen during the incubation period of a particular infectious disease (Chap. 11)

Indigenous microflora (in-dij'-uh-nus my-crow-floor-uh). Microorganisms that live on and in the healthy body; also called *indigenous microbiota*; referred to in the past as normal flora (Chap. 1)

Inducible genes. Genes that are not expressed all the time (Chap. 6)

Infection (in-fek'-shun). The presence and multiplication of a pathogen on or within the body; often used as a synonym for infectious disease (Chap. 14)

Infectious disease (in-fek'-shus di-zeez'). Any disease caused by a microorganism that follows colonization of the body by that microorganism (Chap. 1)

Infestation (in-fes-tay'-shun). The presence of ectoparasites (e.g., lice) on the body (Chap. 18)

Inflammation (in-fluh-may'-shun). A nonspecific pathologic process consisting of a dynamic complex of cytologic and histologic reactions that occur in response to an injury or abnormal stimulation by a physical, chemical, or biologic agent (Chap. 15)

Inflammatory exudate. An accumulation of fluid, cells, and cellular debris at a site of inflammation (Chap. 15)

Inoculation. In microbiology, refers to adding a specimen to some type of culture medium (Chap. 8)

Inorganic (in-or-gan'-ick) chemistry. The science dealing with all types of chemicals except those classified as organic compounds (Chap. 6)

Inorganic compounds. Chemical compounds in which the atoms or radicals consist of elements other than carbon. (Chap. 6)

Interferons (in-ter-fear'-onz). Small, antiviral glycoproteins produced by cells infected with an animal virus; interferons are cell-specific and species-specific, but not virus-specific (Chap. 15)

Interleukins (in-ter-lu'-kinz). Lymphokines and polypeptide hormones; interleukin 1 is produced by monocytes; interleukin 2 is produced by lymphocytes; a category of cytokines (Chap. 15)

Intermediate host. In a parasitic relationship, the host that harbors the larval or asexual stage of a parasite, or the asexual phase of the parasite's life cycle (Chap. 18)

Intraerythrocytic pathogen. A pathogen that lives within erythrocytes (Chap. 14)

Intraleukocytic pathogen. A pathogen that lives within leukocytes (Chap. 14)

Intrinsic resistance. Resistance to a particular drug that is the result of some naturally occurring property of a bacterial cell (Chap. 9)

Ischemia (is-key'-me-uh). Localized anemia as a result of mechanical obstruction of the blood supply (Chap. 17)

Isotonic (eye-soh-tahn'-ick) solution. A solution having the same osmotic pressure as cells placed into that solution; when the concentration of solutes outside the cell equals the concentration of solutes inside the cell (Chap. 8)

K

Keratitis (ker-uh-ty'-tis). Inflammation of the cornea (Chap. 17)

Keratoconjunctivitis (ker'-at-oh-kon-junk'-tuh-vi'-tis). Inflammation of the cornea and conjunctiva (Chap. 17)

Killer cell. A type of cytotoxic T cell involved in cell-mediated immune responses (Chap. 16)

Kinase (ky'-nace). A bacterial enzyme capable of dissolving clots; also known as *fibrinolysin* (Chap. 14)

Koch's postulates. A series of scientific steps, proposed by Robert Koch, that must be fulfilled to prove that a specific microorganism is the cause of a particular disease (Chap. 1)

Krebs cycle. A biochemical pathway that is part of aerobic respiration; also known as the citric acid cycle, tricarboxylic acid, and TCA cycle (Chap. 7)

L

L-forms. Abnormal forms of bacteria that have lost part or all of their rigid cell walls; sometimes the result of exposure of an organism to an antimicrobial agent; also called L-phase variants; the "L" is derived from Lister Institute (Chap. 4)

Lag phase. The part of a bacterial growth curve during which multiplication of the organisms is very slow or scarcely appreciable; the first phase in a bacterial growth curve (Chap. 8)

Laryngitis (lar-in-ji'-tis). Inflammation of the mucous membrane of the larynx (voice box) (Chap. 17)

Latent infection. An asymptomatic infection capable of manifesting symptoms under particular circumstances or if activated (Chap. 14)

Lecithin (less'-uh-thin). A name given to several types of phospholipids that are essential constituents of animal and plant cells (Chap. 14)

Lecithinase (less'-uh-thuh-nace). A bacterial enzyme capable of breaking down lecithin (Chap. 14)

Lethal mutation. A mutation that causes death of the organism possessing the mutation (Chap. 7)

Leukemia (lew-key'-me-uh). A type of cancer in which there is a proliferation of abnormal leukocytes in the blood (Chap. 13)

Leukocidin (lu-koh-sigh'-din). A bacterial exotoxin capable of destroying leukocytes (Chap. 14)

Leukocytes (lu'-koh-sites). White blood cells (Chap. 13)

Leukocytosis (lu'-koh-sigh-toe'-sis). An increased number of leukocytes in the blood (Chap. 15)

Leukopenia (lu-koh-pea'-nee-uh). A decreased number of leukocytes in the blood (Chap. 15)

Lichen (like'-in). An organism composed of a green alga (or a cyanobacterium) and a fungus; an example of a symbiotic relationship known as *mutualism* (Chap. 5)

Life cycle. The generation-to-generation sequence of stages that occur in the history of an organism (Chap. 3)

Light microscope. A type of microscope that uses visible light as a source of illumination; also called a brightfield microscope (Chap. 2)

Lipids (lip'-ids). Organic compounds containing carbon, hydrogen, and oxygen that are insoluble in water but soluble in so-called fat solvents such as diethyl ether and carbon tetrachloride (Chap. 6)

Lipopolysaccharide (lip'-oh-pol-ee-sack'-a-ride). A macromolecule of combined lipid and polysaccharide, found in the cell walls of Gram-negative bacteria (Chap. 4)

Lithotroph (lith'-oh-trof). An organism that uses inorganic molecules as a source of energy; a type of chemotroph (Chap. 7)

Localized infection. An infection that remains localized; that does not spread; also known as a *local infection* or *focal infection* (Chap. 14)

Logarithmic (log'-uh-rith-mik) **growth phase.** The part of a bacterial growth phase during which maximal multiplication is occurring by geometric progression; the second phase in a bacterial growth curve; also known as the *log phase* or *exponential growth phase* (Chap. 8)

Logarithmic (log'-uh-ryth-mik) **scale.** A scale (as on graph paper) in which the values of a variable (e.g., number of organisms at a particular point in time) are expressed as logarithms (Chap. 8)

Lophotrichous (low-fot'-ri-kus) **bacterium.** A bacterium that possesses two or more flagella at one end (pole) of the cell (Chap. 3)

Lymphadenitis (lim'-fad-uh-ny'-tis). Inflammation of a lymph node or lymph nodes (Chap. 17)

Lymphadenopathy (lim-fad-uh-nop'-uh-thee). A disease process affecting a lymph node or lymph nodes (Chap. 17)

Lymphangitis (lim-fan-ji'-tis). Inflammation of lymphatic vessels (Chap. 17)

Lymphocytosis (lim'-foh-sigh-toe'-sis). An increased number of lymphocytes in the blood (Chap. 15)

Lymphokines (lim'-foh-kinz). Soluble proteins released by sensitized lymphocytes; examples include chemotactic factors and interleukins; lymphokines represent one category of *cytokines* (Chap. 16)

Lyophilization (ly-ahf'-eh-leh-zay'-shun). Freeze-drying; a method of preserving microorganisms and foods (Chap. 8)

Lysogenic (lye-so-jen'-ick) **bacterium.** A bacterium in the state of lysogeny (Chap. 7)

Lysogenic conversion. Alteration of the genetic constitution of a bacterial cell due to lysogeny (Chap. 7)

Lysogeny (lye-soj'-eh-nee). A situation in which viral genetic material is integrated into the genome of the host cell (Chap. 7)

Lysosome (lye'-so-som). A membrane-bound vesicle found in the cytoplasm of eucaryotic cells; contains a variety of digestive enzymes, including lysozyme (Chap. 3)

Lysozyme (lye'-so-zyme). A digestive enzyme found in lysosomes, tears, and other body fluids; especially destructive to bacterial cell walls (Chap. 15)

Lytic cycle. When a virus takes over the metabolic machinery of the host cell, reproduces itself, and ruptures (lyses) the host cell so that the newly assembled virions can escape (Chap. 4)

M

Macrophage (mak'-roh-faj). A large phagocytic leukocyte that arises from a monocyte (Chap. 15)

Malaise (muh-laz'). A generalized feeling of discomfort or uneasiness (Chap. 17)

Mast cell. A tissue cell that closely resembles a basophil (Chap. 16)

Mastigophora (mas'-ti-gof'-uh-rah). A subphylum of Protozoa in the phylum Sarcomastigophora; the flagellates; considered a phylum in some classification schemes (Chap. 5)

Mechanical vector. An arthropod vector (e.g., a house fly) that merely transports a pathogen from "point A" to "point B," and within which the pathogen neither multiplies nor matures (Chap. 18)

Medical asepsis (ay-sep'-sis). The absence of pathogens in a patient's environment (Chap. 12)

Medical aseptic (ay-sep'-tick) **techniques.** Procedures followed and steps taken to ensure medical asepsis (Chap. 12)

Meiosis (my-oh'-sis). The type of cell division that results in the formation of haploid gametes; also known as *meiotic division* (Chap. 3)

Meninges (muh-nin'-jez)., sing. *meninx.* As used in this book, the membranes that surround the brain and spinal cord (Chap. 17)

Meningitis (men-in-ji'-tis). Inflammation or infection of the meninges (Chap. 13)

Meningococcemia (meh-ninge'-oh-kok-see'-me-uh). The presence of *Neisseria meningitidis* in the blood (Chap. 13)

Meningococcus (meh-ninge'-oh-kok-us), pl. *meningococci.* A slang term for *Neisseria meningitidis* (Chap. 13)

Meningoencephalitis (muh-ning'-go-en-sef-uh-ly'-tis). Inflammation or infection of the brain and its surrounding membranes (Chap. 13)

Mesophile (meez'-oh-file). A microorganism having an optimum growth temperature between 25°C and 40°C; such an organism is said to be *mesophilic* (Chap. 8)

Messenger RNA (mRNA). The type of RNA that contains the exact same genetic information as a single gene on a DNA molecule; also called *informational RNA* (Chap. 6)

Metabolic (met-uh-bol'-ik) **reactions.** Chemical reactions that occur within cells; of two types—catabolic and anabolic reactions (Chap. 7)

Metabolism (muh-tab'-oh-lizm). The sum of all the chemical reactions occurring in a cell; consists of *anabolism* and *catabolism* (Chap. 3)

Metabolite (muh-tab'-oh-lite). Any chemical product of metabolism (Chap. 7)

Microaerophiles (my-krow-air'-oh-files). Organisms requiring oxygen, but in concentrations lower than the 20—21% found in air; they usually require around 5% oxygen (Chap. 4)

Microbial (my-krow'-be-ul). Pertaining to microorganisms (Chap. 1)

Microbial antagonism (an-tag'-un-izm). The killing, injury, or inhibition of one microbe by substances produced by another (Chap. 10)

Microbial ecology. Study of the interrelationships among microbes and the world around them (other microbes, other living organisms, and the nonliving environment) (Chap. 1)

Microbial intoxication. A disease that results from ingestion of a toxin that was produced by a pathogen in vitro (outside the body) (Chap. 1)

Microbial physiology. The study of the vital life processes of microbes (Chap. 7)

Microbicidal (my-krow'-buh-sigh'-dull) **agent.** A chemical or drug that kills microorganisms; a *microbicide* (Chap. 8)

Microbiologist (my'-crow-by-ol'-oh-jist). One who specializes in the science of microbiology (Chap. 1)

Microbiology (my'-crow-by-ol'-oh-je). The study of microorganisms (Chap. 1)

Microbistatic (my-krow'-buh-stat'-ick) **agent.** A chemical agent or drug that inhibits the growth of microorganisms (Chap. 8)

Microcolonies. Tiny clusters of bacteria within biofilms (Chap. 10)

Micrometer (my-crow'-me-ter). A unit of length, equal to one millionth of a meter and one thousandth of a millimeter (Chap. 2)

Microorganisms (my'-crow-or'-gan-izms). Very small organisms; usually microscopic; also called *microbes;* includes viruses, bacteria, certain algae, protozoa, and certain fungi (Chap. 1)

Microscope (my'-crow-skope). An optical instrument that permits one to observe a small object by producing an enlarged image of the object (Chap. 1)

Microscopic (my-crow-skop'-ik). If an object is microscopic, it is so small that it can only be seen using a microscope (Chap. 2)

Microtubules (my-kro'-two-bules). Cylindrical, cytoplasmic tubules found in the cytoskeleton of eucaryotic cells; may be related to the movement of chromosomes during nuclear division (Chap. 3)

Millimeter (mill'-uh-me-ter). A unit of length equal to one thousandth of a meter (Chap. 2)

Minisystems. Miniaturized biochemical test systems; often used when attempting to speciate microorganisms that have been isolated from clinical specimens (Chap. 13)

Mitochondria (my-toe-kon'-dree-uh), sing. *mitochondrion.* Eucaryotic organelles involved in cellular respiration for the production of energy; energy factories of the cell (Chap. 3)

Mitosis (my-toe'-sis). The type of cell division that results in the formation of two daughter cells, each of which contains exactly the same number of chromosomes as the parent cell; also known as *mitotic division* (Chap. 3)

Molecular epidemiology. Determining relatedness of two microbial isolates in a healthcare setting by genotypic methods (Chap. 12)

Monoclonal (mon-oh-klo'-nul) **antibodies.** Antibodies produced by a clone or genetically identical hybrid cells (Chap. 16)

Monocyte (mon'-oh-site). A relatively large mononuclear leukocyte (Chap. 15)

Monosaccharides (mon-oh-sak'-uh-rides). Carbohydrates that cannot be broken down into any simpler sugar by simple hydrolysis; simple sugars containing three to nine carbon atoms (usually three to seven); the basic units or building blocks of polysaccharides (Chap. 6)

Monotrichous (mah-not'-ri-kus) **bacterium.** A bacterium that possesses only one flagellum (Chap. 3)

Monounsaturated fatty acid. A fatty acid containing only one double bond (Chap. 6)

Morbidity rate. The number of new cases of a particular disease that occurred during a specified time period per a specifically defined population (e.g., per 100,000) (Chap. 11)

Mortality rate. The ratio of the number of people who died of a particular disease during a specified time period per a specified population (e.g., per 100,000); also known as the *death rate* (Chap. 11)

Mucormycosis (mew'-kor-my-koh'-sis). Infection caused by a bread mold; also known as *zygomycosis* (Chap. 17)

Mutagen (myu'-tah-jen). Any agent that can cause a mutation to occur; e.g., radioactive substances, x-rays, or certain chemicals; such an agent is said to be *mutagenic* (Chap. 7)

Mutant (myu'-tant). A phenotype in which a mutation is manifested (Chap. 7)

Mutation (myu-tay'-shun). An inheritable change in the character of a gene; a change in the sequence of base pairs in a DNA molecule (Chap. 7)

Mutualism (myu'-chew-ul-izm). A symbiotic relationship in which both parties derive benefit (Chap. 10)

Mycelium (my-see'-lee-um), pl. *mycelia*. A fungal colony; composed of a mass of intertwined hyphae (Chap. 5)

Mycologist (my-kol'-oh-jist). One who specializes in the science of mycology (Chap. 1)

Mycology (my-kol'-oh-gee). The study of fungi (Chap. 1)

Mycosis (my-ko'-sis), pl. *mycoses*. A fungal disease (Chap. 5)

Mycotoxicosis (my'-ko-tox'-uh-ko-sis), pl. *mycotoxicoses*. A microbial intoxication caused by a mycotoxin (Chap. 5)

Mycotoxins (my'-ko-tox-inz). Toxins produced by fungi (Chap. 5)

Myelitis (my-uh-ly'-tis). Inflammation or infection of the spinal cord (Chap. 17)

Myocarditis (my'-oh-kar-dy'-tis). Inflammation of the myocardium (the muscular walls of the heart) (Chap. 17)

N

Nanobacteria (nah'-no-back-teer'-ee-uh). Especially small bacteria; less than 1 μm in diameter; the sizes of these bacteria are expressed in nanometers (Chap. 4)

Nanometer (nan'-oh-me'-ter). A unit of length, equal to one billionth of a meter and one thousandth of a micrometer (Chap. 2)

Narrow-spectrum antibiotics. Antibiotics that are only effective against a narrow range of bacteria (e.g., perhaps only effective against certain Gram-positive bacteria, or only effective against certain Gram-negative bacteria) (Chap. 9)

Natural active acquired immunity. Active acquired immunity that is acquired naturally (e.g., by being infected with a particular pathogen) (Chap. 16)

Natural (NK) killer cell. A type of cytotoxic human blood lymphocyte (Chap. 16)

Natural passive acquired immunity. Passive acquired immunity that is acquired in a natural manner (e.g., when a fetus receives the mother's antibodies in utero) (Chap. 16)

Necrosis (nuh-kro'-sis). Cell death (Chap. 17)

Negative stain. A staining procedure in which unstained objects can be seen against a stained background (Chap. 3)

Nematodes (nem'-uh-toadz'). Roundworms (Chap. 18)

Nephritis (nef-ry'-tis). Inflammation of the kidneys (Chap. 17)

Neurotoxin (new'-roh-tok'-sin). A bacterial exotoxin that attacks the nervous system (Chap. 14)

Neutralism (new'-trul-izm). A symbiotic relationship in which organisms occupy the same niche but do not affect one another (Chap. 10)

Neutrophil (nu'-tro-fil). A type of granulocyte found in blood; its granules contain neutral substances that attract neither acidic nor basic dyes; also called a *polymorphonuclear cell*, *poly*, or *PMN* (Chap. 15)

Nitrifying bacteria. Bacteria capable of converting ammonia to nitrites and nitrites to nitrates; the process is known as *nitrification* (Chap. 10)

Nitrogen-fixation. The process by which atmospheric nitrogen gas is converted into ammonia (Chap. 4)

Nitrogen-fixing bacteria. Bacteria capable of converting nitrogen gas into ammonia; the process is known as *nitrogen fixation* (Chap. 10)

Nonpathogen (non'-path'-oh-jen). A microorganism that does not cause disease; such an organism is said to be *nonpathogenic* (Chap. 1)

Nonspecific host defense mechanisms. Host defense mechanisms directed against all types of invading pathogens and other foreign substances (Chap. 15)

Nosocomial (nose-oh-koh'-me-ul) **infection.** Any infection acquired while one is hospitalized (or while a patient in some other healthcare facility); also known as a *hospital-acquired infection* (Chap. 12)

Nuclear (new'-klee-er) **membrane.** The membrane that surrounds the chromosomes and nucleoplasm of a eucaryotic cell (Chap. 3)

Nucleic (new-klay'-ick) **acids.** Macromolecules consisting of linear chains of nucleotides; DNA, mRNA, tRNA, and rRNA are examples (Chap. 6)

Nucleolus (new-klee'-oh-lus). A dense portion of the nucleus of a eucaryotic cell; where ribosomal RNA (rRNA) is produced (Chap. 3)

Nucleoplasm (new'-klee-oh-plazm). That portion of a eucaryotic cell's protoplasm that lies within the nucleus (Chap. 3)

Nucleotides (new'-klee-oh-tides). The basic units or building blocks of nucleic acids, each consisting of a purine or pyrimidine combined with a pentose (either ribose or deoxyribose) and a phosphate group (Chap. 6)

Nucleus (new'-klee-us), pl. *nuclei*. That portion of a eucaryotic cell that contains the nucleoplasm and chromosomes (Chap. 3)

O

Obligate aerobe (air'-obe). An organism that requires 20–21% oxygen (the amount found in the air we breathe) to survive (Chap. 4)

Obligate anaerobe (an'-air-obe). An organism that cannot survive in oxygen (Chap. 4)

Obligate intracellular pathogen. A pathogen that must reside within another living cell; examples include viruses, chlamydias, and rickettsias (Chap. 1)

Obligate parasite. An organism that can only exist as a parasite; incapable of a free-living existence (Chap. 18)

Octad. A packet of eight cocci (Chap. 4)

Oncogenic (ong-koh-jen'-ick). An adjective meaning cancer-causing (Chap. 17)

Oncogenic viruses. Viruses capable of causing cancer; also known as *oncoviruses* (Chap. 4)

Oophoritis (oh-of-or-eye'-tis). Inflammation or infection on an ovary (Chap. 17)

Opportunistic pathogen (op-poor-tune'-is-tick path'-oh-jen). A microbe with the potential to cause disease, but does not do so under ordinary circumstances; may cause disease in susceptible persons with lowered resistance; also called an *opportunist* (Chap. 1)

Opsonins (op'-soh-ninz). Substances (such as antibodies or complement fragments) that enhance phagocytosis (Chap. 15)

Opsonization (op'-suh-nuh-zay'-shun). The process by which bacteria (or other particles) are altered so that they may be more readily and more efficiently engulfed by phagocytes; often involves coating the bacteria with antibodies or complement fragments (Chap. 15)

Orchitis (or-ky'-tis). Inflammation or infection of the testes (Chap. 17)

Organelles (or'-guh-nelz). General term for the various and diverse structures contained within a eucaryotic cell (e.g., mitochondria, Golgi complex, nucleus, endoplasmic reticulum, and lysosomes) (Chap. 3)

Organic (or-gan'-ick) **chemistry.** The study of organic compounds; the study of carbon and its covalent bonds (Chap. 6)

Organic compounds. Chemical compounds composed of atoms (some of which are carbon) held together by covalent bonds (Chap. 6)

Osmosis (oz-moh'-sis). The process by which a solvent (e.g., water) moves through a semipermeable membrane from a solution having a lower concentration of solutes (dissolved substances) to a solution having a higher concentration of solutes (Chap. 8)

Osmotic (oz-maht'-ick) **pressure.** A measure of the tendency for water to move into a solution by osmosis; always a positive value (Chap. 8)

Otitis (oh-ty'-tis) **externa.** Inflammation or infection of the outer ear canal (Chap. 17)

Otitis media. Inflammation or infection of the middle ear (Chap. 17)

Oxidation (ok-seh-day'-shun). As used in this book, the loss of one or more electrons, thus making the atom more electropositive (Chap. 7)

Oxidation–reduction reactions. Paired chemical reactions involving the transfer of one or more electrons from one compound to another; reactions which involve both oxidation and reduction; also known as *redox reactions* (Chap. 7)

Oxidative pathways. Metabolic pathways requiring the participation of oxygen (Chap. 7)

Oxygenic photosynthesis (ox'-uh-gen'-ik foe-toe-sin'-thuh-sis). A type of photosynthesis in which oxygen is produced (Chap. 4)

P

Paleomicrobiology (pay'-ee-oh-my'-crow-by-ol'-oh-je). The study of ancient microorganisms (Chap. 1)

Pandemic (pan-dem'-ick) **disease.** A disease occurring in epidemic proportions in several to many countries; sometimes occurring worldwide (Chap. 11)

Parasite (par'-uh-sight). An organism that lives on or in another living organism (called the host) and derives benefit from the host (usually in the form of nutrients) (Chap. 1)

Parasitemia (par'-uh-suh-tee'-me-uh). The presence of parasites in the blood (Chap. 13)

Parasitism (par'-uh-suh-tizm). A symbiotic relationship that is beneficial to one party (the parasite) and detrimental to the other party (the host) (Chap. 10)

Parasitologist (par'-uh-suh-tol'-oh-jist). One who specializes in the science of parasitology (Chap. 1)

Parasitology (par'-uh-suh-tol'-oh-jee). The study of parasites (Chap. 1)

Parenteral (puh-ren'-ter-ul) **injection.** Injection of substances directly into the bloodstream (Chap. 11)

Parotitis (par-oh-ty'-tis). Inflammation of the parotid gland (a salivary gland located near the ear); also known as *parotiditis* (Chap. 17)

Passive acquired immunity. Immunity or resistance acquired as a result of receipt of antibodies produced by another person or by an animal (Chap. 16)

Passive carrier. A person who harbors a particular pathogen without ever having had the infectious disease it causes (Chap. 11)

Pasteurization (pas'-tour-i-zay'-shun). A heating process that kills pathogens in milk, wines, and other beverages (Chap. 1)

Pathogen (path'-oh-jen). Disease-causing microorganism; such an organism is said to be *pathogenic* (Chap. 1)

Pathogenesis (path-oh-jen-uh-sis). The steps or mechanisms involved in the development of a disease (Chap. 14)

Pathogenicity (path'-oh-juh-nis'-uh-tee). The ability to cause disease (Chap. 14)

Pathologist (pah-thol'-oh-jist). A physician who is a specialist in pathology (Chap. 13)

Pathology (pah-thol'-oh-gee). The study of disease, especially structural and functional changes that result from disease processes (Chap. 13)

Pellicle (pel'-uh-kul). As used in this book, a thickened outer membrane possessed by certain protozoa (Chap. 5)

Pelvic inflammatory disease (PID). Acute or chronic inflammation in the pelvic cavity, usually referring to infection of the female genital tract (Chap. 17)

Penicillinase. An enzyme that destroys the β-lactam ring in penicillin molecules; a type of β-lactamase (Chap. 9)

Pentose. A monosaccharide containing five carbon atoms (Chap. 6)

Peptide bond. The name given to the covalent bond that holds amino acids together in protein molecules (Chap. 6)

Peptidoglycan (pep'-tuh-doh-gly'-kan). A complex structure found in the cell walls of bacteria, consisting of carbohydrates and proteins (Chap. 3)

Pericarditis (per'-ee-kar-dy'-tis). Inflammation of the pericardium (the membrane or sac around the heart) (Chap. 17)

Periodontal (purr'-ee-oh-don'-tul) disease. Disease around the teeth (Chap. 17)

Periodontitis (purr'-ee-oh-don-ty'-tis). Inflammation or infection of the *periodontium* (tissues that surround and support the teeth) (Chap. 17)

Peritrichous (peh-rit'-ri-kus) bacterium. A bacterium that possesses flagella over its entire surface (Chap. 3)

Peroxisome (per-ok'-suh-some). A membrane-bound organelle found in eucaryotic cells, within which hydrogen peroxide is both produced and degraded (Chap. 3)

Petri (pea'-tree) dish. A shallow, circular container made of thin glass or clear plastic, with a loosely fitting, overlapping cover; used in microbiology laboratories for cultivation of microorganisms on solid media (Chap. 1)

Phagocyte (fag'-oh-site). A cell capable of ingesting bacteria, yeasts, and other particulate matter by phagocytosis; amebae and certain leukocytes are examples of phagocytic cells (Chap. 3)

Phagocytosis (fag'-oh-sigh-toe'-sis). Ingestion of particulate matter involving the use of pseudopodia to surround the particle (Chap. 3)

Phagolysosome (fag-oh-ly'-soh-sohm). A membrane-bound vesicle formed by the fusion of a phagosome and a lysosome (Chap. 15)

Phagosome (fag'-oh-sohm). A membrane-bound vesicle containing an ingested particle (e.g., a bacterial cell); found in phagocytic cells (Chap. 15)

Pharyngitis (far-in-ji'-tis). Inflammation or infection of the throat; sore throat (Chap. 17)

Phase-contrast microscope. A type of compound light microscope that can be used to observe unstained living microorganisms (Chap. 2)

Phenotype (fee'-no-type). Manifestation of a genotype; all the attributes or characteristics of an individual (Chap. 7)

Phospholipid (fos'-foh-lip'-id). A lipid containing glycerol, fatty acids, a phosphate group, and an alcohol; glycerophospholipids (also called phosphoglycerides) and sphingolipids are examples (Chap. 6)

Photoautotroph (foh'-toe-aw'-toe-trof). An organism that uses light as an energy source and carbon dioxide as a carbon source; a type of autotroph (Chap. 7)

Photoheterotroph (foh'-toe-het'-er-oh-trof). An organism that uses light as an energy source and organic compounds as a carbon source; a type of heterotroph (Chap. 7)

Photomicrograph. Photograph taken through the lens system of a compound light microscope (Chap. 2)

Photosynthesis (foe-toe-sin'-thuh-sis). Chemical process by which light energy is converted into chemical energy; an organism that produces organic substances in this manner is said to be *photosynthetic* (Chap. 3)

Phototroph (foh'-toe-trof). An organism that uses light as an energy source (Chap. 7)

Phycologist (fy-kol'-oh-jist). One who specializes in the science of phycology (Chap. 1)

Phycology (fy-kol'-oh-gee). The study of algae (Chap. 1)

Phycotoxicosis (fy'-koh-tox-uh-coh-sis), pl. *phycotoxicoses*. A microbial intoxication caused by a phycotoxin (Chap. 5)

Phycotoxins (fy'-ko-tox-inz). Toxins produced by algae (Chap. 5)

Phytoplankton (fy'-toh-plank'-ton). Microscopic marine plants and algae that are components of plankton (Chap. 1)

Pili (py'-ly), sing. *pilus*. Hairlike surface projections possessed by some bacteria (called piliated bacteria); most are organelles of attachment; also called *fimbriae;* specialized pili, called *sex pili,* are described below (Chap. 3)

Pinocytosis (pin'-oh-sigh-toe'-sis). A process resembling phagocytosis but used to engulf and ingest liquids rather than solid matter (Chap. 5)

Plankton (plank'-ton). Microscopic organisms in the ocean that serve as the starting point of many food chains (Chap. 1)

Plasma (plaz'-muh). The liquid portion of circulating blood (Chap.13)

Plasma (plaz'-muh) cell. An antibody-secreting cell produced by a stimulated B cell (Chap. 16)

Plasmid (plaz'-mid). An extrachromosomal genetic element; a molecule of DNA that can function and replicate while physically separate from the bacterial chromosome (Chap. 3)

Plasmolysis (plaz-moll'-uh-sis). Cell shrinkage as a result of a loss of water from the cell's cytoplasm (Chap. 8)

Plasmoptysis (plaz-mop'-tuh-sis). The escape of cytoplasm from a ruptured cell (Chap. 8)

Plastid. A membrane-bound organelle containing photosynthetic pigment; plastids are the sites of photosynthesis; a *chloroplast* is a plastid that contains chlorophyll (Chap. 3)

Pleomorphism (plee-oh-more'-fizm). Existing in more than one form; also known as *polymorphism;* an organism that exhibits pleomorphism is said to be *pleomorphic* (Chap. 4)

Pneumonia (new-mow'-nee-uh). Inflammation of one or both lungs (Chap. 17)

Polymer (pol'-uh-mer). A large molecule consisting of repeating subunits; nucleic acids, polypeptides, and polysaccharides are examples (Chap. 6)

Polypeptide (pol-ee-pep'-tide). A protein consisting of more than three amino acids held together by peptide bonds (Chap. 6)

Polyribosomes (pol-ee-ry'-boh-somz). Two or more ribosomes connected by a molecule of messenger RNA (mRNA) (Chap. 3)

Polysaccharide (pol-ee-sack'-uh-ride). Carbohydrate consisting of many sugar units; glycogen, cellulose, and starch are examples (Chap. 6)

Polyunsaturated fatty acid. A fatty acid containing more than one double bond (Chap. 6)

Population growth curve. A graph that represents changes in the number of viable bacteria in a population over time; constructed by plotting the logarithm (log_{10}) of the number of viable bacteria (on the vertical or y axis) against the incubation time (on the horizontal or x axis) (Chap. 8)

Preliminary report. Any report furnished by the laboratory before publication of the final report (Chap. 13)

Prevalence. The number of cases of a particular disease existing in a given population during a specific period of time (period prevalence) or at a particular moment in time (point prevalence) (Chap. 11)

Primary disease. The initial disease; often creates the conditions that lead to a secondary disease; if the primary disease is an infection, it is referred to as a *primary infection* (Chap. 14)

Primary response. The immune response that occurs the first time an antigen enters a person's body (Chap. 16)

Prions (pree'-onz). Infectious protein molecules (i.e., proteins capable of causing certain diseases of animals and humans) (Chap. 4)

Procaryotic (pro'-kar-ee-ah'-tick) cells. Cells lacking a true nucleus; organisms consisting of such cells are referred to as *procaryotes;* can also be spelled prokaryotic (Chap. 3)

Prophage (pro'-faj). During lysogeny, all that remains of the infecting bacteriophage is its DNA; in this form, the bacteriophage is referred to as a prophage (Chap. 7)

Prophylactic (pro'-fuh-lak'-tick) agent. A drug used to prevent a disease (Chap. 17)

Prophylaxis (pro-fuh-lak'-sis). Prevention of a disease or a process that can lead to a disease; e.g., taking antimalarial medication in a malarious area (Chap. 17)

Prostaglandins (pros-tuh-glan'-dinz). Physiologically active tissue substances that cause many effects, including vasodilation, vasoconstriction, and stimulation of smooth muscle (Chap. 15)

Prostatitis (pros-tuh-ty'-tis). Inflammation or infection of the prostate (Chap. 17)

Prostration (pros-tray'-shun). Significant loss of strength; the patient is prostrate (lying flat) (Chap. 13)

Protective antibodies. Antibodies that protect an individual from infection or reinfection (Chap. 16)

Protective isolation. When a patient is placed in isolation to protect him or her from infection; also known as *reverse isolation* and *neutropenic isolation* (Chap. 12)

Proteins (pro'-teens). Macromolecules consisting of two, three, or more amino acids (Chap. 6)

Protists (pro'-tists). Members of the Kingdom Protista; includes algae and protozoa (Chap. 3)

Protoplasm (pro'-toe-plazm). The semifluid matter within living cells; *cytoplasm* and *nucleoplasm* are two types of protoplasm (Chap. 3)

Protozoa (pro-toe-zoe'-uh), sing. *protozoan.* Eucaryotic microorganisms frequently found in water and soil; some are pathogens; usually unicellular (Chap. 5)

Protozoologist (pro'-toe-zoe-ol'-oh-jist). One who specializes in protozoology (Chap. 1)

Protozoology (pro'-toe-zoe-ol'-oh-gee). The study of protozoa (Chap. 1)

Pseudohypha (su-doh-hy-fuh), pl. *pseudohypha*e. An elongated string of yeast buds (Chap. 5)

Pseudomonicidal (su'-doh-moan-uh-side'-ul) agent. A drug or disinfectant that kills *Pseudomonas* spp. (Chap. 8)

Pseudopodium (su-doe-poh'-dee-um), pl. *pseudopodia.* A temporary extension of protoplasm that is extended by an ameba or leukocyte for locomotion or the engulfment of particulate matter; also called a *pseudopod* (Chap. 5)

Psychroduric (sigh-krow-dur'-ick) organisms. Organisms able to endure very cold temperatures (Chap. 8)

Psychrophile (sigh'-krow-file). An organism that grows best at a low temperature (0°C to 32°C), with optimum growth occurring at 15°C to 20°C; such an organism is said to be *psychrophilic* (Chap. 8)

Psychrotroph (sigh'-krow-trof). A psychrophile that grows best at refrigerator temperature (4°C); such an organism is said to be *psychrotrophic* (Chap. 8)

Pure culture. When only one type of organism is growing on or in a culture medium in the laboratory; no other types of organisms are present (Chap. 1)

Purine (pure'-een). A double-ringed nitrogenous base found in certain nucleotides and, therefore, in nucleic acids; adenine and guanine are purines found in both DNA and RNA (Chap. 6)

Purulent exudate. A thick, greenish-yellow exudate that contains many live and dead leukocytes; also known as *pus* (Chap. 15)

Pustule (pus'-chul). A small rounded elevation of the skin that contains purulent material (pus) (Chap. 17)

Pyelonephritis (py'-uh-low-nef-ry'-tis). Inflammation of certain areas of the kidneys, most often the result of bacterial infection (Chap. 17)

Pyogenic (py-oh-jen'-ick). Pus-producing; causing the production of pus (Chap. 15)

Pyogenic microorganisms. Pathogens that cause pus-containing infectious processes (Chap. 15)

Pyrimidine (pi-rim'-uh-deen). A single-ringed nitrogenous base found in certain nucleotides and, therefore, in nucleic acids; thymine and cytosine are pyrimidines found in DNA; cytosine and uracil are pyrimidines found in RNA (Chap. 6)

Pyrogen (py'-roh-jen). A fever-producing substance; also referred to as a *pyrogenic substance* (Chap. 14)

R

R-factor. A plasmid that contains multiple drug resistance genes; a bacterium that possesses an R-factor is multidrug-resistant (i.e., it is a "superbug"); the "R" stands for resistance (Chap. 7)

Receptors. Molecules on the surface of a host cell that a particular pathogen is able to recognize and attach to; also known as *integrins* (Chap. 14)

Reduction (ree-duk'-shun). As used in this book, the gain of one or more electrons, thus making the atom more electronegative (Chap. 7)

Regulatory T cells. T cells that regulate various aspects of immune responses; helper T cells and suppressor T cells are examples (Chap. 16)

Reservoirs (rez'-ev-wars) of infection. Places where pathogens are living and from which they can be transmitted to humans; reservoirs of infection may be living or nonliving; sometimes simply referred to as *reservoirs* (Chap. 11)

Resident microflora. Members of the indigenous microflora that are more or less permanent residents (Chap. 10)

Resistance factor. See *R-factor*

Resolving power. The ability of the eye or an optical instrument to distinguish detail, such as the separation of closely adjacent objects; also called *resolution* (Chap. 2)

Reticuloendothelial (ree-tick'-yu-loh-en-doh-thee'-lee-ul) system (RES). A collection of phagocytic cells that includes macrophages and cells that line the sinusoids of the spleen, lymph nodes, and bone marrow (Chap. 15)

Reverse isolation. See *protective isolation*

Ribonucleic (ry-boe-new-klee'-ick) acid (RNA). A macromolecule of which there are three main types: messenger RNA (mRNA), ribosomal RNA (rRNA), and transfer RNA (tRNA); found in all cells but only in certain viruses (called RNA viruses) (Chap. 3)

Ribosomal (rye-boh-so'-mul) RNA (rRNA). The type of RNA molecule found within ribosomes (Chap. 6)

Ribosomes (ry'-boh-soams). Organelles that are the sites of protein synthesis in both procaryotic and eucaryotic cells (Chap. 3)

RNA nucleotides. The building blocks of RNA; each RNA nucleotide consists of a nitrogenous base, ribose, and a phosphate group (Chap. 6)

RNA polymerase (poh-lim'-er-ace). The enzyme required for transcription (Chap. 6)

Rough endoplasmic reticulum (RER). See *endoplasmic reticulum* (Chap. 3)

S

Salpingitis (sal-pin-jy'-tis). As used in this book, inflammation of the fallopian tube (Chap. 17)

Sanitization (san'-uh-tuh-zay'-shun). The process of making something sanitary (healthful); usually involves reducing the number of microbes present to a safe level (Chap. 8)

Saprophyte (sap'-row-fight). An organism that lives on dead or decaying organic matter; such an organism is said to be *saprophytic* (Chap. 1)

Sarcodina (sar'-ko-dy'-nah). A subphylum of protozoa in the phylum Sarcomastigophora; includes the amebae; considered a phylum in some classification schemes (Chap. 5)

Sarcomastigophora (sar'-ko-mass-ti-gof'-oh-rah). A phylum of protozoa of the subkingdom Protozoa, characterized by flagella, pseudopodia, or both; contains the subphyla *Sarcodina* and *Mastigophora* (Chap. 5)

Saturated fatty acid. A fatty acid containing no double bonds (Chap. 6)

Scanning electron micrograph. Photograph taken through the lens system of a scanning electron microscope (Chap. 2)

Scanning electron microscope. A type of electron microscope; enables the operator to observe the outer surfaces of specimens (i.e., to observe surface detail) (Chap. 2)

Sebaceous (seb-ay'-shous) gland. An oil gland located in the dermis (Chap. 17)

Sebum (see'-bum). The oily secretion produced by sebaceous glands of the skin (Chap. 17)

Secondary disease. A disease that follows an initial disease; if the secondary disease is an infection, it is referred to as a *secondary infection* (Chap. 14)

Secondary response. The immune response that occurs the second time an antigen enters a person's body; also known as a *memory response* or an *anaphylactic response* (Chap. 16)

Selective medium. A culture medium that allows a certain organism or group of organisms to grow while inhibiting growth of all other organisms (Chap. 8)

Selective permeability. An attribute of membranes whereby only certain substances are able to cross the membranes (Chap. 3)

Semisynthetic antibiotic. An antibiotic that has been chemically altered, usually to increase the drug's spectrum of activity (Chap. 9)

Sepsis. The presence of pathogens or their toxins in the bloodstream; often used as a synonym for *septicemia* (Chap. 8)

Septate hyphae. Hyphae that contain septa (cross-walls) (Chap. 5)

Septic shock. A type of shock resulting from sepsis or septicemia (Chap. 14)

Septicemia (sep-tuh-see'-me-uh). A serious disease consisting of chills, fever, prostration, and the presence of pathogens or their toxins in the blood (Chap. 13)

Serologic (ser-oh-loj'-ick) **procedures.** Immunodiagnostic test procedures performed on serum (Chap. 16)

Serology (suh-rol'-oh-jee). That branch of science concerned with serum and serologic procedures (Chap. 13)

Serum (seer'-um), pl. *sera*. The liquid portion of blood that remains after coagulation (clotting) (Chap. 13)

Sex pilus. A specialized pilus through which one bacterial cell (the donor cell) transfers genetic material to another bacterial cell (the recipient cell), in a process called *conjugation* (Chap. 3)

Sexual reproduction. In this type of reproduction, two parents give rise to offspring that have unique combinations of genes inherited from both parents (Chap. 3)

Shock. A sudden, often severe, physical or mental disturbance, usually resulting from low blood pressure and a lack of oxygen in organs (Chap. 14)

Signs of a disease. Abnormalities indicative of disease that are discovered on examination of a patient; objective findings; examples include abnormal laboratory results; abnormal heart or breath sounds; lumps; abnormalities revealed by radiographs, computed tomographic scans, magnetic resonance imaging, electrocardiography, and ultrasound (Chap. 14)

Silent mutation. A mutation that is neither beneficial nor harmful to the mutant organism; the organism is unaware of the mutation; also called a *neutral mutation* (Chap. 7)

Simple microscope. A microscope containing only one magnifying lens (Chap. 2)

Simple stain. A single dye that is used to stain objects (e.g., bacterial cells), enabling scientists to gain information about the objects (e.g., size, shape) (Chap. 4)

Single bond. A type of chemical bond containing one pair of shared electrons (Chap. 6)

Sinusitis (sigh-neu-sigh'-tis). Inflammation of the lining of one or more of the paranasal sinuses (Chap. 17)

Slime layer. An unorganized, loosely attached layer of glycocalyx surrounding a bacterial cell (Chap. 3)

Slime mold. A eucaryotic organism having characteristics of protozoa and fungi; there are two types: cellular and acellular slime molds (Chap. 5)

Smooth endoplasmic reticulum (SER). See *endoplasmic reticulum*

Solute (sol'-yute). The dissolved substance in a solution; for example, sucrose (table sugar) when it is dissolved in water (Chap. 8)

Solution (soh-loo'-shun). A homogeneous molecular mixture; generally, a substance dissolved in water (referred to as an aqueous solution); solute plus solvent (Chap. 8)

Solvent (sol'-vent). A liquid in which another substance dissolves (Chap. 8)

Source isolation. When a patient is isolated to protect other persons from becoming infected (Chap. 12)

Species (spe'-shez), pl. *species*. A specific member of a given genus; e.g., *Escherichia coli* is a species in the genus *Escherichia*; the name of a particular species consists of two parts—the generic name ("the first name") and the specific epithet ("the second name"); singular species is abbreviated sp., and plural species is abbreviated spp. (Chap. 3)

Specific epithet. The second part ("second name") in the name of a species; the specific epithet cannot be used alone (Chap. 3)

Specific host defense mechanisms. Host defense mechanisms directed against a specific invading pathogen; synonym for the immune system or the third line of defense (Chap. 15)

Spirochetes (spy'-roh-keets). Spiral-shaped bacteria; e.g., *Treponema pallidum*, the causative agent of syphilis (Chap. 3)

Splenomegaly (splen-oh-meg'-uh-lee). Enlargement of the spleen (Chap. 17)

Sporadic (spoh-rad'-ick) **disease.** A disease that occurs occasionally, usually affecting only one person; neither endemic nor epidemic (Chap. 11)

Sporicidal (spor-uh-sigh'-dull) **agent.** A chemical agent that kills spores; a *sporicide* (Chap. 8)

Sporozoea (spor-oh-zoh'-ee-uh). A large class of protozoa containing organisms that do not move by cilia, flagella, or pseudopodia; includes the malarial parasites; considered a phylum in some classification schemes; also spelled *Sporozoa* (Chap. 5)

Sporulation (spor'-you-lay'-shun). Production of spores (Chap. 3)

Sputum. Pus that accumulates in the lungs of patients with lower respiratory tract infections such as pneumonia and tuberculosis (Chap. 13)

Standard precautions. Safety precautions taken by healthcare workers to protect themselves and their patients from infection; these precautions are taken for *all* patients and *all* patient specimens (body substances); includes safety precautions previously referred to as universal precautions or universal body substance precautions (Chap. 12)

Staphylococci (staff'-eh-low-kok'-sigh). Cocci arranged in clusters, such as in the genus *Staphylococcus* (Chap. 4)

Staphylokinase (staf'-uh-low-ky'-nace). A kinase produced by *Staphylococcus aureus* (Chap. 14)

Starch. A polysaccharide storage material found in plants (Chap. 6)

Stationary phase. The part of a bacterial growth phase during which organisms are dying at the same rate at which new organisms are being produced; the third phase in a bacterial growth curve (Chap. 8)

STD. Sexually transmitted disease (Chap. 17)

Sterile (stir'-ill). Free of all living microorganisms, including spores (Chap. 8)

Sterile techniques. Techniques used in an attempt to create an environment that is sterile (devoid of microorganisms) (Chap. 8)

Sterilization (stir'-uh-luh-zay'-shun). The destruction of *all* microorganisms in or on something (e.g., on surgical instruments) (Chap. 8)

Stigma. A photosensing (light sensing) organelle; also known as an *eyespot* (Chap. 5)

Streptobacilli (strep'-toh-bah-sill'-eye). Bacilli arranged in chains of varying lengths (Chap. 4)

Streptococci (strep'-toh-kok'-sigh). Cocci arranged in chains of varying lengths, such as in the genus *Streptococcus* (Chap. 4)

Streptokinase (strep'-toh-ky'-nace). A kinase produced by streptococci (Chap. 14)

Structural staining procedures. Staining procedures used to stain bacterial structures such as capsules, flagella, and endospores (Chap. 4)

Sty (stye). Inflammation of a sebaceous gland that opens into a follicle of an eyelash (Chap. 17)

Subclinical disease. See *asymptomatic disease*

Substrate (sub'-strayt). The chemical substance that is acted upon or changed by an enzyme (Chap. 6)

Subunit vaccine. A vaccine that uses antigenic (antibody-stimulating) portions of a pathogen, rather than using the whole pathogen; also known as an *acellular vaccine* (Chap. 16)

Superinfection (sue'-per-in-fek'-shun). An overgrowth or population explosion of one or more particular pathogens; often pathogens that are resistant to an antimicrobial agent that a patient is receiving (Chap. 9)

Surgical asepsis. The absence of microorganisms in a surgical environment (e.g., an operating room) (Chap. 12)

Surgical aseptic techniques. Procedures followed and steps taken to ensure surgical asepsis (Chap. 12)

Symbionts (sim'-bee-ontz). The parties in a symbiotic relationship (Chap. 10)

Symbiosis (sim-bee-oh'-sis). The living together or close association of two dissimilar organisms (usually two different species) (Chap. 10)

Symptomatic disease. A disease in which the patient experiences symptoms (Chap. 14)

Symptoms of a disease. Indications of disease that are experienced by the patient; subjective; examples include aches and pains, chills, blurred vision, nausea (Chap. 14)

Synergism (sin'-er-jiz-um). When two or more drugs work together to accomplish a cure rate that is greater than either drug could accomplish by itself (Chap. 9)

Synergistic (sin-er-jis'-tik) **infection.** An infection caused by the correlated action of two or more microorganisms; also known as a *polymicrobial infection*; examples include trench mouth and bacterial vaginosis (Chap. 10)

Synergistic relationship. A symbiotic relationship in which two or more microorganisms work together to accomplish a task (e.g., to cause a synergistic infection) (Chap. 10)

Systemic infection. An infection that has spread throughout the body; also known as a *generalized infection* (Chap. 14)

T

T cells (T lymphocytes). A category of leukocytes that play a variety of important roles in the immune system (Chap. 16)

T-dependent antigens. Antigens that require T helper cells for their processing in the body (Chap. 16)

T-independent antigens. Antigens that do not require T helper cells for their processing in the body (Chap. 16)

Taxa, sing. *taxon.* The names given to various groups in taxonomy; the usual taxa are kingdoms, phyla (or divisions), classes, orders, families, genera, species, and subspecies (Chap. 3)

Taxonomy (tak-sawn'-oh-me). The systematic classification of living things (Chap. 3)

Teichoic (tie-ko'-ick) **acids.** Polymers found in the cell walls of Gram-positive bacteria (Chap. 4)

Temperate bacteriophage. A bacteriophage whose genome incorporates into and replicates with the genome of the host bacterium; also known as a *lysogenic bacteriophage* (Chap. 4)

Tetanospasmin (tet'-uh-noh-spaz'-min). The neurotoxin produced by *Clostridium tetani*; causes tetanus (Chap. 14)

Tetrad. A packet of four cocci (Chap. 4)

Tetrose. A monosaccharide containing four carbon atoms (Chap. 6)

Thermal death point (TDP). The temperature required to kill all microorganisms in a liquid culture in 10 minutes at pH 7 (Chap. 8)

Thermal death time (TDT). The length of time required to kill all microorganisms in a liquid culture at a given temperature (Chap. 8)

Thermophile (ther'-mow-file). An organism that thrives at a temperature of 50°C or higher; such an organism is said to be *thermophilic* (Chap. 8)

Tinea (tin'-ee-uh) **infections.** Fungal infections of the skin, hair, and nails; ringworm infections; named for the part of the body that is affected (e.g., tinea capitis is a fungal infection of the scalp, tinea pedis is athlete's foot, tinea unguium is a fungal infection of the nails) (Chap. 17)

Toxemia (tok-see'-me-uh). The presence of toxins in the blood (Chap. 13)

Toxigenicity (tok'-suh-juh-nis'-uh-tee) or **toxinogenicity** (tok'-suh-no-juh-nisv-uh-tee). The ability to produce toxin; a microorganism capable of producing a toxin is said to be *toxigenic* (or *toxinogenic*) (Chap. 14)

Toxin (tok'-sin) As used in this book, a poisonous substance produced by a microorganism (Chap. 1)

Toxoid (tok'-soyd). A toxin that has been altered in such a way as to destroy its toxicity but retain its antigenicity; certain toxoids are used as vaccines (Chap. 16)

Toxoid vaccine. A vaccine prepared from a toxoid (Chap. 16)

Transcription (tran-skrip'-shun). Transfer of the genetic code from one type of nucleic acid to another; usually, the synthesis of an mRNA molecule using a DNA template (Chap. 6)

Transduction (trans-duk'-shun). Transfer of genetic material (and its phenotypic expression) from one bacterial cell to another via bacteriophages; in *generalized transduction,* the transducing bacteriophage is able to transfer any gene of the donor bacterium; in *specialized transduction,* the bacteriophage is able to transfer only one or some of the donor bacterium's genes (Chap. 7)

Transfer RNA (tRNA). The type of RNA molecule that is capable of combining with (and thus activating) a specific amino acid; involved in protein synthesis (translation); the anticodon on a tRNA molecule recognizes the codon on an mRNA molecule (Chap. 6)

Transferrin (trans-fer'-in). A glycoprotein, synthesized in the liver, used to store iron and deliver it to host cells (Chap. 15)

Transformation (trans-for-may'-shun). In microbial genetics, transfer of genetic information between bacteria via uptake or absorption of naked DNA; bacteria capable of absorbing naked DNA from their environment are said to be *competent* (Chap. 7)

Transient bacteremia. A temporary bacteremia (Chap. 17)

Transient microflora. Temporary members of the indigenous microflora (Chap. 10)

Translation (trans-lay'-shun). The process by which mRNA, tRNA, and ribosomes effect the production of proteins from amino acids; translation is also known as *protein synthesis* (Chap. 6)

Transmission-based precautions. Safety precautions taken by healthcare workers, in addition to standard precautions, to protect themselves and their patients from infection via airborne, contact, or droplet routes of transmission (Chap. 12)

Transmission electron micrograph. Photograph taken through the lens system of a transmission electron microscope (Chap. 2)

Transmission electron microscope. A type of electron microscope in which electrons are transmitted through very thin sections of specimens; enables the operator to observe internal detail (Chap. 2)

Trematodes (trem'-uh-toadz). A category of flatworms; often referred to as *flukes* (Chap. 18)

Triglyceride (try-glis'-er-ide). A lipid that is composed of glycerol (a three-carbon alcohol) and three fatty acids; fats and oils are examples (Chap. 6)

Triose. A monosaccharide containing three carbon atoms (Chap. 6)

Tripeptide (try-pep'-tide). A protein consisting of three amino acids held together by peptide bonds (Chap. 6)

Triple bond. A type of chemical bond containing three pairs of shared electrons (Chap. 6)

Trophozoite (trof-oh-zoe'-ite). The motile, feeding, dividing stage in a protozoan's life cycle (Chap. 5)

Tuberculocidal (too-bur'-kyu-low-sigh'-dull) agent. A chemical or drug that kills the bacterium that causes tuberculosis (*Mycobacterium tuberculosis*); also known as a *tuberculocide* (Chap. 8)

Tyndallization (tin-dull-uh-zay'-shun). A process of boiling and cooling in which spores are allowed to germinate and then the vegetative bacteria are killed by boiling again (Chap. 3)

U

Ubiquitous (you-bik'-wah-tus). Present everywhere (Chap. 1)

Ureteritis (you-ree-ter-eye'-tis). Inflammation or infection of a ureter (Chap. 17)

Urethritis (you-ree-thry'-tis). Inflammation or infection of the urethra (Chap. 17)

V

Vaccine (vak'-seen). Any preparation which, after injection (or ingestion, in some cases), produces active acquired immunity (Chap. 16)

Vaginitis (vaj-uh-ny'-tis). Inflammation of the vagina (Chap. 10)

Vaginosis (vag-uh-no'-sis). Infection of the vagina, with no influx of leukocytes (Chap. 10)

Vasoconstriction (vay'-so-kon-strik'-shun). A decrease in the diameter of blood vessels (Chap. 15)

Vasodilation (vay'-soh-die-lay'-shun). An increase in the diameter of blood vessels (Chap. 15)

Vectors (vek'-tour). As used in this book, invertebrate animals (e.g., ticks, mites, mosquitoes, fleas) capable of transmitting pathogens among vertebrates (Chap. 4)

Vegetative hyphae. Hyphae that lie above the surface of whatever a fungal mycelium is growing on (Chap. 5)

Viable plate count. A laboratory technique used to determine the number of living bacteria in a milliliter of liquid; involves the use of plated media (Chap. 8)

Viremia (vy-ree'-me-uh). The presence of viruses in the blood (Chap. 13)

Viricidal (vy-ruh-sigh'-dull) agent. A chemical or drug that inactivates a virus, rendering it noninfectious; can also be spelled *virucidal agent;* also known as a *viricide* or a *virucide* (Chap. 8)

Virion (veer'-ee-on). A complete, infectious viral particle (i.e., a virus that contains all of its parts) (Chap. 4)

Viroids (vi'-roydz). Infectious RNA molecules (i.e., RNA molecules capable of causing certain plant diseases) (Chap. 4)

Virologist (vi-rol'-oh-jist). One who studies or works with viruses (Chap. 1)

Virology (vi-rol'-oh-gee). That branch of science concerned with the study of viruses (Chap. 1)

Virulence (veer'-u-lenz). A measure of pathogenicity (i.e., some pathogens are more or less *virulent* than others) (Chap. 14)

Virulence factors. Attributes or properties of a microorganism that contribute to its virulence or pathogenicity (e.g., certain exoenzymes and toxins produced by pathogenic bacteria) (Chap. 14)

Virulent (veer'-yu-lent) **strains.** Strains that are pathogenic; capable of causing disease (Chap. 14)

Virulent bacteriophage. A bacteriophage that regularly causes lysis of the bacteria it infects; causes the lytic cycle to occur (Chap. 4)

Viruses (vi'-rus-ez), sing. *virus.* Acellular microorganisms that are smaller than bacteria; obligate intracellular parasites; sometimes referred to as *infectious agents* or *infectious particles* rather than microorganisms (Chap. 4)

Vulvovaginitis (vul'-voh-vaj-uh-ny'-tis). Inflammation of the vulva (the external genitalia of females) and the vagina (Chap. 17)

W

Wandering macrophages. Macrophages that migrate in the bloodstream and tissues; sometimes called *free macrophages* (Chap. 15)

Waxes. Lipids consisting of a saturated fatty acid and a long-chain alcohol (Chap. 6)

Z

Zoonoses (zoh-oh-no'-seez), sing. *zoonosis.* Infectious diseases transmissible from animals to humans; also known as *zoonotic diseases* (Chap. 1)

Zooplankton (zoh'-oh-plank'-ton). Microscopic marine animals that are components of plankton (Chap. 1)

Page numbers in *italics* denote figures; those followed by a *t* denote tables.